Immunology of the Connective Tissue Diseases

IMMUNOLOGY AND MEDICINE SERIES

IMMUNOLOGY
· SERIES · SERIES · SERIES · SERIES · AND · SERIES · SERIES · SERIES · SERIES ·
MEDICINE

Volume 22

Immunology of the Connective Tissue Diseases

Edited by
G. S. Panayi

ARC Professor of Rheumatology
Guy's Hospital
London, UK

Series Editor: K. Whaley

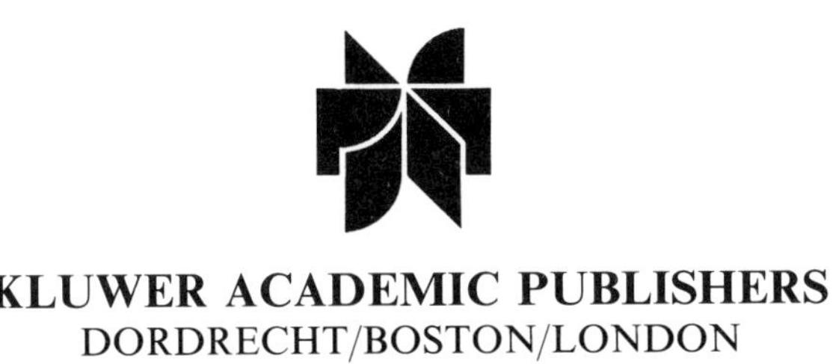

KLUWER ACADEMIC PUBLISHERS
DORDRECHT/BOSTON/LONDON

Distributors

---

for the United States and Canada: Kluwer Academic Publishers, PO Box 358,
Accord Station, Hingham, MA 02018-0358, USA
for all other countries: Kluwer Academic Publishers, Distribution Center, PO Box
322, 3300 AH Dordrecht, The Netherlands

A catalogue record for this book is available from British Library.

ISBN 0-7923-8988-3

Library of Congress Cataloguing in Publication Data

Immunology of the connective tissue diseases / edited by G.S. Panayi.
    p. cm. — (Immunology and medicine series ; v. 22)
    Includes bibliographical references and index.
    ISBN 0-7923-8988-3 (casebound)
    1. Connective tissues—Diseases—Immunological aspects. 2. Rheumatoid
arthritis—Immunological aspects. I. Panayi, Gabriel S. (Gabriel Stavros)
II. Series.
    [DNLM: 1. Connective Tissue Diseases–immunology. WI IM53BI v.22
1993 / WD 375 I33 1993]
RC924.I46   1993
616.7'7079—dc20
DNLM/DLC
for Library of Congress   93-39860
                                            CIP

Published in the United Kingdom by Kluwer Academic Publishers, PO Box 55,
Lancaster, UK.

Kluwer Academic Publishers BV incorporates the publishing programmes of D.
Reidel, Martinus Nijhoff, Dr W. Junk and MTP Press.

Typeset by Lasertext Ltd, Stretford, Manchester, U.K.
Printed and bound in Great Britain by Hartnolls Ltd., Bodmin, Cornwall

Contents

Series Editor's Note

The interface between clinical immunology and other branches of medical practice is frequently blurred and the general physician is often faced with clinical problems with an immunological basis and is expected to diagnose and manage such patients. The rapid expansion of basic and clinical immunology over the past two decades has resulted in the appearance of increasing numbers of immunology journals and it is impossible for a non-specialist to keep apace with this information overload. The *Immunology and Medicine* series is designed to present individual topics of immunology in a condensed package of information which can be readily assimilated by the busy clinician or pathologist.

K. Whaley, Leicester
November 1993

Preface

The connective tissue diseases are an important group of diseases for a variety of reasons: they are relatively frequent, they have a high morbidity and mortality, and they can present in practically any medical specialty. They offer intriguing and interesting challenges in the fields of diagnosis, management and research. Diagnosis has undoubtedly been enormously helped by the description of autoantibodies which define particular clinical syndromes and some of which help in the monitoring of disease activity. Although the role of these autoantibodies in pathogenesis is unclear, some significant advances have been made as witnessed by work on ANCA and anti-cardiolipin antibodies. In the field of cellular immunology, the understanding of the function of cellular subsets, cell membrane structures, cell signalling and activation and the multifaceted activities of cytokines has increased exponentially. Hence, the range of knowledge needed to understand the immunological basis of these diseases is so large that no single individual can master the whole subject.

What is needed is a book which reviews this complex and important area.

Immunology of Connective Tissue Diseases has been written by experts who are either clinical or basic scientists. The aims of the book are to present up-to-date reviews, written by world authorities in their chosen fields, of the immunological basis of connective tissue diseases as it impacts on diagnosis, pathogenetic concepts, disease monitoring and management. The book does not present the clinical features of the diseases in question, leaving that to standard texts, unless they clarify some aspect of the disease of relevance to its aims.

Immunology of Connective Tissue Diseases is aimed at the physician and student interested in understanding the immunological basis of these diseases and at immunologists who are either entering the field for the first time and would like to have a convenient state-of-the-art account of its status or who are already researching in one area and would like to appraise themselves of the developments which have taken place in others. It is hoped that the book will form a convenient resource which brings together knowledge which is widely scattered as reviews and original papers in many journals and books.

List of Contributors

F. BREEDVELD
Department of Rheumatology
Bldg 1 E3-Q, Postbus 9600
2300 RC Leiden, The Netherlands

D. BUSKILA
Department of Medicine 'B'
Soroka Medical Centre
Beer Sheva 84101, Israel

L. J. CROFFORD
Arthritis and Rheumatism Branch NIAMS
National Institutes of Health
Building 10, Room 9N240
Bethesda, MD 20892, USA

R. P. DE VRIES
Department of Immunohaematology and
  Blood Bank
Bldg 1 E3-Q, Postbus 9600
2300 RC Leiden, The Netherlands

G. W. DUFF
Section of Molecular Medicine
Royal Hallamshire Hospital
Glossop Road
Sheffield S10 2JF, UK

Ø. FØRRE
Institute of Immunology and Rheumatology
Rikshospitalet, Fr Qvamsgt. 1
0172 Oslo 1, Norway

G. D. HARKISS
Department of Veterinary Pathology
University of Edinburgh
Summerhall, Edinburgh EH9 1QH, UK

D. O. HASKARD
Rheumatology Unit
Royal Postgraduate Medical School
Hammersmith Hospital, Du Cane Road
London W12 0NN, UK

J. HIGHTON
Wellcome Medical Research Institute
University of Otago Medical School
Dunedin, New Zealand

J. E. HUNT
Department of Immunology
St George Hospital, Kogarah
New South Wales 2217, Australia

G. KINGSLEY
Rheumatology Unit, Division of Medicine
Guy's Hospital
London SE1 9RT, UK

M. D. KRAMER
Institut für Immunologie der Universität
  Heidelberg
Im Neuenheimer Feld 305
D-6900 Heidelberg, Germany

S. A. KRILIS
2 South Street
South Street Centre
St George Hospital, Kogarah
New South Wales 2217, Australia

J. S. LANCHBURY
Rheumatology and Molecular
  Immunogenetics Units
Division of Medicine, UMDS
Guy's Hospital
London SE1 9RT, UK

L. MEAGHER
Rheumatology Unit
Royal Postgraduate Medical School
Hammersmith Hospital, Du Cane Road
London W12 0NN, UK

IMMUNOLOGY OF THE CONNECTIVE TISSUE DISEASES

H. M. MOUTSOPOULOS
The University of Ioannina
School of Medicine
451 10 Ioannina, Greece

J. B. NATVIG
Institute of Immunology and Rheumatology
Rikshospitalet, Fr Qvamsgt. 1
0172 Oslo 1, Norway

D. G. PALMER
Wellcome Medical Research Institute
University of Otago Medical School
Dunedin, New Zealand

G. S. PANAYI
Rheumatology Unit, Division of Medicine
Guy's Hospital
London SE1 9RT, UK

I. RANDEN
Institute of Immunology and Rheumatology
Rikshospitalet, Fr Qvamsgt. 1
0172 Oslo 1, Norway

P. RES
Department of Immunohaematology and
   Blood Bank
Bldg 1 E3-Q, Postbus 9600
2300 RC Leiden, The Netherlands

U. E. SCHAIBLE
Max-Planck-Institut für Immunobiologie
Stubeweg 51
D-7800 Freiburg, Germany

Y. SHOENFELD
Department of Medicine 'B'
Chaim Sheba Medical Centre
Tel Hashomer 52621, Israel

M. M. SIMON
Max-Planck-Institut für Immunobiologie
Stubeweg 51
D-7800 Freiburg, Germany

N. A. STAINES
Division of Life Sciences
King's College London
Campden Hill Road
London W8 7AH, UK

N. TALAL
University of Texas Health Science Center
   at San Antonio
San Antonio, TX 78284, USA

K. M. THOMPSON
Institute of Immunology and Rheumatology
Rikshospitalet, Fr Qvamsgt. 1
0172 Oslo 1, Norway

A. G. TZIOUFAS
University of Ioannina
School of Medicine
45110 Ioannina, Greece

J. THOLE
Department of Immunohaematology and
   Blood Bank
Bldg 1E3-Q, Postbus 9600
2300 RC Leiden, The Netherlands

W. J. VAN VENROOIJ
Department of Biochemistry
University of Nijmegen
PO Box 9101
6500 HB Nijmegen, The Netherlands

T. J. VYSE
Rheumatology Unit
Royal Postgraduate Medical School
Hammersmith Hospital, Du Cane Road
London W12 0NN, UK

R. WALLICH
Angewandte Immunologie am Deutschen
   Krebsforschungszentrum
Im Neuenheimer Feld 280
D-6900 Heidelberg, Germany

M. J. WALPORT
Rheumatology Unit
Royal Postgraduate Medical School
Hammersmith Hospital, Du Cane Road
London W12 0NN, UK

R. L. WILDER
Arthritis & Rheumatism Branch NIAMS
National Institutes of Health
Building 10, Room 9N240
Bethesda, MD 20892, USA

A. G. WILSON
Section of Molecular Medicine
Royal Hallamshire Hospital
Sheffield S10 2JF, UK

P. WOO
Section of Molecular Rheumatology
MRC Clinical Research Centre
Watford Road, Harrow
Middlesex HA1 3UJ, UK

1
The Role of T Cells in the Immunopathogenesis of the Connective Tissue Diseases: Rheumatoid Arthritis as the Paradigm

G. S. PANAYI and G. H. KINGSLEY

INTRODUCTION

Why should we study T cells in the connective tissue diseases? Since the cause of these diseases is unknown, a clear understanding of pathogenesis is not only of intrinsic merit but offers the only avenue for the development of newer, more effective and better-tolerated therapy. There are a number of compelling reasons why the study of the role of T cells is of importance in understanding the pathogenesis of the connective tissue diseases including:

1. T cells are found at the target tissue of the disease, such as the synovial membrane (SM) in rheumatoid arthritis (RA), the salivary glands in Sjögren's syndrome (SS) and the muscles in polymyositis;
2. most of the diseases of interest are linked to the class II major histocompatibility antigens (MHC) whose main, if not sole, function is to present processed antigenic peptides or superantigen to the T cell receptor (TCR) of the specific responding T lymphocyte;
3. experimental models of these diseases have been created by manipulations which involve the activation of disease-inducing T lymphocytes. Examples of such models include the arthritis following the injection of streptococcal cell walls into rats and the development of several connective tissue diseases after the induction of a graft-versus-host response;
4. from some of the experimental models described above, disease can be

transferred to naive, syngeneic animals with lines or clones of T cells. Analysis of the TCR of disease-transferring T lymphocytes has shown these to be of restricted Vβ gene usage. As a consequence, a considerable effort has been invested by many investigators into analysing TCR V gene usage in human diseases, such as RA, in the belief that this would also prove to be oligoclonal in nature;

5. many of the autoantibodies found in the serum of patients with these diseases are of the IgA and IgG isotype, and T cells are involved in isotype switching during the differentiation and maturation of B cells;

6. specific anti-T-cell therapy is effective both in animal models of and in human autoimmune diseases.

The role of T cells in specific diseases is discussed in the Chapters devoted to them. In this Chapter we shall deal with T cell subsets and their function, the organization of the TCR, T cell migration and retention into inflammatory foci and T cell activation. We shall use RA as the paradigm but it should be understood that the mechanisms being discussed are of relevance not only for RA and the connective tissue diseases but also for organ-specific autoimmune diseases, infectious diseases and organ allotransplantation.

T CELL PHYSIOLOGY

T lymphocytes arise from bone marrow progenitors and undergo a series of complex maturational events in the thymus whose details are not of relevance here. As a result of those events, T cells, carrying unique phenotypic markers which are also of functional significance, are released into the circulation. The majority, some 70%, of the cells are CD4 positive and subserve helper functions whilst the remainder are CD8 positive and express suppressor and cytotoxic functions. CD4 T cells recognize antigenic peptides in the context of the class II MHC antigens (HLA-DR, -DQ and -DP) while CD8 cells do so in the context of class I MHC antigens. The antigenic peptides presented by class II MHC are derived from exogenous antigens processed via the lysosomal/endosomal pathway[1] while those presented in the context of class I MHC have been derived from endogenous cytoplasmic proteins and have been processed via the endoplasmic reticulum and the Golgi apparatus[2] (Figure 1). This distinction is of crucial importance as RA and the other connective tissue diseases are linked to class II MHC antigens while ankylosing spondylitis is linked to HLA-B27, a class I MHC antigen; this difference has clear implications in terms of the nature of the antigens driving these diseases although these antigens have not yet been fully characterized in the majority of the conditions in which we are interested. Furthermore, the HLA make-up of an individual influences the T cell repertoire and hence the range of antigens to which the individual responds[3].

The structure of the T cell receptor

The TCR is a heterodimeric structure with which T lymphocytes engage the antigenic peptide in the groove of the MHC molecule on the surface of the

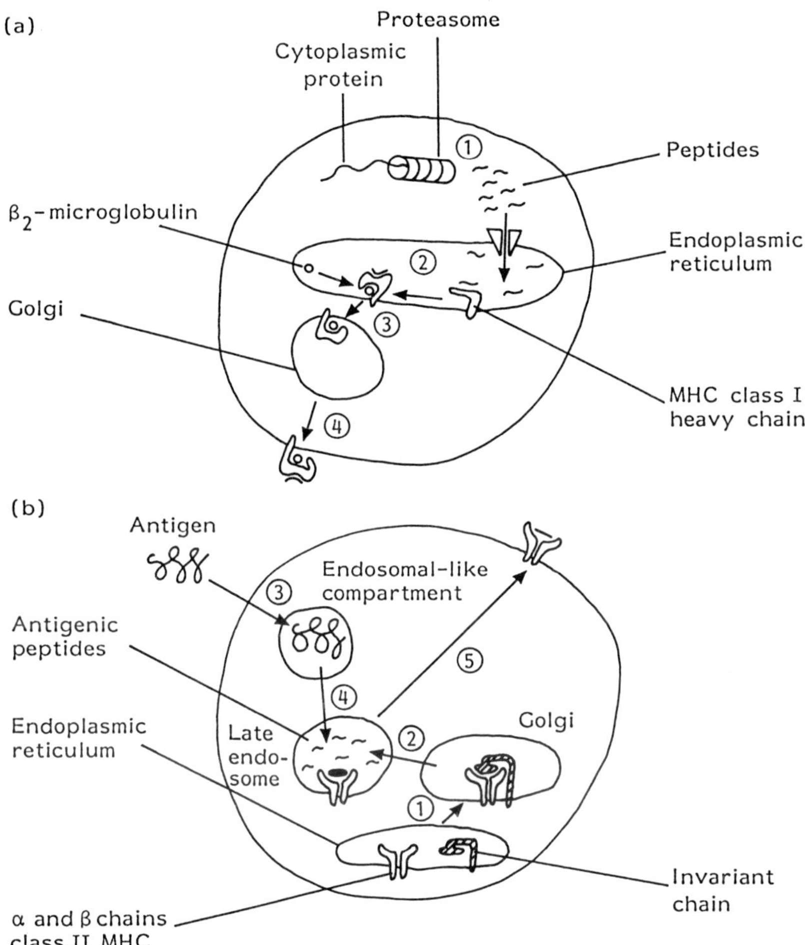

Figure 1 Simplified representation of antigen processing for class I (A) and for class II (B) major histocompatibility molecules (MHC).

In A: (step 1) cytoplasmic proteins are cleaved into peptides by the proteasome enzyme complex; (step 2) the peptides enter the endoplasmic reticulum via a transporter system and there form high affinity stable complexes with the heavy and the light chain ($\beta2$ microglobulin) of class I MHC; the complex is transported to the Golgi apparatus (step 3) for export and insertion into the cell membrane (step 4).

In B: (step 1) the α, β and invariant chains of class II MHC are synthesized in the endoplasmic reticulum and transported to the Golgi where they associate into a trimolecular complex such that the invariant chain occupies the antigen-binding groove formed by the α and β chains; they are then transported into the late endosome (step 2). The antigen is phagocytosed into the endosomal pathway (step 3) and cleaved into antigenic fragments in the late endosome/phagolysosome (step 4). At the same time the invariant chain is degraded thereby opening up the antigen-binding groove on the MHC so that it can be charged with antigenic peptides. The class II MHC/antigenic peptide complex is then exported and inserted into the cell membrane (step 5)

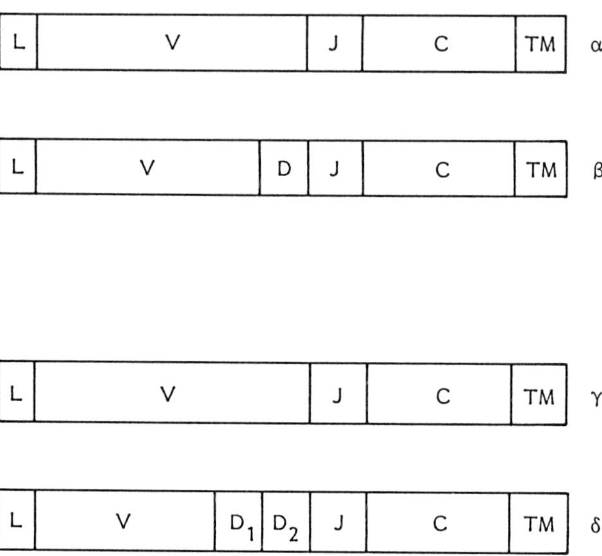

Figure 2 The primary structure of the T cell receptor polypeptides. The leader sequence (L) and the variable (V), diversity (D), joining (J), constant (C) and transmembrane (TM) segments are shown. Between V–J, V–D and D–J there are areas of N region addition and of non-germline encoded nucleotides which further increase T cell receptor combinatorial diversity dependent on V, D and J. More than 10^{16} possible combinations may exist for $\alpha\beta$ and $\gamma\delta$ heterodimers

antigen presenting cell. The majority of T cells in the blood have TCR consisting of α and β chains while only some 5% have TCR composed of γ and δ chains.

The TCR, whether $\alpha\beta$ or $\gamma\delta$, is intimately associated with the CD3 molecule through which the engagement of the TCR and the peptide-MHC complex is signalled to the lymphocyte nucleus to initiate T cell activation. The primary structure of the TCR polypeptides is shown in Figure 2; they consist of the leader sequence (L), the variable region (V), the diversity region (D), the joining region (J), the constant region (C) and the transmembrane region (TM)[4]. The current model of the interaction of the TCR with the peptide-MHC complex proposes that the V domain would interact with determinants on the MHC molecule while the VJ domain (for TCR α) and the VDJ domain (for TCR β) would interact with the peptide within the groove of the MHC[5] (Figure 3). The intracytoplasmic region is extremely short, and this is probably accounted for by the fact that signalling is carried out via the CD3 molecular complex which consists of a group of non-covalently bound, non-polymorphic molecules. The TCR polypeptides belong to the immunoglobulin gene superfamily. The genes for the β and δ chains are found on the short arm of chromosome 7 while those for the α chain are found on chromosome 14 at 14q11; the genes for the δ chain are found in the midst of the α locus lying between Vα and Jα. The enormous diversity of TCR arises from recombinations between the different gene segments V, D and J as well as

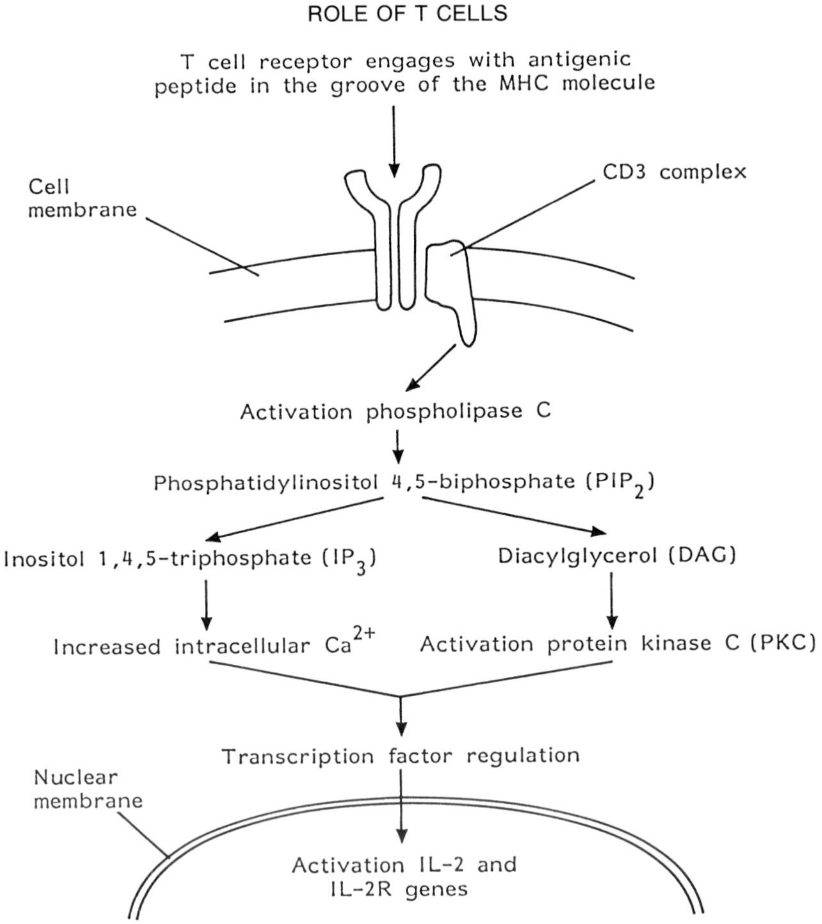

Figure 3 A simplified scheme of the activation of T cells following the binding of the T cell receptor to the complex composed of the antigenic peptide lying in the groove of the MHC molecule. There is perturbation of the CD3 complex which activates phospholipase C leading sequentially to the generation of PIP$_2$, IP$_3$ and, finally, to a rise in intracellular Ca^{2+} (iCa^{2+}). Diacylglycerol is generated from PIP$_2$ and activates protein kinase C (PKC). The combined effect of a rise in iCa^{2+} and activated PKC causes transcription of the interleukin 2 and interleukin 2 receptor genes and T cell proliferation and activation

N region diversity between these segments (Table 1) such that it has been estimated that the number of unique sequences capable of being generated by $\alpha\beta$ or $\gamma\delta$ combinatorial mechanisms are of the order of 10^{15} and 10^{18} respectively.

THE IMMUNOHISTOLOGY OF RA

Large numbers of CD4 positive T cells[6], which are of the CD45RO memory phenotype, accumulate within the RA SM[7]. These T cells are activated as shown by a large number of phenotypic and functional characteristics[8–13].

Table 1 The molecular composition of different T cell receptor genes

	Segments				
TCR Gene	V	D	J	C	Functional diversity
α	50	5	70	1	Present
β	57	2	2	2	Present
γ	8	0	2	2	Present
δ	3	3	3	1	Extensive

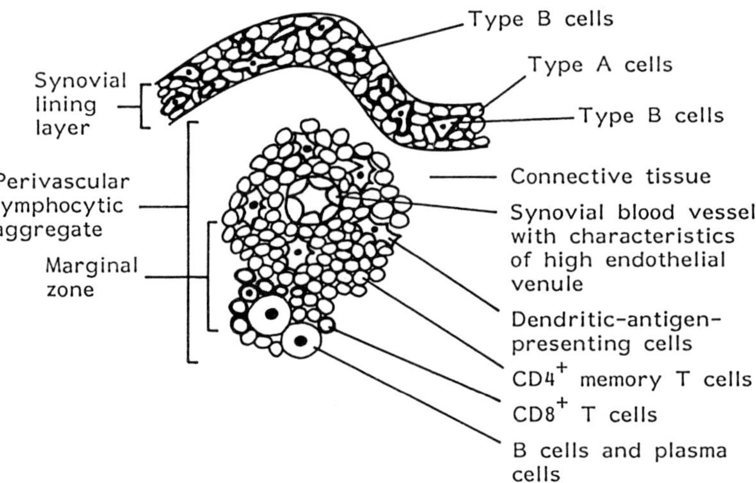

Figure 4 The structure and cellular composition of the rheumatoid synovial membrane. The Type A cells of the synovial lining layer are macrophages whilst the Type B cells are secretory synoviocytes. Both CD4+ and CD8+ T cells belong to the memory pool being CD45RO positive. The location of B lymphocytes and plasma cells in the marginal zone should be noted

Nevertheless, their activation state is unusual since the majority do not express the interleukin 2 (IL-2) receptor and since it has proved extremely difficult to detect the classical T cell lymphokines, interferon-gamma (IFNγ) and IL-2. The presence of IFNγ has proved extremely difficult to demonstrate at both the mRNA and the protein level[14–16] whilst abundant mRNA for IL-2 does not seem to be translated into protein[16–19]. By contrast, it has proved an easy task to demonstrate that synovial T cells do produce interleukin 6 (IL-6) at both the mRNA and the protein level[20]. The T cells within the SM are found within two principal areas: as a perivascular lymphocytic aggregate and as a diffuse infiltrate within the connective tissue (Figure 4). No T cells are found within the synovial lining layer. CD8 positive T cells are sparse and, apart from a diffuse infiltrate in the connective tissue, are found in the periphery of the perivascular lymphocytic aggregate in the so-called marginal zone (Figure 4). B cells and plasma cells are also found but are organized into typical germinal follicles in only some 20% of SM examined. The lymphocytes of the B cell lineage produce IgM, IgA and IgG rheumatoid factors but the specificity of the Ig produced by 47 to 99% of the B cells is unknown[21].

Cells of the monocyte/macrophage series are prominent within the RA SM; they are found in the three principal areas of the SM, namely, the perivascular aggregate, the synovial lining layer (where they are known as the Type A cells) and diffusely within the synovial connective tissue. These cells subserve an important effector function by secreting inflammatory cytokines such as interleukin 1 (IL-1), tumour necrosis factor α (TNFα), granulocyte/macrophage colony-stimulating factor (GM-CSF), interleukin 8 (IL-8), transforming growth factor β (TGFβ) and IL-6[11,15,22-32]. Another crucially important cell from the pathophysiological point of view must be the strongly HLA-DR positive, dendritic cell which has the phenotypic, enzymatic and functional properties of an antigen presenting cell. Since RA is strongly linked to HLA-DR4/DR1 in most populations studied, the processing and presentation of antigen via the class II MHC pathway must be a central and critical feature of the pathogenesis of the disease. This further suggests that the 'rheumatoid antigen or antigens', whether of endogenous or exogenous origin, must be presented via this pathway rather than the class I MHC pathway classically involved in the presentation of cytoplasmic antigens, especially of viral origin, to CD8 positive T cells. Perhaps an answer to this question will be provided when the sequence of peptides eluted from the groove of HLA-DR4 molecules from RA synovial membranes cells has been sequenced and compared to known proteins.

The T and B lymphocytes and cells of the monocyte/macrophage series have been recruited into the SM from the blood stream. Synoviocytes, which are specialized synovial fibroblasts, and endothelial cells increase in numbers by cell division within the tissue rather than by recruitment. Synoviocytes are found throughout the SM but in the lining layer they are known as Type B cells. They have an important effector role within the joint secreting collagen and various enzymes such as neutral proteases and metalloproteinases of which collagenase is the most important[33-35]. Of the cytokines which they secrete, IL-6[31,36] and transforming growth factor β (TGFβ)[29,37,38] may be involved in tissue repair while IL-1 and TNFα are proinflammatory[25]. However, TGFβ has more janus-like pleiotropic properties[29]. It promotes fibrosis, new blood vessel formation and entry of leucocytes into tissues. These properties, although obviously of advantage in wound repair and other acute situations, may be deleterious in the context of chronic inflammation. It is of importance to note that systemically administered TGFβ has anti-inflammatory effects whilst when it is injected directly into the joint it causes a marked synovitis[39,40]. Finally, TGFβ[40] and IL-6[41] may be immunosuppressive; indeed, corticosteroids may exert part of their immuno-suppressive effects by stimulating T cells to secrete TGFβ[42]. IL-6 can form complexes with solubilized IL-6 receptors which then stimulate TGFβ secretion from target cells[43]. The importance of TGFβ in regulating inflammation has received powerful support from genetic recombination experiments in mice in which targeted disruption of the TGFβ gene results in multifocal inflammatory disease including changes in the salivary glands similar to Sjögren's syndrome[44].

The RA SM is grossly hypertrophic and hyperplastic and invades bone and cartilage at the cartilage/pannus junction. The eroding cells are macrophages and synoviocytes, which exert their destructive properties by the release of various cytokines and enzymes[45]. The eroding and invasive characteristics of the synovial pannus are properties which are possessed by tumours. Just like tumours, the RA SM requires new blood vessel formation for an adequate supply of nutrients and oxygen (for review see [46]). A number of angiogenesis promoting factors are present within the rheumatoid synovium including IL-1, epidermal growth factor, basic and acidic fibroblast growth factors, platelet derived growth factor and TGFβ[23,25,29,37,38,47-49]. Recent evidence from experimental models of arthritis suggests that suppression of angiogenesis could prove a novel therapeutic approach for the treatment of RA[50].

THE T CELL HYPOTHESIS FOR THE PATHOGENESIS OF RHEUMATOID ARTHRITIS

Any one of the cells discussed in the preceding section could be the prime mover for the initiation and/or perpetuation of RA. Indeed, experiments with mice transgenic for the transactivating gene *tax* of the HTLV-I virus[51] or for the human TNFα gene[52] have shown that the joint pathology of RA, including joint destruction, can be induced by these procedures; in the former case a number of cytokine genes are activated whilst in the latter TNFα is produced in a dysregulated manner. In the former, expression of the transgene within synovial tissue, and, in the latter, expression within chondrocytes of the articular cartilage, appear to be required for the induction of arthritis. Since a number of viruses, including retroviruses, have been proposed as possible aetiological agents in RA, why could the disease not be due to dysregulated production of one or more cytokines through a mechanism such as transactivation? There are at least three arguments against this scenario. First, it would not explain the HLA-DR4/DR1 association; second, in both the transgenic models a high copy number of the transgene needs to be expressed within the joint; third, the absence of an oligo- or monoclonal T cell population within the RA SM (see below) argues against the possibility that a viral product could be acting as a superantigen.

If RA is initiated and/or perpetuated by T cells how could this come about? RA could be switched on by a virus, endogenous or exogenous, which could directly or indirectly activate a clone of T cells which are programmed by their particular combination of TCR $\alpha\beta$ chains to recognize autoantigenic peptides presented in the context of the groove of the HLA-DR4/DR1 molecule. The antigen itself would be a component unique to the joint such as the articular cartilage; this would account for the restriction of the cellular destructive response to diarthrodial joints. Type II collagen has been proposed as such an autoantigen[53,54] but its candidacy is weakened by the absence of damage to nose, ear and tracheal cartilages which contain this collagen in abundance. By contrast, in relapsing polychondritis, damage is mainly restricted to these cartilages although some inflammation can occur in diarthrodial joints. These observations, which are supported by direct biochemical analyses, suggest that cartilage at different anatomical sites may contain unique component(s)[55]. Furthermore, the individual may not be tolerant to such autologous component(s), as the absence of a vascular and lymphatic supply to articular cartilage could mean that articular components may not have been available for the induction of tolerance during the thymic education of T cells. The evidence for these proposals may be summarized as follows: the first piece of evidence is the differences in the target tissues damaged in patients with RA and in those with relapsing polychondritis, in which the articular cartilage is pre-eminent in the former and non-articular cartilage in the latter. A second piece of evidence supporting the central role of diarthrodial cartilage in driving the immune response is the quiescence of synovitis in knees which have undergone total joint replacement in which all articular cartilage has been removed and the continued presence of synovitis in knees in which patellar cartilage has been left *in situ*[56]. The third is the cloning of T cells responding to type II collagen from the peripheral blood of healthy individuals. The hypothesis that RA is at least maintained by autoimmunity to unique cartilage components leads to the conclusion that RA is an organ-specific autoimmune disease and, as such, could be investigated and manipulated therapeutically by the same procedures which have proved so instructive and productive in experimental models of autoimmune disease including arthritis.

T cell responses to antigen and the pathogenesis of autoimmune disease

An extremely fruitful approach in investigating the contribution of antigen-responsive T cells to the pathogenesis of autoimmune disease has been the cloning of T cells responding to antigenic peptides of the disease-inducing antigen. In experimental arthritis the antigens have been the mycobacterial 65 kD heat shock protein (adjuvant arthritis) and type II collagen (collagen arthritis) whilst in allergic encephalomyelitis the relevant antigen is myelin basic protein. Some of these clones are able to transfer disease to naive recipient animals in the absence of the disease-inducing antigen[57,58]. Analysis of the TCR β chains of these clones has shown them to be oligoclonal[59–61]. As a consequence, the disease-causing T cells themselves or peptides synthesized from unique sequences in CR β chains have been used as vaccines for the prevention or treatment of the disease in question[62–67]. Since the inducing antigen in human connective tissue diseases is unknown, it is not possible to clone the responsive T cells for such studies. Instead efforts have been made, using a variety of techniques, to ascertain whether TCR gene usage by T cells from patients with connective tissues are oligo- or polyclonal in origin.

TCR gene usage in the human connective tissue diseases

This area has been recently and thoroughly reviewed[68,69].

TCR $\alpha\beta$ T cells

Variable results have been reported, with some investigators finding an increased frequency of various TCR, but there is no consensus and no consistency in these findings. Why these disappointing results? There are three possibilities. The first is that the T cells driving the disease are polyclonal and that the polyclonality increases with time from the start of the disease. Hence, there is an increasing emphasis in more recent studies on investigating patients with early disease. The second is that the techniques being used are not sufficiently sensitive to detect the low frequency of disease-causing T cells. The third is that the disease-causing T cells in animal models of arthritis have been derived by expansion and cloning with the disease-inducing antigen; the unavailability of such antigens in human rheumatic diseases clearly means that this approach is not available. The results from some specific diseases are shown below:

1.   In rheumatoid arthritis

The frequency of T cells responding to antigen is a crucial and decisive point as it will determine the success or failure of such efforts. Determination of the frequency of T cells responding to known antigens shows that it varies from 1:300 to 1:3000; although TCR occurring at such frequency could be detected by present techniques, their significance would be difficult to establish. This almost certainly explains the failure to detect a mono- or oligoclonal T cell receptor α/β gene usage amongst T cells within the rheumatoid joint[68-76]. These considerations help to resolve another paradox of rheumatoid research, namely, the difficulty of detecting the classical T cell lymphokines IL-2 and IFNγ, both at the mRNA and at the protein level, in the joints of patients with RA. The probable low frequency of T cells responding to the 'rheumatoid antigen' above resolves this difficulty; more recent experiments using the sensitive quantitative polymerase chain reaction (PCR) have demonstrated the presence of mRNA for both IL2 and IFNγ.

From the foregoing, it may be concluded that only a tiny minority of the T cells accumulating within the RA SM will be directly involved in responding to the 'rheumatoid antigen'. The vast majority of the T cells will be cells recruited into the inflammatory focus but will be antigen non-specific, i.e. will have widely differing specificities but not to the 'rheumatoid antigen'. Thus, T cells responding to the recall antigens tuberculin PPD and tetanus toxoid have been detected within the rheumatoid joint; the presence within the joint of T cells responding to bacterial superantigens could explain the increased frequency of Vβ14 found by some investigators[77]. Hence, it is of crucial importance to understand the mechanisms involved in the accumulation and persistence of T cells within the joint and the role, if any, of such 'rheumatoid antigen' non-responding T cells in the physiology of chronic synovitis.

2.   In juvenile chronic arthritis

No results have been reported.

3.   In systemic lupus erythematosus

There is little work on TCR $\alpha\beta$ gene usage by SLE T cells. In the blood, a RFLP associated with TCR Cα has been found in Caucasian patients but not in Mexican patients[78] but this is not a universal finding[79-81]. There is a Cβ RFLP associated with anti-Ro antibodies[82]. Investigations involving T cells from lesions of the disease are urgently required.

4.   In Sjögren's syndrome

Kay et al[83] found a significant decrease of Vβ6.7 positive T cells in the blood of patients with SS. This decrease was not due to the cells being in the salivary tissue as they were absent from the lesions. This raises the intriguing possibility that the deficit may be due to deletion of these lymphocytes during thymic education. An oligoclonal rearrangement of Vβ was found in lesional T cells from 2 of 9 patients[84,85]. Although Sumida *et al.*[86] did not find a restricted TCR Vβ gene in infiltrating T cells in lips of patients, Vβ2 was found in 6 of 7 lips and Vβ13 in 4 of 7 lips when neither Vβ gene family was found in the blood or lips from control subjects. This finding suggests selectivity in the T cells found in SS lesions.

5.   In progressive systemic sclerosis and polymyositis

No work on TCR $\alpha\beta$ gene usage has been reported.

TCR $\gamma\delta$ cells

1.   In rheumatoid arthritis

Most[87-92] but not all investigators[93,94] have found an increase in TCR $\gamma\delta$ positive T cells in the synovial fluid of patients with RA compared with matched peripheral blood. However, a more important finding is that these cells were enriched in Vδ1 whilst in the blood it is Vδ2 positive cells which form the majority. Molecular analysis revealed variable usage of $\gamma\delta$ T cell receptor transcripts[95]. In the SM $\gamma\delta$ T cells are found mainly in the T lymphocyte rich perivascular lymphoid aggregates[96]. The function of these cells in the pathophysiology of RA is unclear. The excess of Vδ1 cells implies that they may selectively home into or be selectively expanded within the joint.

As a rheumatological control for these findings in RA, there is no change in the proportion or subset distribution of $\gamma\delta$ T cells in the blood or synovial fluid from patients with spondyloarthropathy[88].

2.   In juvenile chronic arthritis

In some children with juvenile chronic arthritis there may be an expansion of $\gamma\delta$ positive T cells within the joint but this is not a universal finding; part of the discrepancy may reside in the nature of the arthritic disease from which the children suffer. However, it seems that the majority of the $\gamma\delta$ T cells are Vδ1[96,97] so that the situation is reminiscent of RA (see above).

3. In systemic lupus erythematosus

When T cells were non-specifically cloned from the blood of patients with SLE, seven of 59 clones were able to stimulate autologous B lymphocytes to augment anti-DNA antibody production. All seven clones were $\gamma\delta$ positive[98], four clones preferentially used Vγ1 and δ chain usage was restricted to Vδ1, Vδ3 and Vδ5[99]. This is striking when one remembers that peripheral blood cells usually express Vγ9/Vδ2. Lunardi *et al.*[100] have reported a relative decrease in the number of peripheral Vγ9/Vδ2 cells with a compensatory increase in Vδ1 cells. The relevance of these observations to the pathogenesis of SLE is at present unknown.

4. In Sjögren's syndrome

Kratz *et al.*[101] have reported a unique RFLP near the TCR γ gene in 41% of PSS patients and 22% of controls; this RFLP may associate with Vδ1. The significance of this finding, if confirmed, is unclear.

5. In polymyositis

A single patient with polymyositis was found to have a $\gamma\delta$ T cell infiltrate within involved muscle but only a low percentage, 2–6%, of infiltrating T cells were $\gamma\delta$ positive in a further four of 28 patients[102].

THE ENTRY AND PERSISTENCE OF T CELLS WITHIN THE RHEUMATOID SYNOVIAL MEMBRANE

The entry and persistence of lymphocytes into any inflammatory lesion, including the rheumatoid synovium, can be conveniently divided into four stages: adhesion to vascular endothelial cells (EC); migration through the blood vessel wall, basement membrane and connective tissue matrix; adhesion to fibrillar components of the connective tissue; and adhesion to cells already present within the lesion. Little is known about the mechanisms involved in the migration of human lymphocytes through tissue and these will not be considered further here[103,104].

Adhesion of lymphocytes to endothelial cells

This is, obviously, the first stage in the complex process beginning with the exit of a lymphocyte from the circulation and ending with its entry into the tissue. This has been extensively reviewed recently[105]. The efficiency of the process is directly dependent on the state of activation of EC and the lymphocyte being greatest for activated T cells binding to activated EC. These interactions may be mutually stimulatory (Figure 5). In addition, memory T cells of the CD45RO positive phenotype bind more efficiently to unactivated as well as cytokine-activated EC *in vitro*[106]; this may be one property of memory T cells which accounts for the overwhelming preponderance of this subpopulation of lymphocytes within inflammatory

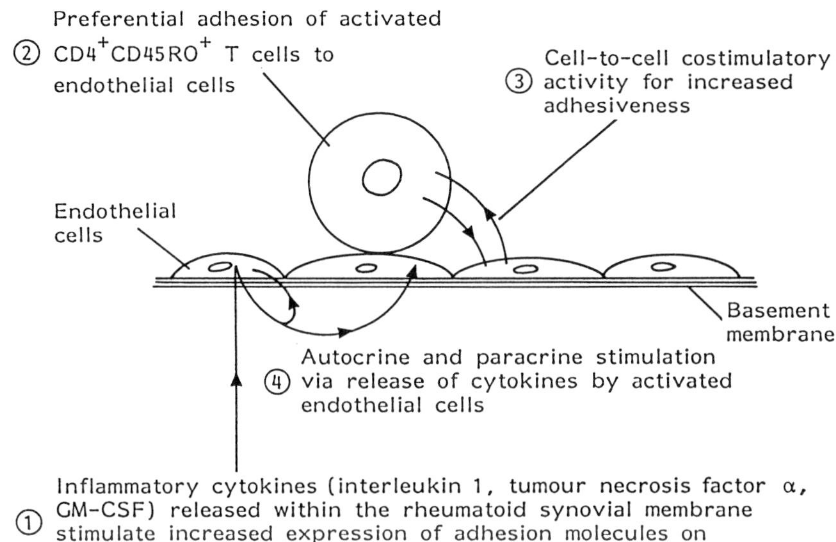

Figure 5 The mechanisms involved in the adhesion of T cells to activated endothelial cells. The numbers refer to a series of sequential events which initiate and amplify adhesion

Table 2 The receptor/ligand pairs involved in the preferential adhesion of CD45RO positive memory T cells to human endothelial cells

Receptor on T lymphocyte	Ligand on endothelial cell
Lymphocyte function associated antigen-1 (LFA-1)	Intercellular adhesion molecule-1 (ICAM-1)
Very late activation antigen-4 (VLA-4)	Vascular cell adhesion molecule-1 (VCAM-1)
?A variant of sialyl Lewis blood group X	Endothelial leucocyte adhesion molecule-1 (ELAM-1)

lesions[107]. The results of these *in vitro* studies have been confirmed by *in vivo* experiments using blisters raised on the forearm of human volunteers following the intradermal injection of tuberculin PPD[108]. The blister fluid contains over 95% of CD45RO positive T cells at a ratio of 4:1 of CD4:CD8 T cells, identical to the characteristics of the lymphocytes found within the RA SM (see above). The molecular basis of these interactions is well understood (Table 2) and is forming the basis of new therapeutic approaches by means of the infusion of blocking monoclonal antibodies directed, for example, against ICAM-1.

As we have already noted above, it is likely that the overwhelming majority of T cells found within the RA SM are 'rheumatoid antigen' non-specific. *In vivo* and *in vitro* experiments suggest that these cells preferentially accumulate within inflammatory foci, such as the rheumatoid joint, because they

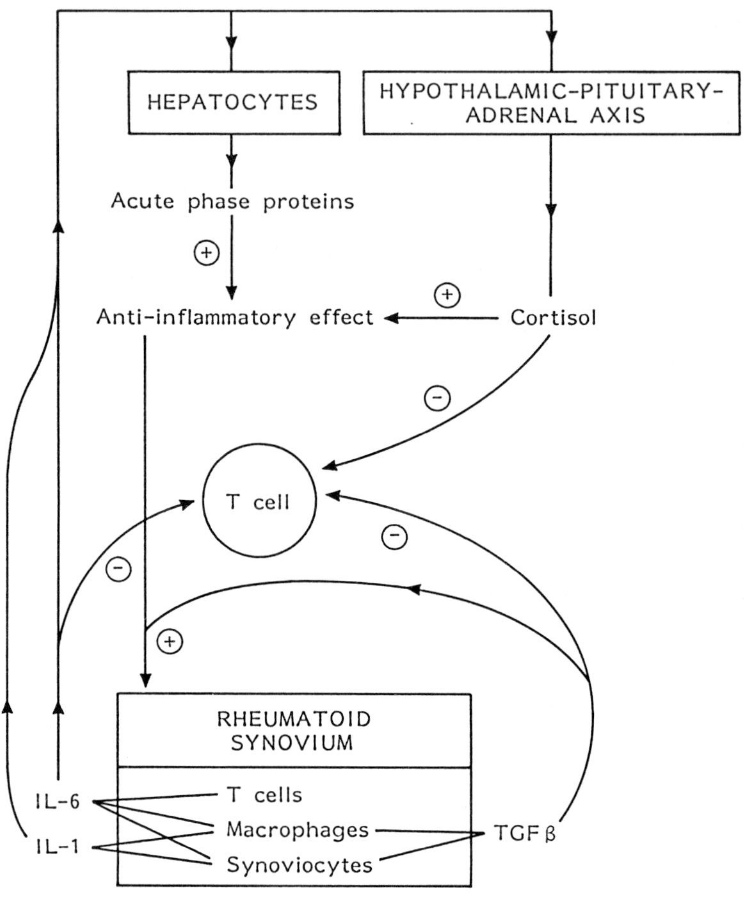

Figure 6 Some of the processes which may be operating to limit the activation of T cells and which exert anti-inflammatory effects in the rheumatoid synovium

have been recently activated and, consequently, show increased adhesive characteristics[104,107,109–111]. The exact contribution of these T cells to the pathophysiology of inflammation has not been determined although it has been established that a proportion of them make IL-6[20,32]. This is of some considerable interest as IL-6 may be considered to be an 'anti-inflammatory' cytokine since it stimulates the secretion of acute phase proteins from hepatocytes[31,112–114], stimulates cortisol secretion by stimulating the hypo-thalamic–pituitary–adrenal axis[115], inhibits T cells involved in cell mediated immune reactions[41,43] and suppresses experimental arthritis[41] probably by stimulating the release of TGFβ. Hence, several mechanisms may be operating to downregulate the function of 'rheumatoid antigen' activated T cells and thus to limit or retard joint damage (Figure 6). It is of interest that stimulation of resting T cells via CD2 leads to IL-6 gene transcription without cell proliferation[116]. We have already noted the paucity of T cell replication within the RA SM.

Adhesion of lymphocytes to fibrillar components of the connective tissue matrix

The major fibrillar components of the connective tissue matrix are fibronectin (FN), collagen (COLL) and laminin (LN). Collectively they form the framework around and between which are organized the non-fibrillar components of the connective tissue matrix and to which cells are attached. This area has been reviewed in great detail[117]. The cells are attached via β_1 integrin receptors, also called very late activation (VLA) antigens, which consist of a common β_1 chain and different α chains. T cells use predominantly the VLA-2 integrin receptor to bind to collagen[118]. Synovial T cells adhere more strongly to FN via the VLA-5 and VLA-4 receptor; a property they share with post-activated memory T cells[119,120]. Thus, the enhanced adhesion of synovial memory T cells to FN is another example of the activated state of these cells and further supports the concept (see above) that an inflammatory focus acts as a 'filter' attracting and retaining T cells activated outside the focus.

The term integrin was coined in order to describe the integrating function of integrin receptors on the surface of fibroblasts with the external milieu. There is evidence that a similar function may be subserved by integrins on the surface of lymphocytes as it has been shown that T cells adhering to FN via VLA-4 receptors transcribe the AP-1 transcription factor which is involved in the transcription of several cytokine genes including IL-2[121]. Other functional consequences of T cell integrin/fibrillar matrix component interaction remain to be elucidated. It may be concluded that these adhesive interactions not only serve the important function of retaining activated synovial T cells within the tissue but may also contribute to the inflammatory events taking place by providing co-stimulatory signals for the production of cytokines.

Adhesion of T lymphocytes to cells found within the synovial membrane

Adhesion of cells of similar phenotype to each other is known as homotypic adhesion while adhesion of cells of different phenotype to each other is known as heterotypic adhesion. As an example of the former may be cited the adhesion of activated memory T cells to each other to form large cellular clusters[106]. One important receptor/ligand pair in this interaction is LFA-1/ICAM-1[122]. It may be that the propensity of CD45RO positive T cells to form large cellular clusters on activation is one mechanism by which the large perivascular aggregates of CD4 CD45RO positive T cells form in the RA SM and other chronic immune-mediated inflammatory foci (see above). An example of heterotypic adhesion is that between T cells and antigen presenting cells during antigen presentation[123] and of T cells to synoviocytes[124].

It may be asked whether these adhesive interactions have any functional consequences. Clearly the heterotypic adhesion of T cells to antigen presenting cells is crucial for the activation of T cells by processed antigenic peptides;

it is the proposed essential first step in the T cell hypothesis for the aetiopathogenesis of RA. No obvious functional consequences have been described after CD4 CD45RO T cell homotypic adhesion or T cell/synoviocyte heterotypic adhesion but no investigations directed to that end have been reported. We have investigated the interaction between CD2 on T cells and LFA-3 on macrophages, as an example of heterotypic adhesion[116], and have found that this leads to increased transcription of the HLA-DRα and IL-6 genes but not the genes for IL-2, IL-2 receptor or IFNγ. It should be remembered that expression of HLA-DR and secretion of IL-6 are two of the activation characteristics of synovial T cells. Thus, adhesive interactions *in situ* within an inflammatory lesion may provide activation signals to T cells which may lead to cytokine production without cellular proliferation. Further analysis of the functional consequences of homo- and heterotypic cellular adhesion is eagerly awaited.

SUMMARY AND CONCLUSIONS

This chapter has presented a synthesis of the consequences of the activation of that small population of T cells specific for the 'rheumatoid antigen' and the functional contribution of the vast majority of T cells which are not specific for the 'rheumatoid antigen' and which are attracted to and retained within the RA SM by non-specific means particularly their pre-activated state. The lessons learnt can be applied to other diseases induced by T cells particularly those linked to the inheritance of HLA-DR genes. In the process, certain molecules have been described which are of crucial importance in these events. It is hoped that interference with the functions of these molecules, for example by the administration of blocking monoclonal antibodies, will be of therapeutic benefit. These possibilities are discussed in the final chapter.

ACKNOWLEDGEMENT

A core support grant (U9) from the Arthritis and Rheumatism Council and the secretarial skills of Mrs Stella Stone are gratefully acknowledged.

References

1. Ploegh HL. Intracellular transport of MHC class II molecules. Immunol Today. 1992; 13: 179–184.
2. Monaco JJ. A molecular model of MHC class I restricted antigen processing. Immunol Today. 1992; 13: 173–179.
3. Gulwani-Akolkaw B, Posnett DN, Janson CH, et al. HLA genes influence the human T cell repertoire. J Exp Med. 1991; 174: 1139–1146.
4. Wilson RK, Lai E, Concannon P, Barth RK, Hood LE. Structure, organisation and polymorphism of murine and human T cell receptor and α and β chain gene families. Immunol Rev. 1988; 101: 149–172.
5. Davis MM, Bjorkman PJ. T cell antigen receptor genes and T cell recognition. Nature. 1988; 334: 395–402.

6. Duke O, Panayi GS, Janossy G, Poulter LW. An immunohistological analysis of lymphocyte subpopulations and their microenvironment in the synovial membranes of patients with rheumatoid arthritis using monoclonal antibodies. Clin Exp Immunol. 1982; 49: 22–30.

7. Pitzalis C, Kingsley GH, Murphy J, Panayi GS. Abnormal distribution of the helper-inducer and suppressor-inducer T lymphocyte subsets in the rheumatoid joint. Clin Immunol Immunopathol. 1987; 45: 252–258.

8. Poulter LW, Duke O, Panayi GS, Hobbs S, Raftery MJ, Janossy G. Activated T lymphocytes of the synovial membrame in rheumatoid arthritis and other arthropathies. Scand J Immunol. 1985; 22: 683–690.

9. Talal N, Tovar S, Dauphinee MJ, Flescher E, Dang H, Galarza D. Abnormalities of T cell activation in the rheumatoid synovium detected with monoclonal antibodies to CD3. Scand J Rheumatol. 1988; 76 (suppl): 175–180.

10. Kirkham BW, Pitzalis C, Kingsley GH, Timms AM, Kyriazis N, Panayi GS. Rheumatoid T lymphocyte MHC Class II expression: in vitro stimulation produces normal MHC Class II expression, independent of proliferation. J Rheumatol. 1989; 16: 270–274.

11. Miyasaka N, Sato K, Goto M, et al. Augmented interleukin 1 production and HLA-DR expression in the synovium of rheumatoid arthritis patients. Arthritis Rheum. 1988; 31: 480–486.

12. Laffon A, Garcia-Vincuna R, Humbria A, et al. Upregulated expression and function of VLA-4 fibronectin receptors on human activated T cells in rheumatoid arthritis. J Clin Invest. 1991; 88: 546–552.

13. Fox DA, Millard JA, Kan L, et al. Activation pathways of synovial T lymphocytes. Expression and function of the UM4D4/CDW60 antigen. J Clin Invest. 1990; 86: 1124–1136.

14. Firestein GS, Zvaifler NJ. Peripheral blood and synovial fluid monocyte activation in inflammatory arthritis. II Low levels of synovial fluid and synovial tissue interferon suggest that gamma-interferon is not the primary macrophage activating factor. Arthritis Rheum. 1987; 30: 864–871.

15. Firestein GS, Alvaro-Garcia JM, Maki R. Quantitative analysis of cytokine gene expression in rheumatoid arthritis. J Immunol. 1990; 144: 3347–3353.

16. Brennan FM, Chantry D, Jackson A, Maini RN, Feldmann M. Cytokine production by cells isolated from the synovial membrane. J Autoimmun. 1989; 2: 177–186.

17. Buchan G, Barrett K, Fujita T, Taniguchi T, Maini RN. Detection of activated T cell products in the RA joint using cDNA probe to IL-2, IL2-R and IFNγ. Clin Exp Immunol. 1988; 71: 295–301.

18. Howell WM, Warren CJ, Cook NJ, Cawley MID, Smith JL. Detection of IL-2 at mRNA and protein levels in synovial infiltrates from inflammatory arthropathies using biotinylated oligonucleotide probes in situ. Clin Exp Immunol. 1991; 86: 393–398.

19. Howell M, Smith J, Cawley M. The rheumatoid synovium: a model for T cell anergy? Immunol Today. 1992; 13: 191 (letter).

20. Wood NC, Symons JA, Dickens E, Duff GW. In situ hybridisation of IL-6 in rheumatoid arthritis. Clin Exp Immunol. 1992; 87: 183–189.

21. Egeland T, Lea T, Saari G, Mellbye OJ, Natvig JB. Quantitation of cells secreting rheumatoid factor of IgG, IgA and IgM class after elution from rheumatoid synovial tissue. Arthritis Rheum. 1982; 25: 1445–1450.

22. Kirkham BW, Navarro FJ, Corkill MM, Barbatis C, Panayi GS. Immunohistological localisation of interleukin-1 in rheumatoid and osteoarthritis synovial membrane. Brit J Rheumatol. 1989; 28: 47.

23. Bucala R, Ritchlin C, Winchester R, Cerami A. Constitutive production of inflammatory and mitogenic cytokines by rheumatoid synovial fibroblasts. J Exp Med. 1991; 173: 569–574.

24. Buchan G, Barrett K, Turner M, Chantry D, Maini RN, Feldmann M. Interleukin 1 and tumour necrosis factor mRNA expression in rheumatoid arthritis: prolonged production of IL1 alpha. Clin Exp Immunol. 1988; 73: 449–455.

25. MacNaul KL, Hutchinson NI, Parsons JN, Bayne EK, Tocci MJ. Analysis of IL-1 and TNF-alpha gene expression in human rheumatoid synoviocytes and normal monocytes by in situ hybridization. J Immunol. 1990; 145: 4154–4166.

26. Brennan FM, Maini RN, Feldmann M. TNF alpha – a pivotal role in rheumatoid arthritis?

Brit J Rheumatol. 1992; 31: 293–298.
27. Haworth C, Brennan FM, Chantry D, Turner M, Maini RN, Feldmann M. Expression of granulocyte-macrophage colony-stimulating factor in rheumatoid arthritis: regulation by tumor necrosis factor alpha. Eur J Immunol. 1991; 21: 2575–2579.
28. Uematsu Y. A novel and rapid cloning method for the T cell receptor variable region sequences. Immunogenetics. 1991; 34: 174–178.
29. Wahl SM, Allen JB, Wong HL, Dougherty SF, Ellingsworth LR. Antagonistic and agonistic effects of transforming growth factor-beta and IL-1 in rheumatoid synovium. J Immunol. 1990; 145: 2514–2519.
30. Miossec P, Naviliat M, Dupuy S, Sany J, Banchereau J. Low levels of interleukin-4 and high levels of transforming growth factor beta in rheumatoid synovitis. Arthritis Rheum. 1990; 33: 1180–1187.
31. Guerne PA, Zuraw BL, Vaughan JH, Carson DA, Lotz M. Synovium as a source of interleukin 6 in vitro. Contribution to local and systemic manifestations of arthritis. J Clin Invest. 1989; 83: 585–592.
32. Hirano T, Matsuda T, Turner M, et al. Excessive production of interleukin-6/B cell stimulatory factor-2 in rheumatoid arthritis. Eur J Immunol. 1988; 18: 1797–1801.
33. Kumkumian GK, Lafyatis R, Remmers EF, Case JP, Kim SJ, Wilder RL. Platelet-derived growth factor and IL-1 interactions in rheumatoid arthritis. Regulation of synoviocyte proliferation, prostaglandin production, and collagenase transcription. J Immunol. 1989; 143: 833–837.
34. Unemori EN, Hibbs MS, Amento EP. Constitutive expression of a 92-kD gelatinase (type V collagenase) by rheumatoid synovial fibroblasts and its induction in normal human fibroblasts by inflammatory cytokines. J Clin Invest. 1992; 88: 1656–1662.
35. Case JP, Lafyatis R, Remmers EF, Kumkumian GK, Wilder RL. Transin/stromelysin expression in rheumatoid synovium. A transformation-associated metalloproteinase secreted by phenotypically invasive synoviocytes. Am J Pathol. 1989; 135: 1055–1064.
36. Tan PL, Farmiloe S, Yeoman S, Watson JD. Expression of the interleukin 6 gene in rheumatoid synovial fibroblasts. J Rheumatol. 1990; 17: 1608–1612.
37. Lafyatis R, Thompson NL, Remmers EF, et al. Transforming growth factor-beta production by synovial tissues from rheumatoid patients and streptococcal cell wall arthritic rats. Studies on secretion by synovial fibroblast-like cells and immunohistologic localization. J Immunol. 1989; 143: 1142–1148.
38. Fara R, Olsen N, Keski-Oja J, Moses H, Pincus T. Active and latent forms of transforming growth factor β activity in synovial effusions. J Exp Med. 1989; 169: 291–296.
39. Brandes ME, Allen JB, Ogawa Y, Wahl SM. Transforming growth factor beta 1 suppresses acute and chronic arthritis in experimental animals. J Clin Invest. 1991; 87: 1108–1113.
40. Wahl SM. The role of transforming growth factor-beta in inflammatory processes. Immunol Res. 1991; 10: 249–254.
41. Mihara M, Ikuta M, Koishihara Y, Ohsugi Y. Interleukin 6 inhibits delayed-type hypersensitivity and the development of adjuvant arthritis. Eur J Immunol. 1991; 21: 2327–2331.
42. Ayanlar Batuman O, Ferrero AP, Diaz A, Jimenez SA. Regulation of transforming growth factor beta-1 gene expression by glucocorticoids in normal human T lymphocytes. J Clin Invest. 1992; 88: 1577–1580.
43. Honda M, Yamamoto S, Cheng S, et al. Human soluble IL-6 receptor: its detection and enhanced release by HIV infection. J Immunol. 1992; 148: 2175–2180.
44. Schull MM, Ormsby I, Kier AB, et al. Targeted disruption of the mouse transforming growth factor-β1 gene results in multifocal inflammatory disease. Nature. 1992; 359: 693–699.
45. Chu CQ, Field M, Allard S, Abney E, Feldmann M, Maini RM. Detection of cytokines at the cartilage/pannus junction in patients with rheumatoid arthritis: implications for the role of cytokines in cartilage destruction and repair. Brit J Rheumatol. 1992; 31: 653–661.
46. Colville-Nash PR, Scott DL. Angiogenesis and rheumatoid arthritis: pathogenetic and therapeutic implications. Ann Rheum Dis. 1992; 51: 919–925.
47. Sano H, Forough R, Maier JA, et al. Detection of high levels of heparin binding growth factor-1 (acidic fibroblast growth factor) in inflammatory arthritic joints. J Cell Biol. 1990; 110: 1417–1426.

48. Shiozawa S, Shiozawa K, Tanaka Y, et al. Human epidermal growth factor for the stratification of synovial lining layer and neovascularisation in rheumatoid arthritis. Ann Rheum Dis. 1989; 48: 820–828.

49. Butler DM, Leizer T, Hamilton JA. Stimulation of human synovial fibroblast DNA synthesis by platelet-derived growth factor and fibroblast growth factor. Differences to the activation by IL-1. J Immunol. 1989; 142: 3098–3103.

50. Ingber D, Fujita T, Kishimoto S, et al. Synthetic analogues of fumagillin that inhibit angiogenesis and suppress tumor growth. Nature. 1990; 348: 555–557.

51. Iwakura I, Tosu M, Yoshida E, et al. Induction of inflammatory arthropathy resembling rheumatoid arthritis in mi

52. Keffer J, Probert L, Cazlaris H, et al. Transgenic mice expressing human tumour necrosis factor: a predictive genetic model of arthritis. EMBO J. 1991; 10: 4025–4031.

53. Londei M, Savill CM, Verhoef A, et al. Persistance of collagen type II specific T-cell clones in the synovial membrane of a patient with rheumatoid arthritis. Proc Natl Acad Sci USA. 1989; 86: 636–640.

54. Klimiuk PS,, Clague RB, Grennan DM, Dyer PA, Smeaton I, Harris R. Autoimmunity to native type II collagen: A distinct genetic subset of rheumatoid arthritis. J Rheumatol. 1985; 12: 865–870.

55. Saxne T, Heinegard D. Involvement of nonarticular cartilage, as demonstrated by release of a cartilage-specific protein, in rheumatoid arthritis. Arthritis Rheum. 1989; 32: 1080–1086.

56. Laskin RS. Total condylar knee replacement in patients who have rheumatoid arthritis. A ten year follow-up study. J Bone Jt Surg (Am). 1991; 72: 529–535.

57. van Eden W, Holoshitz J, Nevo Z, Frenkel A, Klajman A, Cohen IR. Arthritis induced by a T lymphocyte clone that responds to mycobacterium. Proc Natl Acad Sci USA. 1985; 82: 5117–5120.

58. Holoshitz J, Matitiau A, Cohen IR. Arthritis induced in rats by cloned T lymphocytes responsive to mycobacteria. J Clin Invest. 1984; 73: 211–215.

59. Acha-Orbea H, Mitchell DJ, Timmerman L, et al. Limited heterogeneity of T cell receptors from lymphocytes mediating autoimmune encephalomyelitis allows specific immune intervention. Cell. 1988; 54: 263–273.

60. Urban JL, Kumar V, Kono DH, et al. Restricted usage of T cell receptor V genes in murine autoimmune encephalomyelitis raises possibilities for antibody therapy. Cell. 1988; 54: 577–592.

61. Heber-Katz E, Acha-Orbea H. The V-region disease hypothesis: evidence from autoimmune encephalomyelitis. Immunol Today. 1989; 10: 164–169.

62. Howell MD, Winters ST, Olee T, Powell HC, Carlo DJ, Brostoff SW. Vaccination against experimental allergic encephalomyelitis with T cell receptor peptides. Science. 1989; 246: 668–670.

63. Offner H, Hashim GA, Vandenbark AA. T cell receptor peptide therapy triggers autoregulation of experimental encephalomyelitis. Science. 1991; 251: 430–432.

64. Lider O, Karin N, Shinitzky M, Cohen IR. Therapeutic vaccination against adjuvant arthritis using T cells treated with hydrostatic pressure. Proc Natl Acad Sci USA. 1987; 84: 4577–4580.

65. Cohen IR, Weiner HL. T cell vaccination. Immunol Today. 1988; 9: 332–335.

66. Lider O, Reshef T, Beraud E, Ben-Nun A, Cohen IR. Anti-idiotypic network induced by T cell vaccination against experimental autoimmune encephalomyelitis. Science. 1988; 239: 181–193.

67. Cohen PL, Naparstek Y, Ben-Nun A, Cohen IR. Lines of T lymphocytes induce or vaccinate against autoimmune arthritis. Science. 1983; 219: 56–58.

68. Marguerie C, Lunardi C, So A. PCR-based analysis of TCR repertoire in human autoimmune diseases. Immunol Today. 1992; 13: 336–338.

69. Richardson BC. T cell receptor usage in rheumatic disease. Clin Exp Rheumatol. 1992; 10: 271–283.

70. Steinmetz M, Uematsu Y. Heterogeneity of T cell repertoires in human autoimmune disease. Brit J Rheumatol. 1991; 30: 24–27.

71. Uematsu Y, Wege H, Straus A, et al. The T cell receptor repertoire in the synovial fluid of a patient with rheumatoid arthritis is polyclonal. Proc Natl Acad Sci USA. 1991; 88:

8534–8538.
72. Sottini A, Imberti L, Gorla R, Cattaneo R, Primi D. Restricted expression of T cell receptor Vβ but not Vα genes in rheumatoid arthritis. Eur J Immunol. 1991; 21: 461–466.
73. Paliard X, West SG, Lafferty JA, et al. Evidence for the effects of a superantigen in rheumatoid arthritis. Science. 1991; 253: 325–329.
74. Bowness P, Bell J. T cell receptors and rheumatic disease: approaches to repertoire analysis. Brit J Rheumatol. 1992; 31: 3–8.
75. Hylton W, Smith-Burchnell C, Pelton BK, Palmer RG, Denman AM, Malkovsky M. Polyclonal origin of rheumatoid synovial T lymphocytes. Brit J Rheumatol. 1992; 31: 55–57.
76. Williams WV, Fang Q, Demarco D, VonFeldt J, Zurier RB, Weiner DB. Restricted heterogeneity of T cell receptor transcripts in rheumatoid synovium. J Clin Invest. 1992; 90: 326–333.
77. Choi Y, Kotzin B, Herron L, Callahan J, Marrack P, Kappler J. Interaction of *Staphylococcus aureus* toxin 'superantigens' with human T cells. Proc Natl Acad Sci USA. 1989; 86: 8941–8945.
78. Tebbib M, Alcocer-Varela J, Alarcon-Segovia D, Schur PH. Association between a T cell receptor restriction fragment length polymorphism and systemic lupus erythematosus. J Clin Invest. 1990; 86: 1961–1967.
79. Fronek Z, Lentz D, Berliner N, et al. Systemic lupus erythematosus is not genetically linked to the beta chain of the T cell receptor. Arthritis Rheum. 1986; 29: 1023–1025.
80. Wong DW, Bentwich Z, Martinez-Tarquino C, et al. Nonlinkage of the T cell receptor α, β and γ genes to systemic lupus erythematosus in multiplex families. Arthritis Rheum. 1988; 31: 1371–1376.
81. Dunckley H, Gatenby PA, Serjeantson SW. T cell receptor and HLA class II RFLPs in systemic lupus erythematosus. Immunogenetics. 1988; 27: 392–395.
82. Frank MB, McArthur R, Harley JB, Fujisaku A. Anti-Ro (SSA) autoantibodies are associated with T cell receptor β genes in systemic lupus erythematosus patients. J Clin Invest. 1990; 85: 33–39.
83. Kay RA, Hay EM, Dyer PA, et al. An abnormal T cell repertoire in hypergammaglobulinaemic primary Sjögren's syndrome. Clin Exp Immunol. 1991; 85: 262–264.
84. Freimark B, Pickering L, Concannon P, Fox R. Nucleotide sequence of a uniquely expressed human T cell receptor β chain variable region gene (Vβ) in Sjögren's syndrome. Nucleic Acids Res. 1989; 17: 455.
85. Freimark B, Fantozzi R, Bone R, Bordin G, Fox R. Detection of clonally expanded salivary gland lymphocytes in Sjögren's syndrome. Arthritis Rheum. 1989; 32: 859–869.
86. Sumida T, Yonaha F, Maeda T, et al. T cell receptor repertoire of infiltrating T cell in lips of Sjögren's syndrome patients. J Clin Invest. 1992; 89: 681–685.
87. Brennan FM, Londei M, Jackson AM, et al. T cells expressing $\gamma\delta$ chain receptors in rheumatoid arthritis. J Autoimmun. 1988; 1: 319–326.
88. Meliconi R, Pitzalis C, Kingsley GH, Panayi GS. Gamma/delta T cells and their subpopulations in blood and synovial fluid from rheumatoid arthritis and spondyloarthritis. Clin Immunol Immunopathol. 1991; 59: 165–172.
89. Brennan FM, Plater-Zyberk C, Maini RN, Feldmann M. Coordinate expansion of 'fetal type' lymphocytes (TCR $\gamma\delta$ + T and CD5 + B cells) in rheumatoid arthritis and primary Sjögren's syndrome. Clin Exp Immunol. 1989; 77: 175–178.
90. Chaouni I, Radal M, Simony-Lafontaine J, Combe B, Sany J, Reme T. Distribution of T cell receptor-bearing lymphocytes in the synovial membrane from patients with rheumatoid arthritis. J Autoimmun. 1990; 3: 737–745.
91. Reme T, Portier M, Frayssinoux F, et al. T cell receptor expression and activation of synovial lymphocyte subsets in patients with rheumatoid arthritis: phenotyping of multiple synovial sites. Arthritis Rheum. 1990; 33: 485–492.
92. Andreu JL, Trujillo A, Alonso JM, Mulero J, Martinez C. Selective expansion of T cells bearing the $\gamma\delta$ receptor and expressing an unusual repertoire in the synovial membrane of patients with rheumatoid arthritis. Arthritis Rheum. 1991; 34: 808–814.
93. Smith MD, Broker B, Moretta L, et al. T$\gamma\delta$ cells and their subsets in blood and synovial tissues from rheumatoid arthritis patients. Scand J Immunol. 1990; 32: 585–593.
94. Keystone EC, Rittershaus C, Wood N, et al. Elevation of a $\gamma\delta$ T cell subset in peripheral

blood and synovial fluid of patients with rheumatoid arthritis. Clin Exp Immunol. 1991; 84: 78–82.

95. Olive C, Gatenby PA, Serjeantson SW. Variable gene usage of T cell receptor γ- and δ-chain transcripts expressed in synovia and peripheral blood of patients with rheumatoid arthritis. Clin Exp Immunol. 1992; 87: 172–177.

96. Shen Y, Li S, Quayle AJ, Mellbye OJ, Natvig JB, Førre O. TCR γ/δ+ cell subsets in the synovial membranes of patients with rheumatoid arthritis and juvenile rheumatoid arthritis. Scand J Immunol. 1992; 36: 533–540.

97. Kjeldsen-Kragh J, Quayle A, Kalvenes C, et al. T γ/δ cells in juvenile rheumatoid arthritis and rheumatoid arthritis. In the juvenile arthritis synovium the T γ/δ cells express activation antigens and are predominantly Vδ1+ and a significant proportion of these patients have elevated percentages of T γ/δ cells. Scand J Immunol. 1990; 32: 651–660.

98. Rajagopalan S, Zordan T, Tsokos GC, Datta SK. Pathogenic anti-DNA autoantibody-inducing T helper cell lines from patients with active lupus nephritis: isolation of CD4- T helper cell lines that express the $\gamma\delta$ T cell antigen receptor. Proc Natl Acad Sci USA. 1990; 87: 7020–7024.

99. Rajagopalan S, Mao C, Datta SK. Pathogenic autoantibody-inducing $\gamma\delta$ T helper cells in human lupus nephritis express unusual T cell receptors. Arthritis Rheum. 1991; 34: S74.

100. Lunardi C, Marguerie C, Bowness P, Walport MJ, So AK. Reduction in T $\gamma\delta$ cell numbers and alteration in subset distribution in systemic lupus erythematosus. Arthritis Rheum. 1991; 34: S162.

101. Kratz LE, Boughman JA, Pincus T, Cohen DI, White-Needleman B. Association of scleroderma with a T cell antigen receptor γ gene restriction fragment length polymorphism. Arthritis Rheum. 1990; 33: 569–573.

102. Hohfeld R, Engel AG, Ii K, Harper MC. Polymyositis mediated by T lymphocytes that express the γ/δ receptor. N Engl J Med. 1991; 324: 877–881.

103. Oppenheimer-Marks N, Davis LS, Bogue DT, Ramberg J, Lipsky PE. Differential utilization of ICAM-1 and VCAM-1 during the adhesion and transendothelial migration of human T lymphocytes. J Immunol. 1991; 147: 1913–1921.

104. Pietschmann P, Cush JJ, Lipsky PE, Shen C-L, Chou L-J, Jan M-S. Identification of subsets of human T cells capable of enhanced transendothelial migration. J Immunol. 1992; 149: 1170–1178.

105. Shimizu Y, Newman W, Tanaka Y, Shaw S. Lymphocyte interactions with endothelial cells. Immunol Today. 1992; 13: 106–112.

106. Pitzalis C, Kingsley GH, Haskard DO, Panayi GS. The preferential accumulation of helper-inducer T lymphocytes in inflammatory lesions: evidence for regulation by selective endothelial and homotypic adhesion. Eur J Immunol. 1988; 18: 1397–1404.

107. Pitzalis C, Kingsley GH, Costantinides Y, Panayi GS. Predominance of 4B4+ (helper-inducer/memory) T cells within the joint may be partly related to their maturation state. Brit J Rheumatol. 1988; 27: 97.

108. Pitzalis C, Kingsley GH, Covelli M, Meliconi R, Markey A, Panayi GS. Selective migration of the human helper-inducer memory T cell subset: confirmation by in vivo cellular kinetic studies. Eur J Immunol. 1991; 21: 369–376.

109. Damle NK, Doyle LV. Ability of human T lymphocytes to adhere to vascular endothelial cells and to augment endothelial permeability to macromolecules is linked to their state of post-thymic maturation. J Immunol. 1990; 144: 1233–1240.

110. Cush JJ, Lipsky PE, Oppenheimer-Marks N. Phenotypic analysis of T cell with intrinsically different abilities to bind and migrate through endothelium. Arthritis Rheum. 1991; 34: D30.

111. Mackay CR, Marston WL, Dudler L, Spertini O, Tedder TF, Heine WR. Tissue-specific migration pathways by phenotypically distinct subpopulations of memory T cells. Eur J Immunol. 1992; 887: 895.

112. Gauldie J, Richards C, Harnish D, Lansdorp PM, Bauman H. Interferon beta 2/B cell stimulator factor type 2 shares identity with monocyte-derived hepatocyte-stimulating factor and regulates the major acute phase protein response in liver cells. Proc Natl Acad Sci USA. 1987; 84: 7251–7255.

113. Andus T, Geiger T, Hirano T, Kishimoto T, Heinrich PC. Action of recombinant human interleukin 6, interleukin 1 and tumour necrosis factor α on the mRNA induction of acute

phase proteins. Eur J Immunol. 1988; 18: 739–746.
114. Morrone G, Cilberto G, Olivero S, et al. Recombinant interleukin 6 regulates the transcriptional activation of a set of human acute phase genes. J Biol Chem. 1988; 263: 12554–12558.
115. Naitoh Y, Fukata J, Tominaga T, et al. Interleukin-6 stimulates the secretion of adrenocorticotropic hormone in conscious, freely moving rats. Biochem Biophys Res Commun. 1988; 155: 1459–1463.
116. Linardopoulos S, Corrigall V, Panayi GS. Activation of HLA-DR and interleukin 6 gene transcription in resting T cells via the CD2 molecule: relevance to chronic immune-mediated inflammation. Scand J Immunol. 1992; 36: 469–477.
117. Shimizu Y, Shaw S. Lymphocyte interactions with extracellular matrix. FASEB J. 1991; 5: 2292–2299.
118. Goldman R, Harvey J, Hogg N. VLA-2 is the integrin receptor used as a collagen receptor by leukocytes. Eur J Immunol. 1992; 22: 1109–1114.
119. Rodriguez RM, Pitzalis C, Kingsley GH, Henderson EM, Humphries MJ, Panayi GS. T-lymphocyte adhesion to fibronectin: a possible mechanism for T cell accumulation in the rheumatoid joint. Clin Exp Immunol. 1992; 89: 439–445.
120. Garcia-Vicuna R, Humbria A, Postigo AA, et al. VLA family in rheumatoid arthritis: evidence for in vivo regulated adhesion of synovial fluid T cells to fibronectin through VLA-5 integrin. Clin Exp Immunol. 1992; 88: 435–441.
121. Yamada A, Nikaido T, Nojima Y, Schlossman SF, Morimoto C. Activation of human CD4 T lymphocytes. Interaction of fibronectin with VLA-5 receptor on CD4 cells induces the AP-1 transcription factor. J Immunol. 1991; 146: 53–56.
122. Lazarovits AI, White MJ, Karsh J. CD7- T cells in rheumatoid arthritis. Arthritis Rheum. 1992; 35: 615–624.
123. Doyle C, Strominger JL. Interaction between CD4 and class II MHC molecules mediates cell adhesion. Nature. 1987; 330: 256–259.
124. Krzesicki RF, Fleming WE, Winterrowd GE, Hatfield CA, Sanders ME, Chin JE. T lymphocyte adhesion to human synovial fibroblasts. Arthritis Rheum. 1991; 34: 1245–1253.

2

B Cells and Rheumatoid Factors in Rheumatoid Arthritis

K. M. THOMPSON, I. RANDEN, Ø. FØRRE and J. B. NATVIG

INTRODUCTION

B cells and autoantibodies play a significant role in several autoimmune diseases including rheumatoid arthritis (RA)[1], systemic lupus erythematosus (SLE) and many organ specific autoimmune diseases[2]. There is considerable evidence to implicate immunoglobulins and immune complexes in the pathogenesis of RA. The central site of pathology in RA is the synovial tissue. This tissue becomes chronically stimulated in the disease and may increase in weight from 100 to 1000 times normal. Blood vessels proliferate in the tissue, and macrophages, dendritic cells, T and B lymphocytes and plasma cells accumulate (Table 1), such that greater than 50% of the tissue mass can be of lymphoid cells[3]. In contrast to normal peripheral blood, synovial tissue B cells and plasma cells are highly activated, and synovial tissue fragments, or isolated cells, spontaneously secrete significant amounts of immunoglobulin in culture. Unlike peripheral blood lymphocytes, this spontaneous secretion is only very moderately augmented by mitogenic stimulation (Table 2)[4]. The immunoglobulins secreted by synovial plasma cells have been shown to display a restricted electrophoretic mobility and unusual isotype distributions of IgG that may vary from patient to patient[3,5–7]. This suggests that the immunoglobulin secretion may be driven by a single, or restricted number of antigens, rather than by a random polyclonal activation. The nature of this, or these antigens is unknown, and the only specificity of antibody response that is accepted as part of the pathogenic process is that directed to IgG, i.e. rheumatoid factor. Rheumatoid factors are found in the plasma, synovial fluid and synovial tissues of most RA patients. In the synovial tissues, RF and RF secreting plasma cells can be found in considerable quantities and in all major classes of immunoglobulin. They are deposited as complexes in the synovial tissues, where they fix

Table 1 Some characteristics of inflammatory cells in rheumatoid synovitis

Macrophages (5%–10%)
– Activated *in vivo* with phagocytosis and ADCC-type cytotoxic reactions
– Antigen processing and presentation

Lymphoid Dendritic cells (2%–4%)
– CD45+, HLA-DR, DP, DQ+
– Antigen-presenting cells

T cells (70%–80%)
– Mostly CD4+ T helper cells of CD45 RO memory type but also CD8+ T suppressor cells
– T cells activated *in vivo*, HLA-DR+, IL-2R+, TFR+

B cells (10%–15%)
– Activated *in vivo*, develop into plasma cells
– Spontaneously produce Ig and antibodies (e.g. RF)

IL-2R, Interleukin-2 receptor; TfR, transferring receptor; RF, rheumatoid factor; ADCC, antibody-dependent cellular cytotoxicity
Data from [8,89]

Table 2 Immunoglobulin* synthesized by 1×10^6 cells/ml in peripheral blood of normal donors and lymphocytes from rheumatoid arthritis (RA) synovial tissue

	Normal donors (17)	*RA synovial tissue (8)*	P *value*
Without PWM†	244 ng (98–1331)	3019 ng (900–8050)	<0.006
With PWM	1670 ng (440–8976)	4201 ng (850–16 285)	<0.02
Stimulation index	6.8	1.39	

*values of Ig are geometric mean. Values in parenthesis show the ranges. P value by Mann-Whitney test (two-tailed)
†PWM = pokeweed mitogen
Data from[4]

complement and probably contribute to the pathology of the disease by generating inflammatory responses[8]. The largest complexes are found in the synovial tissue. Large, soluble complexes are found in the synovial fluid and these have strong complement binding properties. In serum, complexes are usually small and mostly non-complement-fixing[8]. The presence of larger circulating immune complexes may play a role in extra-articular disease in RA[9].

Rheumatoid factors are found in other conditions than the rheumatic diseases; they appear in the plasma transiently following infection or immunization, and can be frequently seen as M components in lymphoproliferative diseases such as mixed cryoglobulinaemia and Waldenstrom's macroglobulinaemia. In neither case are symptoms of RA apparent. It has been shown that immune complexes and vaccination can trigger the production of RF in normals[10–12], and there is evidence that B cells expressing membrane IgM with RF activity can act as antigen presenting cells for antibody-antigen complexes[13]. One important challenge in understanding the rheumatoid inflammatory process is to discover how and why RF form a pathological process in RA, whereas they are a part of a physiological process in normal individuals.

THE ROLE OF THE CD5-POSITIVE B CELL IN RA

CD5 molecules present on all human T cells are also detectable, but weakly expressed, on some human B cells. From about the 17th week of gestation most foetal splenic and lymph node B cells are CD5 positive[14]. This proportion falls during development to 8–25% of circulating and splenic B cells in the normal adult[15,16]. Based on observations showing self-renewal capacity of such cells in mice and the absence of a substantial change of CD5 phenotype during B cell activation *in vitro*, CD5+ B cells have been considered to represent a separate cell lineage and have attracted much attention in the study of autoimmune responses. CD5 B cells appear enriched in autoantibody producing cells, particularly those producing 'polyreactive' or 'multispecific' antibodies that bind several unrelated auto- and exo-antigens[17,18].

There have been several reports of an elevated proportion of CD5+ B cells in the peripheral blood of some RA patients compared to normals[19–21]. Estimates of the degree of this increase vary; in one study it was found that treatment of the B cells with PMA was necessary before a statistical increase was found[19], whereas one report documented that 100% of peripheral blood B cells in a single RA patient expressed the CD5 marker[22]. There is some evidence of an association between CD5+ B cells and RF production. A significant correlation between IgM RF and the percentage of B cells expressing CD5 in the peripheral blood of RA patients has been reported[20]. EBV stimulation of purified B cell subsets from RA peripheral blood leads to a greater production of IgM RF by CD5+ B cells than by CD5− B cells[21]. CD5+ B cells produce IgM RF when activated by *Staphylococcus aureus in vitro*, and produce similar amounts whether derived from cord blood, adult blood or RA peripheral blood[23].

The role of the CD5+ B cell in RA is still controversial. Examination of RA synovial tissues revealed very few CD5+ B cells[24]. The CD5 molecule may be a marker on B cells for differentiation or activation, as it has been shown that after stimulation *in vitro* with mutagenized thymoma cells and T cell supernatant, 70% of CD5− B cells become CD5+ after three days[25]. CD5 expression can also be induced by TPA, reaching a maximum after 48 hours, then declining[26]. The higher frequency of RF secreting cells among the CD5+ population may just reflect *in vivo* activation of these cells, either in physiological or in pathological conditions[27]. There is no absolute distinction in the properties of immunoglobulins secreted by CD5+ vs CD5− B cells. CD5+ B cells have been reported to secrete both 'monoreactive' and 'polyreactive' RF[27]. IgM antibodies from both CD5+ and CD5− cord blood B cells show polyreactivity and RF activity[28]. Polyreactivity is not restricted to a subset of B cells distinct from those engaged in responses to external antigens[29].

THE SPECIFICITY AND POLYREACTIVITY OF RF

Rheumatoid factors have, by definition, specificity for the Fc region of immunoglobulins of the IgG isotype (IgG Fc). Initially described as a factor in serum of RA patients that agglutinated sheep red blood cells coated with rabbit IgG[30], RF has been shown to bind IgG Fc of a variety of species[31]. Although RF are described that bind to the pFc' fragment (CH3)[32], most determinants for RF binding are located in the $C\gamma2$–$C\gamma3$ interface region[33,34].

Human IgG can be divided into four isotypes and several allotypes. Most allotypes represent only one amino acid interchange and were first discovered using sera from RA patients with restricted RF specificity[35]. Both anti-allotypic sera[36] and a monoclonal anti-allotypic RF have been described[37], but more typically, RF recognize non-genetic epitopes found on several IgG subclass proteins. Common is the Ga antigen that is found on IgG1, IgG2 and IgG4 molecules. IgM antibodies showing Ga specificity are frequently found among synovial tissue derived RF[37,38] and serum polyclonal RF[34]. Interestingly, a variant of the Ga specificity, named 'the Ga related specificity' that includes binding to IgG3 molecules bearing the G3m(s,t) markers, corresponds to the conventional binding site for Staphylococcal protein A (SPA)[39,40]. The first human monoclonal RF isolated from peripheral blood lymphocytes (RFAN) was shown to have Ga related specificity[41].

Monoclonal antibodies particularly, but not exclusively of the multivalent IgM class, can often be shown to be multispecific[42], and it is thought that these correspond to the natural autoantibodies present in the serum. The term 'natural antibody' was first used to describe 'those molecules present in the body fluids of normal animals having the capacity to combine specifically with potential antigens and being distinct to those produced in response to specific antigenic stimulus'[43]. Natural antibodies are usually multispecific and are able to recognize several different self and foreign antigens. They are often termed natural autoantibodies[44]. Natural autoantibodies reacting with IgG, tubulin, actin, myoglobin, thyroglobulin, fetuin, albumin and transferrin are present in normal human sera, and monoclonal immunoglobulins from multiple myeloma and Waldenstrom's macroglobulinaemia may express similar antibody specificities. It has been suggested that natural autoantibodies (multispecific, polyspecific or polyreactive antibodies) originate in humans from the CD5+ subset of B cells[16]. These multispecific antibodies are seen as a distinct population of antibodies from the monospecific antibodies produced in response to external antigens, having a possible role in the first line of defence against invading micro-organisms, the elimination of dead tissues or being part of a primitive interconnecting set of B cells involved in setting up an idiotypic network early in life. It has been suggested that these antibodies may produce high affinity, monospecific antibodies by the process of affinity maturation[45,46]. It seems unlikely that this simple interpretation is correct, as highly mutated antibodies of high affinity, specific for exogenous antigens can display multispecific reactions[29].

There has been much interest over the last few years in using monoclonal antibody technology for studying the autoantibody response in autoimmune diseases, including RA. Many autoantigens that are the targets of pathological autoimmune responses are also frequently recognized by multispecific anti-bodies (e.g. IgG, thyroglobulin, DNA). However, it has been shown that monoclonal antibodies that are the product of immune responses to exogenous antigens can share these specificities against unrelated antigens[29]. This poses some problems in deciding whether monoclonal RF (and other autoantibodies) derived from autoimmune patients are typical of the disease, represent natural autoantibodies or are multispecific antibodies directed to exogenous antigens. There is the possibility that three 'classes' of RF exist:

(i)   antibodies that are apparently monospecific for the IgG Fc;
(ii) antibodies that show multispecific properties, but whose 'primary' antigen is IgG Fc;
(iii) antibodies that show multispecific properties, whose autoreactivity to IgG is unrelated to the 'primary' antigen.

One would clearly have most confidence in studying autoantibodies of the first category, but as multispecificity may be a function of the number of antigens tested and the concentration of antibody, these may be rather few. The use of fixed tissue sections seems particularly sensitive for detecting polyreactivity, although the significance of such interactions is questionable[29]. Monoclonal RF originally designated as 'monoreactive' can be shown to bind several structurally unrelated antigens in these assays (unpublished data). Distinguishing whether a monoclonal RF selected on the basis of an autoreactivity belongs to the second (relevant?) or third (irrelevant?) categories is difficult. To distinguish whether an antibody has RF activity because of its polyreactivity, a minimum requirement should be the demonstration of RF activity in two or more types of assay (e.g. agglutination of IgG coated latex, and ELISA), with the use of appropriate controls in each assay type (irrelevant protein coated latex, irrelevant antigen coated ELISA trays). This review tries to focus on monoclonal RF that meet these criteria.

THE GENETIC ORIGINS OF RF

There are several questions related to the genes coding for autoantibodies such as RF. Are genes coding for rheumatoid factors from RA patients different from those coding for M-component rheumatoid factor? Is there any unusual gene utilization or any genes that are peculiar to RA patients involved in RF production? Do RF genes in RA show evidence of somatic mutations and affinity maturation typical of a product of an antigen driven response? To answer some of these questions, a thorough analysis of the genetic origins of rheumatoid factors as well as an understanding of the organization of IgG genes are important. The human V_H, D and J_H segments map to chromosome 14 and recombine during B cell development. In contrast to the mouse, where V_H gene families are found clustered, the human V_H family members are very interspersed. The number of V_H gene segments is probably less than 100, the number of D segments is approximately 25, and there are six J_H gene segments. The human V_H gene segments can be divided into six or seven families based on nucleotide sequence homology.

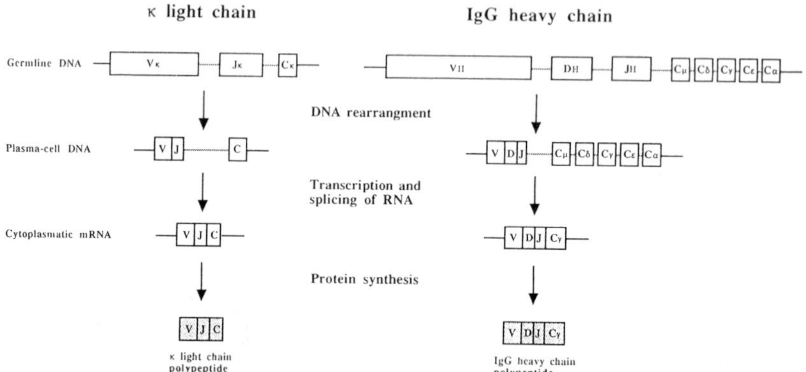

Figure 1 Schematic presentation of the germline DNA segments coding for the production of light-chains (κ-light chain) and heavy chain in mature plasma cells. The various gene segments of the variable gene (V and J for light chain and V-D and J for heavy chains, rearrange first to make a VJ or VDJ transcript and then rearrange with constant gene segments by transcription and splicing of RNA to make RNA coding for a complete polypeptide chain

Members of the same family show greater than 80% sequence identity whereas there is less than 70% homology between families[47–49]. The largest V_H families are V_HI and V_HIII, which contain approximately 20–40 members. Considerable effort has recently been directed to sequencing the germline repertoire of V_H gene segments, such that we can now be fairly confident in ascribing germline counterparts to expressed immunoglobulin sequences[50]. Fewer light chain gene segments have been sequenced. The human Vκ gene repertoire in the human germline contains about 50 potentially functional gene segments and a maximum of 85 all together[51,52]. These gene segments have been divided into six families with sizes ranging from one member (VκIV) to between 20 and 30 (VκI and VκII). There are approximately 15 germline genes belonging to the VκIII family. How many of these are pseudogenes is not known. The Vκ locus is polymorphic and as with the V_H families, the human Vκ gene family members are widely dispersed. There are five Jκ gene segments and a single Cκ gene segment[51].

Although 40% of human light chains belong to the lambda isotype compared with only 5% in the mouse, the Vλ light chain locus in humans is less well characterized than the κ locus. Seven or eight Vλ families have been identified and several polymorphic variants have been detected indicating that the human Vλ locus is considerably more complex than that of the mouse. By analogy with the V_H and Vκ loci, it is reasonable to suggest that the different Vλ families should be interspersed and that extensive polymorphism should be expected. The principle of rearrangement of Ig heavy chain genes and κ light chain genes is shown in Figure 1.

The different rearrangements of the V, D and J segments for heavy chain or V and J for light chains, potentially can produce many different antibody specificities. However, besides specificities that are directly encoded in the germline, additional variability of antigen binding regions can be made by differences in the joining process. Multiple mechanisms participate in the generation of human CDR3 (complementarity determining region) that are particularly important for the generation of the antibody combining site[53]. Somatic mutations add additional variability to the expressed immunoglobulin.

As mentioned above, much interest has been directed to the structure and genetic origins of RF. Such studies may provide insights into the role of 'disease specific' genes in the production of RF in RA, whether RF in the rheumatoid inflammation are antigen driven or the result of a functional dysregulation (polyclonal activation), and whether somatic mutations may result in particularly pathogenic antibodies. The earliest studies relied on serological techniques using the readily available M-components with RF activity. Cross-reactive idiotypes (CRI) were defined on different molecules and these were predicted to be contained in the variable regions of the antibodies[54]. Studies on RF M-components suggested that RF activity was associated with a restricted set of variable region structures. Kunkel and co-workers found that approximately 60% of mixed cryoglobulin RF of the IgM express the Wa CRI[55]. Sequence analyses of Wa positive proteins showed that they use gene segments from the V_HI family, often in combination with light chains of the VκIIIb sub-subgroup[56]. Some mixed cryoglobulin RF (20%) were found to express the Po CRI[54]. A minor group shared a CRI termed Bla, and this was found associated with RF that also showed antihistone activity[57]. Over the last few years, studies on the genetic origins of RF have benefited from the development of rodent monoclonal antibodies to defined variable region structures on human immunoglobulins, and the production of human monoclonal RF secreting cell lines derived from both the peripheral blood and synovial tissues of RA patients. This has allowed a much more detailed analysis of the variable region gene segments involved in the production of RF specificities.

LIGHT CHAIN VARIABLE REGION GENE UTILIZATION BY RF

There is considerable evidence that M-components with RF activity preferentially use a restricted set of kappa light chain gene segments. This is particularly evident in monoclonal RF derived from mixed cryoglobulinaemia patients, where 97% of a panel of IgMκ RF were shown to use light chains of the VκIII family, and 70% of these to use VκIIIb (Figure 2)[58]. In a review of many M-component RF from different sources, 86% of the entire panel used KIII light chains, and more than half these utilized VκIIIb light chains[59]. Evidence that very few gene segments were involved within these two sub-families was provided by using two monoclonal antibodies, 17.109 and 6B6.6, which together recognise 60% of a panel of IgMκ RF M-components[60]. The 17.109 monoclonal antibody recognises the product of two members of the VκIIIb subfamily, Kv325[61,62] and Kv305[63,64], while the 6B6.6 monoclonal antibody recognises the product of a single member of the VκIII subfamily, Kv328[51,65].

The restriction of kappa V region gene segments seen in the M-component RF is not found in RF derived from RA patients. The expression of both the 17.109 and the 6B6.6 idiotopes is low in both RA patients and normals.

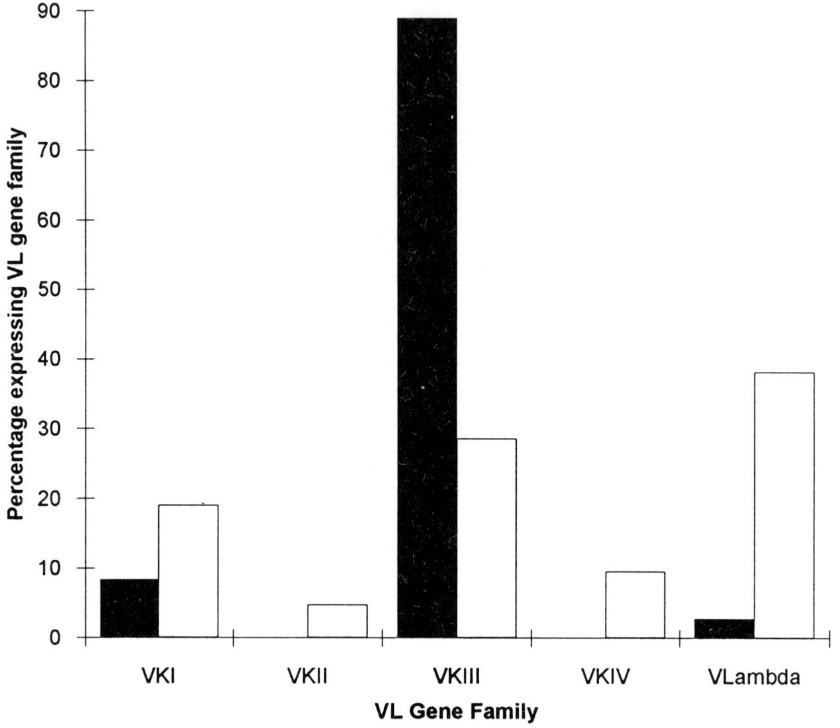

Figure 2 A comparison of V_L gene family usage by RF from M-components (solid bars, $n = 36$), and RF from RA patients (open bars, $n = 21$). The gene families used by RF from RA patients are much more diverse than in the case of M-component RF, where predominantly members of the VκIII family are used. The single lambda M-component RF is of unknown gene family. The lambda RF from RA patients include λ1 (4), λ2 (1), λ3 (2) and λ8 (1). Data from[59] and see legend to Table 3

In a survey of 7200 individuals including both normals and RA patients, the 17.109 idiotope was detected in 13% of the RA group, and 19% of the healthy, non-RA group. The 6B6.6 idiotope was found in 26% of the RA group and 28% of the non-RA group[66]. Studies on monoclonal RF produced from the synovial tissues of RA patients support this view. A panel of 14 monoclonal RF derived from three RA patients included 12 of the kappa isotype. In contrast to the M-component RF, only four of these were of the VκIII family. Three of these were of the VκIIIb subfamily, and all three of these expressed the 17.109 idiotope[63]. One utilized the VκIIIa gene segment with high homology to Kv328, although this was reported not to express the 6B6.6 idiotope. The level of VκIII family expression seems approximately the same as among random immunoglobulins in normals. It has been shown by *in situ* hybridization that approximately 30% of all kappa light chains expressed by normal peripheral blood lymphocytes use the VκIII family[67]. A review of the light chains used by monoclonal RF derived from RA patients shows a lack of restriction of V_L gene segments used. Thus very

Table 3 V-gene usage in RF derived from RA patients

Clone	Donor	V_H	Germline Donor	% homology	VL	Closest gene	% homology
IgM							
RF-TS1	ST	I	HON-1	100.0	κIIIb	325	99.3
RF-TS5	ST	III	22-2B	99.3	κI	HK102	97.9
RF-SJ2	ST	III	GL-SJ2	99.3	λ1	FOG B	96.3
RF-SJ3	ST	III	1.9111	99.3	κIIIb	325	98.7
RF-TS3	ST	I	DP-21	99.3	κII	A23	100
HAF 10	ST	I	DP-7	97.3	λVIII	k6h6	89
RF-TS2	ST	III	1.9111	97.3	κIIIa	328	97
mAb 61	PB	IV	V71-2	96.3	λI	1B9/F2	96.2
RF-SJ1	ST	III	GL-SJ2	96.3	λI	FOG B	93
RF-TS4*	ST	III	1.9111	95.8	κI	Vκ1-02	96.5
RF-SJ4	ST	IV	V71-2	95.4	κIIIb	305	100
YES 8	BM	I	DP-10	94.5	κIIIb	325	98
RF-KL1	ST	III	VH26	94.2	κI	Vd	97.5
RFAN	PB	III	VH26	83.7	λIII	ND	ND
IgA							
mAb 60	PB	III	DP-53	91.4	λIII	?	–
P61B27	PB	I	DP-21	90.1	κIV	HSVK1VR	89.5
IgG							
D1	ST	III	DP-51	99.3	κIII	AE6-5	96.0
RF-TS7	ST	I	Hv1L1R	99.3	λII	HuL2-4A	98.6
RF-KL5	ST	III	DP-31	96.9	κIV/VI	?	–
L1	ST	I	Hv1L1	95.9	λI	Hulv1L1	95.3
RF-SJ5	ST	III	1.9111	93.3	κI	VD	94.7

RF from RA patients shown ranked according to their homologies with closest V_H germline gene segments. Closest V_L gene segments are shown whether they are expressed or germline, D1 and L1 from [81], HAF 10 from [82], Yes 8 from [83], mAb 60 and 61 from [84], RFAN, RF-TS, RF-SJ and RF-KL from [64,85,86]. P61B27 from [87]
*Partial heavy chain variable region sequence
ST = synovial tissue
BM = bone marrow
PB = peripheral blood

many different light chain families can contribute to the generation of RF specificity (Table 3).

HEAVY CHAIN VARIABLE REGION GENE UTILIZATION BY RF

The Wa positive, M-component RF frequently express the V_HI-associated idiotope defined by the G6 monoclonal antibody[68]. In a study of random IgM M-components, 35% of those with RF activity were found to express the idiotope, compared to only 5% of those without RF activity. RF heavy chains expressing the G6 idiotope are frequently, but not exclusively, found expressed with VκIIIb light chains expressing the 17.109 idiotope[60]. Examination of various M-component RF from different sources has revealed V_HI to be the most frequently used variable heavy chain family (41%); the

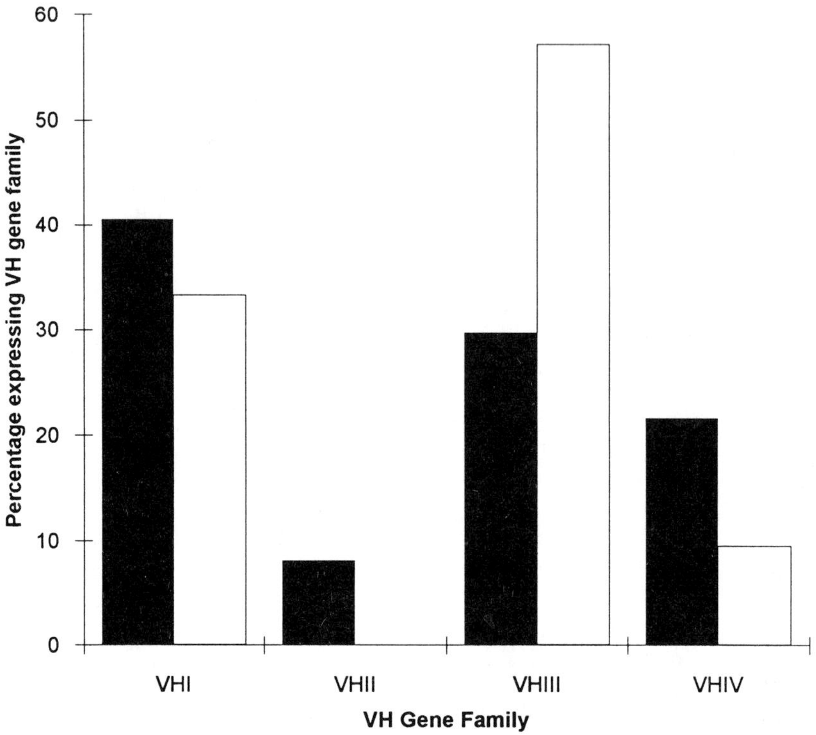

Figure 3 A comparison of V_H gene family usage by RF from M-components (solid bars, $n = 37$) and RF from RA patients (open bars, $n = 21$). Data from[59] and see legend to Table 3

vast majority of these pairing with VκIIIb light chains. V_HIV family gene segments were used by 22% of the M-component RF. Rheumatoid factors of the V_HIV family have been shown to pair highly preferentially with light chains expressing the 6B6.6 idiotope[69]. V_HIII family gene segments were used by 30% of the M-component RF. RF using V_HIII gene segments seem more promiscuous in use of light chain variable region gene segments, and have been found together with lambda, VκI, VκIIIa and VκIIIb light chains.

Studies on the V_H gene family use by monoclonal RF derived from RA patients show a different distribution (Figure 3). Of 17 reported monoclonal RF, 10 (59%) use V_HIII gene family members, compared to only 5 (29%) that use V_HI (Figure 3). Two were found to use V_HIV gene segments. As is true with the M-component RF, the V_HIII monoclonal RF are promiscuous in their pairing with light chain gene segments, and have been shown to pair with VλI, VλIII, VκI, VκIIIa and VκIIIb segments. Of the four V_HI monoclonal IgM RF, only two pair with VκIIIb light chains (both using Kv325), whereas the other two use VλVII and VκII (Table 3). The lower levels of V_HI RF in RA seem borne out in studies on circulating RF. RF bearing the V_HI-related, G6 idiotope have been found to represent 37% of the total RF in normal individuals, but only 27% in RA patients with self-limiting synovitis, and only 3% of those with persistent synovitis[70].

V GENES USED BY RF ARE DIVERSE AND FOUND IN THE GENERAL POPULATION

A restriction in variable region gene structures used in response to some exogenous and auto-antigens has been shown[71-73]. Such restriction is not apparent in RF derived from RA patients, nor is there evidence for the presence of 'RA-specific' variable region gene segments. Nucleotide sequencing of RF of all major isotypes from patients with rheumatoid arthritis shows that a majority use variable heavy chain genes belonging to the V_HIII family (Table 3). Twelve out of twenty-one, sequenced V_H genes belong to this family (57%), whereas seven use V_H gene segments belonging to the V_HI family and two belong to the V_HIV family. Because the number of genes sequenced is small, it is hard to say whether there is an over-representation of V_HIII genes among RF. However, we have found, by making more RF secreting hybridomas from the synovial tissue of patient TS, that $\sim 80\%$ (15/18) V_H genes in these RF belong to the V_HIII family (unpublished observations). If this turns out to be a general feature among RF from RA patients, one may speculate that framework structures, which are conserved among members of a given family more than the hypervariable regions, could be involved in antigen binding. Involvement of family-specific FW regions (FW1 and FW3) in antigen binding has been suggested by Schroeder et al.[74]. These authors base their hypothesis on the high degree of FW sequence conservation, especially in regions that are solvent exposed, in both mice and humans. Four RF display the closest homology with a single member of the V_HIII family, the germline 1.9III gene segment. It is difficult to decide if this prevalence is connected to RF specificity or whether it just reflects the normal repertoire. The fact that this segment is also used in antibodies without RF activity[75] suggests that it may be frequently used in diverse immune responses. Other than this possible reference, RF use a diverse array of V gene segments. The seven antibodies that use genes belonging to the V_HI family display their closest homology to seven different V_HI gene segments. Virtually all V_L families seem able to contribute to the binding of RF to human IgG.

D AND J GENE USAGE BY RF

There is tremendous heterogeneity in the D segments of the RF. Although some of them display homology to known germline D gene segments (Table 4), this is only of limited degree, and indicates that multiple mechanisms of diversification or not yet described germline genes are involved. Except for the clonally related RF-SJ1 and RF-SJ2, which are 75% homologous at the protein level, there is extensive diversity in the D segments among these antibodies sharing the same specificity for IgG Fc (Figure 4). The sequence differences and variations in length may reflect the various fine specificities for Fc epitopes and allotypes.

The J_H usage does not seem to be restricted as all J_H gene segments are represented except J_H2. There is a slight preference for J_H4, however, as close

Table 4 D and J gene segment usage in RF

Clone	V_H	D Germline donor	J_H	V_L	J_L
IgM					
RF-TS1	I	DHFL16	3	κIIIb	κ1
RF-TS3	I	21-05/DK1	1	κII	κ5
HAF 10	I	?	4	λVIII	?
YES 8	I	?	4	κIIIb	κ2
RF-TS5	III	?	4	κI	κ4
RF-SJ2	III	DLR2	6	λl	λ2
RF-SJ3	III	DLR1	6	κIIIb	?
RF-TS2	III	?	3	κIIIa	κ5
RF-SJ1	III	DLR2	6	λI	λ2
RF-TS4	III	?	1	κI	κ2
RF-KL1	III	DN4	4	κI	κ5
RFAN	III	DLR2	4	λIII	?
RF-SJ4	IV	DHFL16	4	κ3IIIb	κ5
mAb 61	IV	DLR1	6	λI	λ2
IgA					
P61B27	I	?	4	κIV	κ2
mAb 60	III	DLR1	5	λIII	λ2
IgG					
RF-TS7	I	DRL4	4	λII	λ2
L1	I	D21-9	3	λI	λ2
D1	III	D21-10/DK4	4	κIII	κ1
RF-KL5	III	?	4	κIV/VI	κ2
RF-SJ5	III	?	3	κI	κ4

The different V_H, D, J_H, V_L and J_L segments used by rheumatoid factors from RA patients. There is only partial homology between the expressed D segments and the germline D segments listed here

to 50% are using this particular J_H gene segment. The J segments in the light chains are diverse for the κ chains, but all λ light chains in this group of RF use $J_\lambda 2$ gene segments. This may indicate some restriction in the J_λ usage.

THE ROLE OF SOMATIC MUTATION AND AFFINITY MATURATION IN RF

Studies on the degree to which RF are somatically mutated will give an indication as to whether RF are the product of an antigen driven response, or the result of a non-driven expansion of germline encoded B cells. In this context it is important to compare sequences with those which are definitely the result of an antigen drive. A number of such studies have been carried out, most comprehensively for the human response to the Rh(D) blood group antigen[76]. The V_H segment of IgM anti-D antibodies were found to be on average approximately 99% homologous to germline segments. IgG anti-D, V_H gene segments differed considerably in their homologies to germline

	ISOTYPE	CDR3 REGION			
RF-SJ2	M	GRFCSGGSCYS	YYYYYY MDV	WGK	JH6
RF-SJ1	M	GVYCSSSSCYS	YYYYHY MDV	WGK	JH6
RF-SJ3	M	WGGYCTNGVCYRGG	YGMDV	WGK	JH6
mAb 61	M	LGPDDYTL	YYYDGMDV	WGQ	JH6
mAb 60	A	TGGGTNW	FDS	WGQ	JH5
RF-KL1	M	LRSGLVPYY	FDS	WGQ	JH4
RF-SJ4	M	GSVGATLGE	FDY	WGQ	JH4
RF-KL5	G	EG	FDY	WGQ	JH4
YES 8	M	GIASAGTLN	YFF Y	WGQ	JH4
RFAN	M	TRSYVVAAEYY	FHY	WGQ	JH4
RF-TS5	M	TPFI	DY	WGQ	JH4
P61B27	A	DRWN	DY	WGQ	JH4
HAF 10	M	DSRGGDLLTGHHCI	DY	WGQ	JH4
D1	G	SGYRGG	DY	WGQ	JH4
RF-TS7	G	GYQMDVN	Y	WGQ	JH4
RF-TS1	M	EDPYGDYVANP	FDI	WGQ	JH3
RF-TS2	M	DRVAVYASVFFIDS	FDI	WGQ	JH3
RF-SJ5	G	LGDYIGSYGGFRA	FDI	WGQ	JH3
L1	G	EYFYDGSDLKPSDV	FDI	WGQ	JH3
RF-TS3	M	EDSNGYKI	FDI	WDQ	JH1
RF-TS4	M	EDAPYCSGGTCNP	Y FQH	WGP	JH1

Figure 4 A comparison of the amino acid sequence of the third hypervariable region (CDR3) of the heavy chains of RF from RA patients. There are extensive differences in length and amino acid composition of these proteins all binding IgG Fc

sequences, varying from almost 92% to 99%, with an average of approximately 97%. Clearly, with 'antigen driven' IgM antibodies demonstrating such lack of somatic mutation in the V_H segments (one had only a single nucleotide difference from germline), it could be very difficult to judge the role of antigen-drive amongst IgM antibodies. However, over half the IgM RF (Table 3) have homologies of less than 97.3% with germline counterparts, and some are considerably further from germline, which suggests they are the product of an antigen driven response. This is strongly supported by the isolation of two clonally related IgM RF, RF-SJ1 and RF-SJ2, from a single donor[77]. Both antibodies use V_HIII genes together with a D segment derived from the DRL-2D germline gene combined with JH6 gene segments. The light chains consist of Vλ1 rearranged to Jλ2. All the joints generated during the rearrangement procedure are identical, including the nucleotides randomly added at the 5' end of the D segments. The V_H of RF-SJ2 has only two nucleotide differences compared to its germline counterpart (GL-SJ2), while RF-SJ1 had accumulated 18 nucleotide differences compared to RF-SJ2. The light chain of RF-SJ1 had also acquired 18 nucleotide differences compared to RF-SJ2. Functional affinity studies showed that the extensively mutated antibody has a hundred times higher affinity for human IgG than the RF which was close to germline. The characteristics of the two clonally related RF are summarized in Table 5. This report of clonally related antibodies in human autoimmune disease may indicate that clonal expansion and affinity maturation is also a feature of RF in RA as it has been shown

Table 5 Characterization of two clonally related rheumatoid factors

	Antibody	
	RF-SJ2	RF-SJ1
Specificity	Ga	Pan
Reactivity with rabbit IgG	No	Yes
Expression of V_HIII associated cross-reacting idiotopes	B6, D12	B6, D12
Variable region of heavy chain	V_HIII, J_H6	V_HIII, J_H6
Variable region of light chain	V λ I, J λ II	V λ I, J λ II
Dissociation constant, K_D	2.7×10^{-6} M	2.4×10^{-8} M

A comparison of two clonally related RF derived from a single synovial tissue. RF-SJ2 is the antibody which is close to germline configuration, while RF-SJ1 is the somatically mutated antibody
Ga: Reaction with IgG1, IgG2 and IgG4
Pan: Reaction with all four human subclasses

to occur in mouse models of autoimmune disease[78,79].

Although affinity measurements of the IgG RF are not available, high replacement versus silent substitution ratios (R/S) and clustering of mutations within CDRs are all strongly suggestive of an antigen driven process. The variable region of the heavy chain of RF-SJ5 shows 18 nucleotide differences compared to the closest identified germline sequence, 1.9III. The nucleotide differences lead to 13 amino acid replacements clustered in the hypervariable regions (CDR) giving a replacement versus silent substitution ratio (R/S) of 9. In the FR this ratio is 1.5. A R/S ratio significantly higher than 3 is very strong evidence for positive selection of replacement substitutions[78]. The same conclusion is supported by the pattern of somatic mutations leading to amino acid replacements in the light chain. The closest homology found was to the germline VD sequence. Compared to this sequence the R/S mutation ratio in the CDR was 4, while in FR it was 2. The V_H gene segment of RF-TS7 is not very mutated compared to the closest germline sequence, showing only two nucleotide differences with Humhv1l1R. Both differences are, however, in the CDR, and lead to amino acid replacements[80].

CONCLUSIONS

The pathogenesis of autoimmune diseases in humans is poorly understood and many investigators have assumed that information about autoantibodies that are characteristic of these diseases would aid in understanding the disease processes. How these autoantibodies compare to antibodies against foreign antigens is only now being elucidated. Structural analyses of IgM RF derived from patients with RA may provide new insights into the pathology of RA. In contrast to paraprotein RF, their structures show a remarkable diversity of V_H and V_L gene families and indeed individual V_H and V_L gene segments. Many of the genes sequenced so far have also been found expressed in antibodies with other specificities than RF. Most of the IgM RF genes are identical or close to germline configuration and exhibit only a limited degree of somatic mutation. Overall these data suggest that RF may be part of the normal B cell repertoire and appear to use a number of genes which are expressed early in B cell ontogeny. There is evidence for an antigen drive in the production of RF in RA. Two clonally related IgM RF show strong evidence of affinity maturation, and the high replacement to silent mutation ratio in the CDRs of IgG RF are characteristic of antigenic selection.

References

1. Smolen JS, Kalden JR, Maini RN. Rheumatoid Arthritis. Berlin: Springer Verlag; 1992.
2. Rose NR, Mackay IR. The Autoimmune Diseases II. San Diego: Academic Press; 1992.
3. Norton WL, Ziff M. Electron microscopic observations on the rheumatoid synovial membrane. Arthritis Rheum. 1966; 9: 589–610.
4. Chattopadhyay C, Chattopadhyay H, Natvig JB, Michaelsen TE, Mellbye OJ. Lack of suppressor cell activity in rheumatoid synovial lymphocytes. Scand J Immunol. 1979; 10: 309–316.
5. Hoffman WL, Goldberg MS, Smiley JD. Immunoglobulin G3 subclass production by rheumatoid synovial tissue cultures. J Clin Invest. 1982; 69: 136–144.
6. Munthe E, Natvig JB. Immunoglobulin classes, subclasses and complexes of IgG rheumatoid factor in rheumatoid plasma cells. Clin Exp Immunol. 1972; 12: 55–70.
7. Hoffman WL, Douglass RR, Smiley JD. Synthesis of electrophoretically restricted IgG by cultured rheumatoid synovium. Arthritis Rheum. 1984; 27: 976.
8. Natvig JB, Randen I, Thompson K, Førre O, Munthe E. The B cell system in the pathogenesis of rheumatoid arthritis using synovial B cell clones. Springer Semin Immunopathol. 1989; 11: 301–313.
9. Mageed RA, Kirwan JR, Thompson PW, McCarthy DA, Holborow EJ. Characterisation of the size and composition of circulating immune complexes in patients with rheumatoid arthritis. Ann Rheum Dis. 1991; 50: 231–236.
10. Wysocki LJ, Margolies MN, Huang B, Nemazee DA, Wechsler DS, Sato VL, Smith JA, Gefter ML. Combinational diversity within variable regions bearing the predominant anti-p-azophenylarsonate idiotype of strain A mice. J Immunol. 1985; 134: 2740–2747.
11. Coulie PG, Van Snick J. Rheumatoid factor (RF) production during anamnestic immune responses in the mouse. III. Activation of RF precursor cells is induced by their interaction with immune complexes and carrier-specific helper T cells. J Exp Med. 1985; 161: 88–97.
12. Stanley SL, Jr., Bischoff JK, Davie JM. Antigen-induced rheumatoid factors. Protein and carbohydrate antigens induce different rheumatoid factor responses. J Immunol. 1987; 139: 2936–2941.
13. Roosnek E, Lanzavecchia A. Efficient and selective presentation of antigen-antibody complexes by rheumatoid factor B cells. J Exp Med. 1991; 173: 487–489.
14. Bofill M, Janossy G, Janossa M, Burford GD, Seymour GJ, Wernet P, Kelemen E. Human B cell development. II. Subpopulations in the human fetus. J Immunol. 1985; 134: 1531–1538.
15. Valente G, Geuna M, Novero D, Arisio R, Palestro G, Stramignoni A. CD5-positive B-cells of the fetal and adult spleen lymphoid tissue: an immunophenotypical study. Verh Dtsch Ges Pathol. 1990; 74: 155–158.
16. Casali P, Notkins AL. CD5+ B lymphocytes, polyreactive antibodies and the human B-cell repertoire. Immunol Today. 1989; 10: 364–368.
17. Broker BM, Klajman A, Youinou P, Jouquan J, Worman CP, Murphy J, Mackenzie L, Quartey Papafio R, Blaschek M, Collins P. Chronic lymphocytic leukemic (CLL) cells secrete multispecific autoantibodies. J Autoimmun. 1988; 1: 469–481.
18. Nakamura M, Burastero SE, Notkins AL, Casali P. Human monoclonal rheumatoid factor-like antibodies from CD5 (Leu-1)+ B cells are polyreactive. J Immunol. 1988; 140: 4180–4186.

19. Youinou P, MacKenzie L, Jouquan J, Le Goff P, Lydyard PM. CD5 positive B cells in patients with rheumatoid arthritis: phorbol ester mediated enhancement of detection. Ann Rheum Dis. 1987; 46: 17–22.
20. Youinou P, MacKenzie L, Katsikis P, Merdrignac G, Isenberg DA, Tuaillon N, Lamour A, Le Goff P, Jouquan J, Drogou A. The relationship between CD5-expressing B lymphocytes and serologic abnormalities in rheumatoid arthritis patients and their relatives. Arthritis Rheum. 1990; 33: 339–348.
21. Plater Zyberk C, Maini RN. Phenotypic and functional features of CD5+ B lymphocytes in rheumatoid arthritis. Scand J Rheumatol Suppl. 1988; 75: 76–83.
22. Smith HR, Olson RR. CD5+ B lymphocytes in systemic lupus erythematosus and rheumatoid arthritis. J Rheumatol. 1990; 17: 833–835.
23. Hardy RR, Hayakawa K, Shimizu M, Yamasaki K, Kishimoto T. Rheumatoid factor secretion from human Leu-1+ B cells. Science. 1987; 236: 81–83.
24. Smith MD, O'Donnell J, Highton J, Palmer DG, Rozenbilds M, Roberts Thomson PJ. Immunohistochemical analysis of synovial membranes from inflammatory and non-inflammatory arthritides: scarcity of CD5 positive B cells and IL2 receptor bearing T cells. Pathology. 1992; 24: 19–26.
25. Werner Favre C, Vischer TL, Wohlwend D, Zubler RH. Cell surface antigen CD5 is a marker for activated human B cells. Eur J Immunol. 1989; 19: 1209–1213.
26. Freedman AS, Freeman G, Whitman J, Segil J, Daley J, Nadler LM. Studies of in vitro activated CD5+ B cells. Blood. 1989; 73: 202–208.
27. Burastero SE, Casali P, Wilder RL, Notkins AL. Monoreactive high affinity and polyreactive low affinity rheumatoid factors are produced by CD5+ B cells from patients with rheumatoid arthritis. J Exp Med. 1988; 168: 1979–1992.
28. Lydyard PM, MacKenzie LE, Youinou PY, Deane M, Jefferis R, Mageed RA. Specificity and idiotope expression of IgM produced by CD5+ and CD5− cord blood B-cell clones. Ann NY Acad Sci. 1992; 651: 527–539.
29. Thompson KM, Sutherland J, Barden G, Melamed MD, Wright MG, Bailey S, Thorpe SJ. Human monoclonal antibodies specific for blood group antigens demonstrate multispecific properties characteristic of natural autoantibodies. Immunology. 1992; 76: 146–157.
30. Waaler E. On the occurrence of a factor in human serum activating the specific agglutination of sheep corpuscles. Acta Pathol Microbiol Scand. 1940; 1: 172–188.
31. Kaplan S, Hyman K, Brooks R, Wakai M, Hashimoto S, Furie R, Chiorazzi N. Monoclonal IgM, IgG and IgA human rheumatoid factors produced by synovial tissue-derived, EBV-transformed B-cell lines. Clin Immunol Immunopathol. 1993; 66: 18–25.
32. Steward MW, Turner MW, Natvig JB. The binding affinities of rheumatoid factors interacting with the C gamma 3 homology region of human IgG. Clin Exp Immunol. 1973; 15: 145.
33. Natvig JB, Gaarder PI, Turner MW. IgG antigens of the C gamma2 and C gamma3 homology regions interacting with rheumatoid factors. Clin Exp Immunol. 1972; 12: 177.
34. Sasso EH, Barber CV, Nardella FA, Yount WJ, Mannik M. Antigenic specificities of human monoclonal and polyclonal IgM rheumatoid factors. The C gamma 2-C gamma 3 interface region contains the major determinants. J Immunol. 1988; 140: 3098–3107.
35. Grubb R, Laurell AB. Hereditary serological human serum groups. Acta Pathol Microbiol Scand. 1956; 39: 390–398.
36. Gaarder PI, Natvig JB. The reaction of anti-Gm antibodies with native and aggregated Gm-negative IgG. Scand J Immunol. 1974; 3: 559.
37. Randen I, Thompson KM, Natvig JB, Førre O, Waalen K. Human monoclonal rheumatoid factors derived from the polyclonal repertoire of rheumatoid synovial tissue: production and characterization. Clin Exp Immunol. 1989; 78: 13–18.
38. Gaarder PI, Natvig JB. Hidden rheumatoid factors reacting with 'non a' and other antigens of native autologous IgG. J Immunol. 1970; 105: 928–937.
39. Recht B, Frangione B, Franklin E, van Loghem E. Structural studies of a human gamma 3 myeloma protein (Goe) that binds staphylococcal protein A. J Immunol. 1981; 127: 917.
40. Nardella FA, Teller DC, Barber CV, Mannik M. IgG rheumatoid factors and staphylococcal protein A bind to a common molecular site on IgG. J Exp Med. 1985; 162: 1811–1824.
41. Jefferis R, Nik Jaafar MI, Steinitz M. Immunogenic and antigenic epitopes of immunoglobulins. VIII. A human monoclonal rheumatoid factor having specificity for a discontinuous

epitope determined by histidine/arginine interchange as residue 435 of immunoglobulin G. Immunol Lett. 1984; 7: 191–194.

42. Ghosh S, Cambell AM. Multispecific monoclonal antibodies. Immunol Today. 1986; 7: 217–222.

43. Boyden SV. Natural antibodies and the immune response. Adv Immunol. 1966; 5: 1–28.

44. Avrameas S, Guilbert B, Dighiero G. Natural antibodies against tubulin, actin, myoglobulin, thyroglobulin, fetuin, albumin and transferrin are present in normal human sera, and monoclonal immunoglobulins from multiple myeloma and Waldenstrom's macroglobulin-emia may express similar antibody specificities. Ann Immunol (Paris). 1981; 132C: 231–236.

45. Dighiero G, Lymberi P, Mazie JC, Rouyre S, Butler Browne GS, Whalen JD, Avrameas S. Murine hybridomas secreting natural monoclonal antibodies reacting with self antigens. J Immunol. 1983; 131: 2267–2272.

46. Avrameas S. Natural autoantibodies: from 'horror autotoxicus' to 'gnothi seauton'. Immunol Today. 1991; 12: 154–159.

47. Kodaira M, Kinashi T, Umemura I, Matsuda F, Noma T, Ono Y, Honjo T. Organization and evolution of variable region genes of the human immunoglobulin heavy chain. J Mol Biol. 1986; 190: 529–541.

48. Lee KH, Matsuda F, Kinashi T, Kodaira M, Honjo T. A novel family of variable region genes of the human imunoglobulin heavy chain. J Mol Biol. 1987; 195: 761–768.

49. Shen A, Humphries C, Tucker P, Blattner F. Human heavy-chain variable region gene family nonrandomly rearranged in familial chronic lymphocytic leukemia. Proc Natl Acad Sci USA. 1987; 84: 8563–8567.

50. Tomlinson IM, Walter G, Marks JD, Llewelyn MB, Winter G. The repertoire of human germline V(H) sequences reveals about 50 groups of V(H) segments with different hypervariable loops. J Mol Biol. 1992; 227: 776–798.

51. Meindl A, Klobeck HG, Ohnheiser R, Zachau HG. The V kappa gene repertoire in the human germ line. Eur J Immunol. 1990; 20: 1855–1863.

52. Marks JD, Tristem M, Karpas A, Winter G. Oligonucleotide primers for polymerase chain reaction amplification of human immunoglobulin variable genes and design of family-specific oligonucleotide probes. Eur J Immunol. 1991; 21: 985–991.

53. Sanz I. Multiple mechanisms participate in the generation of diversity of human H chain CDR3 regions. J Immunol. 1991; 147: 1720–1729.

54. Natvig JB, Kunkel HG. Human immunoglobulins: classes, subclasses, genetic variants and idiotypes. Adv Immunol. 1973; 16: 1–59.

55. Kunkel HG, Agnello V, Joslin FG, Winchester R, Capra JD. Cross idiotypic specificity among monoclonal IgM proteins with anti-gamma-globulin activity. J Exp Med. 1973; 137: 331–342.

56. Newkirk MM, Mageed RA, Jefferis R, Chen PP, Capra JD. Complete amino acid sequences of variable regions of two human IgM rheumatoid factors, BOR and KAS of the Wa idiotypic family, reveal restricted use of heavy and light chain variable and joining region gene segments. J Exp Med. 1987; 166: 550–564.

57. Agnello V, Arbetter A, Ibanez de Kasep G, Powell R, Tan EM, Joslin F. Evidence for a subset of rheumatoid factors that cross-react with DNA-histone and have a distinct cross-idiotype. J Exp Med. 1980; 151: 1514–1527.

58. Ledford DK, Goni F, Pizzolato M, Franklin EC, Solomon A, Frangione B. Preferential association of kappa IIIb light chains with monoclonal human IgM kappa autoantibodies. J Immunol. 1983; 131: 1322–1325.

59. Randen I, Thompson KM, Pascual V, Victor K, Beale D, Coadwell J, Førre O, Capra JD, Natvig JB. Rheumatoid Factor V genes from patients with rheumatoid arthritis are diverse and show evidence of an antigen driven response, In: Moller G, ed. Immunological Reviews. Copenhagen: Munksgaard, 1992; 49–71.

60. Crowley JJ, Goldfien RD, Schrohenloher RE, Spiegelberg HL, Silverman, Mageed RA, Jefferis R, Koopman WJ, Carson DA, Fong S. Incidence of three cross-reactive idiotypes on human rheumatoid factor paraproteins. J Immunol. 1988; 140: 3411–3418.

61. Chen PP, Albrandt K, Kipps TJ, Radoux V, Liu FT, Carson DA. Isolation and characterization of human VkIII germ-line genes. Implications for the molecular basis of human VkIII light chain diversity. J Immunol. 1987; 139: 1727–1733.

62. Radoux V, Chen PP, Sorge JA, Carson DA. A conserved human germline V kappa gene

directly encodes rheumatoid factor light chains. J Exp Med. 1986; 164: 2119–2124.

63. Thompson KM, Randen I, Natvig JB, Mageed RA, Jefferis R, Carson DA, Tighe H, Førre O. Human monoclonal rheumatoid factors derived from the polyclonal repertoire of rheumatoid synovial tissue: incidence of cross-reactive idiotopes and expression of VH and V kappa subgroups. Eur J Immunol. 1990; 20: 863–868.

64. Pascual V, Victor K, Randen I, Thompson K, Steinitz M, Førre O, Fu SM, Natvig JB, Capra JD. Nucleotide sequence analysis of rheumatoid factors and polyreactive antibodies derived from patients with rheumatoid arthritis reveals diverse use of VH and VL gene segments and exensive variability in CDR-3. Scand J Immunol. 1992; 36: 349–362.

65. Liu MF, Robbins DL, Crowley JJ, Sinha S, Kozin F, Kipps TJ, Carson DA, Chen PP. Characterization of four homologous L chain variable region genes that are related to 6B6.6 idiotype positive human rheumatoid factor L chains. J Immunol. 1989; 142: 688–694.

66. Kouri T, Crowley J, Aho K, Palosuo T, Isomaki H, Von Essen R, Heliovaara M, Carson D, Vaughan JH. Occurrence of two germline-related rheumatoid factor idiotypes in rheumatoid arthritis and in non-rheumatoid seropositive individuals. Clin Exp Immunol. 1990; 82: 250–256.

67. Guigou V, Cuisinier AM, Tonnelle C, Moinier D, Fougereau M, Fumoux F. Human immunoglobulin VH and VK repertoire revealed by in situ hybridization. Mol Immunol. 1990; 27: 935–940.

68. Mageed RA, Dearlove M, Goodall DM, Jefferis R. Immunogenic and antigenic epitopes of immunoglobulins. XVII – Monoclonal antibodies reactive with common and restricted idiotopes to the heavy chain of human rheumatoid factors. Rheumatol Int. 1986; 6: 179–183.

69. Silverman GJ, Schrohenloher RE, Accavitti MA, Koopman WJ, Carson DA. Structural characterization of the second major cross-reactive idiotype group of human rheumatoid factors. Association with the VH4 gene family. Arthritis Rheum. 1990; 33: 1347–1360.

70. Shokri F, Mageed RA, Tunn E, Bacon PA, Jefferis R. Qualitative and quantitative expression of VHI associated cross reactive idiotopes within IgM rheumatoid factor from patients with early synovitis. Ann Rheum Dis. 1990; 49: 150–154.

71. Thompson KM, Sutherland J, Barden G, Melamed MD, Randen I, Natvig JB, Pascual V, Capra JD, Stevenson FK. Human monoclonal antibodies against blood group antigens preferentially express a VH4-21 variable region gene-associated epitope. Scand J Immunol. 1991; 34: 509–518.

72. Pascual V, Victor K, Lelsz D, Spellerberg MB, Hamblin TJ, Thompson KM, Randen I, Natvig J, Capra JD, Stevenson FK. Nucleotide sequence analysis of the V regions of two IgM cold agglutinins. Evidence that the VH4-21 gene segment is responsible for the major cross-reactive idiotype. J Immunol. 1991; 146: 4385–4391.

73. Scott MG, Tarrand JJ, Crimmins DL, McCourt DW, Siegel NR, Smith CE, Nahm MH. Clonal characterization of the human IgG antibody repertoire to *Haemophilus influenzae* type b polysaccharide. II. IgG antibodies contain VH genes from a single VH family and VL genes from at least four VL families. J Immunol. 1989; 143: 293–298.

74. Schroeder HW, Jr., Hillson JL, Perlmutter RM. Structure and evolution of mammalian VH families. Int Immunol. 1990; 2: 41–50.

75. Pascual V, Capra JD. Human immunoglobulin heavy-chain variable region genes: organization, polymorphism, and expression. Adv Immunol. 1991; 49: 1–74.

76. Bye JM, Carter C, Cui YC, Gorick BD, Songsivilai S, Winter G, Hughesjones NC, Marks JD. Germline variable region gene segment derivation of human monoclonal anti-Rh(D) antibodies – evidence for affinity maturation by somatic hypermutation and repertoire shift. J Clin Invest. 1992; 90: 2481–2490.

77. Randen I, Brown D, Thompson KM, Hughes Jones N, Pascual V, Victor K, Capra JD, Førre O, Natvig JB. Clonally related IgM rheumatoid factors undergo affinity maturation in the rheumatoid synovial tissue. J Immunol. 1992; 148: 3296–3301.

78. Shlomchik MJ, Marshak Rothstein A, Wolfowicz CB, Rothstein TL, Weigert MG. The role of clonal selection and somatic mutation in autoimmunity. Nature. 1987; 328: 805–811.

79. Shlomchik M, Weigert M. Is the hypothesis alive that IgM anti-IgG1 rheumatoid factor specificity is determined by framework regions? [letter; comment]. Eur J Immunol. 1990; 20: 2529–2531.

80. Randen I, Pascual V, Victor K, Thompson KM, Førre O, Capra JD, Natvig JB. Synovial IgG rheumatoid factors show evidence of an antigen driven immune response and a shift in the V gene repertoire compared to IgM rheumatoid factors. Eur J Immunol. 1993; 23: 1220–1225.
81. Spatz LA, Wong KK, Williams M, Desai R, Golier J, Berman JE, Alt FW, Latov N. Cloning and sequence analysis of the VH and VL regions of an anti-myelin/DNA antibody from a patient with peripheral neuropathy and chronic lymphocytic leukemia. J Immunol. 1990; 144: 2821–2828.
82. Robbins DL, Kenny TP, Coloma MJ, Gavilondo Cowley JV, Soto Gil RW, Chen PP, Larrick JW. Serologic and molecular characterization of a human monoclonal rheumatoid factor derived from rheumatoid synovial cells. Arthritis Rheum. 1990; 33: 1188–1195.
83. Ezaki K, Kanda H, Sakai K, Fukui N, Shingu M, Nobunaga M, Watanabe T. Restricted diversity of the variable region nucleotide sequences of the heavy and light chains of a human rheumatoid factor. Arthritis Rheum. 1991; 34: 343–350.
84. Harindranath N, Goldfarb IS, Ikematsu H, Burastero SE, Wilder RL, Notkins AL, Casali P. Complete sequence of the genes encoding the VH and VL regions of low- and high-affinity monoclonal IgM and IgA1 rheumatoid factors produced by CD5+ B cells from a rheumatoid arthritis patient. Int Immunol. 1991; 3: 865–875.
85. Pascual V, Andris J, Capra JD. Heavy chain variable region gene utilization in human antibodies. Int Rev Immunol. 1990; 5: 231–238.
86. Victor KD, Randen I, Thompson K, Førre O, Natvig JB, Fu SM, Capra JD. Rheumatoid factors isolated from patients with autoimmune disorders are derived from germline genes distinct from those encoding the Wa, Po, and Bla cross-reactive idiotypes. J Clin Invest. 1991; 87: 1603–1613.
87. Mierau R, Gause A, Kuppers R, Michels M, Mageed RA, Jefferis R, Genth E. A human monoclonal IgA rheumatoid factor using the VkIV light chain gene. Rheumatol Int. 1992; 12: 23–31.
88. Pascual V, Victor K, Randen I, Thompson K, Natvig JB, Capra JD. IgM rheumatoid factors in patients with rheumatoid arthritis derive from a diverse array of germline immunoglobulin genes and display little evidence of somatic variation. J Rheumatol. 1992; 19: 50–53.
89. Førre O, Waalen K, Kjeldsen-Kragh J, Sorskaar D, Mellbye OJ, Natvig JB. B cells in autoimmunity; in Rugstad HE, Endresen L, Førre O (eds): Immunopharmacology in autoimmune diseases and transplantation. New York and London: Plenum Press; 1992; 31–43.

3
The Mononuclear Phagocyte and Rheumatoid Arthritis

J. HIGHTON and D. G. PALMER

INTRODUCTION

Rheumatoid arthritis is a systemic inflammatory disease characterized by a destructive arthritis and extra-articular features of which the most typical is the occurrence of granulomas in subcutaneous tissues and other sites. The presence of granulomatous inflammation focuses attention on the involvement of cells of the mononuclear phagocyte series which are the predominant cells found in such lesions. This review discusses the role of monocytes/macrophages in the initiation of rheumatoid arthritis, and in mediating the chronic inflammatory process which results in the destruction of connective tissues in joints and at extra-articular sites. The authors' view that the macrophage is central to these events is emphasized and consequently the importance of discovering the means by which macrophages are activated to understanding the pathogenesis of rheumatoid arthritis. It is proposed that the behaviour of macrophages may determine certain fundamental characteristics of rheumatoid disease such as the symmetry of joint involvement, and that more attention should be given to targeting the activated joint macrophage as a means of therapeutic intervention.

THE ROLE OF THE MACROPHAGE AT THE INITIATION OF JOINT INFLAMMATION

Cells of the monocyte-macrophage series are disseminated from the bone marrow to specific tissue sites where they are adapted to perform specialized local functions by a process involving maturation and differentiation, including selective activation of functions from an enormous potential repertoire[1]. Several of the sites to which monocytes are normally targeted are of potential relevance to rheumatoid arthritis, and include the lungs, sites of tissue repair and of course the joints. Electron microscopic studies established the macrophage-like characteristics of the type A synovial lining cell including its phagocytic capacity[2]. However, the bone-marrow origin of this cell has only been clearly established by more recent studies. Edwards and Willoughby demonstrated that in the beige mouse the type A synoviocytes and circulating monocytes shared a unique identifying feature, a giant granule[3]. Their use of radiation chimeras further demonstrated the gradual replacement of existing host type A synoviocytes with cells containing these giant lysosomal granules identifying them as originating in the donor bone marrow. Estimates based on the rate of replacement suggest that in the mouse complete turnover of type A cells of monocyte origin takes 20 weeks, which is very much faster than the replacement of fibroblast-like type B cells. In humans further evidence of the monocyte origin of the type A synoviocyte comes from the demonstration of macrophage-associated molecules such as CD14 identified by monoclonal antibodies[4–6]. In addition the separate identity of type B synoviocytes may also be distinguished by certain antigens identified by monoclonal antibodies[7]. The differentiation and origin of type A and B synoviocytes and the conclusion that the type A synoviocyte is a tissue macrophage derived from circulating monocytes have been the subject of a recent review[8]. These two cell types form a discontinuous lining unsupported by a basement membrane above a rich supply of capillaries. This surface structure is thought to adapt the synovial lining for free movement over joint surfaces without adherence, and for nutrition of cartilage[9]. The contribution of the type A phagocytic macrophage to the function in the normal synovial membrane has not been defined, but it has been considered to play a housekeeping role in clearing debris through phagocytosis. However, the presence within the normal joint of this monocyte-derived cell indicates the potential for joint inflammation to be initiated by events affecting peripheral blood monocyte precursors, such as infection, with subsequent expression of disease within the joints. In addition, since macrophages are part of the cell population of the normal joint they would be expected to take part in inflammation initiated within the joint.

  Studies of patients with early rheumatoid arthritis have demonstrated the involvement of lining macrophages in the initial inflammatory events. Kulka[10] reported appearances in two membranes studied at 7 days and at 9 days. Both showed intimal proliferation and a perivascular infiltrate of lymphocytes and monocytes described as a focal granulomatous infiltrate. Endothelial cells were thickened and some vessel lumens were filled with lymphocytes and monocytes. In later cases up to a year in duration the thickened lining layer was a prominent feature and was described as showing a granulomatous reaction with palisading of the superficial synoviocytes. There were occasional giant cells and appearances suggesting cell necrosis. Some areas of the lining were noted to be ischaemic. Fibrin was found at the surface and within the synovial tissue. The author commented that the early histological appearances showed a closer resemblance to those of the nodule (where macrophages are the predominant infiltrating cell) and other systemic lesions[10]. In a systematic study of patients within the first month of disease Schumacher confirmed that lining cell 'proliferation' is an early change[11]. The other main feature was the presence of large endothelial cells with obliteration of vessel lumens, infiltration of the vessel walls and a perivascular mononuclear infiltrate as was also noted in the previous study. The presence of fibrin and cell necrosis was again noted. The vascular changes described in the early histological studies are consistent with activation of endothelial cells, a process which is reviewed in detail in another chapter. The synovial vessels would then be adapted for adherence and subsequent transmigration of the lymphocytes and monocytes which were shown to be filling the vessel. These early changes are similar to those noted in clinically uninvolved joints[12] where two-thirds showed lining hyperplasia but only one-third showed a perivascular mononuclear cell infiltrate. Lining cell hyperplasia results in a layer of cells up to ten deep in which the predominant cell type identified using monoclonal antibodies is the macrophage[4-6]. Furthermore the evidence that this accumulation results from local proliferation is lacking, and studies using thymidine incorporation and a monoclonal antibody Ki 67 to identify dividing cells has shown cells in this state to be present in only very low numbers[13,14]. The thickened lining layer which is an early feature of rheumatoid arthritis therefore results mainly from transmigration of monocytes through an altered synovial vasculature and the local accumulation of infiltrating macrophages.

The first changes in the rheumatoid synovial membrane can be compared with those described at the initiation of animal models of arthritis. The MRL mouse has been considered as a model for both SLE and rheumatoid arthritis. The first synovial change is proliferation of synovial lining cells which is most notable in the lateral joint recesses. Projecting villi are formed which adhere to cartilage and intra-articular ligaments and tendons which are subsequently eroded. The synovial lining cells have large nuclei and prominent nucleoli resulting in a transformed appearance. A lymphocytic inflammatory infiltrate is a late feature of this destructive synovitis[15]. By contrast, adjuvant arthritis is an animal model of particular interest because there is evidence that it is mediated by T lymphocytes which recognize a mycobacterial antigen which has identity with a sequence in joint proteoglycan[16]. The first changes in the joints are seen after a delay of nine to ten days following the injection of adjuvant[17]. On the day of onset of joint inflammation there is oedema involving synovial membrane, tendon sheaths, periosteum and para-articular tissues. A sparse mononuclear cell infiltrate is seen. The second to fourth days see the development of lining hyperplasia, fibrin deposition and an intensifying mononuclear cell infiltrate. This process subsequently results in the production of an actively erosive granulation tissue. These two important animal models of erosive arthritis differ in that lymphocytic infiltration is an earlier occurrence in adjuvant arthritis but occurs late in the MRL mouse. A common feature which is prominent in both types of arthritis is thickening of the lining layer which is due to infiltration and accumulation of macrophages suggesting that this is a characteristic feature of different processes which result in joint erosion.

Table 1 Phenotypic changes of monocytes/macrophages in rheumatoid arthritis

	PB	SF	SM	Nodule
MHC class II	↔[23,24,104]	↑[23,24]	↑[19–22]	↑[76–79,81,88]
FcRI	↑[34,104]	↑[34]	↔[33]	↓[81]
FcRII	↑[104]		↔[33]	
FcRIII			↔[33]	
CR1	↔[24]	↓[24]	↓[5]	↓[79]
CR3	↑[34]	↑[34]	↑[35]	↑[79,81]
CR4	↑[34]	↑[34,38]	↑[35]	↑[81]
ICAM-1	↔[38]	↑[38]	↑[37]	
CD14	↔[24,104]	↑[34]	↔[4]	↔[79,88]
Tissue factor			↑[45]	
p8,14			subset macrophages[4]	subset macrophages[85]

Phenotypic changes in monocytes/macrophages in different situations in rheumatoid arthritis. Expression of various markers is indicated as unchanged ↔, decreased ↓, or increased ↑. Adjacent numbers are appropriate references from the text. Changes in synovial membrane and nodules are subjective impressions based on immunohistological methods. Peripheral blood and synovial fluid changes are based on semi-quantitative measurements from fluorescence analysis or immunoassay. The results have been arbitrarily simplified by the authors where conflict exists, but details can be found in the appropriate references

ACTIVATION STATUS OF MACROPHAGES IN THE SYNOVIAL INFILTRATE: PHENOTYPIC CHANGES

Macrophages which are recruited into the inflamed synovial lining show evidence of activation. This term implies the activation of specific effector functions. Which particular functions are recruited from the very large repertoire which the macrophage possesses will depend upon the nature of the stimuli to which the cell has been exposed including both activating and suppressing signals[1,18]. Activation is accompanied by altered expression of various functional molecules. Such considerations have led to investigation of the phenotype of macrophages in rheumatoid arthritis. Antibodies recognizing macrophage-associated molecules have provided evidence of macrophage activation in this disease (Table 1) and have allowed some speculation as to the nature of the stimuli which might have resulted in the changes observed. Molecules studied include MHC class II, Fc gamma receptors, the complement receptor CR1, the β_2 integrins CR3 and p150,95 (CR4), tissue factor and a number of less well characterized molecules including the glycoprotein CD14 and the p8,14 dimer.

Greatly enhanced expression of MHC class II was one of the first features to be noted in immunohistological studies of rheumatoid synovial membrane[19,20]. Many of the cells expressing MHC class II were macrophages and emphasis was given to the potential for enhanced antigen presentation by these cells and interdigitating cells within the rheumatoid synovial membrane[21,22]. These studies were influential in promoting the concept that in rheumatoid arthritis a causative antigen is presented by MHC class II positive cells within the joint. Lymphocytes interacting with these cells would be activated and in turn activate macrophage effector functions responsible for joint inflammation and destruction. Since IFN-gamma is an important mediator of macrophage functions such as arming for the killing of bacteria and in increasing expression of MHC class II[18] it was reasonable to suggest that this mechanism might operate within the rheumatoid joint. However, despite the presence of marked upregulation of MHC class II on synovial fluid macrophages[23] (e.g. Figure 1) we were unable to detect significant levels of IFN-gamma within synovial fluid[24], which was in keeping with the findings of most other groups[25,26]. Interleukin 2 and IFN-gamma were not demonstrable within synovial membrane using immunohistological techniques[27] despite the reported detection of mRNA for IL-2 and IFN-gamma[28]. More recent evidence suggests that GM-CSF, possibly acting in conjunction with TNF-α, may be the main regulator of MHC class II in rheumatoid arthritis[29]. This evidence means that reassessment of the lymphocyte/macrophage model of rheumatoid arthritis is required and that alternative mediators of macrophage activation must be considered[30] as is discussed subsequently.

Another macrophage molecule which is regulated by IFN-gamma is FcRI (CD64)[31,32]. This high affinity receptor for IgG is expressed by macrophages in rheumatoid synovial membrane, together with FcRII (CD32) and FcRIII (CD16)[33]. We have found expression of FcRI to be increased on circulating monocytes in patients with rheumatoid arthritis[34], and in some cases levels are further increased on synovial fluid macrophages (Figure 1). Broker et al.[33] reported concordant expression of FcRI and CD14 in synovial membrane. Since IFN-gamma reduces expression of CD14 they argue that as for MHC class II there may be alternative regulators of FcRI expression in rheumatoid arthritis.

Macrophages within rheumatoid synovial membrane strongly express the β_2 integrins CR3 (CD11b) and p150,95 (CD11c, CR4). Expression is most notable on macrophages within the thickened synovial lining layer[35]. Expression of CR3 is also increased on circulating monocytes in patients with rheumatoid arthritis, and CR4 is further increased on macrophages within synovial fluid[34]. These molecules are stored within monocytes/macrophages and additional molecules can be rapidly deployed to the cell surface in response to chemotactic signals[36]. We have found that whereas normal monocytes show marked increase in surface expression of CR3 and CR4 in response to fMLP, synovial fluid macrophages which already have increased expression are unable to upregulate expression further in response to fMLP (unpublished observation). We have interpreted these findings as suggesting that joint macrophages have depleted internal stores of CR3 and CR4 due to translocation to the cell surface. This is most likely to reflect exposure to chemotactic factors generated within the inflamed joint. Expression of LFA-1 (CD11a), the third member of the β_2 integrin group, and its ligand ICAM-1 (CD54) is also widespread in the rheumatoid synovial membrane[37] and expression of ICAM-1 is increased on synovial fluid macrophages[38] (Figure 1). The adhesive function of the β_2 integrins is regulated from within the cell by an energy dependent mechanism so that the adhesive state of a cell cannot be deduced from the number of integrin molecules expressed[39]. An epitope associated with functional activation of the β_2 integrins[39] is expressed in

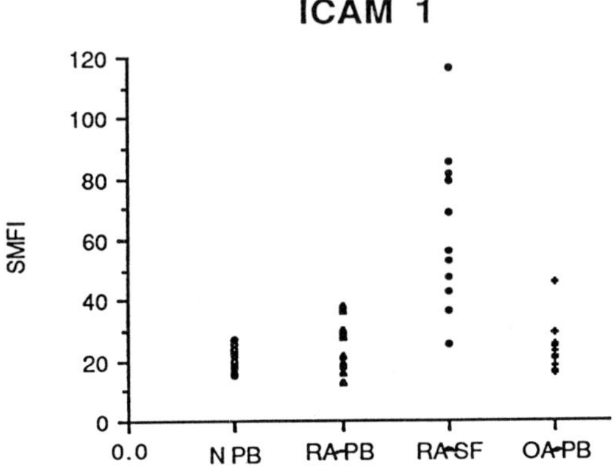

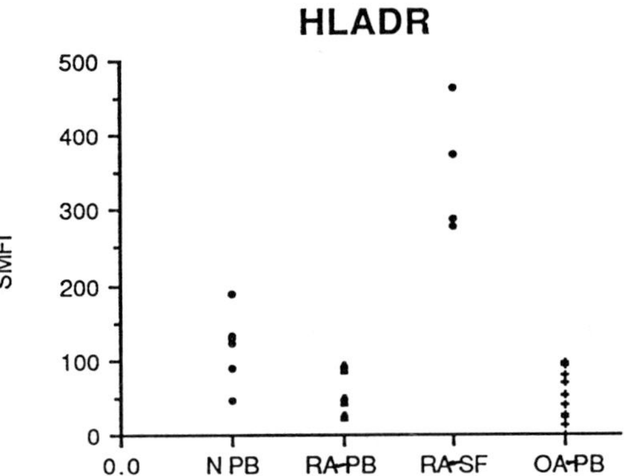

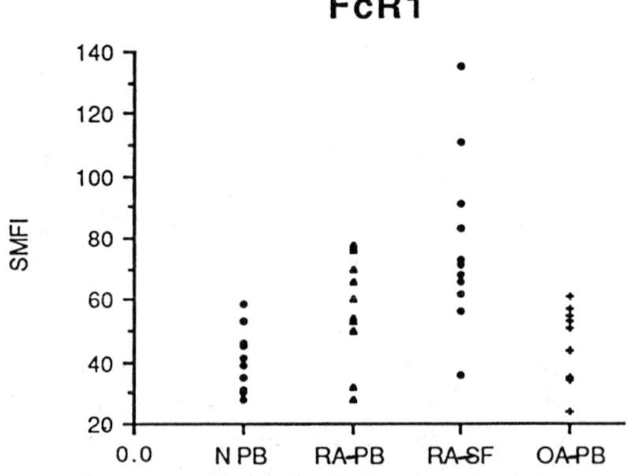

Figure 1 Results are mean fluorescence intensity derived from FACScan analysis of monocytes double-stained with mouse monoclonal antibodies to CD14 in combination with antibodies to ICAM-1, FcR1 and HLA-DR. NPB, normal peripheral blood; RA-PB, rheumatoid peripheral blood; RA-SF, rheumatoid synovial fluid; OA-PB, osteoarthritis peripheral blood

rheumatoid synovial membrane[4]. Expression of this antigen is dependent upon conformational change in the $\beta2$ integrin, however, and it is possible that its expression in synovial membrane might result from conformational changes occurring during processing and fixation of the synovial samples. Thus, although integrin activation, as well as upregulation, might be expected in response to chemotactic stimuli, it cannot necessarily be assumed that these molecules are functionally active until this has been specifically tested.

Another surface functional molecule expressed by activated macrophages is tissue factor. This is a transmembrane glycoprotein[40] which binds factor VII and activates the extrinsic clotting pathway, ultimately leading to fibrin deposition. Tissue factor expression and consequent macrophage pro-coagulant activity can be activated by T lymphocytes[41], immune complexes[42] and bacterial products such as LPS[43]. Interestingly, in view of the increased expression of β_2 integrins by synovial macrophages, engagement of CR3 enhances the tissue factor response[44]. Expression of tissue factor is markedly upregulated in rheumatoid synovial membrane, whereas in osteoarthritis it is only found in the endothelium of synovial vessels[45]. Pro-coagulant features of the rheumatoid synovial membrane correlated with the degree of macrophage infiltration. Thus fibrin deposition is another important aspect of synovitis in rheumatoid arthritis which is a consequence of increased infiltration by activated inflammatory macrophages.

ACTIVATED SYNOVIAL MACROPHAGES ARE A MAJOR SOURCE OF INFLAMMATORY CYTOKINES

Another important result of macrophage activation is their potential to produce cytokines capable of mediating local and systemic effects fundamental to the pathogenesis of arthritis, including the activation of connective tissue cells and induction of the acute phase response. Intra-articular production of cytokines including IL-1, TNF-α, GM-CSF, IL-6, IL-8 and TGF-β has been documented by detection in synovial fluid or demonstration of production from cultured synovial membrane *in vitro*[30,46–50]. A notable feature of these cytokines is that they are predominantly the products of monocytes/macrophages[30,47]. Consequently it has been presumed that the macrophage is an important source of the cytokines relevant to synovial inflammation. This has been borne out by experiments designed to localize cytokine production. Immunohistological studies have demonstrated the presence of the principal pro-inflammatory cytokines IL-1[51] and TNF-α[52] within synovial macrophages. Macrophages are the predominant cell type showing hybridization with probes for IL-1 and TNF[53]. Macrophages also contain mRNA for IL-6[53] and GM-CSF[54], but share production of these cytokines with rheumatoid synovial fibroblasts[55,56] and synovial T cells[57]. *In situ* hybridization studies have also suggested that the main source of cytokines is macrophages in the synovial lining layer and that synovial fluid macrophages contain relatively small amounts of cytokine mRNA[53]. This conclusion is in broad agreement with recent preliminary studies we have

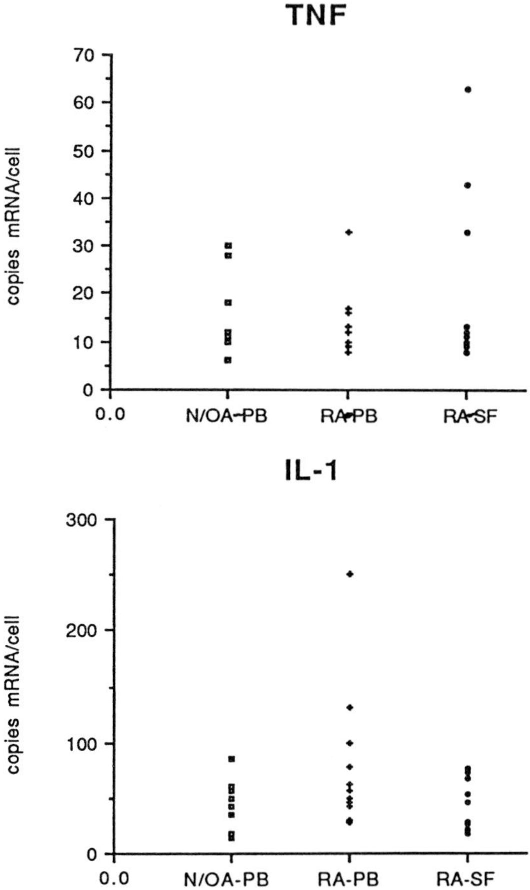

Figure 2 Figures shown are copies mRNA per monocyte/macrophage. Monocytes/macrophages were isolated by adherence to plastic petri dishes, and total RNA extracted from 1×10^5 cells in GTC. Synthetic cRNA was added to the monocytes prior to treatment with GTC. Extracted RNA and cRNA was treated with reverse transcriptase and subjected to 35 cycles of PCR with primers specific for IL-1β, (IL-1α, not shown) and TNFα. The resulting DNA was separated by agarose gel electrophoresis. Copies mRNA per monocyte was calculated from relative amounts of radioactivity in DNA amplified from control and sample RNAs (Wong AM, Doyle MV, Mark DF. Quantitation of mRNA by the polymerase chain reaction. Proc Natl Acad Sci USA, 1989; 86: 9717–9721). N/OA-PB, monocytes from normal and osteoarthritic peripheral blood; RA-PB, rheumatoid arthritis peripheral blood; RA-SF, rheumatoid arthritis synovial fluid

conducted using reverse transcriptase and PCR to obtain semi-quantitative measurements of mRNA for IL-1β and TNF-α in monocytes and macrophages from peripheral blood and synovial fluid of patients with rheumatoid arthritis (unpublished observations) although as can be seen from Figure 2 some synovial fluid monocytes contain increased amounts of mRNA for TNFα. Thus, recent evidence suggests that the activated synovial macrophage within the thickened, hyperplastic synovial lining is responsible for the production of a large proportion of the inflammatory cytokines found within the rheumatoid joint.

INTERACTION OF MACROPHAGES AND FIBROBLASTS IN THE SYNOVIAL LINING TO PRODUCE A DESTRUCTIVE GRANULATION TISSUE

The synovial lining macrophage shares its position both in the normal synovial lining and in the hyperplastic inflamed lining with cells of fibroblastic origin. As has been discussed both cell types contribute to cytokine production in rheumatoid arthritis. Recent studies have also demonstrated that both cell types within the hyperplastic joint lining contain mRNA encoding collagenase and stromelysin[58-61]. Therefore within the synovial lining there is juxtaposition of functionally altered macrophages and fibroblasts, both producing a broad range of cytokines, as well as enzymes capable of destroying connective tissues. This suggests that the synovial lining is the principal site of cell interactions responsible for joint destruction in rheumatoid arthritis. The capacity of IL-1 and TNF to act singly or in concert to induce fibroblast proliferation, and production of prostaglandin E2, collagenase and neutral proteases is well known[46-48,62]. The situation is made more complex by contributions from other relevant cytokines including PDGF, HBGF-1 and TGF-B[63]. What finally results is a complex network in which macrophage cytokines recruit fibroblasts into an activated state. The activated fibroblast is then able to contribute to macrophage activation by the production of cytokines such as GM-CSF. In addition autocrine pathways contribute to what is potentially a self-sustaining interplay of cytokines between these two cell types. Local production of other molecules such as fibronectin[64] and hyaluronan[65] further alter the environment in the hyperplastic synovial lining. The juxtaposition of macrophages and fibroblasts in the synovial lining also indicates the likely importance of direct cell to cell contact in maintaining these interactions. It is through these processes and the medium of the activated joint macrophage that the synovial lining is converted from a structure designed to sustain freedom of movement and nutrition of the joint, to an activated granulation tissue with locally invasive potential.

THE ROLE OF THE MACROPHAGE WITHIN THE PANNUS

Realization of the full destructive potential of the hyperplastic synovial membrane requires an additional step which is adherence to cartilage or other structures within the joint or tendon sheath. It is therefore of interest that monocytes exposed to IL-1 adhere to cartilage, and particularly to damaged cartilage from the joints of patients with rheumatoid arthritis[66]. Extracellular matrix components might also be involved in adhesion[67]. Alternatively, ingrowth of the transformed invasive synovial lining could occur by extension from the normal synovial/cartilage junction. At this site synovial tissue containing macrophages and fibroblastic lining cells overlies cartilage[68]. Tissue removed from established erosive fronts shows variable morphology. Invasive pannus is characterized by a clear junction between damaged cartilage and massed cells of synovial origin. A transitional zone of tissue characterized by the presence of cartilage associated molecules such as chrondroitin and keratan sulphates is characteristic of large joints, and may explain the prevalence of joint space loss rather than erosion which often occurs at these sites[69]. Invasive pannus is characterized by the presence of activated macrophages and cells of fibroblastic origin[70,71]. In addition to exhibiting phenotypic changes of activation, pannus macrophages produce cytokines including TNF-α[52] and TGF-β_1[72]. Fibroblastic cells at the cartilage pannus junction contain proteases such as cathepsin G[73] and cathepsin L[74] and express oncogenes including *jun* and *fos* which are involved in pathways mediating protease production[74,75]. Overall the close association of activated cytokine-producing inflammatory macrophages and functionally altered fibroblasts in pannus conforms closely to the structure of the expanded synovial lining layer. This is consistent with the proposal that joint erosion results either from the adherence of the invasive hyperplastic synovial lining to cartilage or from its extension over cartilage from the cartilage/synovial junction.

THE MACROPHAGE IN SUBCUTANEOUS NODULES

Whereas the hyperplastic synovial lining layer is responsible for erosion of intra-articular tissues, the subcutaneous nodule is characteristic of localized damage to extra-articular tissues. In both lesions there is accumulation of a layer of macrophages either at the joint surface or in the palisade adjacent to the necrotic centre of the nodule. The similarity of these features of the joint lesion on the one hand, and the nodule on the other have been noted in earlier histological studies[10] and subsequently confirmed by immunohistological investigations. The question raised is whether the mechanism of tissue damage is the same in each case.

In the synovial lesion the activated inflammatory macrophage is an important component of the cellular infiltrate: in the nodule, this cell is predominant. The cells of the palisade are HLA-DR positive leukocytes with phenotypic markers such as CD14 which are characteristic of monocytes/macrophages[76–78]. Enumeration of palisade cells bearing these markers showed that 97% expressed the common leukocyte antigen and 87% expressed CD14[79]. In electron microscopic studies a small number of cells with fibroblastic characteristics have been noted amongst the predominant histiocytic cells of the palisade[80]. In the outer vascular zone of established nodules CD14 positive monocytes/macrophages still constitute over 50% of nucleated cells[79]. Even in long-established nodules recruitment of macrophages into the outer vascular zone is an ongoing process. Elongated macrophages can be seen which appear to be migrating from the outer vascular zone towards the centre of the nodule and the central necrotic focus. Phenotypic changes occur during migration which indicate progressive macrophage activation and maturation[79]. Characteristics shared with activated inflammatory macrophages of the synovial membrane include strong expression of MHC class II, and the β_2 integrins CD11b (CR3) and CD11c (p150,95)[76–79,81]. There is variable expression of FcRI[81] and low expression of CR1[79]. Expression of acid phosphatase and not ATPase is a further indication that cells of the palisade layer are inflammatory macrophages[77]. Activated macrophages in nodules secrete angiotensin converting enzyme as has also been demonstrated in synovial membrane[82]. The upregulated expression of the β_2 integrins suggests that sustained recruitment of macrophages to the nodule, and centripetal migration are due to their exposure to a continuing chemotactic stimulus[79].

Although macrophages within nodules and the inflamed synovial membrane show similar characteristics, other cell populations differ between the two lesions. The nodule contains a variable, diffuse infiltrate of T lymphocytes which is relatively unstructured in comparison to synovial membrane. In the nodule the CD4/CD8 ratio is comparable to normal values established for peripheral blood[77,81], rather than increased. A proportion of these lymphocytes are MHC class II positive but expression of the IL-2 receptor is low. B cells and plasma cells either are absent or are present in very low numbers[77,78] and classical lymphoid follicles with germinal centres which can be found in some rheumatoid synovial membranes are not present in nodules. These differences suggest that whereas there is a localized immune response occurring in synovial membrane, this is not the case in the nodule. Consequently, systemic factors are likely to be of greater importance in driving the rheumatoid nodule.

The importance of systemic factors in mediating necrosis within the nodule was perceived by Sokoloff and others in a careful histological study of early rheumatoid nodules[83]. They found that early foci of necrosis were centred around vessels and granulation tissue. A palisade of cells and necrosis was observed to develop along the line of tissue planes around the central vessel, which was postulated to be delivering the 'lethal agent'. They further postulated that the necrosis-producing agent was fluid borne. A recent interpretation by Ziff has envisaged delivery of immune complexes to areas of trauma, and immune-complex mediated activation of macrophages[84]. The activated macrophage would then be the 'lethal agent' responsible for fibrin deposition and tissue necrosis. Such a mechanism is supported by our own observations. We found that the earliest signs of necrosis occurred within small clusters of macrophages[85]. Such macrophages were part of a subset of macrophages within the nodules distinguished by persistent expression of the p8,14 antigen identified by monoclonal antibody 5.5. This calcium binding dimer is abundant within the cytoplasm of circulating monocytes and neutrophils[86], but is reduced upon maturation of monocytes to macrophages *in vitro*[87]. This may explain the low frequency of macrophages expressing this antigen in 'indolent' nodules, and within macrophages of the palisade. In nodules with active tissue necrosis p8,14 positive monocytes can be seen entering the vascular zone and migrating centrally. Migrating p8,14 positive cells are large and show branching pseudopodia. The margins of such cells are often indistinct when stained with mAb 5.5 due to a surrounding halo of released p8,14. When necrosis occurs within a group of 5.5 positive cells, the death of the cells results in a deposit of 5.5 positive material. Such small foci of early necrosis were not surrounded by a macrophage palisade which was only found around larger, established areas of early necrosis. In such larger, and presumably older foci, cell death occurred in two situations. One was associated with collections of 5.5 positive cells at 'breaches' in the palisade. In the other, moribund epitheloid cells are shed from the palisade into the necrotic zone where they undergo progressive disintegration.

These observations establish a connection between collections of a subset of activated inflammatory macrophages and the occurrence of cell death. They do not allow us to draw definite conclusions about the mechanism by which cell death and tissue destruction are produced. The dominance of macrophages within the palisade, with few fibroblasts, suggests that in the nodule there is limited scope for interaction between these two cell types to produce a destructive granulation tissue as occurs in synovial membrane. Thus, despite the documented production of IL-1β by nodule macrophages[88], and the presence of collagenase[89], electron microscopic observation of the central necrotic zone shows that collagen fibres within this zone initially retain their characteristic structure[80]. This suggests that other macrophage-mediated mechanisms of tissue damage such as production of nitric oxide[90] are likely to be responsible for necrobiosis within the rheumatoid nodule. Further study is required to delineate the precise means by which activated macrophages mediate tissue necrosis within these characteristic granulomas.

SYSTEMIC OR 'PRESYNOVIAL' ACTIVATION OF MONOCYTES/MACROPHAGES

Evidence has been presented that a prominent feature of the lesions most typical of rheumatoid arthritis, including synovitis and subcutaneous nodules, is the presence of activated macrophages. Macrophage activation can also be detected at other extra-articular sites such as in the lungs[91,92], and products from activated bone marrow and splenic macrophages appear to be responsible for depressed erythropoiesis and disturbances in iron metabolism which contribute to chronic inflammatory anaemia[93,94]. One consequence of widespread macrophage activation is the manifestations of the acute phase response which is responsible for many of the features of rheumatoid arthritis common to other systemic inflammatory diseases (Chapter 8). Most mechanisms that have been postulated to explain such activation of macrophages in rheumatoid arthritis have concerned local activation at the site of inflammation, for example, by a localized immune response within the synovial membrane[19] or by immune complexes deposited at the site of nodule formation[84]. However, the presence of activated macrophages at diverse systemic sites suggests the alternative possibility that macrophages might be delivered to such sites in a pre-activated state.

A further reason for considering the possibility of activation or priming of macrophages prior to arrival at sites of inflammation ('presynovial activation') is the presence of extensive changes in the maturity, phenotype and function of circulating monocytes in patients with rheumatoid arthritis. It has been demonstrated that in inflammatory disease, including rheumatoid arthritis, there is an increase in large circulating non-phagocytic mononuclear cells[95]. With continued culture such cells develop phagocytic properties. This may be an expansion of the non-adherent, non-specific-esterase (NSE) negative mononuclear cell population of normal blood which matures into NSE-positive macrophages[96]. Expansion of the NSE-negative mononuclear cell population in rheumatoid arthritis has been associated with defective C3b receptor function[97]. These observations suggest that in rheumatoid arthritis monocytopoiesis is stimulated with an increase in cells of relative immaturity within the circulation[98]. Circulating monocytes have an increased ability to bind immunoglobulin complexes which is not simply an expression of bound rheumatoid factor[99–103]. Increased binding may be a consequence of increased expression of Fc receptors for IgG[34,104] (Figure 1). Circulating monocytes also show increased expression of the β_2 integrin CR3 which functions both as an adhesion molecule and as a receptor for iC3b[34,104], and of urokinase receptors[105]. In contrast to upregulated expression of FcR, CR3 and urokinase receptors, MHC class II expression is not increased on circulating monocytes[23] (Figure 1). There is some evidence that circulating monocytes produce angiotensin converting enzyme and IL-1[106,107] and monocytes from patients with rheumatoid arthritis produce factors, including IL-6, which modify glycosylation of acute phase proteins[108]. Our observation of relatively high levels of mRNA for IL-1β in peripheral blood monocytes from some patients with rheumatoid arthritis might be in keeping with these observations (unpublished observation, Figure 2). Thus circulating monocytes from patients with rheumatoid arthritis show evidence of selective activation, which differs from that seen in macrophages within synovial fluid or synovial membrane. Such changes might be the result of demonstrable levels of cytokines present within the circulation of patients with rheumatoid arthritis or changes in bone marrow[109] but could result from other processes of more potential importance to the pathogenesis of rheumatoid arthritis.

MECHANISMS OF MACROPHAGE ACTIVATION

Consideration of the site of macrophage activation in rheumatoid arthritis, and the extent to which this might occur systemically, or locally at sites of inflammation, naturally leads to considering possible mechanisms by which macrophages might be activated in patients with rheumatoid arthritis. Evidence from animal models of arthritis and *in vitro* experiments suggest at least five main possibilities. These include lymphocyte-mediated activation, activation by other synovial cells such as 'transformed' synovial fibroblasts (synoviocytes), activation by interaction with immune complexes, direct activation by bacterial cell wall products and activation mediated by virus infection of monocytes/macrophages. There is also no reason why a single mechanism should operate exclusively, and there is considerable potential for synergistic activation of macrophages, for example by application of stimuli from lymphocytes and synoviocytes as well as immune complexes.

Lymphocyte mediated macrophage activation

The hypothesis that rheumatoid arthritis is a disease driven by activation of macrophages by lymphocytes reacting specifically to a postulated arthritogenic antigen is attractive. It can be argued that the association of rheumatoid arthritis with possession of very specific sequences within the third hypervariable region of the DRβ chain favours recognition of an arthritogenic antigen[110]. Animal models such as adjuvant arthritis and streptococcal cell wall arthritis are mediated by T cells reactive with defined arthritogenic antigens and disease can be transferred by T cells[16,111]. In human arthritis caused by defined organisms such as *Borrelia burgdorferi*, joint T cells react preferentially with the triggering organism[112]. There is some evidence that lymphocytes in rheumatoid synovial membrane are activated, such as expression of MHC class II and limited expression of IL-2R[113,114], and therapies which damage lymphocytes show some efficacy against rheumatoid arthritis[115–117]. Thus there are reasons to believe that lymphocytes triggered by antigen recognition could mediate macrophage activation and consequent joint inflammation and destruction in patients with rheumatoid arthritis. It might be envisaged for example that such activation might follow pathways similar to those demonstrable in lymphocyte-mediated arming of macrophages against mycobacterial organisms in which lymphocyte production of IL-2 and interferon gamma are critical events[118]. However, the use of antibodies and *in situ* hybridization have not convincingly demonstrated production of these two cytokines by lymphocytes within rheumatoid synovial membrane[27,119]. This has led to suggestions such that lymphocyte activation in rheumatoid arthritis might be atypical or 'arrested'[120]. Alternatively, since synovial T lymphocytes express mRNA encoding IL-2, but not IL-2 protein, they may be in a state of anergy such as is found in T cells infiltrating engrafted tissues in tolerant animals[121]. Because there are difficulties in demonstrating direct evidence for lymphocyte-mediated macrophage activation by classical pathways in rheumatoid arthritis, and also because different mechanisms might operate at non-articular sites of inflammation, it is pertinent to consider other mechanisms which could lead to macrophage activation in rheumatoid arthritis[30].

The contribution of synoviocytes to macrophage activation

The juxtaposition of activated fibroblasts and synoviocytes in the thickened lining of the inflamed joint, and the potential for a self-sustaining cycle of mutual stimulation via direct cell contact and cytokine production have been discussed. The view was expressed that such a cycle, which results in production of a destructive locally invasive tissue, was likely to be initiated by the activated macrophage. However, the production of cytokines such as GM-CSF and IL-6, and their sustained production during several cycles of *in vitro* culture[55,56] indicate the possibility that synoviocytes might initiate such a cycle. For this to happen the synoviocyte would have to be activated or 'transformed'. In the mrl/lpr mouse model of arthritis, synoviocytes with a 'transformed' appearance with large nuclei and prominent nucleoli are an early feature, and infiltration with inflammatory cells occurs later[15]. It has been proposed that such activation in the mouse model and in human rheumatoid arthritis could be caused by retroviral infection of synoviocytes, transactivation and upregulated expression of cellular oncogenes, and consequent production of cytokines and matrix-degrading enzymes[122]. In this model attraction of lymphocytes and macrophages, and macrophage activation would be initiated by the transformed synoviocyte.

Immune complex mediated macrophage activation

Immunoglobulin complexes, with or without complement, are still considered to be the likely pathogenic basis for extra-articular lesions in patients with rheumatoid arthritis, including subcutaneous nodules[84]. Less attention has been given in recent times to this aspect of inflammation within the joint. However, it has been established that active synthesis of immunoglobulin occurs within the synovial membrane[123,124]. A significant proportion of this is rheumatoid factor[125], and local production of anticollagen antibodies has also been identified[126]. Immune complexes are deposited in joint tissues and may become sequestered in cartilage[127], and complement activation occurs within the rheumatoid joint[128]. Complement activating complexes are also present in the circulation, and are associated with the presence of extra-articular disease[129]. Self-associating IgG rheumatoid factor may be important in the formation of such complexes[130] and this interaction is enhanced by abnormal glycosylation of the immunoglobulins produced in rheumatoid arthritis[131]. The identification of unknown antigens[132] and the recent finding of CMV viral antigens within such circulating complexes[133] are also of note. Monocytes/macrophages within the rheumatoid joint and nodules possess FcR[33,81] and receptors for activated complement components including iC3b and C5a[35,134] and are therefore equipped to interact with complexes and the products of immune complex mediated complement activation[102]. In addition, the interaction of immunoglobulins with Fc receptors on monocytes/macrophages is enhanced by abnormal glycosylation[135]. Interaction of complexes[136–138] and complement components[139–141] with monocytes/macrophages mediates activation of a number of macrophage effector mechanisms including production of IL-1 and TNF. Consequently immune complexes produced locally within the joints, or derived from the circulation, are likely to contribute to macrophage activation and subsequent inflammation and tissue destruction in patients with rheumatoid arthritis. Furthermore, it has been demonstrated in the collagen induced animal model that such antibody mediated mechanisms and cell mediated immune mechanisms can act synergistically to produce arthritis[142].

Activation of macrophages by bacterial components

Amongst the most potent macrophage activating stimuli are bacterial products. Lipopolysaccharide is in widespread experimental use for activating macrophage effector functions including production of a wide range of cytokines and prostanoids relevant to arthritis. This response is triggered by interaction with macrophage receptors including a 73 kDa LPS-binding protein and CD14[143]. Other bacterial cell wall components are also potent macrophage activators which induce cytotoxicity[144,145] and production of nitrogen intermediates[146]. Bacterial 'superantigens' which bind MHC-class II and preferentially activate T cells carrying receptors with particular Vβ also stimulate macrophages to produce IL-1 and TNF by transmitting a positive signal via MHC-class II[147]. The simultaneous presence of T lymphocyte products such as gamma interferon modifies and augments the response of macrophages to interaction with components of bacteria[148] and other infectious agents such as mycoplasmas[149]. In this complex interplay between infectious agents and the lymphocytes and macrophages of the host it has been considered that 'lymphocytes play the music but the macrophage calls the tune'[150].

Such interactions undoubtedly occur in animal models of arthritis mediated by bacterial components including streptococcal cell walls. Inflammatory processes initiated by streptococcal cell walls which contribute to the early induction phase of arthritis include complement activation, activation of endothelial cells, direct activation of macrophages, and later a T cell mediated component contributing to further macrophage activation[151]. The role of T cells in streptococcal cell wall arthritis, adjuvant arthritis and collagen induced arthritis has been emphasized[152-154]. However, even in these animal models macrophages are critically involved as effector cells in producing joint destruction and in the initiation of arthritis since the initial phase of joint inflammation in streptococcal cell wall arthritis is T cell independent[155]. These animal models are therefore examples of arthritis mediated by macrophage/lymphocyte interaction as has been envisaged in rheumatoid arthritis. It is also known that bacterial components such as endotoxin can directly induce joint inflammation dependent upon production of IL-1 and TNF[156]. Direct activation of macrophages can mediate arthritis in severe combined immunodeficient mice lacking T cells upon infection with *Borrelia burgdorferi*[157,158] and there is evidence that macrophages are important mediators of experimental arthritis induced by fragmented *Streptococcus agalacticae*[159].

That aseptic inflammatory arthritis can be produced by intra-articular bacterial components in humans is now established beyond reasonable doubt in patients with reactive arthritis. Intra-articular chlamydial antigen has been detected using monoclonal antibodies by some but not all investigators[160,161]. *Chlamydia trachomatis* has been shown by electron microscopy within macrophages in synovial tissue[162,163]. Similarly chlamydia associated DNA was not found by initial investigators[164,165] but the presence of RNA has now been detected[166]. In the case of *Chlamydia trachomatis* the presence of elementary bodies and reticular bodies in macrophages[162] and the presence of chlamydial RNA argue for productive infection within affected joints despite the fact that joints are culture negative. In bacterially mediated reactive arthritis the presence of fragments of *Salmonella* and *Yersinia* organisms has been shown[167-169]. This has included the demonstration of intra-articular lipopolysaccharide[170,171]. Thus, although the exact role of the macrophage in human reactive arthritis has not been established, there are indications that it is likely to play a critical part in pathogenesis[172].

First, since many of the organisms are intracellular with the potential to grow within macrophages, the ability of the host macrophages to control the growth of intracellular organisms is relevant to containment of the initial infection. It has also been suggested that dissemination of bacterial fragments could take place within the host's macrophages. The presence of lipopolysaccharide and the known sensitivity of macrophages to LPS-mediated activation imply that this is likely to make a contribution to joint inflammation in reactive arthritis by a direct action upon macrophages. The increased severity of experimental arthritis induced by chlamydiae in mice which have been pre-immunized[173,174], the presence in reactive joints of antigen-reactive T cells[175,176], and in human reactive synovial membrane of lymphocytes producing IL-2 and IFN-gamma[121] suggest that lymphocyte-mediated mechanisms of macrophage activation contribute to more prolonged and severe arthritis associated with destructive changes.

Could bacteria also trigger destructive arthritis in rheumatoid arthritis? It has been strongly argued that this is a possible mechanism[151] and more particularly since Lyme arthritis was demonstrated to be caused by a spirochaete present in very low numbers. Recent attention has been focused upon the presence within the human gut of multiple organisms capable of mediating arthritis[177,178], proteus species in the urinary tract[179], mycobacteria and other slow bacterial infections[180,181]. However, whilst such possibilities remain no more substantial than a twinkle in the eye of the ardent researcher one can only point to the likely ways that macrophages might be involved in such a process.

Activation of macrophages by viruses, and other interactions

Another credible cause for rheumatoid arthritis is viral infection. Candidate viruses have included Epstein-Barr virus, cytomegalovirus, parvovirus, and rubella[182]. The potential of non-AIDS retroviruses such a HTLV-1 to be the cause of as yet unexplained diseases has been recognized[183]. Mice transgenic for HTLV-1 develop arthritis[184], and HTLV-1 infection in humans is associated with an inflammatory arthritis[185]. Proteins associated with HTLV-1 have been detected in rheumatoid synovial membrane[186]. Thus, despite the failure so far to provide direct experimental evidence for a retroviral aetiology for rheumatoid arthritis[187] many are still attracted to this possibility. First, HIV infection may result in articular disease[188]. Second, the lentiviruses caprine arthritis-encephalitis virus (CAEV) and Visna cause arthritis in goats and sheep[189]. In both cases macrophages play an important role in maintaining and disseminating the infection. In HIV the macrophage acts as a reservoir for persistent infection[190,191]. The lentiviruses responsible for arthritis in animals are also macrophage-tropic[192,193]. Furthermore, although CAEV is present in monocytes productive infection only occurs on maturation of the monocyte to a tissue macrophage[192]. In lentivirus arthritis in animals inflammatory arthritis develops in infected animals only after a latency of some two years[189]. The evolution of inflammatory changes in synovial membrane parallel those of rheumatoid arthritis[194], and of particular interest is the observation that in some synovial samples taken at an early stage of the disease synovial membrane 'hypertrophy' was a finding[195]. Synovial fluid macrophages from sheep with Visna virus arthritis show changes indicative of activation including upregulated expression of MHC-class II[196]. Syncytial giant cell formation from infected macrophages in tissue culture is a conspicuous cytopathic change[197]. Similar syncytia develop when rheumatoid synovial macrophages are cultured[198–200] and there have been reports of virus-like particles seen in such cultured macrophages from the rheumatoid joint[201,202]. Other authors have argued that the formation of giant cells in cultured synovial fluid from other forms of inflammatory arthritis suggests that the phenomenon is more general and is likely to be a consequence of cell-mediated immune mechanisms rather than viral infection[203]. In addition to infectious retroviruses it is also possible that endogenous retroviruses could cause arthritis. Mechanisms include encoding endogenous superantigens and immunomodulating proteins, and activation of genes such as those encoding cytokines through transactivation[204]. Recently an endogenous retroviral gene has been associated with rheumatoid arthritis[205]. Thus retroviruses of either exogenous or endogenous origin are capable of mediating arthritis. Expression of infection can be specific to certain cells, especially macrophages, and dependent upon specific stages in the development of these cells.

Because infection with macrophage-tropic retroviruses can result in arthritis, and because they are carried to sites of infection in monocytes, it is relevant to consider the possible consequences of monocyte mediated dissemination of infection. Similar considerations might also apply to dissemination of monocytes pre-activated by other means. Since recruitment of monocytes to joints is a normal process in the turnover of the macrophages within the synovial lining layer, infected or pre-activated macrophages would inevitably be delivered to joints. In either case joint inflammation would occur mediated either as a result of infection and a subsequent immune response, or as a result of recruitment of other inflammatory cells by activated macrophages releasing cytokines within the joint. It might be expected that arthritis mediated in this way would be of symmetrical form. Further, if the rate of monocyte turnover in joints were reflected in their use then it might be expected that the joints most affected would be the small joints of the hands and feet. Such considerations suggest that one means by which the pattern of arthritis typical of rheumatoid arthritis could be determined is by the ongoing physiological recruitment of monocytes to replenish the population of macrophages within the normal joint.

THERAPEUTIC TARGETING OF ACTIVATED JOINT MACROPHAGES

Although the mechanisms by which macrophages are activated in rheumatoid arthritis remain unknown, it is clear that these cells are activated, and that this results in joint inflammation and destruction. This information provides good reasons for therapeutic targeting of activated joint macrophages and their products. Despite this most strategies which have been developed for novel treatment of rheumatoid arthritis have targeted the lymphocyte, with relatively little attention to macrophages[117]. One indirect approach has been to inhibit pro-inflammatory macrophage products, and particularly IL-1 and TNF-α because of their demonstrable importance to destructive mechanisms in arthritis. The naturally occurring IL-1 receptor antagonist (IL-1ra) acts through competitive binding to IL-1 receptors[206,207], including those on rheumatoid synovial cells[208]. Consequently blocking the effect of IL-1 using IL-1ra and TNF using soluble TNF receptor molecules has been proposed for treatment of arthritis and other inflammatory diseases[209,210], and there is already some experimental support for the effectiveness of this therapeutic approach[211,212]. Some drugs may also reduce production of IL-1[213] and TNF in macrophages[214]. Another approach might be to 'deactivate' macrophages, for example by using cytokines such as transforming growth factor beta-1 (TGF-β_1)[215]. Intra-articular injection of TGF-β_1 causes an influx of macrophages, production of inflammatory cytokines, and synovitis[216]. By contrast, systemic administration of TGF-β_1 to animals with experimental arthritis is therapeutically effective[217–219] possibly through reducing leukocytosis and consequently recruitment of inflammatory cells into joints. Monoclonal antibodies can also be used to deplete circulating phagocytic cells[220] but this method has been much more extensively applied to lymphocytes, although it is known that use of anti CD4 antibodies also causes depletion of monocytes. Macrophages can also be selectively targeted for delivery of therapeutic substances by exploiting their surface receptors to promote internalization. For example, it has been shown that derivatization with mannose can be used to deliver enzyme to macrophage lysosomes by exploiting the mannose receptor[221]. This mechanism has been used to deliver glucocerebrosidase to deficient macrophages in patients with Gaucher's disease[222]. Thus therapeutic strategies for selectively targeting macrophages are already in use. Furthermore, since activated macrophages accumulate at the joint surface they are vulnerable to intra-articular injection of macrophage-targeted therapeutic agents. Such treatment strategies warrant consideration and might well make a contribution in expanding our therapeutic options in treating erosive arthritis.

CONCLUSIONS

In conclusion, macrophages are normal components of the synovial membrane which is a structure that is adapted for freedom of movement and sustaining joint structures. Continuing recruitment of monocytes to the joint means that they are vulnerable to infectious agents carried by macrophages such as CAEV, and to systemic activation of monocytes subsequently directed as a consequence of their normal function to the joints in the course of replacing lining macrophages. The presence within the joint of macrophages also sets the scene for local antigen processing and presentation and a localized, articular immune response.

Whether these mechanisms contribute to the pathogenesis of rheumatoid arthritis has not been clearly established. There is certainly evidence of presynovial activation and functional changes within circulating monocytes. Recruitment of macrophages into inflamed joints and to extra-articular lesions such as nodules is a prominent feature of the disease. Accumulation of macrophages within these lesions results in synovial lining 'hyperplasia' and formation of a palisade of cells surrounding centres of necrosis within the nodule. These macrophages are activated and produce prostanoids, pro-inflammatory cytokines and proteolytic enzymes. In the joint, activated macrophages interact with fibroblasts to convert the synovial lining into a tissue with locally invasive potential. Activated macrophages may contribute to adherence of the inflamed synovial surface to joint structures and therefore permit full expression of the invasive potential of the inflamed synovial lining. In the nodule, macrophages are probably themselves responsible for necrobiosis. In fact mediation of destructive changes by activated macrophages is a feature of diverse forms of experimental and naturally occurring arthritis in animals and humans.

Different mechanisms are responsible for such activation, and synergistic interactions may occur. The most favoured model in rheumatoid arthritis is lymphocyte-mediated activation of macrophages within the affected joints, but direct evidence for this mechanism has yet to be established. Difficulties in demonstrating production of classical macrophage-activating lymphokines mean that more direct mechanisms of macrophage activation must be considered. Complexed immunoglobulins and activated complement components can activate macrophages and have been considered as prime candidates for inducing macrophage activation within extra-articular lesions. However, activation by bacteria, bacterial fragments and other infectious agents such as mycoplasmas and viruses cannot be excluded on our present inadequate data. Thus, even at this stage, determination of the site at which macrophage activation occurs in rheumatoid arthritis, and the mechanism(s) of activation are still issues which require resolution.

Present data on the importance of the activated macrophage in producing the granulomatous destructive inflammation characteristic of rheumatoid arthritis amply justify a search for therapeutic strategies which might inhibit macrophage function. Although measures for blocking the effect of macrophage products such as IL-1 and TNFα are under active investigation with promising preliminary results, much less effort has been applied to means of directly targeting macrophages than has been applied to the elimination of lymphocytes. Mechanisms for systemic delivery of macrophage-targeted therapeutic agents have been established and applied in other clinical settings. In addition activated synovial lining macrophages are exposed to therapeutic agents administered by intra-articular injection. It therefore seems entirely possible that novel therapeutic approaches based on the elimination of activated macrophages and their products could be developed and could usefully extend our ability to treat rheumatoid arthritis.

References

1. Witsell AL, Schook LB. Macrophage heterogeneity occurs through a developmental mechanism. Proc Natl Acad Sci USA. 1991; 88: 1963–1967.
2. Barland P, Novikoff AB, Hamerman D. Electron microscopy of the human synovial membrane. J Cell Biol. 1962; 14: 207–220.
3. Edwards JCW, Willoughby DA. Demonstration of bone marrow derived cells in synovial lining using giant lysosomal granules as genetic markers. Ann Rheum Dis. 1982; 41: 177–182.
4. Hogg N, Palmer DG, Revell PA. Mononuclear phagocytes of normal and rheumatoid synovial membrane identified by monoclonal antibodies. Immunology. 1985; 56: 673–681.
5. Palmer DG, Selvendran Y, Allen C, Revell PA, Hogg N. Features of synovial membrane identified with monoclonal antibodies. Clin Exp Immunol. 1985; 59: 529–538.
6. Burmester GR, Dimitriou-Bona A, Waters SJ, Winchester RJ. Identification of 3 major synovial lining cell populations by monoclonal antibodies directed to Ia antigens and antigens associated with monocytes/macrophages and fibroblasts. Scand J Immunol. 1983; 17: 69–82.
7. Stevens CR, Mapp PI, Revell PA. A monoclonal antibody (MAb 67) marks type B synoviocytes. Rheumatol Int. 1990; 10: 103–106.
8. Revell PA. Synovial lining cells. Rheumatol Int. 1989; 9: 49–51.
9. Henderson B, Edwards JCW. Functions of synovial lining. In: The Synovial Lining in Health and Disease. London: Chapman and Hall; 1987; 41–74.
10. Kulka JP, Bocking D, Ropes MW, Bauer W. Early joint lesions of rheumatoid arthritis. Arch Pathol. 1955; 59: 129–150.
11. Schumacher HR, Kitridou RC. Synovitis of recent onset. A clinicopathologic study during the first month of disease. Arthritis Rheum. 1972; 15: 465–485.
12. Soden M, Rooney M, Cullen A, Whelan A, Feighery C, Bresnihan B. Immunohistological features in the synovium obtained from clinically uninvolved knee joints of patients with rheumatoid arthritis. Br J Rheumatol. 1989; 28: 287–292.
13. Lalor PA, Mapp PI, Hall PA, Revell PA. Proliferative activity of cells in the synovium as demonstrated by a monoclonal antibody, Ki 67. Rheumatol Int. 1987; 7: 183–186.
14. Mohr W, Beneke G, Mohing W. Proliferation of synovial lining cells and fibroblasts. Ann Rheum Dis. 1975; 34: 219–224.
15. O'Sullivan FX, Fassbender H-G, Gay S, Koopman WJ. Etiopathogenesis of the rheumatoid arthritis-like disease in MRL/l mice. I. The histomorphologic basis of joint destruction. Arthritis Rheum. 1985; 28: 529–536.
16. van Eden W, Holoshitz J, Nevo Z, Frenkel A, Klajman A, Cohen IR. Arthritis induced by a T-lymphocyte clone that responds to *Mycobacterium tuberculosis* and to cartilage proteoglycans. Proc Natl Acad Sci USA. 1985; 82: 5117–5120.
17. Pearson CM, Wood FD. Studies of arthritis and other lesions induced in rats by the injection of mycobacterial adjuvant. VII. Pathologic details of the arthritis and spondylitis. Am J Pathol. 1963; 42: 73–86.
18. Adams DO. Molecular interactions in macrophage activation. Immunology Today. 1989; 10: 33–35.
19. Janossy G, Panayi G, Duke O, Bofill M, Poulter LW, Goldstein G. Rheumatoid arthritis: a disease of T-lymphocyte macrophage immunoregulation. Lancet. 1981; 2: 839–842.
20. Klareskog L, Forsum U, Scheynius A, Kabelitz D, Wigzell H. Evidence in support of a self-perpetuating HLA-DR dependent delayed-type cell reaction in rheumatoid arthritis. Proc Natl Acad Sci USA. 1982; 79: 3632–3636.
21. Klareskog L, Forsum U, Kabelitz D, Ploem L, Sundstrom C, Nilsson W, Wigren A, Wigzell H. Immune functions of human synovial cells. Phenotypic and T cell regulatory properties of macrophage-like cells that express HLA-DR. Arthritis Rheum. 1982; 25: 488–501.
22. Poulter LW, Duke O, Hobbs S, Janossy G, Panayi G, Seymour G. The involvement of interdigitating (antigen-presenting) cells in the pathogenesis of rheumatoid arthritis. Clin Exp Immunol. 1983; 51: 247–254.
23. Ridley MG, Kingsley G, Pitzalis C, Panayi GS. Monocyte activation in rheumatoid arthritis: evidence for *in situ* activation and differentiation in joints. Br J Rheumatol. 1990; 29: 84–88.

24. Hessian PA, Highton J, Palmer DG. Quantification of macrophage cell surface molecules in rheumatoid arthritis. Clin Exp Immunol. 1989; 77: 47–51.
25. Ridley M, Panayi G, Nicholas N, Murphy J. Mechanisms of macrophage activation in rheumatoid arthritis: the role of gamma interferon. Clin Exp Immunol. 1986; 63: 587–593.
26. Firestein GS, Zvaifler NJ. Peripheral blood and synovial fluid monocyte activation in inflammatory arthritis. II. Low levels of synovial fluid and synovial tissue interferon suggest that gamma interferon is not the primary macrophage activating factor. Arthritis Rheum. 1987; 30: 864–871.
27. Husby G, Williams RC. Immunohistochemical studies of interleukin-2 and gamma-interferon in rheumatoid arthritis. Arthritis Rheum. 1985; 28: 174–181.
28. Buchan G, Barrett K, Fujita T, Taniguchi T, Maini R, Feldmann M. Detection of activated T cell products in the rheumatoid joint using cDNA probes to interleukin-2 (IL-2) IL-2 receptor and IFN-gamma. Clin Exp Immunol. 1988; 71: 295–301.
29. Alvaro-Garcia JM, Zvaifler NF, Firestein GS. Cytokines in chronic inflammatory arthritis. IV. GM-CSF mediated induction of class II MHC antigen on human monocytes: a possible role in rheumatoid arthritis. J Exp Med. 1989; 170: 865–876.
30. Firestein GS, Zvaifler NJ. How important are T cells in chronic rheumatoid synovitis? Arthritis Rheum. 1990; 33: 769–773.
31. Guyre PM, Morganelli PM, Miller R. Recombinant immune interferon increases immunoglobulin G Fc receptors on cultured human mononuclear phagocytes. J Clin Invest. 1983; 72: 393–397.
32. Perussia B, Dayton ET, Lazarus R, Fanning V, Trinchieri G. Immune interferon induces the receptor for monomeric IgG on human monocytic and myeloid cells. J Exp Med. 1983; 158: 1092–1113.
33. Broker BM, Edwards JCW, Fanger MW, Lydyard PM. The prevalence and distribution of macrophages bearing $Fc\gamma RI$, $Fc\gamma RII$ and $Fc\gamma RIII$ in synovium. Scand J Rheumatol. 1990; 19: 123–135.
34. Highton J, Smith M, Bradley J. Cells of the Monocyte-Macrophage series in peripheral blood and synovial fluid in inflammatory arthritis. A preliminary study of cellular phenotype. Scand J Rheumatol. 1989; 18: 393–398.
35. Allen CA, Highton J, Palmer DG. Increased expression of p150,95 and CR3 leukocyte adhesion molecules by mononuclear phagocytes in rheumatoid synovial membranes. Arthritis Rheum. 1989; 32: 947–954.
36. Miller LJ, Bainton DF, Borregaard N, Springer TA. Stimulated mobilization of monocyte Mac-1 and p150,95 adhesion proteins from an intracellular vesicular compartment to the cell surface. J Clin Invest. 1987; 80: 535–544.
37. Hale LP, Martin ME, McCollum DE, Nunley JA, Springer TA, Singer KH, Haynes BF. Immunohistologic analysis of the distribution of cell adhesion molecules within the inflammatory synovial microenvironment. Arthritis Rheum. 1989; 32: 22–30.
38. Kingsley G, Pitzalis C, Constantinides Y, Panayi GS. Pathways of monocyte–macrophage (Mo) maturation and migration in chronic inflammatory arthritis. Br J Rheumatol. 1989; 38 (suppl 2): 65, abstract 113.
39. Dransfield I, Hogg N. Regulated expression of Mg^{2+} binding epitope on leukocyte integrin alpha subunits. EMBO J. 1989; 12: 3759–3765.
40. Wildgoose P, Berkner KL, Kisiel W. Synthesis, purification and characterization of an Arg 152-Glu site-directed mutant of recombinant human blood clotting factor VII. Biochemistry. 1990; 29: 3413–3420.
41. Tsao BP, Fair DS, Curtiss LK, Edgington TS. Monocytes can be induced by lipopolysaccharide-triggered T lymphocytes to express functional factor VII/VIIa protease activity. J Exp Med. 1984; 159: 1042–1057.
42. Uchman B, Bang NU, Rathbun MJ, Fineberg NS, Davidson JK, Fineberg SE. Effect of insulin immune complexes on human blood monocyte and endothelial cell procoagulant activity. J Lab Clin Med. 1988; 112: 652–659.
43. Gregory SA, Morrissey JH, Edgington TS. Regulation of tissue factor gene expression in the monocyte procoagulant response to endotoxin. Mol Cell Biol. 1989; 9: 2752–2755.
44. Fan S-T, Edgington TS. Coupling of the adhesive receptor CD 11b/CD18 to functional enhancement of effector macrophage tissue factor response. J Clin Invest. 1991; 87: 50–57.
45. Weinberg JB, Pippen AM, Greenberg CS. Extravascular fibrin formation and dissolution

in synovial tissue of patients with osteoarthritis and rheumatoid arthritis. Arthritis Rheum. 1991; 34: 996–1005.

46. Kirkham B. Interleukin-1, immune activation pathways, and different mechanisms in osteoarthritis and rheumatoid arthritis. Ann Rheum Dis. 1991; 50: 395–400.

47. Brennan FM, Field M, Chu CQ, Feldmann M, Maini RN. Cytokine expression in rheumatoid arthritis. Br J Rheumatol. 1991; 30 (suppl 1): 76–80.

48. Arend WP, Dayer J-M. Cytokines and cytokine inhibitors or antagonists in rheumatoid arthritis. Arthritis Rheum. 1990; 33: 305–315.

49. Perchl P, Ceska M, Effenberger F, Haberhauer G, Broell H, Lundley IJ. Presence of NAP-1/IL-8 in synovial fluids indicates a possible pathogenic role in rheumatoid arthritis. Scand J Immunol. 1991; 34: 333–339.

50. Koch AE, Kunkel SL, Burrows JC, Evanoff HL, Haines GK, Pope RM, Strieter RM. Synovial tissue macrophage as a source of the chemotactic cytokine IL-8. J Immunol. 1991; 147: 2187–2195.

51. Kirkham BW, Navarro FJ, Corkill MM, Barbatis C, Panayi GS. Immunohistochemical localisation of interleukin 1 in rheumatoid and osteoarthritis synovial membrane. J Rheumatol. 1989; 28 (suppl 2): 47, abstract 82.

52. Chu CQ, Field M, Feldmann M, Maini RN. Localization of tumor necrosis factor α in synovial tissues and at the cartilage-pannus junction in patients with rheumatoid arthritis. Arthritis Rheum. 1991; 34: 1125–1132.

53. Firestein GS, Alvaro-Garcia JM, Maki R. Quantitative analysis of cytokine gene expression in rheumatoid arthritis. J Immunol. 1990; 144: 3347–3353.

54. Alvaro-Garcia JM, Zvaifler NJ, Brown CB, Kaushansky K, Firestein GS. Cytokines in chronic inflammatory arthritis. VI. Analysis of the synovial cells involved in granulocyte-macrophage colony-stimulating factor production and gene expression in rheumatoid arthritis and its regulation by IL-1 and tumor necrosis factor-α. J Immunol. 1991; 146: 3365–3371.

55. Bucala R, Ritchlin C, Winchester R, Cerami A. Constitutive production of inflammatory and mitogenic cytokines by rheumatoid synovial fibroblasts. J Exp Med. 1991; 173: 569–574.

56. Rosenbaum JT, Cugnini R, Tara DC, Hefeneider S, Ansel JC. Production and modulation of interleukin 6 synthesis by synoviocytes derived from patients with arthritic disease. Ann Rheum Dis. 1992; 51: 198–202.

57. Wood NC, Symons JA, Dickens E, Duff GW. *In situ* hybridization of IL-6 in rheumatoid arthritis. Clin Exp Immunol. 1992; 87: 183–189.

58. Gravallese EM, Darling JM, Ladd AL, Katz JN, Glimcher LH. *In situ* hybridization studies of stromelysin and collagenase messenger RNA expression in rheumatoid synovium. Arthritis Rheum. 1991; 34: 1076–1084.

59. McCachren SS. Expression of metalloproteinases and metalloproteinase inhibitor in human arthritic synovium. Arthritis Rheum. 1991; 34: 1085–1093.

60. Firestein GS, Paine MM, Littman BH. Gene expression (collagenase, tissue inhibitor of metalloproteinases, complement, and HLA-DR) in rheumatoid arthritis and osteoarthritis synovium. Quantitative analysis and effect of intra-articular corticosteroids. Arthritis Rheum. 1991; 34: 1094–1105.

61. Brickerhoff CD. Joint destruction in arthritis: metalloproteinases in the spotlight. Arthritis Rheum. 1991; 34: 1073–1075.

62. Vassali P. The pathophysiology of tumor necrosis factors. Ann Rev Immunol. 1992; 10: 411–452.

63. Wilder RL, Remmers EF, Sano H, Case JP, Lafayatis R. The cytokine networks in rheumatoid arthritis. Br J Rheumatol. 1991; 30 (suppl 2): 44–47.

64. Waller HA, Butler MG, McClean JGB, Dowd GSE, Scott DL. Localisation of fibronectin mRNA in the rheumatoid synovium by *in situ* hybridisation. Ann Rheum Dis. 1992; 51: 735–740.

65. Wells AF, Klareskog L, Lindblad S, Laurent TC. Correlation between increased hyaluronan localised in arthritic synovium and the presence of proliferating cells. A role of macrophage-derived factors. Arthritis Rheum. 1992; 35: 391–396.

66. Ishikawa H, Ohno O, Saura R, Matsubara T, Kuroda T, Hirohata K. Cytokine enhancement of monocyte/synovial cell attachment to the surface of cartilage: a possible trigger of pannus formation in arthritis. Rheumatol Int. 1991; 11: 31–36.

67. Wolf J, Carsons S. Synovial extracellular matrix: partial characterization of matrix components and identification of type VI collagen molecular forms. Clin Exp Rheumatol. 1991; 9: 51–54.
68. Allard SA, Bayliss MT, Maini RN. The synovium-cartilage junction of the normal human knee. Implications for joint destruction and repair. Arthritis Rheum. 1990; 33: 1170–1179.
69. Allard SA, Muirden KD, Maini RN. Correlation of histopathological features of pannus with patterns of damage in different joints in rheumatoid arthritis. Ann Rheum Dis. 1991; 50: 278–283.
70. Salisbury AK, Duke O, Poulter L-W. Macrophage-like cells of the pannus area in rheumatoid arthritic joints. Scand J Rheumatol. 1987; 16: 263–272.
71. Allard SA, Muirden KD, Hogg N, Maini RN. Differential expression of MHC class II antigens and macrophage sub-populations in rheumatoid pannus. Br J Rheumatol. 1987; 26 (suppl 2): 124 (abstract 207).
72. Chu CQ, Field M, Abney E, Zheng RQH, Allard S, Feldman M, Maini RN. Transforming growth factor-β_1 in rheumatoid synovial membrane. Clin Exp Immunol. 1991; 86: 380–386.
73. Trabant A, Gay RE, Fassbender H-G, Gay S. Cathepsin B in synovial cells at the site of joint destruction in rheumatoid arthritis. Arthritis Rheum. 1991; 34: 1444–1451.
74. Trabant A, Archer WK, Gay R, Sukhatme VP, Nilson-Hamilton M, Hamilton RT, Fassbender HG, McGhee JR, Gay S. Expression of the collagenolytic and ras-induced cysteine proteinase cathepsin L and proliferation-associated oncogenes in synovial cells of MRL/l mice and patients with rheumatoid arthritis. Matrix. 1990; 10: 349–361.
75. Gay S, Gay RE. Cellular basis and oncogene expression of rheumatoid joint destruction. Rheumatol Int. 1989; 9: 105–113.
76. Hedfors E, Klareskog L, Lindblad S, Forsum U, Lindahl G. Phenotypic characterization of cells within subcutaneous rheumatoid nodules. Arthritis Rheum. 1983; 26: 1333–1339.
77. Duke OL, Hobbs S, Panayi GS, Poulter LW, Rasker JJ, Janossy G. A combined immunohistological and histochemical analysis of lymphocyte and macrophage subpopulations in the rheumatoid nodule. Clin Exp Immunol. 1984; 56: 239–246.
78. Athanasou NA, Quinn J, Woods CG, McGee JO'D. Immunohistology of rheumatoid nodules and rheumatoid synovium. Ann Rheum Dis. 1988; 47: 398–403.
79. Palmer DG, Hogg N, Highton J, Hessian PA, Denholm I. Macrophage migration and maturation within rheumatoid nodules. Arthritis Rheum. 1987; 30: 729–736.
80. Cochrane W, Davies DV, Dorling J, Bywaters EGL. Ultramicroscopic structure of the rheumatoid nodule. Ann Rheum Dis. 1964; 23: 345–363.
81. Highton J, Palmer DG, Smith M, Hessian PA. Phenotypic markers of lymphocyte and mononuclear phagocyte activation within rheumatoid nodules. J Rheumatol. 1990; 17: 1130–1136.
82. Goto M, Sasano M, Fuzisawa M, Okabe T, Nishizawa K. Constitutive production of angiotensin converting enzyme from rheumatoid nodule cells under serum free conditions. Ann Rheum Dis. 1992; 51: 741–742.
83. Sokoloff L, McCluskey RT, Bunim JJ. Vascularity of the early subcutaneous nodule of rheumatoid arthritis. Arch Pathol. 1953; 55: 475–495.
84. Ziff M. The rheumatoid nodule. Arthritis Rheum. 1990; 33: 761–767.
85. Palmer DG, Hogg N, Allen CA, Highton J, Hessian PA. A mononuclear phagocyte subset associated with cell necrosis in rheumatoid nodules: identification with monoclonal antibody 5.5. Clin Immunol Immunopathol. 1987; 45: 17–28.
86. Edgeworth J, Gorman M, Bennett R, Freemont P, Hogg N. Identification of p8,14 as a highly abundant heterodimeric calcium binding protein complex of myeloid cells. J Biol Chem. 1991; 266: 7706–7713.
87. Zwaldo G, Bruggen J, Gerhards G, Schlegel R, Sorg C. Two calcium-binding proteins associated with specific stages of myeloid cell differentiation are expressed by subsets of macrophages in inflammatory tissues. Clin Exp Immunol. 1988; 72: 510–515.
88. Miyasaka N, Sato K, Yamamoto K, Goto M, Nishioka K. Immunological and immunohisto-chemical analysis of rheumatoid nodules. Ann Rheum Dis. 1989; 48: 220–226.
89. Harris ED. A collagenolytic system produced by primary cultures of rheumatoid nodule tissue. J Clin Invest. 1972; 51: 2973–2976.
90. Kolb H, Kolb-Bachofen V. Nitric oxide: a pathogenetic factor in autoimmunity. Immunol Today. 1992; 13: 157–160.

91. Perez T, Farre JM, Gossett P, Wallaert B, Duquesnoy B, Voisin C, Delcambre B, Tonnel AB. Subclinical alveolar inflammation in rheumatoid arthritis: superoxide anion, neutrophil chemotactic activity and fibronectin generation by alveolar macrophages. Eur Respir J. 1989; 2: 7–13.

92. Gosset P, Perez T, Lasalle P, Duquesnoy B, Farre JM, Tonnel AB, Capron A. Increased TNF-α secretion by alveolar macrophages from patients with rheumatoid arthritis. Am Rev Respir Dis. 1991; 143: 593–597.

93. Roodman DG, Johnson RA, Clibon U. Tumor necrosis factor alpha and the anaemia of chronic disease: effects of chronic exposure to TNF on erythropoiesis *in vivo*. Adv Exp Med Biol. 1989; 271: 185–196.

94. Bharadqaj M, Khanna N, Mathur A, Chaturvedi UC. Effect of macrophage-derived factor on hypoferraemia induced by Japanese encephalitis virus in mice. Clin Exp Immunol. 1991; 83: 215–218.

95. Horwitz DA, Steagall RV. The development of macrophages from large mononuclear cells in the blood of patients with inflammatory disease. J Clin Invest. 1972; 51: 760–768.

96. Horwitz DA, Allison AC, Ward P, Knight N. Identification of human mononuclear phagocyte populations by esterase staining. Clin Exp Immunol. 1977; 30: 289–298.

97. Hurst NP, Nuki G, Wallington T. Functional defects of monocyte C3b receptor-mediated phagocytosis in rheumatoid arthritis: evidence for an association with the appearance of a circulating population of non-specific esterase-negative mononuclear phagocytes. Ann Rheum Dis. 1983; 42: 487–493.

98. Buchan GS, Palmer DG, Gibbins BL. The response of human peripheral blood mononuclear phagocytes to rheumatoid arthritis. J Leuk Biol. 1985; 37: 221–230.

99. Katayama S, Chia D, Nasu H, Knutson DW. Increased Fc receptor activity in monocytes from patients with rheumatoid arthritis: a study of monocyte binding and catabolism of soluble aggregates of IgG *in vitro*. J Immunol. 1981; 127: 643–647.

100. Moller-Rasmussen J, Brandslund I, Rasmussen GG, Svehag S-E. Increased number of IgG Fc receptors in monocyte-enriched peripheral blood leucocytes from patients with rheumatoid arthritis. Scand J Immunol. 1982; 16: 279–285.

101. Carter SD, Bourne JT, Elson CJ, Hutton CW, Gzudek R, Dieppe PA. Mononuclear phagocytes in rheumatoid arthritis: Fc-receptor expression by peripheral blood monocytes. Ann Rheum Dis. 1984; 43: 424–429.

102. Mackinnon SK, Starkebaum G. Monocyte Fc receptor function in rheumatoid arthritis: enhanced cell binding of IgG induced by rheumatoid factors. Arthritis Rheum. 1987; 30: 498–506.

103. Heurkens AHM, Westedt ML, Breedveld FC, Jonges E, Cats A, Stijner TH, Daha MR. Uptake and degradation of soluble aggregates of IgG by monocytes of patients with rheumatoid arthritis: relation to disease activity. Ann Rheum Dis. 1991; 50: 284–289.

104. Shinohara S, Hirohata S, Inoue T, Ito K. Phenotypic analysis of peripheral blood monocytes isolated from patients with rheumatoid arthritis. J. Rheumatol. 1992; 19: 211–215.

105. Kirchheimer JC, Remold HG, Wanivenhaus A, Binder BR. Increased proteolytic activity on the surface of monocytes from patients with rheumatoid arthritis. Arthritis Rheum. 1991; 34: 1430–1433.

106. Shore A, Jaglal S, Keystone EC. Enhanced interleukin-1 generation by monocytes *in vitro* is temporally linked to an early event in the onset of exacerbation of rheumatoid arthritis. Clin Exp Immunol. 1986; 65: 293–302.

107. Goto M, Fujisawa M, Yamada Y, Okabe T, Takaku F, Sasano M, Mishioka K. Spontaneous release of angiotensin converting enzyme and interleukin-1β from peripheral blood monocytes from patients with rheumatoid arthritis under serum free conditions. Ann Rheum Dis. 1990; 49: 172–176.

108. Mackiewicz A, Sobieska M, Kapcinska M, Mackiewicz SH, Wiktorowicz KE, Pawlowski T. Different capabilities of monocytes from patients with systemic lupus erythematosus and rheumatoid arthritis to induce glycosylation alterations of acute phase proteins *in vitro*. Ann Rheum Dis. 1992; 51: 67–72.

109. Hayashida K, Ochi T, Fujimoto M, Owaki H, Shimaoka Y, Ono K, Matsumoto K. Bone marrow changes in adjuvant-induced and collagen-induced arthritis. Interleukin-1 and interleukin-6 activity and abnormal myelopoiesis. Arthritis Rheum. 1992; 35: 241–245.

110. Nepom GT, Erlich H. MHC class II molecules and autoimmunity. Ann Rev Immunol. 1991; 9: 493–525.
111. de Joy SQ, Ferguson KM, Sapp TM, Zabriskie JB, Oronsky AS, Kerwar SS. Streptococcal cell-wall arthritis: passive transfer of disease with a T cell line and cross reactivity of streptococcal cell wall antigens with *Mycobacterium tuberculosis*. J Exp Med. 1989; 170: 369–382.
112. Sigal LH, Steere A, Freeman DH, Dwyer JM. Proliferative responses of mononuclear cells in Lyme disease. Reactivity to *Borrelia burgdorferi* antigens is greater in joint fluid than in blood. Arthritis Rheum. 1986; 29: 761–769.
113. Cush JJ, Lipsky PE. Phenotypic analysis of synovial tissue and peripheral blood lymphocytes isolated from patients with rheumatoid arthritis. Arthritis Rheum. 1988; 31: 1230–1238.
114. Cush JJ, Lipsky PE. The cellular basis for rheumatoid inflammation. Clin Orthopaedics. 1991; 265: 9–22.
115. Pearson CM, Paulus HE, Machleder HI. The role of the lymphocyte and its products in the propagation of joint disease. Ann NY Acad Sci. 1975; 256: 150–168.
116. Tanay A, Field EH, Hoppe RT, Strober S. Long term follow-up of rheumatoid arthritis patients treated with total lymphoid irradiation. Arthritis Rheum. 1987; 30: 1–10.
117. Kingsley G, Panayi G, Lanchbury J. Immunotherapy of rheumatic diseases – practice and prospects. Immunol Today. 1991; 12: 177–179.
118. Beschin A, Brijs L, de Baetselier P, Cocito C. Mycobacterial proliferation in macrophages is prevented by incubation with lymphocytes activated *in vitro* with a mycobacterial antigen complex. Eur J Immunol. 1991; 21: 793–797.
119. Warren CJ, Howell WM, Bambhani M, Cawley MID, Smith JL. An investigation of T-cell subset phenotype and function in the rheumatoid synovium using *in situ* hybridization for IL-2 mRNA. Immunology. 1991; 72: 250–255.
120. Pitzalis C, Kingsley G, Lanchbury JSS, Murphy J, Panayi GS. Expression of HLA-DR, DQ and DP antigens and interleukin 2 receptor on synovial T lymphocyte subsets in rheumatoid arthritis: evidence for 'frustrated' activation. J Rheumatol. 1987; 114: 662–666.
121. Howell M, Smith J, Cawley M. The rheumatoid synovium: a model for T cell anergy? Immunol Today. 1992; 13: 191.
122. Stransky G, Gay RE, Trabant A, Aicher WK, Barnum S, Gay S. Oncogenes and retroviruses in rheumatoid arthritis. In: Smolen JS, Kalden JR, Maini RN, eds. Rheumatoid arthritis, recent research advances. Berlin: Springer Verlag; 1992.
123. Smiley JD, Sachs C, Ziff M. *In vitro* synthesis of immunoglobulins by rheumatoid synovial membrane. J Clin Invest. 1968; 47: 624–632.
124. Carpenter AB, Huczko E, Eisenbeis CH, Kelly RH. Evidence for locally synthesized and clonally restricted immunoglobulin in the synovial fluid from rheumatoid arthritis patients. Clin Chim Acta. 1990; 193: 1–12.
125. Wernick RM, Lipsky PE, Marban-Arcos E, Maliakkal JJ, Edelbaum D, Ziff M. IgG and IgM rheumatoid factor synthesis in rheumatoid synovial membrane cell cultures. Arthritis Rheum. 1985; 28: 742–752.
126. Tarkowski A, Klareskog L, Carlsten H, Herberts P, Koopman WJ. Secretion of antibodies to types I and II collagen by synovial tissue cells in patients with rheumatoid arthritis. Arthritis Rheum. 1989; 32: 1087–1091.
127. Jasin HE. Autoantibody specificities of immune complexes sequestered in articular cartilage of patients with rheumatoid arthritis. Arthritis Rheum. 1985; 28: 241–248.
128. Mosley G, Ruddy S. Elevated C3 anaphylotoxin levels in synovial fluids from patients with rheumatoid arthritis. Arthritis Rheum. 1985; 28: 1089–1095.
129. Bourke BE, Moss IK, Mumford PA, Horsfall AC, Maini RN. The complement fixing ability of putative circulating complexes in rheumatoid arthritis and its relationship to extra-articular disease. Clin Exp Immunol. 1982; 48: 726–732.
130. Mageed RA, Kirwan JR, Thompson PW, McCarthy DA, Holborow EJ. Characterisation of the size and composition of circulating immune complexes in patients with rheumatoid arthritis. Ann Rheum Dis. 1991; 50: 231–236.
131. Hay FC, Jones MG, Bond A, Soltys AJ. Rheumatoid factors and complex formation. The role of light-chain framework sequences and glycosylation. Clin Orthopaedics. 1991; 265: 54–61.

132. Melsom RD, Smith PR, Maini RN. Demonstration of an unidentified 48 kD polypeptide in circulating immune complexes in rheumatoid arthritis. Ann Rheum Dis. 1987; 46: 104–109.
133. McCormick JN, Wojtacha D, Edmond E. Detection of cytomegalovirus antigens in phagocytosed serum complexes from a patient with rheumatoid arthritis, vasculitis, peripheral neuropathy, cutaneous ulceration and digital gangrene. Ann Rheum Dis. 1992; 51: 553–555.
134. Katona IM, Ohura K, Allen JB, Wahl LM, Chenoweth DE, Wahl SM. Modulation of monocyte chemotactic function in inflammatory lesions. Role of inflammatory mediators. J Immunol. 1991; 146: 708–714.
135. Malaise MG, Franchimont P, Gomez F, Bouillene C, Mahieu PR. The spontaneous ability of human IgG to inhibit the Fc receptors of normal human monocytes is related to their binding capacity to lectins. Clin Immunol Immunopathol. 1987; 45: 1–16.
136. Vissens MCM, Fantone JC, Wiggins R, Kunkel SL. Glomerular basement membrane-containing immune complexes stimulate tumor necrosis factor and interleukin-1 production by human monocytes. Am J Pathol. 1989; 134: 1–6.
137. Chantry D, Winearls CG, Maini RN, Feldman M. Mechanism of immune complex-mediated damage: induction of interleukin-1 by immune complexes and synergy with interferon gamma and tumour necrosis factor-alpha. Eur J Immunol. 1989; 19: 189–192.
138. Nardella FA, Dayer J-M, Roelke M, Krane SM, Mannik M. Self-associating IgG rheumatoid factors stimulate monocytes to release prostaglandins and mononuclear cell factor that stimulates collagenase and prostaglandin production by synovial cells. Rheumatol Int. 1983; 3: 183–186.
139. Goodman MG, Chenoweth DE, Weigle WO. Induction of interleukin-1 secretion and enhancement of humoral immunity by binding of human C5a to macrophage surface C5a receptors. J Exp Med. 1982; 156: 912–917.
140. Haeffner-Cavaillon N, Cavaillon J-M, Lande M, Cazatchkine MD. C3a (C34a des Arg) induces production and release of interleukin 1 by cultured human monocytes. J Immunol. 1987; 139: 794–799.
141. Okusawa S, Dinarello CA, Yancey KB, Endres S, Lawley TJ, Frank MM, Burke JF, Gelfand JA. C5a induction of human interleukin-1. J Immunol. 1987; 139: 2635–2640.
142. Seki N, Sudo Y, Yoshioka T, Sugihara S, Fujitsu T, Sakuma S, Ogawa T, Hamaoka T, Senoh H, Fujiwara H. Type II collagen-induced immune arthritis. I. Induction and perpetuation of arthritis require synergy between humoral and cell-mediated immunity. J Immunol. 1988; 140: 1477–1484.
143. Lynn WA, Galenbock DT. Lipopolysaccharide antagonists. Immunol Today. 1992; 13: 271–276.
144. Utsugi T, Nii A, Tan D, Pak CC, Denkins Y, van Hoogevest P, Fidler IJ. Comparative efficacy of liposomes containing synthetic bacterial cell wall analogues for tumoricidal activation of monocytes and macrophages. Cancer Immunol Immunother. 1991; 33: 285–292.
145. Furukawa M, Ohtsubo Y, Sugimoto M, Katoh Y, Dohi Y. Induction of tumoricidal activated macrophages by a liposome-encapsulated glycolipid, trehalose 2,3,6'-trimycolate from Gordana aurantiaca. FEMS Microbiol Immunol. 1990; 2: 83–88.
146. Keller R, Gehri R, Keist R, Huf E, Kayser FH. The interaction of macrophages and bacteria: a comparative study of the induction of tumoricidal activity and reactive nitrogen intermediates. Cell Immunol. 1991; 134: 249–256.
147. Grossman D, Cooke G, Sparrow JT, Mollick JA, Rich RR. Dissociation of the stimulatory activities of staphylococcal enterotoxins for T cells and monocytes. J Exp Med. 1991; 172: 1831–1841.
148. Yu SF, Koerner TJ, Adams DO. Gene regulation in macrophage activation: differential regulation of genes encoding for tumor necrosis factor, interleukin-1, JE and KC by interferon gamma and lipopolysaccharides. J Leuk Biol. 1990; 48: 412–419.
149. Takema M, Oka S, Uno K, Nakamura S, Arita H, Tawara K, Inaba K, Muramatsu S. Macrophage-activating factor extracted from mycoplasmas. Cancer Immunol Immunother. 1991; 33: 39–44.
150. Solbach W, Moll H, Rollinghoff M. Lymphocytes play the music but the macrophage calls the tune. Immunol Today. 1991; 12: 4–6.

151. Wilder RL, Crofford LJ. Do infectious agents cause rheumatoid arthritis. Clin Orthopaedics. 1991; 265: 36–41.
152. Wooley PH. Animal models of arthritis. Curr Opin Rheumatol. 1991; 3: 407–420.
153. Brahn E. Animal models of rheumatoid arthritis. Clues to etiology and treatment. Clin Orthopaedics. 1991; 265: 42–53.
154. Williams RO, Plater-Zyberk C, Williams DG, Maini RN. Successful transfer of collagen-induced arthritis to severe combined immunodeficient (SCID) mice. Clin Exp Immunol. 1992; 88: 455–460.
155. Allen JB, Malone DG, Wahl SM, Calandra GB, Wilder RL. The role of the thymus in streptococcal cell wall-induced arthritis and hepatic granuloma formation. Comparative studies of pathology and cell wall distribution in athymic and euthymic rats. J Clin Invest. 1985; 76: 1042–1056.
156. Salz-Florens X, Jafari HS, Olsen KD, Narinchi H, Hansen EJ, McCracken GH. Induction of suppurative arthritis in rabbits by Haemophilus endotoxin, tumor necrosis factor-alpha and interleukin-1 beta. J Infect Dis. 1991; 163: 1267–1272.
157. Schaible UE, Kramer MD, Museteanu C, Zimmer G, Mossman H, Simon MM. The severe combined immunodeficiency (SCID) mouse. A laboratory model for analysis of Lyme arthritis and carditis. J Exp Med. 1989; 170: 1427–1432.
158. Simon MM, Schaible UE, Wallech R, Kramer MD. A mouse model for *Borrelia burgdorferi* infection: approach to a vaccine against Lyme disease. Immunol Today. 1991; 12: 11–16.
159. Abd AH, Savage NW, Halliday WJ, Hume DA. The role of macrophages in experimental arthritis induced by *Streptococcus agalactiae* sonicate: actions of macrophage colony-stimulating factor (CSF-1) and other macrophage modulating agents. Lymphokine Cytokine Res. 1991; 10: 43–50.
160. Keat A, Thomas B, Dixey J, Osborn M, Sonnex C, Taylor-Robinson D. *Chlamydia trachomatis* and reactive arthritis: the missing link. Lancet. 1987; 1: 72–74.
161. Wong ML, Poole ES, Williams G, Highton J. A prospective and retrospective study of *Chlamydia trachomatis* in affected tissues of patients with reactive arthritis using a specific monoclonal antibody. Proc Univ Otago Med Sch. 1989; 64: 77–78.
162. Ishikawa H, Ohno O, Yamasaki K, Ikuta S, Hirohata K. Arthritis presumably caused by chlamydia in Reiter's syndrome. J Bone Jt Surg (Am). 1986; 68: 777–779.
163. Schumacher HR, Magge S, Cherian PV, Sleckman J, Rothfuss S, Clayburne G, Sieck M. Light and electron microscope studies on the synovial membranes in Reiter's syndrome. Arthritis Rheum. 1988; 31: 937–946.
164. Wordsworth BP, Hughes RA, Allan I, Keat A, Bell JI. Chlamydial DNA is absent from the joints of patients with sexually acquired reactive arthritis. Br J Rheumatol. 1990; 29: 208–210.
165. Poole ES, Highton J, Wilkins RJ, Lamont IL. A search for *Chlamydia trachomatis* in synovial fluids from patients with reactive arthritis using the polymerase chain reaction and antigen detection methods. Br J Rheumatol. 1992; 31: 31–34.
166. Rahman MU, Cheema MA, Schumacher HR, Hudson AP. Molecular evidence for the presence of Chlamydia in the synovium of patients with Reiter's syndrome. Arthritis Rheum. 1992; 35: 521–529.
167. Granfors K, Jalkanen S, von Essen R, Lahesmaa-Rantala R, Isomaki O, Pekkola-Heino K, Merilahti-Palo R, Saano R, Isomaki H, Toivanen A. Yersinia antigens in synovial fluid cells from patients with reactive arthritis. N Engl J Med. 1989; 320: 216–222.
168. Merilahti-Palo R, Soderstrom K-O, Lahesmaa-Rantala R, Granfors K, Toivanen A. Bacterial antigens in synovial biopsy specimens in *Yersinia* triggered reactive arthritis. Ann Rheum Dis. 1991; 50: 87–90.
169. Viitanen A-M, Arstila TP, Lahesmaa R, Granfors K, Skurnik M, Toivanen P. Application of the polymerase chain reaction and immunofluorescence techniques to the detection of bacteria in *Yersinia*-triggered reactive arthritis. Arthritis Rheum. 1991; 34: 89–96.
170. Granfors K, Jalkanen S, Tendberg AA, Maki-Isola O, von Essen R, Lahesmaa-Rantala R, Isomaki H, Saario R, Arnold WJ, Toivanen A. Salmonella lipopolysaccharide in synovial cells from patients with reactive arthritis. Lancet. 1990; 335: 685–688.
171. Salih A, Aucken H, Pitt T, Hughes R, Hyder E, Keat A. Detection of bacterial lipopolysaccharide in synovial fluid using an amplified ELISA assay. Br J Rheumatol. 1992; 31 (suppl 1): 2 (abstract).

172. Wuorela M, Jalkanen S, Toivanen P, Granfors K. Intracellular pathogens and professional phagocytes in reactive arthritis. Pathobiology. 1991; 59: 162–165.
173. Hough AJ, Rank RG. Induction of arthritis in C57Bl/6 mice by chlamydial antigen. Effect of prior immunisation or infection. Am J Pathol. 1988; 130: 163–172.
174. Hough AJ, Rank RG. Pathogenesis of acute arthritis due to viable *Chlamydia trachomatis* (mouse pneumonitis agent) in C57Bl/6 mice. Am J Pathol. 1989; 134: 903–912.
175. Keat AC, Knight SC. Do synovial fluid cells indicate the cause of reactive arthritis? J Rheumatol. 1990; 17: 1257–1259.
176. Hassell AB, Pilling D, Reynolds D, Fife PF, Bacon PA, Gaston JSH. MHC restriction of synovial fluid lymphocyte responses to the triggering organism in reactive arthritis. Absence of a Class I-restricted response. Clin Exp Immunol. 1992; 88: 442–447.
177. Severijnen AJ, van Kleef R, Hayenberg MP, van de Merwe JP. Cell wall fragments from major residents of the human intestinal flora induce chronic arthritis in rats. J Rheumatol. 1989; 16: 1061–1068.
178. Phillips PE. How do bacteria cause chronic arthritis. J Rheumatol. 1989; 16: 1017–1019.
179. Ebringer A. Rheumatoid arthritis as an infectious disease. Br Med J. 1991; 303: 524 (letter).
180. Rook GAW, Stanford JL. Slow bacterial infection or autoimmunity? Immunol Today. 1992; 13: 160–164.
181. Crick FD, Gatenby PA. Limiting dilution analysis of T cell reactivity to mycobacterial antigens in peripheral blood and synovium from rheumatoid arthritis patients. Clin Exp Immunol. 1992; 88: 424–429.
182. Harris ED. Rheumatoid arthritis. Pathophysiology and implications for therapy. N Engl J Med. 1990; 322: 1277–1289.
183. McFarlin DE. Non-AIDS retroviral infections in humans. Ann Rev Med. 1991; 42: 97–105.
184. Iwakura Y, Tosu M, Yoshida E, Takiguchi M, Sato K, Kitajima I, Nishioka K, Yamamoto K, Takeda T, Hatanaka M. Yamamoto H, Sekiguchi T. Induction of inflammatory arthropathy resembling rheumatoid arthritis in mice transgenic for HTLV-1. Science. 1991; 253: 1026–1028.
185. Sato K, Ikuro M, Maruyama Y, Kitajima I, Nakajima Y, Higaki M, Yamamoto K, Miyasaka N, Osame M, Nishioka K. Arthritis in patients infected with human T lymphotropic virus type I. Clinical and immunopathologic features. Arthritis Rheum. 1991; 34: 714–721.
186. Ziegler B, Gay RE, Huang GQ, Fassbender HG, Gay S. Immunohistochemical localization of HTLV-1 p19 and p24-related antigens in synovial joints of patients with rheumatoid arthritis. Am J Pathol. 1989; 135: 1–5.
187. Kalden JR, Winkler T, Krapf F. Are retroviruses involved in the aetiology of rheumatic diseases. Br J Rheumatol. 1991; 30 (suppl 1): 63–69.
188. Calabrese LH, Kelley DM, Myers A, O'Connell M, Easley K. Rheumatic symptoms and human immunodeficiency virus infection. The influence of clinical and laboratory variables in a longitudinal cohort study. Arthritis Rheum. 1991; 34: 257–263.
189. Crawford TB, Adams DS, Cheevers WP, Cork LC. Chronic arthritis in goats caused by a retrovirus. Science. 1980; 207: 997–999.
190. Koenig S, Gendelman HE, Orenstein JM, Dal Canto MC, Pezeshkpour GH, Yungbluth M, Janotta F, Aksamit A, Martin MA, Fauci AS. Detection of AIDS virus in macrophages in brain tissue from AIDS patients with encephalopathy. Science. 1986; 233: 1089–1093.
191. Rosenberg ZF, Fauci AS. Immunopathogenesis of HIV infection. FASEB J. 1991; 5: 2382–2390.
192. Gendelman HE, Narayan O, Kennedy-Stoskopf S, Kennedy PG, Ghotbi Z, Clements JE, Stanley J, Pezeshkpour G. Tropism of sheep lentiviruses for monocytes: susceptibility to infection and virus gene expression increases during maturation of monocytes to macrophages. J Virol. 1986; 58: 67–74.
193. Gorrell MD, Brandon MR, Sheffer D, Adams RJ, Narayan O. Ovine lentivurs is macrophage tropic and does not replicate productively in lymphocytes-T. J Virol. 1992; 66: 2679–2688.
194. Crawford TB, Adams DS, Sande RD, Gorham JR, Henson JB. The connective tissue component of the caprine arthritis-encephalitis syndrome. Am J Pathol. 1980; 100: 443–454.

195. Adams DS, Crawford TB, Klevjer-Anderson P. A pathogenetic study of the early connective tissue lesions of viral caprine arthritis-encephalitis. Am J Pathol. 1980; 99: 257–278.
196. Harkiss GD, Watt NJ, King TJ, Williams J, Hopkins J. Retroviral arthritis: phenotypic analysis of cells in the synovial fluid of sheep with inflammatory synovitis associated with Visna virus infection. Clin Immunol Immunopathol. 1991; 60: 106–117.
197. Thormar A. An electron microscope study of tissue cultures infected with Visna virus. Virology. 1961; 14: 463–475.
198. Palmer DG. Polykaryocytes and rheumatoid disease. J Roy Coll Physns Lond. 1971; 6: 33–40.
199. Palmer DG. Dispersed cell cultures of rheumatoid synovial membrane. Acta Rheum Scand. 1970; 16: 261–270.
200. MacKay JMK, Panayi G, Neill WA, Robinson NA, Smith W, Marmion BP, Duthie JJR. Cytology of rheumatoid synovial cells in culture. I. Composition and sequence of cell populations in cultures of rheumatoid synovial fluid. Ann Rheum Dis. 1974; 33: 225–233.
201. Clarris BJ, Fraser JRE, Moran CJ, Muirden KD. Rheumatoid synovial cells from intact joints. Ann Rheum Dis. 1977; 36: 293–301.
202. Highton TC, Palmer DG. Electron-microscopic appearances of cultured rheumatoid synovial cells. Proc Univ Otago Med Sch. 1971; 49: 46–47.
203. Panayi GS, MacKay JMK, Neill WA, McCormick JN, Marmion BP, Duthie JJR. Cytology of rheumatoid synovial cells in culture. II. Association of polykaryocytes with rheumatoid and other forms of arthritis. Ann Rheum Dis. 1974; 33: 234–239.
204. Krieg AM, Gourley MF, Perl A. Endogenous retroviruses: potential etiologic agents in autoimmunity. FASEB J. 1992; 6: 2537–2544.
205. Rubin LA, Siminovitch KA, Shi MH, Cohen M. A novel retroviral gene associated with rheumatoid arthritis. Arthritis Rheum. 1991; 34 (suppl): p S60, abstract 168.
206. Dinarello CA. Interleukin-1 and interleukin-1 antagonism. Blood. 1991; 77: 1627–1652.
207. Granowitz EV, Clark BD, Manciela J, Dinarello CA. Interleukin-1 receptor antagonist competitively inhibits the binding of interleukin-1 to the type II interleukin-1 receptor. J Biol Chem. 1991; 266: 14147–14150.
208. Arend WP, Coll BP. Interaction of recombinant monocyte-derived interleukin 1 receptor antagonist with rheumatoid synovial cells. Cytokine. 1991; 3: 407–413.
209. Dayer JM. Chronic inflammatory joint diseases: natural inhibitors of interleukin 1 and tumor necrosis factor alpha. J Rheumatol. 1991; 27 (suppl): 71–75.
210. Dinarello CA, Thompson RC. Blocking IL-1: interleukin 1 receptor antagonist *in vivo* and *in vitro*. Immunol Today. 1991; 12: 404–410.
211. Henderson B, Thompson RC, Hardingham T, Lewthwaite J. Inhibition of interleukin-1 induced synovitis and articular cartilage proteoglycan loss in the rabbit knee by recombinant interleukin-1 receptor antagonist. Cytokine. 1991; 3: 246–249.
212. Smith RJ, Chin JE, Sam LM, Justen JM. Biologic effects of an interleukin-1 receptor antagonist protein on interleukin-1 stimulated cartilage erosion and chondrocyte responsiveness. Arthritis Rheum. 1991; 34: 78–83.
213. Otterness IG, Bliven ML, Downs JT, Natoli EJ, Hanson DC. Inhibition of interleukin 1 synthesis by tenidap: a new drug for arthritis. Cytokine. 1991; 3: 277–283.
214. Sampaio EP, Sarno EN, Galilly R, Cohn ZA, Kaplan G. Thalidomide selectively inhibits tumor necrosis factor α production by stimulated human monocytes. J Exp Med. 1991; 173: 699–703.
215. Nathan C. Mechanisms and modulation of macrophage activation. Behring Inst Mitt. 1991; 88: 200–207.
216. Hand AR, Ohura K, Ellingsworth L, Wahl SM. Rapid onset synovial inflammation and hyperplasia induced by transforming growth factor *β*. J Exp Med. 1990; 171: 231–247.
217. Brandes ME, Allen JB, Ogawa Y, Wahl SM. Transforming growth factor beta 1 suppresses acute and chronic arthritis in experimental animals. J Clin Invest. 1991; 87: 1108–1113.
218. Wahl SM, Allen JB, Brandes ME. Cytokine modulation of bacterial cell wall-induced arthritis. Agents Actions. 1991; suppl 35: 29–34.
219. Kuruvilla AP, Shah R, Hochwald GM, Liggitt HD, Palladino MA, Thorbecke GJ. Protective effect of transforming growth factor beta 1 on experimental autoimmune diseases in mice. Proc Natl Acad Sci USA. 1991; 88: 2918–2921.
220. Nakanishi M, Yagawa K, Aida Y, Hayashi S, Ichinose Y, Yoshida M. The *in vivo* and *in*

vitro use of monoclonal antibody for the deletion of phagocytic cells in guinea pigs. Hybridoma. 1990; 9: 443–451.
221. Doebber TW, Wu MS, Bugianesi RL, Ponpipom MM, Furbish FS, Barranger JA, Brady RO, Shen TY. Enhanced macrophage uptake of synthetically glycosylated human placental β-glucocerebrosidase. J Biol Chem. 1982; 257: 2193–2199.
222. Barton NW, Brady RO, Dambrosia JM, Di Bisceglie AM, Doppelt SH, Hill SC, Mankin HJ, Murray GJ, Parker RI, Argoff CE, Grewal RP, Yu K-T. Replacement therapy for inherited enzyme deficiency – macrophage-targeted glucocerebrosidase for Gaucher's disease. N Engl J Med. 1991; 324: 1464–1470.

4
The HLA Association with Rheumatoid Arthritis

J. S. LANCHBURY

INTRODUCTION

Enormous efforts have been devoted to investigating HLA associations with a large number of diseases, many of which have an autoimmune basis or component. Rheumatoid arthritis (RA), in particular, has received considerable attention. Few people would now dispute the role of inherited factors in the development of rheumatoid arthritis although it has been estimated that the overall genetic contribution may be only in the order of 30%. Of this probably only one-third to a half is accounted for by genes in the HLA region. Despite this the HLA component is the best understood. This chapter will concentrate on recent developments in molecular biology and immunology which have provided a framework for understanding the role of MHC (major histocompatibility complex) in the development of RA.

MHC ORGANIZATION AND POLYMORPHISM IN MAN

The human MHC maps to the short arm of chromosome 6 in the region designated 6p21.3 which represents the most intensively studied area of the human genome. This region occupies approximately 4 megabases of DNA and contains more than 70 genes including HLA[1]. The pace of investigation means that new genes are added to the map almost on a weekly basis. Previously the MHC has been operationally divided into the class I, class II and class III regions which encode the classical transplantation antigens, the immune response gene products and a diverse grouping of genes including several complement components, respectively. The location of genes of similar function to particular areas of the MHC is probably a legacy of gene duplication during evolution. This distinction, although still useful, is breaking down as more genes with novel functions are described such as the peptide transporter and proteosome genes which map to the HLA class II region but are apparently involved in delivering peptides to HLA class I molecules[2].

Immunological interest in the MHC stems from its role in controlling the specificity of immune responses to protein antigens. Many HLA class I and class II genes and their products are highly polymorphic with loci such as HLA-DRβ1 associated with over 50 alleles. The extent of polymorphism has proved useful in uncovering relationships between specific alleles and predisposition to disease but this process is hampered by the phenomenon of linkage disequilibrium. That is the existence at the population level of particular combinations of alleles which tend to be inherited as blocks called haplotypes. This often leads to difficulties in identifying the precise locus of susceptibility within a linkage group of positively associated alleles. One solution is to examine these disease associations in a variety of ethnic groups where the haplotypes carrying susceptible alleles may be distinct.

EARLY STUDIES IN RA

Improvements in tissue typing technology often stimulated by a desire to improve matching for organ grafts have been beneficial in exploring the HLA association with RA. Positive associations of both HLA class I and class II alleles with RA have been reported. HLA class I associations have been defined serologically and it likely that the majority such as B44, B60 and Bw62 are accounted for by linkage disequilibrium to HLA-DR4. Analysis of polymorphism encoded by the HLA class II region in RA was first stimulated by the description of association between RA and a mixed leucocyte specificity (MLC) later named Dw4[3]. This functionally detected sharing of an HLA-D region polymorphism was closely followed by the use of alloantisera to detect a B cell antigen, HLA-DR4, which represented a broader specificity and was more strongly associated with the disease[4,5]. These findings have been confirmed in numerous studies and provided the springboard for the molecular studies.

MOLECULAR POLYMORPHISM OF HLA-DR4

The relationship between Dw and DR specificities has been of key interest. The serological specificity HLA-DR4 was present on cells which were positive for a range of MLC types which were designated Dw4, Dw10, Dw13, Dw14, Dw15 and DwKT2. It was unclear whether each of these represented a subtype of DR4 itself or the effect of a single DR4 entity plus other polymorphic HLA-D region components in linkage disequilibrium with DR4. The elucidation of this relationship has been achieved by biochemical studies of HLA-DR and DQ molecules immunoprecipitated with specific monoclonal antibodies and by nucleotide sequencing of cDNAs. HLA class II antigens are α–β heterodimers with DR products distinguished from DQ and DP by virtue of the non-polymorphic DR α chain. Allelic variability between these molecules locates mainly to the first protein domain. Polymorphism among DR4 Dw subtypes maps to the HLA-DRβ1 chain and in particular to positions 37, 57, 70–74 and 86. The stretch of amino acids between positions 70 and 74 is part of an arbitrary defined area which has been termed the third hypervariable region (HVR3). Each MLC variant is associated with a unique DR4β1 primary sequence[6,7]. A total of 11 DR4 primary sequences have been officially confirmed so far.

HLA-DR4, DR1 AND RA

The elucidation of the molecular basis of DR4 subtype polymorphism has had important consequences for our understanding of the nature of the HLA association with RA. In particular, two important points have been addressed. The first is the observation that although the DR4 association was widespread in a variety of ethnic groups, a number of populations demonstrated either much weaker associations or no association at all. Thus surveys of Greeks, Yakima Indians and Israeli Jews failed to record significant increases in DR4 frequency. Interestingly, some populations such as Asian Indians and Israeli Jews showed stronger DR1 associations but these findings were variable (reviewed in [8]). Analysis of north European derived populations also showed that often a secondary increase in HLA-DR1 was masked by a stronger DR4 association. Related to this was the problem of the incomplete association of HLA-DR4 with RA in a particular population. Typically in northern Europe 70% of hospital-ascertained RA patients are positive for DR4 versus 30% of healthy controls. Was the DR4 the same in both cases and how did HLA influence the 30% of RA patients who are DR4 negative?

In 1987 the struggle to answer these points was taken up by Gregersen and colleagues who pointed out that DR1 and certain DR4β1 variants shared a region of sequence homology in their third hypervariable regions (see Table 1)[9]. In particular it was suggested that the basic unit of association with RA was a stretch of five amino acids (QRRAA between positions 70 and 74) shared between DR1, Dw14 and Dw15 with the latter two alleles implicated in MLC studies in Caucasoids and Orientals, respectively. The other major RA associated allele, DR4 Dw4, carried the related sequence QKRAA at a similar position. Gregersen also pointed out that in the Israeli Jewish population the DR4 Dw10 variant was particularly common. Since the Dw10 HVR3 carried non-conservative amino acid substitutions compared to Dw4 and Dw14, it was suggested that these polymorphisms might render Dw10 a non-susceptibility allele for RA and thus account for the lack of DR4 association in Jewish populations. Furthermore, the association with RA could not be accounted for in a similar fashion by polymorphism of linked HLA-DQβ. The second component of the hypothesis was that the shared third hypervariable region motifs could act as immunologically functional 'epitopes' and predispose to RA via triggering of an as yet undefined T cell response.

Table 1 Summary of HLA-DRβ1 allelic associations with rheumatoid arthritis together with third hypervariable region pentapeptide sequences. Official WHO nomenclature is given for each allele, e.g. HLA-DRβ1*0401 refers to the HLA-DRβ1 allele associated with the Dw4 HLA-D specificity

Serological specificity	Allele HLA-DRβ1*	Previous equivalent	HVR3 (70–74) pentapeptide[a]	Association with RA
DR4	0401	Dw4	QKRAA	Positive
DR4	0404	Dw14.1	QRRAA	Positive
DR4	0405	Dw15	QRRAA	Positive
DR4	0408	Dw14.2	QRRAA	Positive
DR1	0101	Dw1	QRRAA	Positive
DRw14	1402	Dw16	QRRAA	Positive
DRw10	1001	–	RRRAA	Positive
DR4	0402	Dw10	DERAA	Negative
DR4	0403	Dw13.1	QRRAE	Negative
DR4	0407	Dw13.2	QRRAE	Negative
DR2(w15)	1501	Dw2	DRRAA	Negative
DR5(w11)	1101	Dw5	DRRAA	Negative
DR4	0406	DwKT2	QRRAE	Unknown[b]
DR4	0409	–	QKRAA	Unknown

[a]Amino acid sequences are given in single letter code. Underlining indicates a non-conservative substitution compared to the QRRAA template
[b]Indicates insufficient population data exist to estimate RA association

HLA-DRβ1 SEQUENCES AND RA

It has taken several years to test this hypothesis in its simplest form. Evidence for the importance of these HVR3 sequences has been based on the direct examination of HLA-DRβ1 sequences in large groups of RA patients and controls from a number of independent centres. This has been achieved by the use of oligonucleotide probes capable of distinguishing single base changes hybridized either to polymerase chain reaction (PCR) amplified DRβ1 second exons or to restriction digested genomic DNA[10,11]. A number of groups have sequenced DRβ1 alleles from RA patients and found them to be identical to the equivalent allele from normals. The differences between RA and control populations lie in frequency differences of naturally occurring variants rather than the presence of disease specific alleles. RA is associated with the Dw4 (0401), Dw14.1 and 14.2 (0404 and 0408) and Dw15 (0405) subtypes of DR4 while the closely related DR4 subtypes Dw10 (0402) and Dw13.1 and 13.2 (0403 and 0407) do not confer enhanced risk[12–15]. Of the non-DR4 alleles, DR1 (0101), DRw10 (1001) and DRw14 Dw16 (1402) are associated with RA. Four digit numbers refer to the WHO official nomenclature for HLA alleles. The DR1 and DRw14 Dw16 alleles share the QRRAA third hypervariable region motif with Dw14 and Dw15. DRw10 carries a third related sequence RRRAA in its HVR3. Several other alleles including DR2(w15) and DR5(w11) have been consistently shown to be negatively associated with RA and may confer protection against development of RA. Again, these alleles contain radical substitutions in HVR3 compared to the QRRAA template. These data are summarized in Table 1. Although several alleles confer enhanced risk for development of RA, they are by no means equivalent with important differences between ethnic groups and between subsets of patients. In northern Europe Dw4 is the most strongly associated allele[12] whereas in Japanese, Jewish and Greek populations where Dw4 is relatively uncommon, Dw15 is the most common DR4 subtype among RA patients[14,16,17]. Interestingly, although rare in north European controls, this allele was found in 5% of UK RA patients. Significant association of a particular susceptibility allele in an RA population appears to be related to the frequency of that allele in the gene pool.

HLA CLASS II STRUCTURE AND RA

Recently it has been possible to begin to place these correlates of genetic predisposition to RA in an immunological context. HLA class I and class II molecules function by presenting short peptides to the T cell receptors of effector T lymphocytes. In the case of class I molecules the peptides appear to be 8 or 9 amino acids long and derived from proteins synthesized by the cell's own apparatus. In contrast, class II molecules present peptides of 13–17 amino acids in length which may be derived from the cell's interior or exterior. The nature of the interaction of HLA class I molecules and peptides has been revealed by X-ray crystallography which shows that the majority of polymorphic residues are clustered around the floor and sides of a peptide binding groove[18]. Homology between HLA class I and class II enabled construction of a putative class II three-dimensional model in which a deep peptide binding groove is the main feature[19]. If the RA associated HVR3 sequences are positioned on this model, the 70–74 region occupies one part of one of the two α helical regions which form the sides of the peptide binding cleft. As far as the model goes it suggests that the majority of differences between RA associated and non-associated HLA-DRβ alleles occur at positions where the amino acid side chains should make contact with peptide. Dw10 and Dw13, the two DR4 alleles not positively associated with RA, carry substitutions at positions 70 and 71 (Dw10) and 74 (Dw13). These observations are consistent with the possibility that the RA associated HLA alleles selectively interact with a peptide or group of peptides which play a role in predisposition to RA. The substitutions in non-susceptibility alleles such as Dw10 and Dw13 may be sufficient to abrogate an arthritogenic peptide interaction. One caveat is that amino acid position 71 may represent a peptide or T cell receptor contact. Substitutions at this point might therefore affect RA predisposition via a direct effect on the T cell repertoire.

FUTURE CONSIDERATIONS

Considerable genetic epidemiological evidence exists for the importance of the QRRAA, QKRAA and RRRAA motifs in predisposition to RA. However, a number of questions remain to be answered. First is the reason for the enhanced role of the Dw4 variant in predisposition to RA in a number of populations. This is particularly evident in the subset of RA with Felty's syndrome, 90% of whom are positive for the Dw4 allele which may hinge upon a distinct role for the lysine residue at position 71 of the HLA-DRβ1 chain[20]. There is a need for further investigation of the relationship between class II allelic sequences and disease subsets, severity of RA and clinical parameters and a role for other linked genes should not be dismissed. It is clearly crucial to establish the mechanism by which HLA class II molecules influence the pathogenesis of RA and to investigate whether the three motifs exert their effects in similar ways. Recent data suggest that certain of the RA associated alleles act exclusively within particular HLA class II genotypes, especially when the arthritis has progressed to a severe or complicated form[20,21]. Thus maximum risk for DR1 and Dw14 (both 0404 and 0408) alleles is observed when the alleles are in combination with Dw4 suggesting that some form of complementation is taking place. The mechanism by which this might be effected is obscure but may involve two distinct HLA-DR mediated events which could be simultaneous or temporally distinct. Subtleties of peptide binding and T cell receptor repertoire selection are attractive candidates.

From the above it is obvious that although we have gone some way towards simplifying the HLA association with RA, fresh levels of complexity can be found in the details of association. It may be that these genetic studies prove to be of most use by providing a rationale for the design of novel HLA-DR allele or motif-specific blocking peptides for use in therapy, rather than directly exposing the mechanisms involved. Such an approach will require that the HLA molecule is still active in disease predisposition and clinical improvement will be the ultimate test of HLA susceptibility locus assignment.

References

1. Trowsdale J, Campbell RD. Complexity in the major histocompatibility complex. Eur J Immunogenetics. 1992; 19: 45.
2. Trowsdale J, Hanson I, Mockridge I, Beck S, Townsend A, Kelly A. Sequences encoded in the class II region of the MHC related to the 'ABC' superfamily of transporters. Nature. 1990; 348: 741.
3. Stastny P. Mixed lymphocyte culture typing cells from patients with rheumatoid arthritis. Tissue Antigens. 1974; 4: 572.
4. Panayi GS, Wooley P, Batchelor JR. Genetic basis of rheumatoid disease: HLA antigens, disease manifestations, and toxic reactions to drugs. Br Med J. 1978; 2: 1326.
5. Stastny P. Association of the B-cell alloantigen DRw4 with rheumatoid arthritis. N Engl J Med. 1978; 298: 869.
6. Cairns JS, Curtsinger JM, Dahl CA, Freeman S, Alter BJ, Bach FH. Sequence polymorphism of HLA DRβ1 alleles relating to T-cell-recognised determinants. Nature. 1985; 317: 166.
7. Gregersen PK, Shen M, Song Q-L, Merryman P, Degar S, Seki T, Maccari J, Goldberg D, Murphy H, Schwenzer J, Wang CY, Winchester RJ, Nepom GT, Silver J. Molecular diversity of HLA-DR4 haplotypes. Proc Natl Acad Sci USA. 1986; 83: 2642.
8. Woodrow JC. Analysis of the HLA association with rheumatoid arthritis. Dis Markers. 1986; 4: 7.
9. Gregersen PK, Silver J, Winchester RJ. The shared epitope hypothesis. An approach to understanding the molecular genetics of susceptibility to rheumatoid arthritis. Arthritis

Rheum. 1987; 30: 1205.

10. Lanchbury JSS, Hall MA, Welsh KI, Panayi GS. Sequence analysis of HLA-DRβ1 subtypes: additional first domain variability is detected by oligonucleotide hybridization and nucleotide sequencing. Hum Immunol. 1990; 27: 136.

11. Nepom GT, Seyfried CE, Holbeck SL, Wilske KR, Nepom BS. Identification of HLA-Dw14 genes in DR4+ rheumatoid arthritis. Lancet. 1986; 2: 1002.

12. Wordsworth BP, Lanchbury JSS, Sakkas LI, Welsh KI, Panayi GS, Bell JI. HLA-DR4 subtype frequencies in rheumatoid arthritis indicate that DRβ1 is the major susceptibility locus within the HLA class II region. Proc Natl Acad Sci USA. 1989; 86: 10049.

13. Nepom GT, Byers P, Seyfried C, Healey LA, Wilske KR, Stage D, Nepom BS. HLA genes associated with rheumatoid arthritis. Identification of susceptibility alleles using specific oligonucleotide probes. Arthritis Rheum. 1989; 32: 15.

14. Watanabe Y, Tokunga K, Matsuki K, Takeuchi F, Matsuta K, Maeda H, Omoto K, Juji T. Putative amino acid sequence of HLA-DRB chain contributing to rheumatoid arthritis. J Exp Med. 1989; 169: 2263.

15. Gao X, Olsen NJ, Pincus T, Stastny P. HLA-DR alleles with naturally occurring amino acid substitutions and risk for development of rheumatoid arthritis. Arthritis Rheum. 1990; 33: 939.

16. Gao X, Brautbar C, Gazit E, Segal R, Naparstek Y, Livneh A, Stastny P. A variant of HLA-DR4 determines susceptibility to rheumatoid arthritis in a subset of Israeli Jews. Arthritis Rheum. 1991; 34: 547.

17. Boki KA, Vaughan RW, Drosos AA, Moutsopoulos HM, Panayi GS, Lanchbury JSS. HLA class II sequence polymorphisms and susceptibility to rheumatoid arthritis in Greece. Arthritis Rheum. 1992; 35: 749.

18. Bjorkman PJ, Saper MA, Samraoui B, Bennett WS, Strominger JL, Wiley DC. The foreign antigen binding site and T cell recognition regions of class I histocompatibility antigens. Nature. 1987; 329: 512.

19. Brown JH, Jardetzky T, Saper MA, Samraoui B, Bjorkman PJ, Wiley DC. A hypothetical model of the foreign antigen binding site of class II histocompatibility molecules. Nature. 1988; 332: 845.

20. Lanchbury JSS, Jaeger EEM, Sansom DM, Hall MA, Wordsworth BP, Stedeford J, Bell JI, Panayi GS. Strong primary selection for the Dw4 subtype of DR4 accounts for the HLA-DQw7 association with Felty's syndrome. Hum Immunol. 1991; 32: 56.

21. Wordsworth BP, Buckley J, Lanchbury JS, Pile K, Ollier W, Bell JI. HLA heterozygosity contributes to susceptibility to rheumatoid arthritis. Am J Hum Genetics. 1992; 51: 585.

5
Cytokines and Inflammatory Arthritis

A. G. WILSON and G. W. DUFF

INTRODUCTION

Cytokines are peptide mediators of cell growth, differentiation and activation. In inflammatory joint disease their effects include bone and cartilage resorption, induction of inflammatory prostanoids, and lymphocyte, monocyte and endothelial cell activation. Systemic effects include pyrexia, altered sleep patterns, anorexia, cachexia and induction of the acute phase proteins[1,2].

The classification of cytokines includes the 14 interleukins (IL): IL-1α and β and IL-2 to IL-13, growth factors (including transforming growth factor (TGF) and epidermal growth factor (EGF)), colony stimulating factors and others, including tumour necrosis factor (TNF) α and β.

Different cell types produce different cytokines: IL-1, IL-6, IL-8, interferon α and TNFα are produced at high levels by macrophages and IL-2, 3, 4, 5, 9, 10, interferon γ and TNFβ mainly by activated T cells.

Cytokines act via specific cell-surface receptors. There are at least two distinct receptors each for IL-1 and TNF. Binding of ligand to receptor leads to increased concentration of intracellular second messengers, such as $Ca++$, cyclic nucleotides and protein kinases which in turn activate transcription factors such as NFkB, which bind to specific sequences of DNA in the nucleus and effect gene expression in response to the initial cytokine/receptor interaction. This process of specific effects on gene expression in particular cell types results in the many actions of each individual cytokine.

Cytokine receptors are expressed on different cell types. Thus the IL-1 type 1 receptor (IL1Rt1) is found on T cells and the IL-1 type 2 receptor (IL1Rt2) predominates on B cells and macrophages. The receptors are composed of three domains: extracellular, transmembrane and intracellular. The extracellular domain binds ligand and this is followed by activation of second messenger molecules by the intracellular domain. In some cases (e.g.

IL1Rt2) there is a short intracellular tail and no second messenger signalling appears to occur.

Naturally occurring inhibitors of cytokines have been described in several biological fluids such as synovial fluid, urine and serum. These may be non-specific and interfere with several cytokines, such as lipoproteins, lipids and alpha-2 macroglobulin which inhibit IL-1, IL-2 and IL-6. Specific cytokine inhibitors are also found. The most common form is the soluble receptor, which may be generated, as in the case of the soluble IL-2 receptor, by proteolytic cleavage of the cell surface receptor, resulting in release of the extracellular domain. Soluble receptors can also be generated by alternative splicing of pre-messenger RNA so that a truncated protein consisting of the extracellular domain only is generated, as is the case with soluble receptors of IL-4 and IL-7. The resulting soluble molecule is able to bind ligand and thus inhibits the biological activity of the ligand. Another mechanism of inhibition is seen in the case of the IL-1 receptor antagonist which binds to the IL-1 receptors but does not result in signal transduction intracellularly[3].

This chapter will review those cytokines which have been most implicated in the initiation and maintenance of inflammatory joint disease and discuss improved therapy based on what we know of their biology.

INTERLEUKIN-1

IL-1 is the term for two proteins (IL-1α and IL-1β) that possess a wide range of inflammatory, metabolic, physiological and immunological properties[4].

The observation, made in the late 1960s, of the pyrogenic properties of inflammatory synovial exudates[5] was almost certainly, at least in part, due to the presence of IL-1. Since then the diversity of the effects of IL-1 have become apparent[6]. IL-1α and IL-1β have very different primary structures but act through similar receptors[2]. It is widely believed that IL-1β is a soluble mediator while IL-1α is more cell associated and important in cell–cell contact but this distinction is not absolute.

The best-studied and possibly major source of IL1 is the activated macrophage following stimulation by agents such as lipopolysaccharide, TNF, viruses and complement components[4]. In inflammatory joint conditions where the aetiology is known, such as gout and sepsis, it has been shown that the causative agents are themselves potent direct inducers of IL-1[7,8].

The production of IL-1 is controlled mainly at the level of transcription and mRNA stability. Resting mononuclear cells do not contain IL-1 mRNA, but this can be detected within 15 minutes of stimulation of the cells with lipopolysaccharide and IL-1 is detected intracellularly within 45 minutes[9]. Northern Blot analysis of synovial tissue shows a single 1.6 kb band that hybridizes with IL-1β cDNA and a 2.2 kb band that hybridizes with IL-1α cDNA[10].

Using *in situ* hybridization, cells containing IL-1β mRNA are more numerous than those containing IL-1α in most tissue sections[10] but analysis of extracted mRNA has indicated that there may be greater production of IL-1α mRNA in some cases[11]. By immunostaining these sections with monoclonal antibodies it has been shown that the predominant IL-1β producing cell type is the CD14 positive macrophage[12].

Pro-IL-1β, a 31 kD protein, is cleaved by a converting enzyme to the mature 17 kD form by a recently cloned enzyme[13,14]. It has also been shown that certain virulent cowpox viruses encode an inhibitor of this protein leading to decreased IL-1 production and a poor inflammatory response. This may have implications for future therapeutic ideas; in addition it argues for the biological importance of IL-1[15].

A problem with defining the role for a particular cytokine in rheumatoid arthritis is the interactions with other pro-inflammatory and anti-inflammatory cytokines. Thus IL-1 induces gene expression of TNFα, IL-6, IL-8, colony stimulating factors, transforming growth factors and epidermal growth factor, several of which, especially TNFα, have properties very similar to IL-1. A further complicating issue is the auto-induction and auto-suppression that IL-1 demonstrates, at least *in vitro*.

While many of the effects of IL-1 such as the induction of prostaglandins, and neutrophil and endothelial cell activation are typical of the acute inflammatory response, many of its effects are also immunoactivating and are relevant to the chronic inflammation typical of rheumatoid arthritis. Of particular interest in this respect is the induction of IL-2 and its receptor by IL-1[16]. In RA the sIL-2R is raised and the level in synovial fluid correlates with the concentration of IL-1β. Levels of sIL-2R in sera have been shown to correlate with, and to predict, changes in inflammatory disease in RA[17]. Immunolocalization of IL-1β and IL-2R using monoclonal antibodies in rheumatoid synovia has shown both to be localized to the same cellular aggregates[18]. IL-1 also acts as a co-factor in conjunction with IL-4 to stimulate B cells to produce immunoglobulins. This appears to be in addition to its ability to stimulate production of several B cell growth factors such as IL-2, IL-4 and IL-6[4].

Injection of IL-1 into the joints of rabbits induces cartilage resorption and polymorphonuclear cell accumulation in the joint space[19]. This *in vivo* action strongly supports the evidence that IL-1 is important in the induction of inflammatory arthritis. IL-1β levels in plasma and synovial fluid have been measured by immunoassay, in patients with rheumatoid arthritis. The mean plasma level of IL-1β was significantly higher than in normal age-matched individuals. Using standard clinical and laboratory measurements of disease activity, significant cross-sectional positive correlations were observed with erythrocyte sedimentation rate, pain score and joint tenderness, and a negative correlation existed between IL-1β levels and haemoglobin concentration[20]. No correlation was found between IL-1α levels and any of these indices[21].

IL-1β levels in synovial fluid seem to correlate with local activity. In rheumatoid patients with bilateral knee joint inflammation there were no significant differences between IL-1β levels. However, in patients with asymmetric knee joint disease the levels of IL-1β were significantly increased in the more inflamed joint[22].

These findings indicate that the important pro-inflammatory and immuno-potentiating properties of IL-1 are likely to play a role in the immunopathogenic mechanisms of RA.

INTERLEUKIN-1 RECEPTOR ANTAGONIST (IL-1ra)

The IL-1ra is a naturally occurring specific IL-1 inhibitor which may prove to be of considerable therapeutic benefit in inflammatory conditions such as RA. Its actions are due to its high affinity for the IL-1 receptor, but it has no agonist activity even at concentrations 1000 times greater than biologically active concentrations of IL-1. The structure of the genes for IL-1α, IL-1β and IL-ra (which have been present for at least 75 million years) indicates that IL-1ra diverged from the common ancestral gene before IL-1α diverged from IL-1β, implying an important role for the antagonist[3]. The protein sequence shows 19% and 26% homology with IL-1α and IL-1β respectively[23]. Despite this, the genes for IL-1β and IL-1ra appear to be regulated differently – monocytes activated with LPS produce both proteins whereas adherent IgG stimulates only IL-1ra production[24]. The anti-inflammatory properties of IL-4 are, at least in part, due to its ability to inhibit IL-1β production but also to increase IL-1ra production[25]. The protein was originally identified in the urine of patients with pyrexia[26], and can be detected in the urine of children with systemic juvenile chronic arthritis. Initial studies indicated that IL-1ra bound to the IL-1 type 1 receptor with much greater affinity than to the type 2 receptor. However, it has become clear that the affinity for the two receptors is similar.

In a rat model of recurrent arthritis, caused by intra-articular streptococcal cell wall injection, treatment with IL-1ra has been shown to reduce joint swelling by 60% and reduce cartilage erosion[27]. Interestingly, from the aspect of its possible use as a therapeutic agent, intravenous IL-1ra was effective in protecting against IL-1 induced synovitis in rabbits[28].

It seems likely that naturally produced IL-1ra serves to down regulate the inflammatory response and, given the likely role of IL-1 in chronic inflammatory arthritis, the IL-1ra may be of significant clinical significance.

TUMOUR NECROSIS FACTOR ALPHA

TNF derived its name from the observation that endotoxic mice produced a factor that caused necrosis in certain sarcomatous tumours[29]. The other name for TNF is cachectin, because of its ability to induce cachexia and wasting. It is an inducible, secretory protein with very similar actions to IL-1[30]. The main source is the activated macrophage, although T cells and some B cells are also producers. The gene for TNFα lies within the class III region of the MHC beside TNFβ in a 7 kb stretch of DNA[31]. Their close physical linkage and homology suggest that they have arisen as a genetic duplication event. Stable inter-individual production of TNFα has been demonstrated[32] and this shows association with HLA DR alleles: DR2 with low production and DR3 and 4 with high production[33].

TNF shares with IL-1 the ability to induce cartilage and joint destruction and also to activate bone resorption and mediators of tissue destruction such as collagenase. As with IL-1, TNF is an immunopotentiating molecule which activates T and B cells, and upregulates MHC class I expression, adhesion molecules and other cytokines. TNFα downregulates the IFNγ induced expression of MHC class II molecules on differentiate cells, such as skin fibroblasts and activated macrophages[34].

In the rheumatoid synovium TNF mRNA has been localized to the perivascular areas and the cartilage-pannus junction[35]. TNF can induce and synergize with IL-1 in many pro-inflammatory activities. This action appears to be effected at the second messenger level rather than at the receptor level; indeed IL-1 reduces TNF receptor expression[4]. This synergism may be of major pathogenic significance.

TNF has been demonstrated in synovial exudates[36,37]. No correlation has been found between immunoactive or bioactive levels of TNF and disease activity in cross-sectional studies[38]. This may be due to the presence of biological inhibitors, such as soluble receptors, or to the interindividual variation in TNF production mentioned above[32]. No longitudinal studies in patients with RA have been reported.

Intra-articular injection of recombinant TNFα induces monocyte accumulation and synergy with the effects of IL-1. The potential importance of TNF in RA has recently been shown using transgenic mice, in which the transgene consists of a modified human TNF gene. The resulting mice express high levels of TNFα and some develop inflammatory polyarthritis which is preventable by administering monoclonal antibodies against TNF[39]. A soluble form of the 80 kD TNF receptor is encoded by a member of the poxvirus family; the protective effect of such a molecule would certainly confer a selective advantage to this pathogen and, again, suggests the importance of TNF in inflammation[40].

INTERLEUKIN-6

IL-6 is produced by macrophages, endothelial cells, keratinocytes and activated T cells and has several important actions in common with IL-1 and TNF; it is a pyrogen and an inducer of acute phase proteins such as C-reactive protein, serum amyloid A, C3, alpha-2 macroglobin and fibrinogen. It is a potent stimulator of immunoglobulin production by B cells, and it is probably a major stimulus for rheumatoid factor production. However, it differs from these cytokines in several important respects. Most importantly it seems to suppress production of IL-1, TNF, IL-6 and IL-8[41] and therefore has weak anti-inflammatory properties and does not affect cartilage or bone metabolism.

Production of IL-6, like that of many other cytokines, is controlled mainly at the transcriptional level, and mRNA is not present in unstimulated cells[42]. Inducing agents include bacterial and viral products, IL-1 and TNF.

The role of IL-6 in inflammatory arthritis is unclear. It has been reported that IL-6 is produced *in vitro* by RA synoviocytes. Correlation has been found between synovial fluid IL-6 levels and clinical parameters of joint inflammation[43]. Serum IL-6 levels have also been correlated with disease activity in systemic onset juvenile chronic arthritis[44]. However IL-6 has been shown to be protective against adjuvant arthritis in rats[45].

Some of the systemic features of inflammation, such as the acute phase response, are IL-6 related; however, its role in the pathogenesis of osteoarticular disease is unclear and warrants further study.

INTERLEUKIN-8

IL-8 or neutrophil activating factor displays powerful chemotactic properties and is thought to be the major mediator of leukocyte chemotaxis and granulocyte activation during inflammation[46]. Indeed, the chemotactic properties attributed previously to IL-1 and TNF may well be mediated by IL-8. In an *in vitro* system, using synovial cells and anti-IL-8 antiserum, neutrophil-stimulating activity was reduced by over 90%[47]. IL-8 is produced by monocytes, lymphocytes, fibroblasts and endothelial cells by direct actions of IL-1 and TNF. Production from mononuclear cells can be inhibited using the IL-1ra[48]. IL-8 has no effect on proteoglycan metabolism[49]. However, levels are elevated in rheumatoid synovial fluid and this has been correlated with severe joint disease, with the number and proportion of neutrophils in the joint and with circulating CRP[50]. It therefore seems likely that this cytokine is central to the neutrophil-mediated cartilage damage typically seen in RA.

INTERLEUKIN-10

IL-10 was initially named cytokine synthesis inhibitory factor because of its apparent ability to prevent mouse T_H1 cells from producing IL-2, IFNγ and TNFβ. It is produced by the T_H0 and T_H2 subsets of T cells and by macrophages and B cells[51]. IL-10 displays remarkable homology to an open reading frame, BCRF1, within the Epstein-Barr virus (EBV) genome[52]. The BCRF1 protein displays partial IL-10 activity, and it seems likely that EBV has captured the gene which may therefore confer a selection advantage[53].

The T-helper subset phenotypes in humans are probably similar to those of mice and it is interesting to note the relative deficiency of IL-2, IFNγ and TNFβ in RA and the evidence implicating EBV in the aetiology of RA[54].

INTERLEUKIN-3 AND COLONY-STIMULATING FACTORS (CSFs)

This group of cytokines was named after their effects on haemopoietic progenitor cells *in vitro*. IL-3 is produced by activated T cells and stimulates proliferation of pluripotent stem cells including the production of bone-marrow derived osteoclasts. CSFs stimulate granulocyte and monocyte phagocytosis, superoxide production, cytotoxicity and production of IL-1 and TNF. GM-CSF is produced by macrophages, endothelial cells, T cells and fibroblasts, and acts on stem cells to produce either granulocytes or monocytes. G-CSF and M-CSF stimulate granulocyte and monocyte precursors respectively.

In addition to the above actions, GM-CSF is a potent stimulator of macrophages and neutrophils and MHC class II expression. Studies of CSFs in RA have demonstrated most of the CSF activity to be due to M-CSF[55], although GM-CSF mRNA can be detected in synovial tissue[56].

TRANSFORMING GROWTH FACTOR BETA (TGFβ)

TGFβ exists in at least four dimeric forms. In the RA joint, synoviocytes produce mainly the beta-1 type of which more than 90% exists in an immature form (requiring proteolytic cleavage for full biological activity). Using immunohistochemical techniques on RA joint sections, it has been shown that TGFβ is expressed at the cartilage/pannus junction and in the perivascular region[57]. In animal models of arthritis, systemic administration of TGFβ-1 protected against streptococcal wall arthritis in rats[58] and against collagen induced arthritis in mice[59]. However, when human recombinant TGFβ was injected into rat knee joints extensive recruitment of PMNs and synovial hypertrophy were observed[60]. Further investigation of the role of this cytokine in RA is urgently needed.

EPIDERMAL GROWTH FACTOR

Epidermal growth factor (EGF) is a 53 amino acid, 6 kD protein produced by mesenchymal cells. Its actions include tissue remodelling, growth of epithelial cells, bone resorption and prostaglandin synthesis[61]. EGF has recently been detected in the RA synovium and it has been proposed as being important in synovial hyperplasia. In RA, EGF was found in the synovial lining cells but not at the cartilage-pannus junction. Correlation has been demonstrated between EGF staining in the synovial lining cells and the degree of neovascularization in the rheumatoid synovial sections[62].

CONCLUSIONS

Although the aetiology of diseases such as RA is unknown, cytokines, such as IL-1 and TNF, are probably very important mediators in the chronic inflammatory reaction and are found at very high levels in synovial exudates. A recent report of transgenic mice in which overproduction of human TNFα caused a symmetrical polyarthritis underlined the role of cytokine over-production as a key contributory factor in the pathogenesis of RA.

Polymorphism within regulatory[63–66] or protein coding regions[67] of several of the major cytokines has recently been demonstrated. A polymorphism within the region of the TNFα gene that controls transcription has been shown to be tightly linked with the autoimmune haplotype HLA A1 B8 DR3[68]. In addition, alleles of IL-α and IL-1β and the IL-1 receptor antagonist, all of which lie on chromosome 2, have been found to be associated with autoimmune rheumatic diseases including SLE, scleroderma and juvenile chronic arthritis. It is not yet possible to say whether these polymorphisms of cytokine genes may be important susceptibility or severity factors for chronic inflammatory diseases.

Much present research is directed at the use of cytokine inhibitors, such as the IL-ra, soluble receptors or monoclonal antibodies, as antirheumatic therapies and good results are anticipated. In the long term, the molecular recognition events within the cytokine system should provide excellent structural models for the development of small molecular weight drugs with specific effects on inflammation and its accompanying processes.

References

1. Duff G. Immune diseases. Many roles for interleukin-1. Nature. 1985; 313: 352–353.
2. Bendtzen K. Immune hormones (cytokines); pathogenic role in autoimmune rheumatic and endocrine diseases. Autoimmunity. 1989; 2: 177–189.
3. Dinarello CA, Thompson RC. Blocking IL-1: interleukin 1 receptor antagonist *in vivo* and *in vitro*. Immunol Today. 1991; 12: 404–410.
4. Dinarello CA. Interleukin-1 and Interleukin Antagonism. Blood. 1991; 77: 1627–1652.
5. Bodel P, Hollingsworth JW. Pyrogen release from human synovial exudate cells. Br J Exp Path. 1969; 49: 11–19.
6. di Giovine FS, Duff GW. Interleukin 1: the first interleukin. Immunol Today. 1990; 11: 13–20.
7. di Giovine FS, Malawista SE, Nuki G, Duff GW. Interleukin 1 (IL 1) as a mediator of crystal arthritis. Stimulation of T cell and synovial fibroblast mitogenesis by urate crystal-induced IL 1. J Immunol. 1987; 138: 3213–3218.
8. Wallis RS, Fujiwara H, Ellner JJ. Direct stimulation of monocyte release of interleukin 1 by mycobacterial protein antigens. J Immunol. 1986; 136: 193–196.
9. di Giovine FS, Symons JA, Duff GW. Kinetics of IL-1 beta mRNA and protein induction in human blood mononuclear cells. Immunol Lett. 1991; 29: 211–218.
10. Duff GW, Dickens E, Wood NC, et al. Immunoassay, bioassay and *in situ* hybridization of monokines in human arthritis. In: Powanda MC, Oppenheim JJ, Kluger MJ, Dinarello CA, eds. Monokines and other non-lymphocytic cytokines. New York: Alan R. Liss; 1988; 387–392.
11. Buchan G, Barrett K, Turner M, Chantry D, Maini RN, Feldmann M. Interleukin-1 and tumour necrosis factor mRNA expression in rheumatoid arthritis: prolonged production of IL-1 alpha. Clin Exp Immunol. 1988; 73: 449–455.
12. Wood NC, Dickens E, Symons JA, Duff GW. *In situ* hybridization of interleukin-1 in CD 14-positive cells in rheumatoid arthritis. Clin Immunol Immunopathol. 1992; 62: 295–300.
13. Thornberry NA, Bull HG, Calaycay JR, et al. A novel heterodimeric cysteine protease is required for interleukin-1β processing in monocytes. Nature. 1992; 356: 768–774.
14. Cerretti DP, Kozlosky CJ, Mosley B, et al. Molecular cloning of the interleukin-1β converting enzyme. Science. 1992; 256: 97–100.
15. Ray CA, Black RA, Kronheim SR, et al. Viral inhibition of inflammation: Cowpox virus encodes an inhibitor of the interleukin-1β converting enzyme. Cell. 1992; 69: 597–604.
16. Symons JA, Wood NC, di Giovine FS, Duff GW. Soluble IL-2 receptor in rheumatoid arthritis. Correlation with disease activity, IL-1 and IL-2 inhibition. J Immunol. 1988; 141: 2612–2618.
17. Wood NC, Symons JA, Duff GW. Serum interleukin-2 receptor in rheumatoid arthritis: a prognostic indicator of disease activity? J Autoimmun. 1988; 1: 353–361.
18. Duff G. Interleukin-1 in inflammatory joint disease. In: Bomford R, Henderson B, eds. Interleukin-1, Inflammation and Disease. Amsterdam: Elsevier, 1989; 243–255.
19. Pettipher ER, Higgs GA, Henderson B. Interleukin 1 induces leukocyte infiltration and cartilage proteoglycan degradation in the synovial joint. Proc Natl Acad Sci USA. 1986; 83: 8749–8753.
20. Eastgate JA, Symons JA, Wood NC, Grinlinton FM, di Giovine FS, Duff GW. Correlation

of plasma interleukin 1 levels with disease activity in rheumatoid arthritis. Lancet. 1988; 2: 706–709.

21. Eastgate JA, Symons JA, Wood NC, Capper SJ, Duff GW. Plasma levels of interleukin-1-alpha in rheumatoid arthritis. Br J Rheumatol. 1991; 30: 295–297.

22. Rooney M, Symons JA, Duff GW. Interleukin 1 beta in synovial fluid is related to local disease activity in rheumatoid arthritis. Rheumatology Int. 1990; 10: 217–219.

23. Eisenberg EP, Evans RJ, Arend WP, et al. Primary structure and functional expression from complementary DNA of a human interleukin-1 receptor antagonist. Nature. 1990; 343: 341–346.

24. Arend AP, Smith MF, Janson RW, Joslin FG. IL-1 receptor antagonist and IL-1b production in human monocytes are regulated differently. J Immunol. 1991; 147: 1530–1536.

25. Vannier E, Miller LC, Dinarello CA. Coordinated antiinflammatory effects of interleukin 4: Interleukin 4 suppresses interleukin 1 production but up-regulates gene expression and synthesis of interleukin 1 receptor antagonist. Proc Natl Acad Sci USA. 1992; 89: 4076–4080.

26. Seckinger P, Lowenenthal JW, Williamson K, Dayer JM, MacDonald HR. A urine inhibitor of IL-1 activity that blocks ligand binding. J Immunol. 1987; 139: 1546–1549.

27. Schwab JH, Anderle SK, Brown RR, Dalldorf FG, Thompson RC. Pro-inflammatory and antiinflammatory roles of interleukin-1 in recurrence of bacterial-cell wall-induced arthritis in rats. Infection and Immunity. 1991; 59: 4436–4442.

28. Henderson B, Thompson RC, Hardingham T, Lewthwaite J. Inhibition of interleukin-1-induced synovitis and articular cartilage proteoglycan loss in the rabbit knee by recombinant human interleukin-1 receptor antagonist. Cytokine. 1991; 3: 246–249.

29. Starnes SO. Coley's toxins in perspective. Nature. 1992; 357: 11–12.

30. Beutler B, Cerami A. The biology of cachetin/TNF – a primary mediator of the host response. Ann Rev Imm. 1989; 7: 625–655.

31. Nedospasov SA, Shakov AN, Turetskaya RL, et al. Tandem arrangement of genes coding for tumor necrosis factor (TNFα) and lymphotoxin (TNFβ) in the human genome. Cold Spring Harbor Symp Quant Biol. 1986; L1: 611–624.

32. Molvig J, Baek J, Christensen P, et al. Endotoxin-stimulated human monocytes secretion of Interleukin-1, Tumour Necrosis Factor alpha and Prostaglandin E2 shows stable interindividual differences. Scand J Immunol. 1988; 27: 705–716.

33. Jacob CO, Fronek Z, Lewis GD, Koo M, Hansen JA, McDevitt. Heritable major histocompatibility complex class II-associated differences in production of tumor necrosis factor α: Relevance to genetic predisposition to systemic lupus erythematosus. Proc Natl Acad Sci USA. 1990; 87: 1233–1237.

34. Jacob CO. Tumor necrosis factor α in autoimmunity: pretty girl or old witch? Immunol Today. 1992; 13: 122–125.

35. Chu CQ, Field M, Feldmann M, Maini RN. Localization of tumor necrosis factor alpha in synovial tissues and at the cartilage-pannus junction in patients with rheumatoid arthritis. Arthritis Rheum. 1991; 34: 1125–1132.

36. di Giovine FS, Nuki G, Duff GW. Tumour necrosis factor in synovial exudates. Ann Rheum Dis. 1988; 47: 668–772.

37. Saxne TM, Palladino MA Jr, Heinegard D, Talal N, Wollheim FA. Detection of tumor necrosis factor alpha but not tumor necrosis factor beta in rheumatoid arthritis synovial fluid and serum. Arthritis Rheum. 1988; 31: 1041–1044.

38. di Giovine FS, Meager A, Leung H, Duff GW. Immunoreactive tumour necrosis factor alpha and biological inhibitor(s) in synovial fluids from patients with rheumatic disease. Int J Immunopathol Pharmacol. 1988; 1: 17–26.

39. Keffer J, Probert L, Cazlaris H, Georgopoulos S, Kaslaris E, Kioussis D, Kollias G. Transgenic mice expressing human tumour necrosis factor: a predictive genetic model of arthritis. EMBO J. 1991; 10: 4025–4031.

40. Smith CA, Davis T, Anderson D, et al. A receptor for tumor necrosis factor defines an unusual family of cellular and viral proteins. Science. 1990; 248: 1019–1023.

41. Schindler R, Mancilla J, Endres S, Ghorbani R, Clark SC, Dinarello CA. Correlations and interactions in the production of IL-6, IL-1 and TNF in human mononuclear cells: IL-6 suppresses IL-1 and TNF. Blood. 1990; 75: 40–47.

42. Ray A, Tatter SB, May LT, Sehgal PB. Activation of the human 'beta-2-interferon/hepatocyte stimulating factor/interleukin 6' promoter by cytokines, viruses and second messenger agonists. Proc Natl Acad Sci USA. 1988; 85: 6701–6705.

43. Miltenburg AM, van Laar JM, de Kuiper R, Daha MR, Breedveld FC. Interleukin-6 activity in paired samples of synovial fluid. Correlation of synovial fluid interleukin-6 levels with clinical and laboratory parameters of inflammation. Br J Rheumatol. 1991; 30: 186–189.

44. de Benedetti F, Massa M, Robbioni P, Ravelli A, Burgio, Martini A. Correlation of serum interleukin-6 levels with involvement and thrombocytosis in systemic juvenile rheumatoid arthritis. Arthritis Rheum. 1991; 34: 1158–1163.

45. Mihara M, Ikuta M, Koishihara Y, Ohsugi Y. Interleukin 6 inhibits delayed-type hypersensitivity and the development of adjuvant arthritis. Eur J Immunol. 1991; 21: 2327–2331.

46. Elford PR, Cooper PH. Induction of neutrophil-mediated cartilage degradation by interleukin-8. Arthritis Rheum. 1991; 34: 325–332.

47. Seitz M, Deweld B, Gerber N, Baggiolini M. Enhanced production of neutrophil-activating peptide-1/interleukin-8 in rheumatoid arthritis. J Clin Invest. 1991; 87: 463–469.

48. Porat R, Poutsiaka DD, Miller LC, Granowitz EV, Dinarello CA. Interleukin-1 (IL-1) receptor blockade reduces endotoxin and *Borrelia burgdorferi*-stimulated IL-8 synthesis in human mononuclear cells. FASEB J. 1992; 6: 2482–2486.

49. Endo H, Akahoshi T, Takagishi K, Kashiwazaki S, Matsushima K. Elevation of interleukin-8 (IL-8) levels in joint fluids of patients with rheumatoid arthritis and the induction by IL-8 of leukocyte infiltration and synovitis in rabbit joints. Lymphokine Cytokine Res. 1991; 10: 245–252.

50. Peichl P, Ceska M, Effenberger F, Haberhauer G, Broell H, Lindley IJ. Presence of NAP-1/IL-8 in synovial fluids indicates a possible pathogenic role in rheumatoid arthritis. Scand J Immunol. 1991; 34: 333–339.

51. Mossman TR, Moore KW. The role of IL-10 in crossregulation of T_H1 and T_H2 responses. Immunol Today. 1991; 12: A49–A53.

52. Moore KW, Vieira P, Fiorentino DF, Trounstine ML, Khan TA, Mosmann TR. Homology of cytokine synthesis inhibitory factor (IL-10) to the Epstein-Barr virus gene BCRF1. Science. 1990; 248: 1230–1234.

53. Howard M, O'Garra A. Biological properties of interleukin 10. Immunol Today. 1992; 13: 198–200.

54. Harris ED Jr. Pathogenesis of rheumatoid arthritis. In: Kelley WN, Harris ED Jr, Ruddy S, Sledge CB, eds. Textbook of Rheumatology. Philadelphia: W B Saunders; 1989: 905–942.

55. Firestein GS, Alvaro-Garcia JM, Maki R. Quantitative analysis of cytokine gene expression in rheumatoid arthritis. J Immunol. 1990; 144: 3347–3353.

56. Alvaro-Garcia JM, Zvaifler NJ, Brown CB, Kaushansky K. Cytokines in chronic inflammatory arthritis. VI. Analysis of the synovial cells involved in granulocyte-macrophage colony-stimulating factor production and gene expression in rheumatoid arthritis and its regulation by IL-1 and tumor necrosis factor. J Immunol. 1991; 146: 3365–3371.

57. Chu CQ, Field M, Abney E, Zheng RQ, Allard S, Feldmann M, Maini RN. Transforming growth factor-beta 1 in rheumatoid arthritis synovial membrane and cartilage/pannus junction. Clin Exp Immunol. 1991; 86: 380–386.

58. Fava RA, Olsen NJ, Postlethwaite AE, et al. Transforming growth factor beta 1 (TGF-beta 1) induced neutrophil recruitment to synovial tissues: implications for TGF-beta-driven synovial inflammation and hyperplasia. J Exp Med. 1991; 173: 1121–1132.

59. Kuruvilla AP, Shah R, Hochwald GM, Liggitt HD, Palladino MA, Thorbecke GJ. Protective effects of transforming growth factor beta 1 on experimental autoimmune diseases in mice. Proc Natl Acad Sci USA. 1991; 88: 2918–2921.

60. Brandes ME, Allen JB, Ogawa Y, Wahl SM. Transforming growth factor beta 1 suppresses acute and chronic arthritis in experimental animals. J Clin Invest. 1991; 87: 1108–1113.

61. Waterfield MD. Epidermal growth factors and related molecules. In: A Lancet series. Peptide Regulatory Factors. London: E. Arnold, 1989; 81–90.

62. Shiozawa S, Shiozawa K, Tanaka Y, Morimoto I, et al. Human epidermal growth factor for the stratification of synovial lining layer and neovascularization in rheumatoid arthritis. Ann Rheum Dis. 1989; 48: 820–828.

63. Wilson AG, di Giovine FS, Blakemore AIF, Duff GW. A single base polymorphism in the human tumour necrosis factor alpha (TNFα) gene detectable by Ncol digestion of PCR product. Human Mol Genet. 1992; 1: 353.
64. di Giovine FS, Takash E, Blakemore AIF, Duff GW. Single base polymorphism at -511 in the human interleukin-1β gene (IL1β). Human Mol Genet. 1992; 1: 450.
65. Bailly S, di Giovine FS, Duff GW. Polymorphic tandem repeat sequence region in interleukin-1α intron 6. Human Genetics. 1993; 91: 85–86.
66. Tarlow JK, Blakemore AIF, Lennard A, Solari R, Hughes HN, Steinkasser A, Duff GW. Polymorphism in human IL-1 receptor antagonist gene intron 2 is due to variable number of an 86 bp repeat sequence. Human Genetics. 1993; 91: 403–404.
67. Messer G, Sprengler U, Jung MC, Honold G, Blomer K, Pape GR, Riethmuller G, Weiss EH. Polymorphic structures of the human tumor necrosis factor locus: An Ncol polymorphism in the first intron of the human TNF-β gene correlates with a variant amino acid in position 26 and a reduced level of TNF-β production. J Exp Med. 1991; 173: 209–219.
68. Wilson AG, de Vries N, Pociot F, di Giovine FS, van de Putte LBA, Duff GW. A polymorphism within the human tumor necrosis factor alpha promoter region is strongly associated with HLA A1 B8 DR3 alleles. J Exp Med. 1993; 177: 557–560.

6
Adhesion Molecules involved in Leukocyte–Endothelial Cell Interactions

L. MEAGHER and D. HASKARD

INTRODUCTION

It has long been recognized that the successful extravasation of leukocytes through blood vessel walls into perturbed tissues is central to the progression of inflammatory reactions. The last decade has seen a growing awareness of the basic mechanisms underlying leukocyte emigration and, in particular, the importance of the adhesion molecules which facilitate interactions between leukocytes and vascular endothelial cells (EC). The considerable efforts expended in understanding cell adhesion have yielded not only a rich harvest of new molecules but have also revealed a complex web of interactions between them. The molecules involved in inflammation are reviewed in detail elsewhere[1], and this chapter will concentrate upon those molecules of particular relevance to interactions between leukocytes and EC.

THE ENDOTHELIUM

Vascular endothelium provides a barrier which contains the proteins and formed elements within the blood[2,3]. Under appropriate circumstances EC, which have a role which is by no means passive, make an important contribution to the control of leukocyte traffic, haemostasis, permeability to proteins and the regulation of vascular tone. The majority of studies investigating the activities of human EC *in vitro* have employed human umbilical vein endothelial cells (HUVEC) which are comparatively easy to isolate and culture[4]. More recently techniques have been described for the culture of human microvascular EC[5,6] and it is hoped that comparison

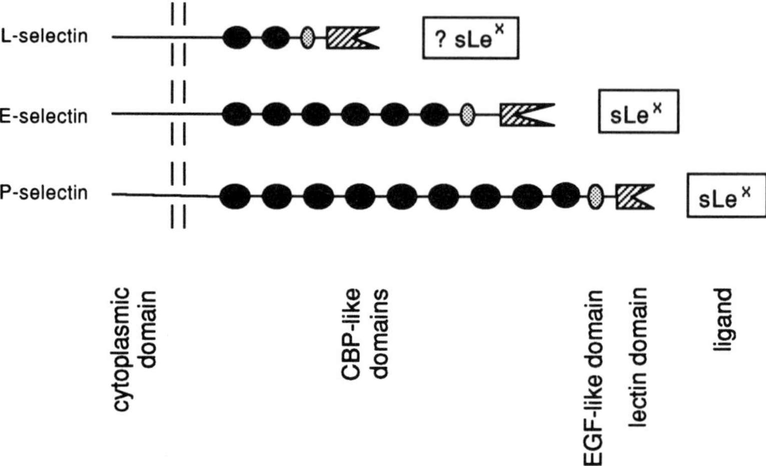

Figure 1 Selectins

between EC from different sources will allow greater understanding of the contribution that EC heterogeneity makes to patterns of inflammation.

MOLECULES INVOLVED IN LEUKOCYTE–ENDOTHELIUM INTERACTIONS

The molecules involved in leukocyte adhesion to EC can be grouped into families in which members show similarities of structure and function.

Selectins

The selectin family comprises three molecules designated L-selectin, E-selectin and P-selectin. The gene for each of these molecules is located within a small area of chromosome 1 and it has been suggested that the three genes have arisen as a result of duplications and mutations of a single gene[7]. The selectins are single chain glycoproteins, with a lectin-like N-terminal domain, an epidermal growth factor-like motif and a variable number of repeated units homologous to the short consensus repeats of complement binding proteins (CBP), such as CR1, CD2 and decay accelerating factor (Figure 1). The most proximal CBP unit adjoins a transmembrane region and a short cytoplasmic tail. One of the most obvious differences between the three molecules is the number of CBP repeats which results in the three molecules being of quite different size. These size differences between the three selectin molecules may be functionally relevant in influencing the distance that the ligand-binding lectin domain can protrude from the cell membrane and hence the efficiency by which the molecule can bind opposing cells under conditions of flow.

P-selectin

P-selectin (GMP-140, PADGEM, CD62) is the largest of the selectins with nine CBP repeats and a relative molecular mass of 140 kD. It was originally identified as a platelet antigen which is stored in α granules and expressed on the platelet surface following activation[8–11]. P-selectin is now known also to be synthesized constitutively by EC and to be stored within Weibel-Palade bodies[12–14].

Stimulation of EC with agents such as thrombin or histamine or with C5b-9 complexes results in the translocation of Weibel-Palade bodies to the cell surface and expression of P-selectin on the luminal membrane[15–17]. P-selectin expression is linked to Weibel-Palade body degranulation and secretion of von Willebrand factor into the extra-cellular environment[15]. This response occurs within minutes of stimulation and is independent of gene transcription and *de novo* protein synthesis. Although P-selectin expression by EC *in vitro* tends to be transient in response to most stimuli, Patel and colleagues have observed a more prolonged expression following activation of EC by oxidants such as hydrogen peroxide[18], suggesting a role for this molecule in chronic as well as acute inflammatory responses.

Judging from immunocytochemical staining with monoclonal antibodies, P-selectin has a wide organ distribution and is particularly expressed by small veins and venules[13]. P-selectin promotes the adhesion of neutrophils and monocytes to activated platelets and EC[17,19–21]. Recent evidence indicates that this molecule also binds natural killer cells and a subset of memory CD4+ and CD8+ T cells[22,23].

E-selectin

E-selectin (Endothelial leukocyte adhesion molecule-1, ELAM-1) is a smaller molecule than P-selectin, with six CBP repeats and a molecular mass of approximately 112 kD[24,25]. Expression of E-selectin is limited to EC and only occurs after activation. The best-characterized activating factors that stimulate EC to express E-selectin are tumour necrosis factor (TNF), interleukin-1 (IL-1) or bacterial lipopolysaccharide (LPS)[26,29]. E-selectin expression by activated EC is dependent upon gene transcription and *de novo* protein synthesis and is maximal after 4–6 hours, declining *in vitro* to near basal levels by 24 hours following stimulation. Experiments using monoclonal antibodies and transfected cells indicate that E-selectin can bind neutrophils[24,25], eosinophils[30,31], basophils[31], monocytes[32,33] and a subpopulation of memory T cells[34–37].

The T cells which are able to bind E-selectin carry an antigen recognized by mAb HECA 452[37]. This structure, which was initially identified as an EC antigen[38], has been designated the Cutaneous Lymphocyte Antigen (CLA) on account of the propensity of T cells carrying the antigen to migrate to the skin[39]. It is possible, however, that E-selectin may also be involved in the migration of T cells to other tissues as T cells able to bind E-selectin have been isolated from rheumatoid synovial membrane and fluid[40]. The overlap between lymphocytes able to bind E-selectin and P-selectin has not yet been defined.

E-selectin has been identified on endothelium in a number of pathological settings, including the vascular leak syndrome due to systemic administration of interleukin-2[41], Kawasaki disease[42], psoriasis[43], the cutaneous late-phase response to allergen[30,44], scleroderma[45], inflammatory bowel disease[46], bronchial mucosa in asthma[47], and synovium in rheumatoid arthritis[48,49]. In experimentally induced inflammation in human skin there is a clear relationship between E-selectin expression and the presence of neutrophils in the tissues[50].

L-selectin

In contrast to E- and P-selectin, L-selectin (LECAM-1, MEL-14 antigen, LAM-1, Leu-8) is expressed on leukocytes rather than EC. Although L-selectin was first characterized as a lymphocyte antigen involved in recirculation through peripheral lymph nodes[51], it is now clear that the same molecule is present on most other populations of peripheral blood leukocytes[52,53]. Monoclonal antibodies against L-selectin inhibit the adhesion of lymphocytes to peripheral lymph node high endothelial venules (HEV)[51] and the adhesion of neutrophils, monocytes and lymphocytes to cytokine activated cultured EC[54-57].

Carbohydrate ligands for selectins

As might be expected from the N-terminal lectin motifs, there is evidence that each of the selectins binds carbohydrate residues. Whilst some carbohydrate determinants such as sialyl-Lewis x (sLe^x) and sialyl-Lewis a (sLe^a) are recognized by each of the three selectins[58,59], there are other structures to which one or sometimes two of the selectins show preferential adhesion[59].

The first carbohydrate ligand to be identified for E-selectin was sLe^x[60-63]. Although there are probably many cell surface glycoproteins and glycolipids that express sLe^x, Picker and colleagues have proposed that E-selectin and P-selectin may selectively bind the sLe^x on neutrophils which decorates L-selectin, perhaps by virtue of the clustering of L-selectin on neutrophil microvillous processes[64,65]. There is also evidence that CD66 nonspecific cross-reacting antigens related to carcinoembryonic antigen may present sLe^x on neutrophils to E-selectin[66]. The ligand for E-selectin on T cells appears to be CLA, which is a carbohydrate determinant related to sLe^x[67]. The ligands for P-selectin on leukocytes are probably broadly the same as those for E-selectin[68-70]. However myeloid and tumour cell sulphatides have been reported to bind P-selectin but not E-selectin[71].

The counter-receptor(s) for L-selectin have not been fully elucidated. Recently Lasky et al.[72] have reported the cloning of a mucin-like glycoprotein which acts as a peripheral lymph node HEV ligand for L-selectin[73]. The ligand(s) responsible for L-selectin mediated leukocyte binding of cytokine-activated cultured EC is still unknown.

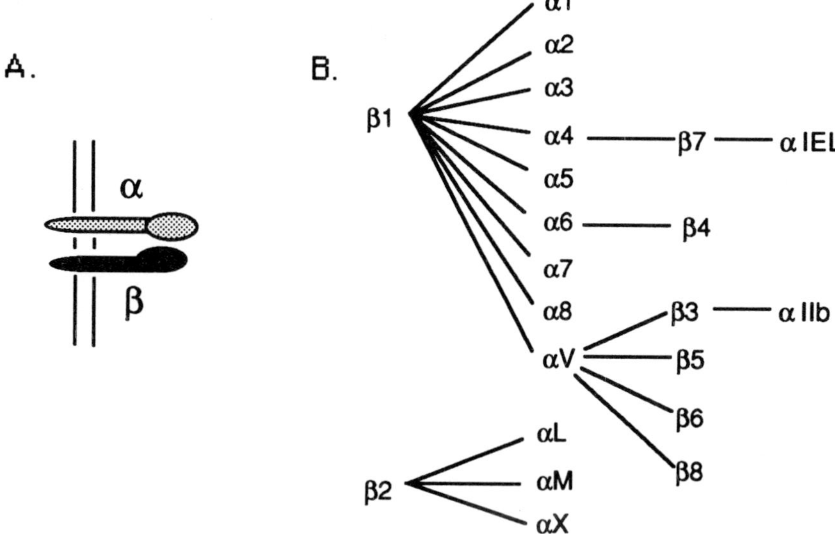

Figure 2 Integrins: (A) heterodimeric conformation, and (B) associations of subunits

Integrins

The integrins are a widely distributed group of cell surface adhesion molecules, involved in both cell–cell and cell–matrix interactions[74]. Each integrin is a heterodimer composed of a large α subunit (120–180 kD) and a non-covalently associated smaller β subunit (90–110 kD) (Figure 2A). Judging from chemical cross-linking experiments, the N-terminal domains of α and β subunits are thought to combine to determine the ligand binding region and hence the specificity for the ligand(s)[75–78].

Integrin α subunits contain repeated segments which putatively act as cation binding determinants and which are important not only for the association of α and β subunits but also in influencing the avidity with which the ligand can be bound (see below). Some α subunits (α_L, α_M, α_x, α_1, α_2) contain an extra or inserted domain (I domain) before the final five homologous repeats of the cation binding region. This region is homologous to complement proteins, cartilage matrix protein and the collagen binding region of von Willebrand factor, suggesting a role in ligand binding. Beta subunits characteristically contain four repeats of a region rich in cystine residues and which probably determine the structure of the molecule through internal disulphide bonds. A tightly folded β subunit N-terminal region is believed to interact with the α subunit in forming the ligand binding domain.

Integrins involved in leukocyte interactions with EC

The number of known integrins is not a simple product of the number of identified α and β subunits, and it is possible to group integrins based upon associations involving particular α or β chains (Figure 2B). Of these groups, the integrins best characterized as being involved in leukocyte-EC interactions are those involving β_2 or α_4 chains.

β_2 integrins

The β_2 integrins consist of LFA-1 ($\alpha_L\beta_2$, CD11a/CD18), Mac-1 ($\alpha_M\beta_2$, CD11b/CD18) and p150,95 ($\alpha_x\beta_2$, CD11c/CD18)[79,80]. β_2 integrins are not only central to the migratory capacity of leukocytes but also play key roles in many other leukocyte functions.

The importance of the β_2 integrins is demonstrated by the widespread abnormalities of leukocyte migration and function in Leukocyte Adhesion Deficiency (LAD) in which β_2 integrins are absent or markedly reduced on account of genetic abnormalities in processing the β_2 subunit[81,82]. This syndrome is typified by the inability of neutrophils to migrate from the bloodstream into inflamed tissues resulting in greatly enhanced susceptibility to bacterial infections.

The effects of LAD can be reproduced *in vitro* and *in vivo* using monoclonal antibodies against the common β_2 subunit or against individual α chains[80]. Using this approach, it is possible to demonstrate a role of β_2 integrins in the adhesion to EC of neutrophils[83,84], eosinophils[85], basophils[86], monocytes[87,88] and lymphocytes[89,90].

$\alpha4$ integrins

The integrins that make up the VLA subfamily mainly bind components of extracellular matrix such as fibronectin, laminin and collagens[91]. An exception is VL-4 ($\alpha_4\beta_1$) which in addition to binding fibronectin can also adhere to the cell surface molecule VCAM-1 (see below)[92]. Recent evidence indicates that a novel integrin composed of α_4 and another β chain, β_7, can also bind VCAM-1[93]. The relative roles of $\alpha_4\beta_1$ and $\alpha_4\beta_7$ in mediating leukocyte adhesion to EC are not yet clear.

Immunoglobulin superfamily

Several members of the immunoglobulin gene superfamily play an important role in the mediation of cell–cell adhesion events[94]. These include intercellular adhesion molecules 1, 2 and 3 (ICAM-1, ICAM-2), vascular cell adhesion molecule 1 (VCAM-1) and PECAM-1 (CD31). Each are single chain glycoproteins containing a variable number of repeats of an immunoglobulin-like domain (Figure 3).

ICAM-1

ICAM-1 is a widely distributed molecule appearing on many cell types including leukocytes, lymphocytes, fibroblasts, keratinocytes and dendritic cells as well as EC[95]. It has five immunoglobulin (Ig) domains, each containing 90–100 amino acids, and which are arranged in linear fashion[96]. ICAM-1

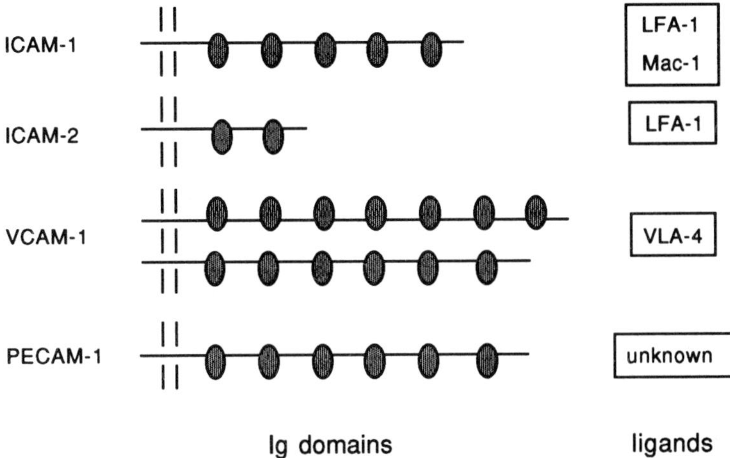

Figure 3 Immunoglobulin-like molecules on EC

binds the leukocyte integrin LFA-1 via the two Ig domains (1 and 2) nearest the N-terminal[96] and binds the integrin Mac-1 by a distinct site on the third Ig domain[97].

ICAM-1 binding is not the exclusive preserve of LFA-1 and Mac-1 as a number of other ligands have been described including the surface glyco-protein sialophorin (also called leukosialin or CD43)[98], major group rhino-virus serotypes[99,100], and *Plasmodium falciparum* infected erythrocytes[101]. The binding sites for LFA-1, rhinovirus and *P. falciparum* infected erythro-cytes are distinct but overlap[96,102–103].

Although ICAM-1 is modestly expressed on unstimulated EC, expression can be upregulated by IL-1, TNF, LPS or interferon gamma[26,29]. In normal tissues endothelial cells are the predominant cell type expressing ICAM-1[95,104,105]. In inflamed tissues ICAM-1 is found on infiltrating macrophages and lymphocytes as well as on specialized resident cells. For example, in inflamed synovium ICAM-1 is widely expressed by synovial fibroblasts[106], whereas chronically inflamed skin is characterized by expres-sion of ICAM-1 on keratinocytes and dermal interstitial cells[50,107,108].

ICAM-2

ICAM-2 is a smaller molecule than ICAM-1, having two rather than five Ig domains. These two domains have a high (34%) homology with the terminal domains 1 and 2 of ICAM-1[109], and bind LFA-1 but probably not Mac-1. ICAM-2 has a higher constitutive expression on EC than ICAM-1 and may therefore be the predominant LFA-1 ligand on endothelium in uninflamed tissues. However, unlike with ICAM-1, the expression of ICAM-2 does not appear to be regulated by cytokines and the upregulation of ICAM-1 expression is sufficient to make ICAM-1 the more abundant molecule on cytokine activated endothelium[109–111].

VCAM-1

Although vascular cell adhesion molecule-1 (VCAM-1, also designated INCAM-110) was originally described as containing six Ig domains[112], the majority of VCAM-1 transcripts have an additional Ig domain placed between domains three and four of the six domain form[113–115]. Whilst N-terminal determinants on both six domain (6D) and seven domain (7D) VCAM-1 can bind the α_4 integrin VLA-4, the 7D form has an additional VLA-4 binding site on the extra central Ig domain[116,117]. As either the N-terminal binding site or the central binding site can function in the absence of the other, both sites must be blocked in order fully to inhibit VLA-4–VCAM-1 interaction. This observation is of obvious importance in interpreting the results of mAb inhibition experiments involving anti-VCAM-1 monoclonal antibodies.

Expression of VCAM-1 on cultured EC is barely detectable on unstimulated EC, but is induced following stimulation with IL-1, TNFa, LPS and, to a lesser extent, IL-4[29,118,119]. As with cultured EC, there is little VCAM-1 expression on uninflamed vessels *in vivo*[120] but vascular expression can be found in inflamed skin[50,121], synovium[49,122], heart[123,124] and rectum[125]. Other cells that can be induced to express VCAM-1 include germinal centre and interdigitating dendritic cells, Kuppfer cells, renal epithelial and proximal tubular cells, bone marrow stromal cells and synovial lining type B cells[120,122,126–129].

By virtue of the restricted distribution of VLA-4 on lymphocytes and monocytes but not on neutrophils, VCAM-1 has been implicated as an EC determinant that may be particularly relevant to the evolution of chronic inflammatory infiltrates. This premise is supported by the relatively normal recruitment into inflammatory sites of β_2 integrin deficient monocytes and lymphocytes in LAD[130]. In contrast to E-selectin expression, there is also some evidence that VCAM-1 expression in skin may not be a ubiquitous manifestation of inflammation, but may be dependent upon cytokines released during immune-mediated inflammation[50,131].

PECAM-1

Platelet endothelial cell adhesion molecule-1 (PECAM-1, endoCAM, CD31) has six Ig domains and a molecular mass of approximately 135 kD[132–134]. It is expressed on a number of cell types including EC, platelets, neutrophils, monocytes and a subpopulation of T cells[135–137]. The expression of PECAM-1 is concentrated at junctions between adjacent EC[138,139], suggesting an important function in mediating intercellular interactions within endothelium. In support of this hypothesis, culture of EC in the presence of anti-CD31 monoclonal antibodies can inhibit the formation of tight intercellular junctions[138]. It has also been proposed that PECAM-1 may be involved in interactions between EC and migrating lymphocytes[137].

CD44

CD44 (HCAM, Pgp-1) is a highly polymorphic integral membrane protein of 90–260 kD with wide distribution on lymphocytes, monocytes, fibroblasts and epithelial cells as well as cells in the nervous system[140,141]. There is evidence emerging that CD44 can exist in a number of isoforms dependent both on alternative splicing of the gene[142–145] and on differential post-translational modification[146]. Isoforms of this molecule may therefore have a number of different functions. Ligands known to bind CD44 include hyaluronate, fibronectin and collagen type I[147–149].

Appreciation of the involvement of CD44 in lymphocyte–EC interactions stems from the characterization of the Hermes antigen in mediating binding of lymphocytes to endothelium of high endothelial venules (HEV) in the Stamper-Woodruff frozen section assay[150]. Jalkanen and colleagues have proposed that different epitopes on CD44 mediate organ-specific adhesion of lymphocytes to HEV in peripheral lymph nodes, mucosal lymph nodes and rheumatoid synovium[151]. There is evidence that CD44 can directly bind an endothelial 'addressin' with restricted distribution on mucosal lymph node HEV[152].

CONTROL OF LEUKOCYTE ADHESION AND MIGRATION

Current models of how adhesion molecules interact to mediate leukocyte-EC interactions invoke the cooperation of a number of the molecules outlined above, acting like relay runners on the road to leukocyte extravasation.

Role of selectins

Each of the selectins mediates early contact events between leukocytes and EC. Selectin-carbohydrate interactions, which do not require leukocyte activation, are thought to occur rapidly but to be of low-avidity. They probably therefore account for leukocyte rolling on the vessel wall under conditions of flow[153,154]. This process slows the passage of circulating leukocytes through inflammatory lesions and thereby exposes cells to activating signals delivered either by contact with EC or as soluble mediators. Rolling of neutrophils on P-selectin has been modelled under shear conditions by incorporation of P-selectin into lipid bilayers[155]. In this model, activation of leukocytes during rolling leads to immobilization of the leukocyte through the secondary involvement of leukocyte integrins (see below). It should be recognized that this sequence of events is better characterized for neutrophils than other leukocytes and that it is not yet established whether or not all leukocytes 'roll'. Furthermore, selectin-mediated leukocyte adhesion is not a prerequisite for transmigration through endothelium *in vitro*[156], suggesting that under pathological conditions of low blood flow this step may be by-passed.

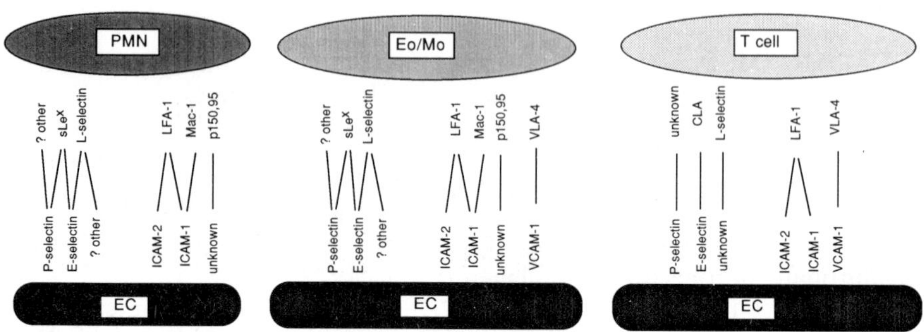

Figure 4 Comparison of molecules on neutrophils (PMN), eosinophils (Eo), monocytes (Mo) and T cells involved in adhesion to EC

Role of integrins

Antibodies against β_2 integrins do not inhibit leukocyte 'rolling' on endothelium under flow conditions either *in vitro* or *in vivo*[157,158]. Furthermore even under static conditions unstimulated freshly isolated lymphocytes show little integrin mediated adhesion to EC[159]. It is likely therefore that integrin mediated adhesion is a secondary event dependent upon appropriate stimulation of the avidity of leukocyte integrins during early contacts with EC.

A hallmark of leukocyte integrins is that they are expressed on the resting leukocyte in a low avidity state that does not effectively bind ligand. Leukocyte activation results in enhanced adhesiveness due in large part to an upregulation in integrin avidity[160–162]. This alteration in integrin avidity is thought to reflect an alteration in the conformation of the α and β subunits, probably in association with a change in the divalent cations bound to the metal binding domains close to the ligand binding sites[163–165]. Integrin avidity can be enhanced in this way by factors that stimulate the cell generally, implying a form of 'inside-out' signalling[160,166]. However, the avidity of LFA-1, Mac-1 and VLA-4 can also be stimulated directly by certain monoclonal antibodies, suggesting that contact of the adhesion molecules with their ligands may also lead to the appropriate conformational change for enhanced ligand binding[163,167–170].

Whilst there are a large number of ways of stimulating the function of leukocyte integrins *in vitro*, the actual factors responsible for this putative event *in vivo* are still poorly established. Besides differing in terms of phenotype of adhesion molecule expression (Figure 4), leukocytes show differences in responsiveness to activating factors, providing an additional way in which leukocytes can be selected into an inflammatory focus from the heterogeneous circulating pool within peripheral blood[171,172]. As discussed below, many factors capable of stimulating integrin function are synthesized by activated EC.

Role of endothelial cell activation

Perhaps the most central event in localizing an inflammatory event is the activation of endothelium. *In vitro* experiments indicate that EC can undergo different forms of activation each associated with increased expression of adhesion ligands for leukocytes.

As described above, the rapid translocation of P-selectin to the cell surface following stimulation of EC with histamine, thrombin or C5b-9 may be the first change in EC adhesivity during the evolution of an inflammatory response. Sub-acute and chronic inflammation is orchestrated by the effects of cytokines on EC, with IL-1 and TNF inducing or upregulating expression of E-selectin, VCAM-1 and ICAM-1[26,29]. It is also likely that in immune-mediated inflammation the effects of TNF and IL-1 are further regulated by the lymphokines interferon gamma and IL-4 which differentially alter the expression of E-selectin, VCAM-1 and ICAM-1[173-175]. For example, co-stimulation of EC with TNFα and IL-4 preferentially induces expression of VCAM-1[175] and enhances the relative adhesiveness of EC for lymphocytes compared to neutrophils[176].

In both rapid protein synthesis independent and delayed protein synthesis dependent forms of EC activation, the altered expression of adhesion molecules can be seen as part of more general pro-inflammatory responses which also include surface expression or secretion of factors capable of modulating the function of leukocyte integrins during the process of adhesion and migration[177,178].

Platelet activating factor (PAF) is expressed on the EC surface after stimulation with the same agonists which stimulate P-selectin expression and has been shown to upregulate neutrophil LFA-1 and Mac-1 avidity and increase responses to chemotactic agents[179,180]. A delayed expression of PAF is seen following *in vitro* stimulation of endothelial cells with IL-1 and TNF with production occurring after 2–8 hours in parallel with increased expression of E-selectin, VCAM-1 and ICAM-1[181,182].

Besides PAF, IL-1 or TNF stimulate EC to synthesize a number of other factors capable of regulating leukocyte function and survival in the tissues including macrophage chemotactic and activating factor, colony stimulating factors (G-CSF, M-CSF and GM-CSF), interleukin-6, and interleukin-8 (IL-8)[177,183,184]. IL-8 may be released into the fluid phase or deposited on the abluminal surface of the endothelium[185,186]. This pattern of deposition has lead to the proposal that IL-8 plays a key role in the directional movement of neutrophils into the tissues[186].

The mechanisms whereby endothelial cell activation is downregulated are largely unknown. There is, however, evidence that transforming growth factor β (TGFβ) has the capacity to inhibit the IL-1 or TNF enhanced adhesiveness for neutrophils and lymphocytes[187,188]. In view of the abundance of this cytokine in chronic inflammatory lesions, this may be an important mechanism for the suppression of acute inflammatory processes.

TRANSMIGRATION

Following adhesion to the luminal surface of EC, leukocytes pass between EC into the tissues. This transmigration process can be studied *in vitro* using EC monolayers cultured on synthetic filters, on collagen gels or on amniotic membranes[189-192]. Two lines of evidence point to the particular importance of CD18-dependent mechanisms in leukocyte transmigration. Firstly, transmigration is inhibited in the presence of anti-β_2 integrin monoclonal antibodies and, secondly, β_2 integrin deficient leukocytes from patients with LAD fail to transmigrate *in vitro* or *in vivo*[193-195]. Inhibition of β_2 integrin function also inhibits migration of monocytes[33] and T lymphocytes[196,197]. During transmigration, leukocyte β_2 integrins are believed to interact with ICAM-1 molecules located on the luminal, lateral and basal surfaces of EC[198]. In contrast, VCAM-1 expression is restricted to the luminal surface of EC and this molecule may be less involved in transmigration than in initial adhesion events[33,198].

ACCESSORY CELL FUNCTION OF ENDOTHELIAL CELLS

A specialized function of particular interest to the immunologist is the possible involvement of EC in the activation of lymphocytes either as fully competent antigen presenting cells (APC) or as accessory cells capable of co-stimulating lymphocyte proliferation in response to other initiating signals. To date most of the evidence in support of EC acting in either way comes from *in vitro* experiments, and many of these have been criticized for utilizing T cell and/or EC cultures in which the presence of small but significant numbers of contaminating monocytes or dendritic cells has not been rigorously excluded. This subject has recently been reviewed in detail elsewhere[199].

The expression of histocompatibility antigens by EC is obviously a prerequisite for their putative role as APC. Cultured EC express HLA class I antigens constitutively, with expression being upregulated by TNF, by interferon gamma or by interferon α/β[200,201]. In contrast, HLA Class II molecules are not expressed by resting cultured HUVEC but are inducible by interferon gamma[202,203]. In contrast to the lack of constitutive expression of HLA Class II by cultured EC, immunocytochemical staining shows constitutive expression of HLA-DR expression in the microcirculation of many organs including skin, kidney and heart[124,204,205]. It has been proposed that this 'constitutive' expression is dependent upon on-going activation by lymphokines[206].

CONCLUSION

Clearly the molecules involved in leukocyte migration present potentially important targets for therapeutic intervention in autoimmune disease[207,208]. It is worth stressing that inhibition of leukocyte adhesion molecules may be therapeutically effective not only in inhibiting leukocyte traffic into inflammatory lesions but also in suppressing leukocyte activation. In the case of lymphocytes, it is also possible that inhibition of adhesion molecule function may critically reduce the co-stimulation required for activation and result in tolerance to antigen[209,210].

Studies are currently in progress in a number of laboratories exploring ways of inhibiting each of the molecules discussed in this chapter, *in vivo* using animal models. There are already very encouraging results both with monoclonal antibodies[210-215] and with recombinant proteins[216]. Data obtained from these studies can be expected to lead the way to inhibiting leukocyte traffic in the clinical setting.

References

1. Springer TA. Adhesion receptors of the immune system. Nature. 1990; 346: 425–434.
2. Jaffe EA. Endothelial Cells. In: Gallin JI, Goldstein IM, Snyderman R, eds. Inflammation: Basic Principles and Clinical Correlates. New York: Raven Press; 1988; 559–576.
3. Cotran RS. Endothelial Cells. In: Kelley WN, Harris EDJ, Ruddy S, Sledge CB, eds. Textbook of Rheumatology. Philadelphia: WB Saunders; 1989: 389–415.
4. Jaffe EA, Nachman RL, Becker CG, Minick CR. Culture of human endothelial cells derived from umbilical veins. J Clin Invest. 1973; 52: 2745–2756.
5. Jackson CJ, Garbett PT, Marks RM, Chapman G, Sonnabend DH, Potter SR, Brooks PM, Schrieber L. Isolation and propagation of endothelial cells derived from rheumatoid synovial microvasculature. Ann Rheum Dis. 1989; 48: 733–736.
6. Jackson CJ, Garbett PK, Nissen B, Schrieber L. Binding of human endothelium to Ulex europeus 1-coated Dynabeads: application to the isolation of microvascular endothelium. J Cell Sci. 1990; 96: 257–262.
7. Watson ML, Kingsmore SF, Johnston GI, Siegelman MH, Le Beau MM, Lemons RS, Bora NS, Howard TA, Weissman IL, McEver RP, Seldin MF. Genomic organization of the selectin family of leukocyte adhesion molecules on human and mouse chromosome 1. J Exp Med. 1990; 172: 263–272.
8. Hsu-Lin S-C, Berman CL, Furie BC, August D, Furie B. A platelet membrane protein expressed during platelet activation and secretion. Studies using a monoclonal antibody specific for thrombin-activated platelets. J Biol Chem. 1984; 259: 9799.
9. McEver RP, Martin MN. A monoclonal antibody to a membrane glycoprotein binds only to activated platelets. J Biol Chem. 1984; 259: 9799.
10. Stenberg PE, McEver RP, Shuman MA, Jacques YV, Bainton DF. A platelet alpha-granule membrane protein (GMP-140) is expressed on the plasma membrane after activation. J Cell Biol. 1985; 101: 880–886.
11. Berman CL, Yeo EL, Wencel-Drake JD, Furie BC, Ginsberg MH, Furie B. A platelet alpha granule membrane protein that is associated with the plasma membrane after activation. J Clin Invest. 1986; 78: 130–137.
12. Bonfanti R, Furie BC, Furie B, Wagner DD. PADGEM (GMP-140) is a component of Weibel-Palade bodies of human endothelial cells. Blood. 1989; 73: 1109.
13. McEver RP, Beckstead JH, Moore KL, Marshall-Carlson L, Bainton DF. GMP-140, a platelet α-granule membrane protein, is also synthesized by vascular endothelial cells and is localized in Weibel-Palade bodies. J Clin Invest. 1989; 83: 92–99.
14. Koedam JA, Cramer EM, Briend E, Furie B, Furie BC, Wagner DD. P-Selectin, a granule membrane protein of platelets and endothelial cells, follows the regulated secretory pathway in AtT-20 cells. J Cell Biol. 1992; 116: 617–625.
15. Hattori R, Hamilton KK, Fugate RD, McEver RD, Sims PJ. Stimulated secretion of endothelial von Willebrand factor is accompanied by rapid redistribution to the cell surface of the intracellular granule membrane protein GMP-140. J Biol Chem. 1989; 264: 7768–7771.
16. Hattori R, Hamilton KK, McEver RP, Sims PJ. Complement proteins C5b-9 induce secretion of high molecular weight multimers of endothelial von Willebrand factor and translocation of granule membrane protein GMP-140 to the cell surface. J Biol Chem. 1989; 264: 9053–9060.
17. Geng J-G, Bevilacqua MP, Moore KL, McIntyre TM, Prescott SM, Kim JM, Bliss GA, Zimmerman GA, McEver RP. Rapid neutrophil adhesion to activated endothelium mediated by GMP-140. Nature. 1990; 343: 757–760.

18. Patel KD, Zimmerman GA, Prescott SM, McEver RP, McIntyre TM. Oxygen radicals induce human endothelial cells to express GMP-140 and bind neutrophils. J Cell Biol. 1991; 112: 749–759.
19. Larsen E, Celi A, Gilbert GE, Furie BC, Erban JK, Bonfanti R, Wagner DD, Furie B. PADGEM protein: a receptor that mediates the interaction of activated platelets with neutrophils and monocytes. Cell. 1989; 59: 305–312.
20. Toothill VJ, van Mourik JA, Niewenhuis HK, Metzelaar MJ, Pearson JD. Characterization of the enhanced adhesion of neutrophil leukocytes to thrombin-stimulated endothelial cells. J Immunol. 1990; 1450: 283–291.
21. Hamburger SA, McEver RP. GMP-140 mediates adhesion of stimulated platelets to neutrophils. Blood. 1990; 75: 550–554.
22. Moore KL, Thompson LF. P-Selectin (CD62) binds to subpopulations of human memory T lymphocytes and natural killer cells. Biochem Biophys Res Commun. 1992; 186: 173–181.
23. Damle NK, Klussman K, Dietsch MT, Mohagheghpour N, Aruffo A. GMP-140 (P-selectin/CD62) binds to chronically stimulated but not resting CD4+ T lymphocytes and regulates their production of proinflammatory cytokines. Eur J Immunol. 1992; 22: 1789–1793.
24. Bevilacqua MP, Pober JS, Mendrick DL, Cotran RS, Gimbrone MA. Identification of an inducible endothelial-leukocyte adhesion molecule. Proc Natl Acad Sci USA. 1987; 84: 9238–9242.
25. Bevilacqua MP, Stengelin S, Gimbrone MA, Seed B. Endothelial leukocyte adhesion molecule 1: an inducible receptor for neutrophils related to complement regulatory proteins and lectins. Science. 1989; 243: 1160–1164.
26. Pober JS, Gimbrone MA, Lapierre LA, Mendrick DL, Fiers W, Rothlein R, Springer TA. Overlapping patterns of activation of human endothelial cells by interleukin 1, tumour necrosis factor, and immune interferon. J Immunol. 1986; 137: 1893–1896.
27. Pober JS, Bevilacqua MP, Mendrick DL, Lapierre LA, Fiers W, Gimbrone MA. Two distinct monokines, interleukin 1 and tumor necrosis factor, each independently induce the biosynthesis and transient expression of the same antigen on the surface of cultured human vascular endothelial cells. J Immunol. 1986; 136: 1680–1687.
28. Pober JS, Lapierre LA, Stolpen AH, Brock TA, Springer TA, Fiers W, Bevilacqua MP, Mendrick DL, Gimbrone MA. Activation of cultured human endothelial cells by recombinant lymphotoxin: comparison with tumour necrosis factor and interleukin-1 species. J Immunol. 1987; 138: 3319–3324.
29. Wellicome SM, Thornhill MH, Pitzalis C, Thomas DS, Lanchbury JSS, Panayi GS, Haskard DO. A monoclonal antibody that detects a novel antigen on endothelial cells that is induced by tumor necrosis factor, IL-1 or lipopolysaccharide. J Immunol. 1990; 144: 2558–2565.
30. Kyan-Aung U, Haskard DO, Poston RN, Thornhill MH, Lee TH. Endothelial leukocyte adhesion molecule-1 and intercellular adhesion molecule-1 mediate the adhesion of eosinophils to endothelial cells in vitro and are expressed by endothelium in allergic cutaneous inflammation in vivo. J Immunol. 1991; 146: 521–528.
31. Bochner BS, Luskinskas GW, Fimbrone MAJ, Newman W, Sterbinsky SA, Derse-Anthony CP, Klunk D, Schleimer RP. Adhesion of human basophils, eosinophils, and neutrophils to IL-1-activated human vascular endothelial cells: contributions of endothelial cell adhesion molecules. J Exp Med. 1991; 173: 1553–1556.
32. Carlos T, Kovach N, Schwartz B, Rosa M, Newman B, Wayner E, Benjamin C, Osborn L, Lobb R, Harlan J. Human monocytes bind to two cytokine-induced adhesive ligands on cultured human endothelial cells: Endothelial-leukocyte adhesion molecule-1 and vascular cell adhesion molecule-1. Blood. 1991; 77: 2266–2271.
33. Hakkert BC, Kuijpers TW, Leeuwenberg JFM, van Mourik JA, Roos D. Neutrophil and monocyte adherence to and migration across monolayers of cytokine-activated endothelial cells: The contribution of CD18, ELAM-1, and VLA-4. Blood. 1991; 78: 2721–2726.
34. Graber N, Gopal TV, Wilson D, Beall LD, Polte T, Newman W. T cells bind to cytokine-activated endothelial cells via a novel, inducible sialoglycoprotein and endothelial leukocyte adhesion molecule-1. J Immunol. 1990; 145: 819–830.
35. Lobb RR, Chi-Rosso G, Leone DR, Rosa MD, Bixler S, Newman BM, Luhowskyj S, Benjamin CD, Dougas IG, Goelz SE, Hession C, Chow EP. Expression and functional

characterization of a soluble form of endothelial-leukocyte adhesion molecule 1. J Immunol. 1991; 147: 124–129.

36. Shimizu Y, Shaw S, Graber N, Gopal TV, Horgan KJ, Van Seventer GA, Newman W. Activation-independent binding of human memory T cells to adhesion molecule ELAM-1. Nature. 1991; 349: 799–802.

37. Picker LJ, Kishimoto TK, Smith CW, Warnock RA, Butcher EC. ELAM-1 is an adhesion molecule for skin-homing T cells. Nature. 1991; 349: 796–799.

38. Duijvestijn AM, Horst E, Pals ST, Rouse BN, Steere AC, Picker LJ, Meijer CJLM, Butcher EC. High endothelial differentiation in human lymphoid and inflammatory tissues defined by monoclonal antibody HECA-452. Am J Pathol. 1988; 130: 147–155.

39. Picker LJ, Michie SA, Rott LS, Butcher EC. A unique phenotype of skin-associated lymphocytes in humans. Preferential expression of the HECA-452 epitope by benign and malignant T cells at cutaneous sites. Am J Pathol. 1990; 136: 1053–1068.

40. Postigo AA, Garcia-Vicuña R, Diaz-Gonzalez F, Arroyo AG, De Landázuri MO, Chi-Rosso G, Lobb RR, Laffon A, Sánchez-Madrid F. Increased binding of synovial T lymphocytes from rheumatoid arthritis to endothelial-leukocyte adhesion molecule-1 (ELAM-1) and vascular cell adhesion molecule-1 (VCAM-1). J Clin Invest. 1992; 89: 1445–1452.

41. Cotran RS, Pober JS, Gimbrone MA, Springer TA, Wiebke EA, Gaspari AA, Rosenberg SA, Lotze MT. Endothelial activation during interleukin 2 immunotherapy: a possible mechanism for the vascular leak syndrome. J Immunol. 1987; 139: 1883–1888.

42. Leung DYM, Cotran RS, Kurt-Jones E, Burns JC, Newburger JW, Pober JS. Endothelial activation and high interleukin-1 secretion in the pathogenesis of acute Kawasaki disease. Lancet. 1989; 2: 1298–1302.

43. Groves RW, Allen MH, Haskard DO, Barker JNWN, MacDonald DM. Endothelial leukocyte adhesion molecule-1 (ELAM-1) expression in cutaneous inflammation. Br J Dermatol. 1991; 124: 117–123.

44. Leung DYM, Pober JS, Cotran RS. Expression of endothelial-leukocyte adhesion molecule-1 in elicited late phase allergic reactions. J Clin Invest. 1991; 87: 1805–1809.

45. Sollberg S, Peltonen J, Uitto J, Jimenez SA. Elevated expression of β_1 and β_2 integrins, intercellular adhesion molecule 1, and endothelial leukocyte adhesion molecule 1 in the skin of patients with systemic slcerosis of recent onset. Arthritis Rheum. 1992; 35: 290–298.

46. Ohtani H, Nakamura S, Watanabe Y, Fukushima K, Mizoi T, Kimura M, Hiwatashi N, Nagura H. Light and electron microscopic immunolocalization of endothelial leucocyte adhesion molecule-1 in inflammatory bowel disease. Morphological evidence of active synthesis and secretion into vascular lumen. Virchows Arch A Pathol Anat Histopathol. 1992; 420: 403–409.

47. Montefort S, Roche WR, Howarth PH, Djukanovic R, Gratziou C, Carroll M, Smith L, Britten KM, Haskard DO, Lee TH, Holgate ST. Intercellular adhesion molecule-1 (ICAM-1) and endothelial leukocyte adhesion molecule-1 (ELAM-1) expression in the bronchial mucosa of normal and asthmatic subjects. Eur Resp J. 1992; 5: 815–823.

48. Corkill MM, Kirkham BW, Haskard DO, Barbatis C, Gibson T, Panayi GS. Gold treatment of rheumatoid arthritis decreases synovial expression of the endothelial leukocyte adhesion receptor ELAM-1. J Rheumatol. 1991; 18: 1453–1460.

49. Koch AE, Burrows JC, Haines GK, Carlos TM, Harlan JM, Leibovich SJ. Immunolocalization of endothelial and leukocyte adhesion molecules in human rheumatoid and osteoarthritic synovial tissues. Lab Invest. 1991; 64: 313–320.

50. Norris P, Poston RN, Thomas DS, Thornhill M, Hawk J, Haskard DO. The expression of endothelial leukocyte adhesion molecule-1 (ELAM-1), intercellular adhesion molecule-1 (ICAM-1) and vascular cell adhesion molecule-1 (VCAM-1) in experimental cutaneous inflammation: a comparison of ultraviolet-B erythema and delayed hypersensitivity. J Invest Dermatol. 1991; 96: 763–770.

51. Gallatin WM, Weissman JL, Butcher EC. A cell-surface molecule involved in organ-specific homing of lymphocytes. Nature. 1983; 304: 30–34.

52. Lewinsohn DM, Bargatze RF, Butcher EC. Leukocyte-endothelial cell recognition: evidence of a common molecular mechanism shared by neutrophils, lymphocytes, and other leukocytes. J Immunol. 1987; 138: 4313–4321.

53. Tedder TF, Penta AC, Levine HB, Freedman AS. Expression of the human leukocyte

adhesion molecule, LAM1: Identity with the TQ1 and Leu-8 differentiation antigens. J Immunol. 1990; 144: 532–540.

54. Hallmann R, Jutila MA, Smith CW, Anderson DC, Kishimoto TK, Butcher EC. The peripheral lymph node homing receptor, LECAM-1, is involved in CD18-independent adhesion of human neutrophils to endothelium. Biochem Biophys Res Commun. 1991; 174: 236–243.

55. Smith CW, Kishimoto TK, Abbass O, Hughes B, Rothlein R, McIntire LV, Butcher E, Anderson DC. Chemotactic factors regulate lectin adhesion molecule 1 (LECAM-1)-dependent neutrophil adhesion to cytokine-stimulated endothelial cells in vitro. J Clin Invest. 1991; 87: 609–618.

56. Spertini O, Luscinskas FW, Kansas GS, Munro JM, Griffin JD, Gimbrone MA, Jr., Tedder TF. Leukocyte adhesion molecule-1 (LAM-1, L-selectin) interacts with an inducible endothelial cell ligand to support leukocyte adhesion. J Immunol. 1991; 147: 2565–2573.

57. Spertini O, Luscinskas FW, Gimbrone MA, Jr., Tedder TF. Monocyte attachment to activated human vascular endothelium in vitro is mediated by leukocyte adhesion molecule-1 (L-selectin) under nonstatic conditions. J Exp Med. 1992; 175: 1789–1792.

58. Foxall C, Watson SR, Dowbenko D, Fennie C, Lasky LA, Kiso M, Hasegawa A, Asa D, Brandley BK. The three members of the selectin receptor family recognize a common carbohydrate epitope, the sialyl Lewis^x oligosaccharide. J Cell Biol. 1992; 117: 895–902.

59. Berg EL, Magnani J, Warnock RA, Robinson MK, Butcher EC. Comparison of L-selectin and E-selectin ligand specificities: The L-selectin can bind the E-selectin ligands sialyl Le^x and sialyl Le^a. Biochem Biophys Res Commun. 1992; 184: 1048–1055.

60. Walz G, Aruffo A, Kolanus W, Bevilacqua M, Seed B. Recognition of ELAM-1 of the Sialyl-Le^x determinant on myeloid and tumour cells. Science. 1990; 250: 1132–1135.

61. Phillips ML, Nudelman E, Gaeta FCA, Perez M, Singhal AK, Kakomori S-I, Paulson JC. ELAM-1 mediates cell adhesion by recognition of a carbohydrate ligand, Sialyl-Le^x. Science. 1990; 250: 1130–1132.

62. Lowe JB, Stoolman LM, Nair RP, Larsen RD, Berhend TL, Marks RM. ELAM-1 dependent cell adhesion to vascular endothelium determined by a transfected human fucosyltransferase cDNA. Cell. 1990; 63: 475–484.

63. Goelz SE, Hession C, Goff D, Griffiths B, Tizard R, Newman B, Chi-Rosso G, Lobb R. ELFT: A gene that directs the expression of an ELAM-1 ligand. Cell. 1990; 61: 1303–1313.

64. Kishimoto TK, Warnock RA, Jutila MA, Butcher EC, Lane C, Anderson DC, Smith CW. Antibodies against human neutrophil LECAM-1 (LAM-1/Leu-8/DREG-56 antigen) and endothelial cell ELAM-1 inhibit a common CD18-independent adhesion pathway in vitro. Blood. 1991; 78: 805–811.

65. Picker LJ, Warnock RA, Burns AR, Doerschuk CM, Berg EL, Butcher EC. The neutrophil selectin LECAM-1 presents carbohydrate ligands to the vascular selectins ELAM-1 and GMP-140. Cell. 1991; 66: 921–933.

66. Kuijpers TW, Hoogerwerf M, van der Laan LJW, Nagel G, van der Schoot CE, Grunert F, Roos D. CD66 nonspecific cross-reacting antigens are involved in neutrophil adherence to cytokine-activated endothelial cells. J Cell Biol. 1992; 118: 457–466.

67. Berg EL, Yoshino T, Rott LS, Robinson MK, Warnock RA, Kishimoto TK, Picker LJ, Butcher EC. The cutaneous lymphocyte antigen is a skin lymphocyte homing receptor for the vascular lectin endothelial cell-leukocyte adhesion molecule 1. J Exp Med. 1991; 174: 1461–1466.

68. Handa K, Nudelman ED, Stroud MR, Shiozawa T, Hakomori S. Selectin GMP-140 (CD62; PADGEM) binds to sialosyl-Le^a and sialosyl-Le^x, and sulfated glycans modulate this binding. Biochem Biophys Res Commun. 1991; 181: 1223–1230.

69. Polley MJ, Phillips ML, Wayner E, Nudelman E, Singhal AK, Hakomori S, Paulson JC. CD62 and endothelial cell-leukocyte adhesion molecule 1 (ELAM-1) recognize the same carbohydrate ligand, sialyl-Lewis x. Proc Natl Acad Sci USA. 1991; 88: 6224–6228.

70. Zhou Q, Moore KL, Smith DF, Varki A, McEver RP, Cummings RD. The selectin GMP-140 binds to sialylated, fucosylated lactosaminoglycans on both myeloid and nonmyeloid cells. J Cell Biol. 1992; 115: 557–564.

71. Aruffo A, Kolanus W, Walz G, Fredman P, Seed B. CD62/P-Selectin recognition of myeloid and tumour cell sulfatides. Cell. 1991; 67: 35–44.

72. Lasky LA, Singer MS, Dowbenko D, Imai Y, Henzel WJ, Grimley C, Fennie C, Gillett N,

Watson SR, Rosen SD. An endothelial ligand for L-selectin is a novel mucin-like molecule. Cell. 1992; 69: 927–938.

73. Lasky LA. Lectin cell adhesion molecules (LEC-CAMs): A new family of cell adhesion proteins involved with inflammation. J Cell Biochem. 1991; 45: 139–146.

74. Hynes RO. Integrins: Versatility, modulation, and signaling in cell adhesion. Cell. 1992; 69: 11–25.

75. D'Souza SE, Ginsberg MH, Burke TA, Plow EF. The ligand binding site of the platelet integrin receptor GPIIb-IIIa is proximal to the second calcium binding domain of its α subunit. J Biol Chem. 1990; 265: 3440–3446.

76. D'Souza SE, Ginsberg MH, Burke TA, Lam SC-T, Plow EF. Localization of an Arg-Gly-Asp recognition site within an integrin adhesion receptor. Science. 1988; 242: 91–93.

77. Smith JW, Cheresh DA. The Arg-Gly-Asp binding domain of the vitronectin receptor. Photoaffinity cross-linking implicates amino-acid residues 61-203 of the β subunit. J Biol Chem. 1988; 263: 18726–18731.

78. Smith JW, Cheresh DA. Integrin ($\alpha_v\beta_3$)-ligand interaction. J Biol Chem. 1990; 265: 2168–2172.

79. Kishimoto TK, Larson RS, Corbi AL, Dustin ML, Staunton DE, Springer TA. The leukocyte integrins. Adv Immunol. 1989; 46: 149–182.

80. Arnaout MA. Structure and function of the leukocyte adhesion molecules CD11/CD18. Blood. 1990; 75: 1037–1050.

81. Anderson DC, Schmalstieg F, Finegold MJ, Hughes BJ, Rothlein R, Miller LJ, Kohl S, Tosi MF, Jacobs RL, Waldrop TC, Goldman AS, Shearer WT, Springer TA. The severe and moderate phenotypes of heritable Mac-1, LFA-1 deficiency: their quantitative definition and relation to leukocyte dysfunction and clinical features. J Infect Dis. 1985; 152: 668–689.

82. Arnaout MA. Leukocyte adhesion molecules deficiency: its structural basis, pathophysiology and implications for modulating the inflammatory response. Immunological reviews. 1990; 114: 145–179.

83. Harlan JM, Killen PD, Senecal FM, Schwartz BR, Yee EK, Taylor RF, Beatty PG, Price TH, Ochs HD. The role of neutrophil membrane glycoprotein GP-150 in neutrophil adherence to endothelium in vitro. Blood. 1985; 66: 167–178.

84. Tonneson MG, Anderson DC, Springer TA, Knedler A, Avdi N, Henson PM. Adherence of neutrophils to cultured human microvascular endothelial cells. J Clin Invest. 1989; 83: 637–646.

85. Lamas AM, Mulroney CM, Schleimer RP. Studies on the adhesive interaction between purified human eosinophils and cultured vascular endothelial cells. J Immunol. 1988; 140: 1500–1505.

86. Bochner BS, Peachell PT, Brown KE, Schleimer RP. Adherence of basophils to cultured umbilical vein endothelial cells. J Clin Invest. 1988; 81: 1355–1364.

87. Wallis WJ, Beatty PG, Ochs HD, Harlan JM. Human monocyte adherence to cultured vascular endothelium: monoclonal antibody-defined mechanisms. J Immunol. 1985; 135: 2323–2330.

88. Keizer GD, Te Velde A, Schwarting R, Figdor CG, De Vries JE. Role of p150,95 in adhesion, migration, chemotaxis and phagocytosis of human monocytes. Eur J Immunol. 1987; 17: 1317–1322.

89. Mentzer SJ, Burakoff SJ, Faller DV. Adhesion of T lymphocytes to human endothelial cells is regulated by the LFA-1 membrane molecule. J Cell Physiol. 1986; 126: 285–290.

90. Haskard DO, Cavender DE, Beatty P, Springer TA, Ziff M. T cell adhesion to endothelial cells: mechanisms demonstrated by anti-LFA-1 monoclonal antibodies. J Immunol. 1986; 137: 2901–2906.

91. Hemler ME. VLA proteins in the integrin family: Structures, functions, and their role on leukocytes. Ann Rev Immunol. 1990; 8: 365–400.

92. Elices MJ, Osborn L, Takada Y, Crouse C, Luhowsky S, Hemler ME, Lobb RR. VCAM-1 on activated endothelium interacts with the leukocyte integrin VLA-4 at a site distinct from the VLA-4/fibronectin binding site. Cell. 1990; 60: 577–584.

93. Rüegg C, Postigo AA, Sikorski EE, Butcher EC, Pytela R, Erle DJ. Role of integrin $\alpha_4\beta_7/\alpha_4\beta_P$ in lymphocyte adherence to fibronectin and VCAM-1 and in homotypic cell clustering. J Cell Biol. 1992; 117: 179–189.

94. Williams AF, Barclay AN. The immunoglobulin superfamily-domains for cell surface recognition. Ann Rev Immunol. 1988; 6: 381–405.
95. Dustin ML, Rothlein R, Bhan AK, Dinarello CA, Springer TA. Induction by IL-1 and interferon gamma: tissue distribution, biochemistry, and function of a natural adherence molecule (ICAM-1). J Immunol. 1986; 137: 245–254.
96. Staunton DE, Dustin ML, Erickson HP, Springer TA. The arrangement of the immunoglobulin-like domains of ICAM-1 and the binding sites for LFA-1. Cell. 1990; 61: 243–254.
97. Diamond MS, Staunton DE, Marlin SD, Springer TA. Binding of the integrin Mac-1 (CD11b/CD18) to the third immunoglobulin-like domain of ICAM-1 (CD54) and its regulation by glycosylation. Cell. 1991; 65: 961–971.
98. Rosenstein Y, Park JK, Hahn WC, Rosen FS, Bierer BE, Burakoff SJ. CD43, a molecule defective in Wiskott-Aldrich syndrome, binds ICAM-1. Nature. 1991; 354: 233–235.
99. Staunton DE, Merluzzi VJ, Rothlein R, Barton R, Marlin SD, Springer TA. A cell adhesion molecule, ICAM-1, is the major surface receptor for rhinoviruses. Cell. 1989; 56: 849–853.
100. Greve JM, Davis G, Meyer AM, Forte CP, Yost SC, Marlor CW, Kamarck ME, McClelland A. The major human rhinovirus receptor is ICAM-1. Cell. 1989; 56: 839–847.
101. Berendt AR, Simmons D, Tansey J, Newbold CI, Marsh K. Intercellular adhesion molecule-1 is an endothelial cell adhesion receptor for *Plasmodium falciparum*. Nature. 1989; 341: 57–59.
102. Berendt AR, McDowall A, Craig AG, Bates PA, Sternberg MJE, Marsh K, Newbold CI, Hogg N. The binding site on ICAM-1 for *Plasmodium falciparum*-infected erythrocytes overlaps, but is distinct from, the LFA-1-binding site. Cell. 1992; 68: 71–81.
103. Ockenhouse CF, Betageri R, Springer TA, Staunton DE. *Plasmodium falciparum*-infected erythrocytes bind ICAM-1 at a site distinct from LFA-1, Mac-1 and human rhinovirus. Cell. 1992; 68: 63–69.
104. Smith MEF, Thomas JA. Cellular expression of lymphocyte function associated antigens and the intercellular adhesion molecule-1 in normal tissue. J Clin Pathol. 1990; 43: 893–900.
105. Fairburn K, Kunaver M, Wilkinson LS, Cambridge G, Haskard DO, Edwards JCW. Intercellular adhesion molecules in normal synovium. Br J Rheumatol. 1992; 32: 302–306
106. Hale LP, Martin ME, McCollum DE, Nunley JA, Springer TA, Singer KH, Haynes BF. Immunohistologic analysis of the distribution of cell adhesion molecules within the inflammatory synovial microenvironment. Arthritis Rheum. 1989; 32: 22–30.
107. Vejlsgaard GL, Ralfkiaer E, Avnstorp C, Czajkowski M, Marlin SD, Rothlein R. Kinetics and characterization of intercellular adhesion molecule-1 (ICAM-1) expression on keratinocytes in various inflammatory skin lesions and malignant cutaneous lymphomas. J Am Acad Dermatol. 1989; 20: 782–790.
108. Barker JNWN, Allen MH, MacDonald DM. The effect of in vivo interferon-gamma on the distribution of LFA-1 and ICAM-1 in normal human skin. J Invest Dermatol. 1989; 93: 439–442.
109. Staunton DE, Dustin ML, Springer TA. Functional cloning of ICAM-2, a cell adhesion ligand for LFA-1 homologous to ICAM-1. Nature. 1989; 339: 61–64.
110. De Fougerolles AR, Stacker SA, Schwarting R, Springer TA. Characterization of ICAM-2 and evidence for a third counter-receptor for LFA-1. J Exp Med. 1991; 174: 253–267.
111. Nortamo P, Li R, Renkonen R, Timonen T, Prieto J, Patarroyo M, Gahmberg CG. The expression of human intercellular adhesion molecule-2 is refractory to inflammatory cytokines. Eur J Immunol. 1991; 21: 2629–2632.
112. Osborn L, Hession C, Tizard R, Vassallo C, Luhowskyj S, Chi-Rosso G, Lobb R. Direct expression cloning of vascular cell adhesion molecule 1 (VCAM1), a cytokine-induced endothelial protein that binds to lymphocytes. Cell. 1989; 59: 1203–1211.
113. Polte T, Newman W, Raghunathan G, Venkat Gopal T. Structural and functional studies of full-length vascular cell adhesion molecule-1: Internal duplication and homology to several adhesion proteins. DNA Cell Biol. 1991; 10: 349–357.
114. Hession C, Tizard R, Vassallo C, Schiffer SB, Goff D, Moy P, Chi-Rosso G, Luhowskyj S, Lobb R, Osborn L. Cloning of an alternate form of vascular cell adhesion molecule-1 (VCAM1). J Biol Chem. 1991; 266: 6682–6685.
115. Cybulsky MI, Fries JWU, Williams AJ, Sultan P, Davis VM, Gimbrone MA, Jr., Collins T. Alternative splicing of human VCAM-1 in activated vascular endothelium. Am J Pathol.

1991; 138: 815–820.
116. Vonderheide RH, Springer TA. Lymphocyte adhesion through very late antigen 4: Evidence for a novel binding site in the alternatively spliced domain of vascular cell adhesion molecule 1 and an additional α_4 integrin counter-receptor on stimulated endothelium. J Exp Med. 1992; 175: 1433–1442.
117. Osborn L, Vassallo C, Benjamin CD. Activated endothelium binds lymphocytes through a novel binding site in the alternately spliced domain of vascular cell adhesion molecule-1. J Exp Med. 1992; 176: 99–107.
118. Rice GE, Bevilacqua MP. An inducible endothelial cell surface glycoprotein mediates melanoma adhesion. Science. 1989; 246: 1303–1306.
119. Thornhill M, Kyan-Aung U, Haskard DO. Interleukin-4 increases human endothelial cell adhesiveness for T cells but not for neutrophils. J Immunol. 1990; 144: 3060–3065.
120. Rice GE, Munro JM, Corless C, Bevilacqua MP. Vascular and nonvascular expression of INCAM-110: A target for mononuclear leukocyte adhesion in normal and inflamed human tissues. Am J Pathol. 1991; 138: 385–393.
121. Rice GE, Munro JM, Bevilacqua MP. Inducible cell adhesion molecule 110 (INCAM-110) is an inducible endothelial cell receptor for lymphocytes. J Exp Med. 1990; 171: 1369–1374.
122. Wilkinson LS, Poston RN, Edwards J, Haskard DO. Expression of vascular cell adhesion molecule-1 (VCAM-1) in normal and inflamed synovium. Lab Invest. 1992; 68: 82–88
123. Briscoe DM, Schoen FJ, Rice GE, Bevilacqua MP, Ganz P, Pober JS. Induced expression of endothelial-leukocyte adhesion molecules in human cardiac allografts. Transplantation. 1991; 51: 537–539.
124. Page C, Rose M, Yacoub M, Pigott R. Antigenic heterogeneity of vascular endothelium. Am J Pathol. 1992; 141: 673–683.
125. Norton J, Sloane JP, Al-Saffar N, Haskard DO. Expression of adhesion molecules in human gastrointestinal graft-versus-host disease. Clin Exper Immunol. 1992; 87: 231–236.
126. Freedman AS, Munro JM, Rice GE, Bevilacqua MP, Morimoto C, McIntyre BW, Rhynhart K, Pober JS, Nadler LM. Adhesion of human B cells to germinal centers in vitro involves VLA-4 and INCAM-110. Science. 1990; 249: 1030–1032.
127. Seron D, Cameron JS, Haskard DO. Expression of VCAM-1 in the normal and diseased kidney. Nephrology Dialysis Transplantation. 1991; 6: 917–922.
128. Ruco LP, Pomponi D, Pigott R, Gearing AJH, Baiocchini A, Baroni CD. Expression and cell distribution of the intercellular adhesion molecule, vascular cell adhesion molecule, endothelial leukocyte adhesion molecule, and endothelial cell adhesion molecule (CD31) in reactive human lymph nodes and in Hogdkin's disease. Am J Pathol. 1992; 140: 1337–1344.
129. Miyake K, Medina K, Ishihara K, Kimoto M, Auerbach R, Kincade PW. A VCAM-like adhesion molecule on murine bone marrow stromal cells mediates binding of lymphocyte precursors in culture. J Cell Biol. 1991; 114: 557–565.
130. Anderson DC, Springer TA, Leukocyte adhesion deficiency: an inherited defect in the Mac-1, LFA-1, and p150,95 glycoproteins. Annu Rev Med. 1987; 38: 175–194.
131. Pelletier RP, Ohye RG, Vanbuskirk A, Sedmak DD, Kincade P, Ferguson RM, Orosz CG. Importance of endothelial VCAM-1 for inflammatory leukocytic infiltration in vivo. J Immunol. 1992; 149: 2473–2481.
132. Newman PJ, Berendt MC, Gorski J, White GC, Lyman S, Paddock C, Muller WA. PECAM-1 (CD31) cloning and relation to adhesion molecules of the immunoglobulin gene superfamily. Science. 1990; 247: 1219–1222.
133. Simmons DL, Walker C, Power C, Pigott R. Molecular cloning of CD31, a putative intercellular adhesion molecule closely related to carcinoembryonic antigen. J Exp Med. 1990; 171: 2147–2152.
134. Stockinger H, Gadd SJ, Eher R, Majdic O, Schreiber W, Kasinrerk W, Strass B, Schnabl E, Knapp W. Molecular characterization and functional analysis of the leukocyte surface protein CD31. J Exp Med. 1990; 145: 3889–3897.
135. Ohto H, Maeda H, Shibata Y, Chen R-F, Ozaki Y, Higashihara M, Takeuchi A, Tohyama H. A novel leukocyte differentiation antigen: two monoclonal antibodies TM2 and TM3 define a 120-kD molecule prsent on neutrophils, monocytes, platelets, and activated lymphoblasts. Blood. 1985; 66: 873–881.

136. Cabanas C, Sanchez-Madrid F, Bellon T, Figdor CG, Te Velde AA, Fernandez JM, Acevedo A, Bernabeu C. Characterization of a novel myeloid antigen regulated during differentiation of monocytic cells. Eur J Immunol. 1989; 91: 1373–1378.
137. Tanaka Y, Albelda SM, Horgan KJ, Van Seventer GA, Shimizu Y, Newman W, Hallam J, Newman PJ, Buck CA, Shaw S. CD31 expressed on distinctive T cell subsets is a preferential amplifier of β1 integrin-mediated adhesion. J Exp Med. 1992; 176: 245–253.
138. Albelda SM, Muller WA, Buck CA, Newman PJ. Molecular and cellular properties of PECAM-1 (endoCAM/CD31): A novel vascular cell-cell adhesion molecule. J Cell Biol. 1991; 114: 1059–1068.
139. Muller WA, Ratti CM, McDonnell SL, Cohn ZA. A human endothelial cell-restricted, externally disposed plasmalemmal protein enriched in intercellular junctions. J Exp Med. 1989; 170: 399–414.
140. Picker LJ, Nakache M, Butcher EC. Monoclonal antibodies to human lymphocyte homing receptors define a novel class of adhesion molecules on diverse cell types. J Cell Biol. 1989; 109: 927–937.
141. Haynes BF, Telen MJ, Hale LP, Denning SM. CD44 – A molecule involved in leukocyte adherence and T-cell activation. Immunology Today. 1989; 10: 423–428.
142. Stamenkovic I, Amiot M, Pesando JM, Seed B. A lymphocyte molecule implicated in lymph node homing is a member of the cartilage link protein family. Cell. 1989; 56: 1057–1062.
143. Dougherty GJ, Lansdorp PM, Cooper DL, Humphries RK. Molecular cloning of CD44R1 and CD44R2, two novel isoforms of the human CD44 lymphocyte 'homing' receptor expressed by hemopoietic cells. J Exp Med. 1991; 174: 1–5.
144. Hofmann R, Rudy W, Zoller M, Tolg C, Ponta H, Herrlich P, Gunthert U. CD44 splice variants confer metastatic behaviour in rats: homologous sequences are expressed in human tumor cell lines. Cancer Research. 1991; 51: 5292–5297.
145. Jackson DG, Buckley J, Bell JI. Multiple variants of the human lymphocyte homing receptor CD44 generated by insertions at a single site in the extracellular domain. J Biol Chem. 1992; 267: 4732–4739.
146. Jalkanen S, Jalkanen M, Bargatze R, Tammi M, Butcher EC. Biochemical properties of glycoproteins involved in lymphocyte recognition of high endothelial venules in man. J Immunol. 1988; 141: 1615–1623.
147. Aruffo A, Stamenkovic I, Melnick M, Underhill CB, Seed B. CD44 is the principal cell surface receptor for hyaluronate. Cell. 1990; 61: 1303–1313.
148. Carter WG, Wayner EA. Characterization of the class III collagen receptor, a phosphorylated, transmembrane glycoprotein expressed in nucleated human cells. J Biol Chem. 1988; 263: 4193–4201.
149. Jalkanen S, Jalkanen M. Lymphocyte CD44 binds the COOH-terminal heparin-binding domain of fibronectin. J Cell Biol. 1992; 116: 817–825.
150. Jalkanen S, Bargatze RF, Herron LR, Butcher EC. A lymphoid cell surface glycoprotein involved in endothelial recognition and lymphocyte homing in man. Eur J Immunol. 1986; 16: 1195–1202.
151. Jalkanen S, Bargatze RF, Toyos Jde los, Butcher EC. Lymphocyte recognition of high endothelium: antibodies to distinct epitopes of an 85–95 kD glycoprotein antigen differentially inhibit lymphocyte binding to lymph node, mucosal, or synovial endothelial cells. J Cell Biol. 1987; 105: 983–990.
152. Culty M, Miyake K, Kincade PW, Silorski E, Butcher EC, Underhill C. The hyaluronate receptor is a member of the CD44 (H-CAM) family of cell surface glycoproteins. J Cell Biol. 1990; 111: 2765–2774.
153. Atherton A, Born GVR. Quantitative investigations of the adhesiveness of circulating polymorphonuclear leukocytes to blood vessel walls. J Physiol. 1972; 222: 447–474.
154. Williams AF. Out of equilibrium. Nature. 1991; 352: 473–474.
155. Lawrence MB, Springer TA. Leukocytes roll on a selectin at physiologic flow rates: distinction from and prerequisite for adhesion through integrins. Cell. 1991; 65: 859–873.
156. Furie MB, Burns MJ, Tancinco MCA, Benjamin CD, Lobb RR. E-selectin (endothelial-leukocyte adhesion molecule-1) is not required for the migration of neutrophils across IL-1-stimulated endothelium in vitro. J Immunol. 1992; 148: 2395–2404.
157. Arfors KE, Lundberg C, Lindbom L, Lundberg K, Beatty PG, Harlan JM. A monoclonal

antibody to the membrane glycoprotein complex CD18 inhibits polymorphonuclear leukocyte accumulation and plasma leakage in vivo. Blood. 1987; 69: 338.

158. Lawrence MB, Smith CW, Eskin SG, McIntyre LV. Effect of venous shear stress on CD18-mediated neutrophil adhesion to cultured endothelium. Blood. 1990; 75: 227–237.

159. Oppenheimer-Marks N, Davis L, Lipsky PE. Human T lymphocyte adhesion to endothelial cells and transendothelial migration: alteration of receptor use relates to the activation status of both the T cell and the endothelial cell. J Immunol. 1990; 145: 140–148.

160. Dustin ML, Springer TA. T-cell receptor cross-linking transiently stimulates adhesiveness through LFA-1. Nature. 1989; 341: 619–624.

161. van Kooyk Y, van de Wiel-van Kemenade P, Weder P, Kuijpers TW, Figdor CG. Enhancement of LFA-1-mediated cell adhesion by triggering through CD2 or CD3 on T lymphocytes. Nature. 1988; 342: 811–813.

162. Dransfield I, Buckle A-M, Hogg N. Early events of the immune response mediated by leukocyte integrins. Immunol Rev. 1990; 114: 29–44.

163. Altieri DC. Occupancy of CD11b/CD18 (Mac-1) divalent ion binding site(s) induces leukocyte adhesion. J Immunol. 1991; 147: 1891–1898.

164. Dransfield I, Cabañas C, Craig A, Hogg N. Divalent cation regulation of the function of the leukocyte integrin LFA-1. J Cell Biol. 1992; 116: 219–226.

165. Dransfield I, Cabañas C, Barrett J, Hogg N. Interaction of leukocyte integrins with ligand is necessary but not sufficient for function. J Cell Biol. 1992; 116: 1527–1535.

166. Shimizu Y, Van Seventer GA, Horgan KJ, Shaw S. Regulated expression and binding of three VLA (beta 1) integrin receptors on T cells. Nature. 1990; 345: 250–253.

167. van Kooyk Y, Weder P, Hogervorst F, Verhoeven AJ, Van Seventer G, Te Velde AA, Borst J, Keizer GD, Figdor CG. Activation of LFA-1 through a Ca^{2+}-dependent epitope stimulates lymphocyte adhesion. J Cell Biol. 1991; 112: 345–354.

168. Robinson MK, Andrew D, Rosen H, Brown D, Ortlepp S, Stephens P, Butcher EC. Antibody against the Leu-CAM β-chain (CD18) promotes both LFA-1 and CR3-dependent adhesion events. J Immunol. 1992; 148: 1080–1085.

169. Bednarczyk JL, McIntyre BW. A monoclonal antibody to VLA-4 α-chain (CDw49d) induces homotypic lymphocyte aggregation. J Immunol. 1990; 144: 777–784.

170. Campanero MR, Pulida R, Ursa MA, Rodriguez-Moya M, Landazuri MO, Sanchez-Madrid F. An alternative leukocyte homotypic adhesion mechanism, LFA-1/ICAM-1-independent, triggered through human VLA-4. J Cell Biol. 1990; 110: 2157–2165.

171. Butcher EC. Leukocyte-endothelial cell recognition: Three (or more) steps to specificity and diversity. Cell. 1991; 67: 1033–1036.

172. Shimizu Y, Newman W, Tanaka Y, Shaw S. Lymphocyte interactions with endothelial cells. Immunol Today. 1992; 13: 106–112.

173. Leeuwenberg JFM, von Asmuth EJU, Jeunhomme TMAA, Buurman WA. Interferon-gamma regulates the expression of an adhesion molecule ELAM-1 and IL-6 by human endothelial cells in vitro. J Immunol. 1990; 145: 2110–2114.

174. Doukas J, Pober JS. IFNy enhances endothelial activation induced by tumor necrosis factor but not IL-1. J Immunol. 1990; 145: 1727–1733.

175. Thornhill MH, Haskard DO. IL-4 regulates endothelial activation by IL-1, tumor necrosis factor or IFNy. J Immunol. 1990; 145: 865–872.

176. Thornhill M, Wellicome SM, Mahiouz DL, Lanchbury JSS, Kyan-Aung U, Haskard DO. Tumor necrosis factor combines with IL-4 or IFN-y to selectively enhance endothelial cell adhesiveness for T cells: the contribution of VCAM-1 dependent and independent binding mechanisms. J Immunol. 1991; 146: 592–598.

177. Pober JS, Cotran RS. Cytokines and endothelial cell biology. Physiological Reviews. 1990; 70: 427–451.

178. Mantovani A, Bussolino F. Endothelium-derived modulators of leukocyte function. In: Gordon JL, ed. Vascular Endothelium: Interactions with Circulating Cells. Amsterdam: Elsevier, 1991: 129–140.

179. Zimmerman GA, McIntyre TM, Mehra M, Prescott SM. Endothelial cell-associated platelet-activating factor: A novel mechanism for signaling intercellular adhesion. J Cell Biol. 1990; 110: 529–540.

180. Lorant DE, Patel KD, McIntyre TM, McEver RP, Prescott SM, Zimmerman GA. Coexpression of GMP-140 and PAF by endothelium stimulated by histamine or thrombin:

A juxtacrine system for adhesion and activation of neutrophils. J Cell Biol. 1991; 115: 223–234.

181. Bussolino F, Breviario F, Tetta C, Aglietta M, Mantovani A, Dejana E. Interleukin 1 stimulates platelet-activating factor production in cultured human endothelial cells. J Clin Invest. 1986; 77: 2027–2033.

182. Breviario F, Bertocchi F, Dejana E, Bussolino F. IL-1-induced adhesion of polymorphonuclear leukocytes to cultured human endothelial cells: role of platelet-activating factor. J Immunol. 1988; 141: 3391–3397.

183. Sica A, Matsushima K, van Damme J, Wang JM, Polentarutti N, Dejana E, Colotta F, Mantovani A. IL-1 transcriptionally activates the neutrophil chemotactic factor/IL-8 gene in endothelial cells. Immunology. 1990; 69: 548–553.

184. Sironi M, Breviario F, Proserpio P, Biondi A, Vecchi A, Damme JV, Dejana E, Mantovani A. IL-1 stimulates IL-6 production in endothelial cells. J Immunol. 1989; 142: 549–553.

185. Strieter RM, Kunkel SL, Showell HJ, Remick GD, Phan SH, Ward PA, Marks RM. Endothelial cell gene expression of a neutrophil chemotactic factor by TNF, IL-1 and LPS. Science. 1989; 243: 1467–1469.

186. Huber AR, Kunkel SL, Todd RF, III, Weiss SJ. Regulation of transendothelial neutrophil migration by endogenous interleukin-8. Science. 1991; 254: 99–102.

187. Gamble JR, Vadas MA. Endothelial adhesiveness for blood neutrophils is inhibited by transforming growth factor beta. Science. 1988; 242: 97–99.

188. Gamble JR, Vadas MA. Endothelial cell adhesiveness for human T lymphocytes is inhibited by transforming growth factor-β1. J Immunol. 1991; 146: 1149–1154.

189. Territo M, Berliner JA, Fogelman AM. Effect of monocyte migration on low density lipoprotein transport across aortic endothelial monolayers. J Clin Invest. 1984; 74: 2279–2284.

190. Migliorisi G, Folkes E, Pawlowski N, Cramer EB. In vitro studies of human monocyte migration across endothelium in response to Leukotriene B4 and f-Met-Leu-Phe. Am J Pathol. 1987; 127: 157–167.

191. Pawlowski NA, Kaplan G, Abraham E, Cohn ZA. The selective binding and transmigration of monocytes through the junctional complexes of human endothelium. J Exp Med. 1988; 168: 1865–1882.

192. Hakkert BC, Rentenaar JM, van Aken WG, Roos D, van Mourik JA. A three-dimensional model system to study the interactions between human leukocytes and endothelial cells. Eur J Immunol. 1990; 20: 2775–2781.

193. Smith CW, Rothlein R, Hughes B, Mariscalco M, Schmalstieg F, Anderson DC. Recognition of an endothelial determinant for CD18-dependent neutrophil adherence and transendothelial migration. J Clin Invest. 1988; 82: 1746–1756.

194. Smith CW, Marlin SD, Rothlein R, Toman C, Anderson DC. Cooperative interactions of LFA-1 and Mac-1 with intercellular adhesion molecule-1 in facilitating adherence and transendothelial migration of human neutrophils in vitro. J Clin Invest. 1989; 83: 2008–2017.

195. Furie MB, Tancinco MCA, Smith CW. Monoclonal antibodies to leukocyte integrins CD11a/CD18 and CD11b/CD18 or intercellular adhesion molecule-1 inhibit chemoattractant-stimulated neutrophil transendothelial migration in vitro. Blood. 1991; 78: 2089–2097.

196. Van Epps DE, Potter J, Vachula M, Smith CW, Anderson DC. Suppression of human lymphocyte chemotaxis and transendothelial migration by anti-LFA-1 antibody. J Immunol. 1989; 143: 3207–3210.

197. Kavanaugh AF, Lightfoot E, Lipsky PE, Oppenheimer-Marks N. Role of CD11/CD18 in adhesion and transendothelial migration of T cells: Analysis utilizing CD18-deficient T cell clones. J Immunol. 1991; 146: 4149–4156.

198. Oppenheimer-Marks N, Davis LS, Bogue DT, Ramberg J, Lipsky PE. Differential utilization of ICAM-1 and VCAM-1 during the adhesion and transendothelial migration of human T lymphocytes. J Immunol. 1991; 147: 2913–2921.

199. Pober JS, Cotran RS. Immunologic interactions of T lymphocytes with vascular endothelium. Adv Immunol. 1991; 50: 261–288.

200. Collins T, Lapierre LA, Fiers W, Strominger JL, Pober JS. Recombinant human tumor necrosis factor increases mRNA levels and surface expression of HLA-A,B antigens in vascular endothelial cells and dermal fibroblasts in vitro. Proc Natl Acad Sci USA. 1986;

83: 446–450.

201. Johnson DR, Pober JS. Tumor necrosis factor and immune interferon synergistically increase transcription of HLA class I heavy- and light-chain genes in vascular endothelium. Proc Natl Acad Sci USA. 1990; 87: 5183–5187.

202. Pober JS, Collins T, Gimbrone MA, Cotran RS, Gitlin JD, Fiers W, Clayberger C, Krensky AM, Burakoff SJ, Reiss CS. Lymphocytes recognize human vascular endothelial and dermal fibroblast Ia antigens induced by recombinant immune interferon. Nature. 1983; 305: 726–729.

203. Lapierre LA, Fiers W, Pober JS. Three distinct classes of regulatory cytokines control endothelial MHC antigen expression. J Exp Med. 1988; 167: 794–804.

204. Natali PG, De-Martino C, Quaranta V, Nicotra MR, Frezza F, Pellegrino MA, Ferrone S. Expression of Ia-like antigens in normal human nonlymphoid tissues. Transplantation. 1981; 31: 75–78.

205. Messadi DV, Pober JS, Murphy GF. Effects of recombinant γ-interferon on HLA DR and DQ expression in skin cells in short-term organ culture. Lab Invest. 1988; 58: 61–67.

206. Groenewegen G, Buurman WA, Van der Linden CJ. Lymphokine dependence of in vivo expression of MHC class II by endothelium. Nature. 1985; 316: 361–363.

207. Carlos TM, Harlan JM. Membrane proteins involved in phagocyte adherence to endothelium. Immunol Rev. 1990; 114: 5–29.

208. Keelan E, Haskard DO. CAMs and anti-CAMs: The clinical potential of leukocyte adhesion molecules. J Roy Coll Phys. 1992; 26: 17–24.

209. Benjamin RJ, Qin S, Wise MP, Cobbold SP. mechanisms of monoclonal antibody-facilitated tolerance induction: a possible role for the CD4 (L3T4) and CD11a (LFA-1) molecules in self–non-self discrimination. Eur J Immunol. 1988; 18: 1079–1088.

210. Isobe M, Yagita H, Okumura K, Ihara A. Specific acceptance of cardiac allograft after treatment with antibodies to ICAM-1 and LFA-1. Science. 1992; 255: 1125–1127.

211. Mulligan MS, Varani J, Dame MK, Lane CL, Smith CW, Anderson DC, Ward PA. Role of endothelial-leukocyte adhesion molecule 1 (ELAM-1) in neutrophil-mediated lung injury in rats. J Clin Invest. 1991; 88: 1396–1406.

212. Yednock TA, Cannon C, Fritz LC, Sanchez-Madrid F, Steinman L, Karin N. Prevention of experimental autoimmune encephalomyelitis by antibodies against $\alpha_4\beta_1$ integrin. Nature. 1992; 356: 63–66.

213. Iigo Y, Takashi T, Tamatani T, Miyasaka M, Higashida T, Yagita H, Okumura K, Tsukada W. ICAM-1-dependent pathway is critically involved in the pathogenesis of adjuvant arthritis in rats. J Immunol. 1991; 147: 4167–4171.

214. Jasin HE, Lightfoot E, Davis LS, Rothlein R, Faanes RB, Lipsky PE. Amelioration of antigen-induced arthritis in rabbits treated with monoclonal antibodies to leukocyte adhesion molecules. Arthritis Rheum. 1992; 35: 541–549.

215. Harning R, Pelletier J, Van G, Takei F, Merluzzi VJ. Monoclonal antibody to MALA-2 (ICAM-1) reduces acute autoimmune nephritis in kdkd mice. Clin Immunol Immunopathol. 1992; 64: 129–134.

216. Watson SR, Fennie C, Lasky LA. Neutrophil influx into an inflammatory site inhibited by a soluble homing receptor-IgG chimaera. Nature. 1991; 349: 164–167.

7
The Complement System and Connective Tissue Disease

T. J. VYSE and M. J. WALPORT

INTRODUCTION

Complement comprises a complex system of proteins incorporating a triggered enzyme cascade, regulatory proteins and complement receptors. The activities of complement include: promotion of the inflammatory response; opsonization of pathogens; opsonization and clearance of immune complexes; target cell lysis; and the development of antibody responses. These diverse activities, bridging the inflammatory and adaptive immune systems, are compatible with an important role for the complement system in the pathogenesis of the connective tissue diseases. At the heart of these disorders is immunologically generated inflammation, and complement participates both in the induction of disease and in the expression of tissue injury. Thus complement can operate within the disease process at both the inducer and the effector stages.

In this chapter we shall briefly discuss the normal function of the complement system and how this is regulated. We will then review complement deficiencies, including the clinical and molecular features of the genetic disorders of the complement system. Complement deficiencies can be clinically manifest by immune complex syndromes, particularly the development of systemic lupus erythematosus (SLE). The relationship between complement and SLE gives insights into the mechanisms of immune complex clearance and how disturbances of these may relate to the pathogenesis of disease. We will consider the role of complement as a source of inflammatory mediators, and review evidence for local synthesis of some complement components at sites of inflammation, such as synovial tissue.

The serum concentration of certain complement proteins, e.g. C3 and C4, is known to fall in some rheumatic diseases in which immune complexes play a role. Hence complement estimation can be used as a diagnostic aid and in monitoring disease activity. Since complement is an important source of mediators in the inflammatory and immune responses, it may be possible to use complement regulatory proteins to treat disease. The potential therapeutic value of soluble, engineered regulatory proteins in the treatment of the connective tissue diseases is reviewed at the end of the chapter.

A REVIEW OF THE COMPLEMENT CASCADE

Complement may be activated by two pathways: the classical and alternative pathways. These converge to activate C3, cleavage of which is the pivotal step of the complement cascade. The activation of C3 is achieved by the cleavage of a small fragment, C3a, from the end of the C3 α chain by a C3 convertase. The remaining C3b portion contains an internal thioester bond which is now highly reactive, being susceptible to nucleophilic attack. Although the bulk of this unstable C3b is inactivated by hydrolysis in the fluid phase, a small proportion binds covalently to neighbouring hydroxyl or amino groups (via its thioester bond) on the surface of pathogens or immune complexes[1]. The bound C3b acts as an opsonin and to initiate the terminal part of the complement cascade.

The alternative pathway (see Figure 1)

This pathway is in effect a positive feedback loop and relies on the input of a small amount of C3b which is used to generate a C3 convertase, C3bBb, which in turn splits C3 into C3a and more C3b[2]. The initial C3b may be derived from several sources: i) classical pathway activation; ii) a low level of spontaneous hydrolysis of the thioester bond of native C3 to form C3i, an alternative factor B binding site; iii) proteolysis of C3 by microbial proteases. Activation of this pathway can therefore be independent of the adaptive immune system and it forms part of the innate defence system.

The classical pathway (see Figure 1)

It is by virtue of the classical pathway that complement activation is linked with the adaptive humoral immune system. This pathway is initiated by the binding of the C1 complex through the globular domains of its C1q subcomponent to the constant regions of IgM or aggregated IgG[3]. As well as C1q, the C1 complex comprises two C1r-C1s dimers, and two C1-inhibitor molecules. Multivalent antibody-C1q binding induces a conformational change in the C1 complex with the release of C1 inhibitor and consequent autocatalytic cleavage of C1r; the active form of the latter then generates an active form of C1s (reviewed in [4]). There then follows a cascade (shown in Figure 1) in which C1s, a serine esterase, first splits C4, and then splits C2 – together the cleaved products form the classical pathway C3 convertase, C4b2a. It is of note that C4 is homologous to C3, both containing a reactive

Alternative Pathway

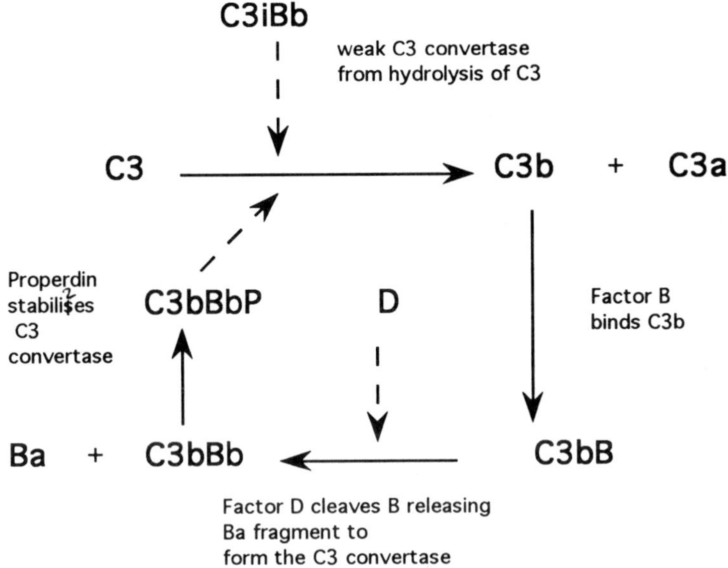

Classical Pathway

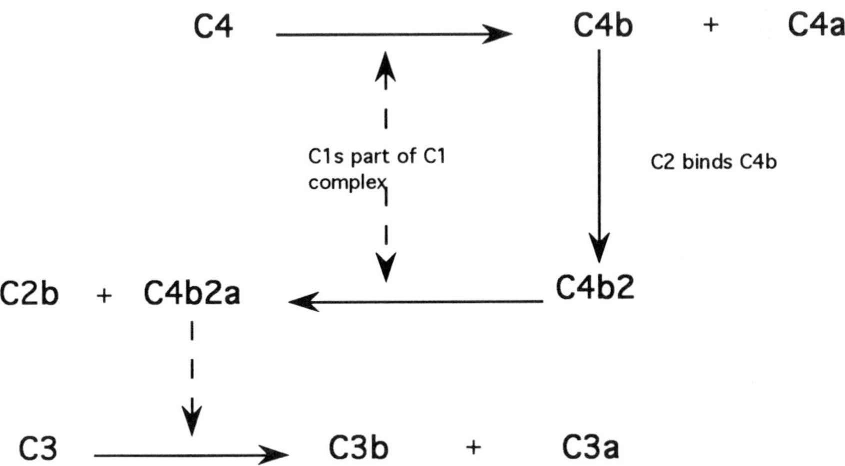

Figure 1 The formation of the classical and alternative pathway C3 convertases

internal thioester bond which undergoes nucleophilic attack, thereby allowing covalent binding to surfaces[5].

Terminal pathway

After the formation of bound C3b there is a final pathway that results in the production of a large, multimolecular membrane attack complex (MAC) with the capacity to insert into cell membranes to cause cell lysis or cellular activation. The only enzymic step in the terminal sequence is the initial one in which the classical or alternative pathway C3 convertase forms a tetramolecular complex with bound C3b and C5. Then either the Bb or C2a of the C5 convertase cleaves a small N-terminal fragment, C5a, from C5, to form C5b. Thereafter C6 and C7 bind C5b, detaching it from the convertase complex. The lipophilic C5b67 now inserts into a membrane where it binds a single molecule of C8 and at least six molecules of C9 to become fully effective[6].

REGULATORS OF COMPLEMENT ACTIVATION AND COMPLEMENT RECEPTORS

Classical and alternative pathways

Once C3b has been formed there is the potential for uncontrolled complement activation because of the positive feedback loop within the alternative pathway. At least ten control proteins exist, both in the fluid-phase, and on cell membranes to prevent inappropriate complement fixation.

In the fluid-phase and on cell surfaces the alternative pathway is regulated by a circulating glycoprotein, factor H, which competes with factor B to bind C3b (and C3i). Factor H then acts as a cofactor for the serine esterase factor I that degrades C3b. The importance of factors H and I can be appreciated when one considers that if there is complete genetic deficiency of either, the consequent uncontrolled alternative pathway activation produces a secondary C3 and factor B deficiency by virtue of consumption. The classical pathway has its own specialized fluid-phase inhibitor, C4-binding protein (C4BP). C4BP is a cofactor for factor I in the cleavage of C4b, in an analogous fashion to the cofactor activity of factor H.

The surface regulatory complement proteins (see Table 1) act to delineate self from non-self so that inappropriate C3 fixation to host tissue is minimized. The classical and alternative pathways share three proteins: decay acceleration factor (DAF)[7], membrane cofactor protein (MCP)[8]; and complement receptor type 1 (CR1)[9]. These inhibitors have three modes of operation:

(i)   to inhibit the association of C3b and factor B or of C4b and C2b: – DAF and CR1

(ii) to promote the dissociation of the C3 convertase: – DAF and CR1

(iii) to promote catabolism of C3b or C4b by factor I: – MCP and CR1.

The classical pathway has its own specific fluid-phase inhibitor, C1 inhibitor.

Table 1 Cell-surface complement regulators and complement receptors

Name/ CD number	Structure	Ligands	Gene localization	Cellular distribution
DAF CD56	Single chain Glycoprotein GPI anchor MWt 70 kD	C3b, C4b	RCA cluster*	Erythrocytes, neutrophils, monocytes, platelets, lymphocytes, widespread on epithelia and endothelia
MCP CD46	Single chain Transmembrane Glycoprotein MWt 60–70 kD†	C3b, C4b	RCA cluster*	Neutrophils, monocytes, lymphocytes, platelets, macrophages
CR1 CD35	Single chain Transmembrane Glycoprotein MWt 210–290 kD§	C3b, C4b, iC3b	RCA cluster*	Erythrocytes, neutrophils, monocytes, macrophages, lymphocytes (mainly B), follicular dendritic cells (FDC)
CR2 CD21	Single chain Glycoprotein MWt 145 kD	iC3b, C3dg	RCA cluster*	B lymphocytes and some T lymphocytes, FDC, nasopharyngeal epithelium
CR3 α CD11b β CD 18 (Mac-1)	Heterodimer Glycoprotein α 165 kD β 95 kD	iC3b, ICAM-1	β on 21q22 α on 16p11-11.2	Neutrophils, macrophages, NK – natural killer cells, FDC
CR4 α CD11c β CD 18 (p150/95)	Heterodimer Glycoprotein α 150 kD β 95 kD	iC3b	β on 21q22 α on 16p11-11.2	Neutrophils, macrophages, NK cells, some B lymphocytes
CD59 (HRF 20)	Single chain GPI anchor MWt ∼20 kD	C8, C9	11p	Erythrocytes, T lymphocytes, Widespread on epithelia, endothelia, connective tissue
C8BP (HRF)	MWt ∼65 kD Protein sequence not known GPI anchor	C8, C9	Not known	Erythrocytes, neutrophils, monocytes, lymphocytes

*The RCA (regulators of complement activation) cluster is a group of structurally related complement genes on chromosome 1 at q3.2. They comprise: CR1, CR2, MCP, DAF, C4BP and factor H.
†Variation in MCP size is due to alternative RNA splicing and variable glycosylation
§There is allotypic variation in the size of CR1 (see text for further details)

This serpin (serine protease inhibitor) is mentioned above as part of the C1 complex in which it inhibits C1r[10].

Terminal pathway

Because the terminal pathway components are lipophilic and are released from sites of C3b fixation they have the potential to injure bystander cells in the vicinity of the site of complement activation, a process termed reactive lysis. There are both fluid-phase and cell surface molecules that are designed to restrict this potential self-injurious process. In the fluid-phase vitronectin, also known as S protein, binds C5b67 to block its insertion into lipid bilayers[11]. On the cell surface two inhibitors have been described. A glycoprotein, CD59, acts by binding to C8 and C9 and thereby prevents the unfolding of the latter through the target cell membrane which is necessary for mature MAC formation[12]. A less well characterized protein, C8-binding protein (C8BP), which is also called homologous restriction factor (HRF), binds C8 and thereby halts MAC assembly[13]. Both CD 59 and C8BP are anchored to the cell membrane by a glycolipid tail (a glycosylphosphatidylinositol or GPI anchor) in a similar way to DAF. The deficiency of such molecules with a GPI anchor underlies the complement sensitivity seen in paroxysmal nocturnal haemoglobinuria (PNH)[14].

Complement receptors

CR1 is another important regulator of complement activation. It has the facility to bind to both C3b and C4b and in doing so acts both as a cofactor for factor I in the cleavage of C3b to iC3b and C3dg, and also as a receptor mediating endocytosis and phagocytosis of opsonized particles. The CR1 on neutrophils and macrophages potentiates Fcγ-mediated phagocytosis of microbes and immune complexes that have fixed C3b (and C4b). CR1 has an additional function in transporting immune complexes in the circulation – in primates there is a large CR1 reservoir on erythrocytes[9]. In this instance CR1 is acting as a receptor mediating immune adherence, whereby immune complexes are bound to the erythrocyte surface and are not phagocytosed.

The second complement receptor, CR2, is homologous to CR1. They both consist of multiple repeating subunits of 60–70 amino acids called short consensus repeats (SCRs). SCRs are also found in other complement components, predominantly those that bind C3b and/or C4b (review [15]). In CR2 there are 16 consecutive SCRs, whilst in the commonest allotype of CR1 there are 30 repeats. Variation in the number of SCRs gives rise to the allotypic size variants of CR1. There are two common allotypes with molecular weights of 250 kD and 290 kD (review [16]). This has been shown to be due to partial gene duplication at the molecular level[17].

CR2 binds iC3b and C3dg, derivatives that are products of the cleavage of C3b by factor I. Both these C3 fragments remain surface bound since they include the thioester region of C3. CR2 is mainly found on B lymphocytes where it also serves as the receptor for the Epstein-Barr virus[18]. This receptor is particularly strongly expressed by B cells within germinal centres and its potential role in the immune response of localizing antigen is illustrated by the inhibition of the primary immune response in mice by anti-CR2 monoclonal antibody[19]. The maintenance of B cell memory requires continued antigen presentation to B cells by the follicular dendritic cells in germinal centres[20]. This has been shown to be complement dependent in mice, since C3-depleted mice neither localize immune complexes to follicular dendritic cells nor form B memory cells in response to T-dependent antigens[21].

Two other complement receptors have been described, CR3 and CR4, although there is variation in nomenclature. Both of these molecules belong to the β2 integrin family of receptors. They are all heterodimers which share a common β chain, CD18, and have distinct α chains, CD11: CR3 (CD11b), and CR4 (CD11c). The third member of the β2 integrin family is leucocyte functional antigen 1 (LFA-1 or CD11a/CD18). CR3 and CR4 are expressed on both neutrophils and macrophages and bind iC3b (reviewed in [22]). Their major role appears to be the phagocytosis of iC3b-coated particles. CR3 also binds intercellular adhesion molecule 1 (ICAM-1) which is an important ligand for LFA-1. Since ICAM-1 is present on endothelial cells and both T and B lymphocytes, CR3 has a role in transendothelial migration of phagocytic cells[23] and in the generation of the immune response.

COMPLEMENT DEFICIENCY AND DISEASE

The clinical sequelae of complement deficiency are very variable (see Table 2): a substantial number of individuals with certain complement protein deficiencies are clinically unaffected (presumably as a result of alternative mechanisms available within the innate and adaptive immune systems)[24]. When they do occur, the clinical consequences of deficiency relate to the various functions of the complement system. The complement system has a vital role in immune complex handling as may be inferred by the increased prevalence of immune complex disease, most commonly SLE, in patients with genetic deficiencies of the classical pathway and C3 deficiency. These deficiency states, although very rare in most instances, provide fascinating insights into the *in vivo* functioning of the complement system and provide clues as to the pathogenesis of conditions such as SLE. Patients with complement deficiencies are susceptible also to pyogenic infection with organisms such as *Staphylococci* and *Streptococci*, presumably because of defective opsonization, and *Neisseria* because of the role of complement-mediated cytolysis in the host defence against such pathogens.

Classical pathway deficiencies

Of the classical pathway deficiency states, C1q deficiency shows the closest association with SLE, almost all patients with homozygous C1q deficiency are affected; individuals suffer recurrent pyogenic infections too. C1q is comprised of three chains, A, B and C. The genes encoding all three chains have been shown to be located on the short arm of chromosome 1[25]. Approximately 30 cases of genetic C1q deficiency have been described. The majority of these are the result of a complete inability to synthesise C1q[26]; the remainder are due to a dysfunctional protein[27]. The molecular basis of C1q deficiency is unknown in most cases, but in one instance of complete deficiency there was a nonsense mutation of the B chain gene at a point which corresponds to the middle of the globular head. In this situation no A or C chain could be detected, implying that a complete B chain is essential

Table 2 Hereditary complement deficiencies

Component	Number of cases	Chromosome location	Disease association
Classical pathway proteins			
C1q	>25	A, B and C chains 1p.34.1 - 36.3	SLE in majority Pyogenic infection
C1r/C1s	10	Tightly linked - 12p13	As for C1q
C4A and C4B	17	MHC locus - 6p21.3	As for C1q
C2	>100	MHC locus - 6p21.3	SLE in ~50% Pyogenic infection
Alternative pathway proteins			
Factor D	1	Unknown	*Neisseria* infection
Properdin	>50	Xp11.23-21.1	*Neisseria* infection
C3	16	19pter-p13.2	Pyogenic infection SLE, immune complex disease
Factor H	12	RCA cluster - 1q3.2	As for C3 and haemolytic-uraemic syndrome
Factor I	15	4q25	As for C3
Terminal pathway proteins			
C5	19	9q32-q34	*Neisseria* infection, rarely SLE
C6	>50	5 close to C7	As for C5
C7	26	5 close to C6	As for C5
C8	32	α,β -closely linked on 1p γ-9pq32	As for C5
C9	5 (Caucasian) 1 in 1000 (Japanese)	5p13	Mostly asymptomatic, *Neisseria* infection

for C1q assembly and secretion[28]. Deficiencies of C1r or C1s are rare with only about ten cases having been published. Almost all of these are of combined deficiency of both molecules. The molecular pathology is unknown, but the two genes are only about 10 kilobases apart on chromosome 12[29]. The clinical consequences of absent C1r and C1s are, as expected, similar to those of C1q deficiency.

The C4 and C2 (and factor B) genes are located within the class III region of the MHC on chromosome 6. C4 has two isotypes, C4A and C4B, encoded by the genes which are very tightly linked. Complete absence of C4 occurs when all four loci contain null alleles, termed C4AQ*0 and C4BQ*0 at the C4A and C4B loci respectively. Complete homozygous deficiency of C4 is rare, only 16 cases being identified to date, most of whom have severe SLE. Single null alleles, however, are surprisingly common in normal populations. Estimates of the gene frequency of null alleles vary, but for C4AQ*0 it is about 0.1, and for C4BQ*0 about 0.15 in Caucasians, but occur with similar frequencies in both Mongoloid and African-American populations[30]. Alleles with both C4 genes null are considerably underrepresented in normal populations, presumably because of the disease association with complete

C4 deficiency. Because of the high incidence of SLE in total C4 deficiency, and the association of other hereditary classical pathway disorders with lupus, it has been postulated that partial deficiencies, in the form of single C4 null alleles, might act as disease susceptibility genes for SLE. Investigation of C4 null haplotypes has been complicated by the linkage disequilibrium that exists between C4AQ*0 and HLA-DR3 in Caucasians, this class II allele is observed to have an association with SLE. Evidence that the C4 null allele is the relevant disease susceptibility gene comes from studies of Caucasians with SLE who do not possess HLA-DR3[31], and non-Caucasians who carry different MHC extended haplotypes[32]. In contrast, there is no clear association with C4BQ*0 and SLE. C4A and C4B show physiological differences; the internal thioester bond of C4A is more susceptible to nucleophilic differences; the internal thioester bond of C4A is more susceptible to nucleophilic attack by amine groups, whereas the B isotype tends to form ester bonds with hydroxyl groups. Because amine groups are frequent on proteins and hydroxyl groups more prevalent on carbohydrates, C4B is more active in haemolysis than C4A, but C4A is more able to bind protein-containing immune complexes[33]. This may explain the association of partial C4A deficiency with immune complex disease. Despite this plausible pathophysiological explanation it must be stressed that C4A deficiency is only part of the genetic susceptibility to lupus. The gene frequency of C4AQ*0 in Caucasian patients with SLE is about 0.4 (and as stated above it is 0.1 in the normal population)[34]. Within the class III region there are other genes: including those for tumour necrosis factor (TNF) α and TNFβ and heat shock protein 70, there are also about 20 other genes currently under investigation. Polymorphism at these loci in the class III region may also influence disease susceptibility to SLE as may polymorphism at other loci within the MHC region. Indeed, in a murine model of SLE – NZW × NZB FI1 – there is evidence that one of the disease-susceptibility genes contributed by the NZW strain may be one that is associated with low TNFα production. A restriction fragment length polymorphism that correlates with the synthetic rate has been described using a TNFα exonic probe[35]. It is possible that low TNFα synthesis has a role in disease susceptibility in human SLE, or perhaps in the type of disease expression. The haplotype DR2, DQw1 has been associated with lupus nephritis and is also associated with low TNFα production[36].

The molecular basis of C4 deficiency is understood in part. Approximately one-half of null alleles at either C4 locus are caused by three different, large deletions of about 28 kilobases, each removing all, or almost all of a C4 gene. These deletions occur in linkage disequilibrium with other MHC products as part of extended haplotypes; the commonest one in Caucasians is: B8, C2C, BfS, C4AQ*0, C4B1, DR3 (the complement components are followed by a description of their allotype)[37]. Detection of partial deficiencies with a non-deleted basis is difficult because of the considerable overlap of C4 concentrations from different genotypes making it difficult to predict null alleles on the basis of serum C4 measurement. It is also of note that there is considerable polymorphism at both C4 alleles. Approximately 40 different allotypes have been described[38]. The relationship, if any, between C4 allotypic variation and disease awaits elucidation. Although polymorphism exists in the C2 and factor B genes there is considerably less variation at these loci when compared to C4.

Partial deficiency of both C4 isotypes has been reported to occur at a higher than expected frequency in several autoimmune diseases besides SLE. These include: diabetes mellitus, Graves' disease, Sjögren's syndrome, systemic sclerosis and IgA nephropathy[39]. The validity of these associations is uncertain. There have been recent reports of an association between Felty's syndrome and C4BQ*0. Felty's syndrome occurs in association with HLA-DR4, particularly with the haplotype: B44, C2C, BfS, C4A3, C4BQ*0, DR4 (Dw4), DQw7. The relationship of Felty's syndrome to complement deficiency is complex. The haplotype described contains two functioning C4A genes (probably as a result of gene conversion of a C4B gene)[40].

C2 deficiency is the commonest homozygous complement deficiency in Caucasians. The prevalence is estimated at 1 in 10 000. About one-third of those with this genetic disorder develop connective tissue disease, predominantly SLE, and there are sporadic reports of associations between C2 deficiency and other connective tissue diseases such as: discoid lupus, juvenile chronic arthritis, Henoch–Schonlein purpura, and dermatomyositis[41]. They are also susceptible to pyogenic bacterial infection. In an analogous fashion to C4 deficiency, heterozygous C2 deficiency may be associated with connective tissue disease as well as homozygous C2 deficiency. The association has been documented in one survey of patients with rheumatic disease: 5.9% of those with SLE, and 3.7% of patients with juvenile chronic arthritis, had partial genetic C2 deficiency[42]. The commonest C2Q*0 gene occurs in linkage disequilibrium with the MHC haplotype: A25, B18, C2Q*0, BfS, C4A4, C4B2, DR2, in Caucasians, which suggests a common molecular pathology. Recently, a small 28 base-pair deletion within the C2 gene has been reported in eight different families with this haplotype. The deletion removes a splice site and causes premature C2 mRNA termination[43].

Certain clinical features appear to be characteristic of C4 and C2 deficient SLE. These include early onset of disease, prominent skin involvement and photosensitivity, marked Raynaud's phenomenon and mild renal disease. Serologically, antinuclear antibodies are in a low titre, but autoantibodies that recognize the extractable nuclear antigen Ro (SSA) are common although antibodies to La (SSB) are unusual[39]. C1q deficiency is notable not only in that it has the closest association with SLE, when compared to C4 and C2, but in that the SLE is clinically more severe with a higher incidence of nephritis and anti-double stranded DNA antibodies.

C1-inhibitor acts on the enzymes C1r and C1s, together with kallikrein and plasmin. An autosomal dominant inherited form of C1-inhibitor deficiency causes angioedema. It is clinically manifest by recurrent attacks of painless swelling in the skin and the mucosa of the gastrointestinal tract and pharynx[44]. The lack of functioning C1-inhibitor means that there is consumption of C1r and C1s, and degradation of C2 and C4. Serum C3 levels are preserved, however, as is the C1q concentration. In view of the consumption of C2 and C4 it is of note that about 2% of affected individuals develop SLE[45]. This association emphasizes the fact that depressed C4 and/or C2 functionally predispose to the development of immune complex disease and that the association of immune complex disease with the genetic deficiencies of C4 and C2 is a causal one.

Deficiency of alternative pathway components and C3

Sixteen patients with homozygous C3 deficiency have been described, 12 of whom have a susceptibility to a range of pyogenic organisms including *Neisseria*. There is evidence of glomerulonephritis and immune complex disease in five. A splice site mutation at an intron–exon boundary[46] and a genomic deletion[47] have been shown to be the molecular lesions in two cases. Complete deficiencies of factor I and factor H produce a secondary C3 deficiency. Their clinical manifestations are as expected similar to those of C3 deficiency. In both instances the molecular basis is unknown. Although numbers are small, factor H deficiency appears unusual in that there is a prominent association with renal disease including haemolytic–uraemic syndrome[48].

Homozygous factor B deficiency has not been described (although absent factor B is a consequence of factor I deficiency) and only one homozygous case of factor D deficiency is recorded in an individual with recurrent *Neisseria* infections. Properdin deficiency, which was thought to be very rare, has been the subject of a number of recent reports from Holland, Scandinavia and Israel suggesting that it is not uncommon. More than 50 cases are known, all of which are in males, due to the location of the properdin gene on the X chromosome. Individuals with properdin deficiency usually present with infection due to *N. meningitidis* or *N. gonorrhoeae*[49].

Deficiency of membrane attack complex proteins

Because each of the terminal pathway components is essential for functional MAC assembly, the loss of any one of them inhibits the ability of the MAC to cause cytolysis. The consequences of all these complement deficiencies is similar, that is recurrent infection with *Neisseriae*[50]. There is a slight increase in the incidence of immune complex syndromes with terminal pathway deficiencies[51]. For further details of the genetics of the terminal pathway deficiencies see Table 2.

Deficiency of membrane-associated regulatory proteins

Although complete CR1 deficiency has not been described, the total number of receptors expressed on red cells is subject to both genetic and acquired influences. There is an inherited polymorphism in the number of CR1 expressed on the erythrocyte surface[52] which vary between individuals from 100 to 1200 per cell. The molecular basis of the genetic influence on erythrocyte CR1 numbers is not fully known although there is an informative restriction fragment polymorphism at the CR1 locus which corresponds with high or low expression[53]. In contrast to red cells, there is less evidence for genetic influence on CR1 expression on the surface of neutrophils and B lymphocytes.

A low level of expression of CR1 on erythrocytes and leucocytes is associated with immune complex diseases such as SLE[54]. Because of the role of CR1 in immune complex transport this was viewed as a possible genetic risk factor for lupus. The bulk of the evidence, however, favours the view that CR1 deficiency is acquired rather than inherited in SLE (reviewed in [55]). The evidence includes the observations that CR1 loss in the circulation *in vivo* can be demonstrated on transfused erythrocytes in patients with active SLE; and that low CR1 numbers occur in other conditions such as: RA, autoimmune haemolytic anaemia, PNH, AIDS, and congenital factor I deficiency. CR1 numbers in SLE also show variation within a given patient and appear to inversely mirror disease activity. The mechanism by which CR1 numbers are lowered in active lupus is unclear although they may be removed as immune complexes are delivered to the liver when bound to erythrocyte CR1 (see further discussion below on immune complex clearance).

Acquired complement deficiencies

Complement deficiency may be acquired either as a result of complement activation or as a result of autoantibodies against complement components. Many such autoantibodies have been described; for example, immunoconglutinins which bind to neoantigens on iC3b, C3 nephritic factor, anti-C1q antibodies, antibodies to C1-inhibitor, MAC and CR1. However, only a few of these autoantibodies appear to play a direct role in immunopathogenesis.

C3 nephritic factor (C3NeF) is an IgG autoantibody[56]. It binds to the alternative pathway C3 convertase, C3bBb, and acts in a similar fashion to properdin to stabilize the enzyme complex. C3 is therefore consumed. C3NeF is associated with type II mesangiocapillary glomerulonephritis in which there are characteristic electron-dense deposits within the basement membrane. The antibody also occurs in association with partial lipodystrophy, both with and without glomerulonephritis[57]. The mechanism of the link between C3 nephritic factor and nephritis or lipodystrophy is not yet elucidated. The effects of the acquired hypocomplementaemia include an increased susceptibility to meningococcal infection. There is also a rare association of C3 nephritic factor and SLE – one may speculate that the hypocomplementaemia is the basis for this latter association. Classical pathway 'nephritic factors' have also been described[58] in patients with SLE. They stabilize the C4b2a convertase enzyme. Their role, if any, in lupus pathogenesis remains to be established.

Recently, autoantibodies to C1q have been described in association with hypocomplementaemic urticarial vasculitis. This may occur as a manifestation of connective tissue disease, in particular SLE, or as a primary syndrome. Some patients with primary urticarial vasculitis have an associated hypocomplementaemia and may have other clinical manifestations such as uveitis, glomerulonephritis, and peripheral neuropathy; the hypocomplementaemic urticarial vasculitis syndrome (HUVS)[59]. Autoantibodies to C1q bind to a neoepitope on the collagen-like tail of C1q which becomes exposed on C1q after the dissociation of C1s and C1r by C1 inhibitor. The demonstration, *in vitro*, of the anti-C1q antibody is difficult because of the potential for confusion due to the physiological binding of the globular head of C1q to the Fc antibody region. The methodological difficulties can be reduced by using the purified collagen-like stalk of C1q as the substrate for an ELISA to detect anti-C1q. Indeed, by using this system it is apparent that these antibodies are common in the plasma of patients with SLE[60,61]. The presence of anti-C1q antibodies in SLE has implications for the use of the C1q-binding assay for immune complexes, in that they are probably responsible for false positive results, rendering the assay unreliable. Anti-C1q is associated with a marked depression in serum classical pathway components; in particular C1q and C4 levels are very low. Thus in SLE a persistently low C4 (and C1q) is an indicator of the possible presence of the autoantibody. The strong association between anti-C1q and hypocomplementaemia suggests a causal link between the autoantibody and SLE, but this has not been proven. The mechanism by which anti-C1q is associated with HUVS has not been unravelled. More recently anti-C1q antibodies have been reported in a number of other conditions such as: Felty's syndrome, polyarteritis nodosa, membranoproliferative glomerulonephritis and antiglomerular basement membrane disease[62]. Because of variation in assay system and incomplete characterization it is uncertain whether the anti-C1q found in these latter conditions is identical to that described in SLE and HUVS.

IMMUNE COMPLEX HANDLING, DISEASE AND COMPLEMENT

The role of complement

The physiological role of the complement system in relation to immune complex clearance is attested to by the high prevalence of immune complex-mediated diseases in both acquired and hereditary complement deficiency. Immune complexes may activate the classical pathway of complement by binding C1q; following C1 activation, C4b and C3b are covalently bound to the complex. The consequence of this is that the tendency for immune complexes to precipitate is inhibited. The mechanism by which this inhibition occurs is now largely understood (reviewed in [63]). When immune complexes form, large aggregates can be generated by two means: as a result of antibody binding to multiple epitopes on the antigen; and because of Fc–Fc interactions between the binding antibodies. The importance of the latter can be inferred by the retardation of immune complex formation when F(ab)$_2$ IgG fragments are used instead of whole antibody[64]. By fixing C4b/C3b to the immune complex the Fc–Fc interactions are impeded, thus reducing one means by which large aggregates arise. The second mechanism of inhibition of large immune complex lattice formation is the effective reduction in valency of the antigen/antibody interaction by C3b and C4b binding to the complex. The role of the classical pathway can be shown by the inability of serum that is deficient in C1q, C4, or C2 to produce this inhibition of precipitation[65]. If immune complexes do precipitate then any small amount of fixed C3b on them can be amplified by the alternative pathway and complement fixation can further disrupt the immune complex lattice. Thus a process of solubilization exists which is dependent on the alternative pathway. Inhibition of precipitation is the more effective of the two methods employed to maintain immune complexes in solution. The end result, that is the solubilization of complexes, removes these potentially tissue-damaging products from their site of formation into the fluid phase where they can interact with complement receptors. Immune complexes within the vasculature bind predominantly to CR1 on erythrocytes rather than leucocytes owing to the red cell's numerical superiority and the clustering of CR1 on the erythrocyte's surface[66]. Immune complexes formed in the extravascular compartment can bind to leucocyte complement and Fc receptors.

Complexes bound to erythrocyte CR1 are delivered to the liver and spleen where they are removed. Catheterization of the hepatic and portal veins of baboons has shown that this process is very efficient in that it occurs during a single transit of complexes through the hepatic circulation[67]. Studies on complement-deficient baboons[68] and in humans with varying CR1 numbers[69] testify to the conclusion that deficiency of complement or of erythrocyte CR1 produces reduced binding of immune complexes to cells and an accelerated clearance from the circulation.

Immune complexes and the connective tissue diseases

The unequivocal demonstration of immune complexes in serum is very difficult in human disease. The presence of cryoglobulins provides good evidence but is useful in only a minority of cases, although it is clearly of relevance in mixed essential cryoglobulinaemia. Other frequently employed assays are: polyethylene glycol precipitation and the C1q binding assay (reviewed in [70]). There are poor correlations between results obtained using different immune complex assays on the same specimens of serum. Results of the solid-phase C1q binding assay for immune complexes have been largely discredited by the discovery that the anti-C1q autoantibody is responsible for the majority of positive results[71]. More recently, experimental assays for immune complexes use monoclonal antibodies to neoantigens on C3b[72].

Immune complexes can be considered to be pathogenic under two circumstances: either circulating immune complexes are deposited in tissues, or they are formed *in situ*. Although immune complex deposition from the circulation is frequently cited as a disease mechanism, confirmatory data is often lacking. Conditions for which the evidence is strongest for immune complex deposition are: essential mixed cryoglobulinaemia, experimental serum sickness, and infectious endocarditis.

Essential mixed cryoglobulinaemia (EMC) is associated with a profound depression in C4 concentrations. The circulating cryoglobulins contain both IgG and IgM; the IgM component has anti-IgG activity and the complex can fix complement[73]. Immune deposits containing both IgG and complement can be demonstrated in the cutaneous blood vessels and in the glomerular basement membrane. In infectious endocarditis and serum sickness, circulating complexes are generated as a consequence of chronic antigenic stimulation. In both instances immune complexes can be demonstrated in the circulation and at the site of tissue damage. Other connective tissue diseases (excluding SLE and RA) in which immune complexes may be involved in pathogenesis include: post-viral arthritis, polyarteritis nodosa (PAN), Henoch–Schonlein purpura (HSP), and hypersensitivity vasculitis.

A self-limiting polyarthritis is described following hepatitis B infection. The development of joint disease is associated with the following: a rapid rise and high titres of anti-HBs antibodies; cryoprecipitates containing HBs, anti-HBs, C3 and C4; and hypocomplementaemia (reviewed in [74]). Similar syndromes are described in association with other viral infections, e.g. hepatitis C and parvovirus.

In PAN circulating immune complexes have been described but are not reliably demonstrable. There is a subset of PAN patients that have serological evidence of previous hepatitis B infection. It has been suggested that PAN is an immune complex disease following viral hepatitis; however, the exact nature of the relationship between hepatitis B infection and PAN remains unsettled. Hepatitis B surface antigen (HBsAg) and anti-HBs together with complement have been demonstrated in the arterial lesions[75]. However, hypocomplementaemia is a feature of active polyarteritis in only about 25% of cases[76].

Circulating immune complexes, containing IgA, are implicated in the aetiology of HSP and IgA nephropathy. Both are characterized by an elevated level of serum IgA and normal complement values. Cryoglobulins isolated from the sera of patients with acute HSP show a preponderance of IgA, the antigen component of the putative complex remains unidentified[77]. Immunofluorescence of involved renal tissue in both conditions shows mesangial IgA together with C3 and properdin. This is accounted for by the fact that IgA complexes do activate the alternative pathway.

Immune complexes and the pathogenesis of SLE

There is strong evidence that immune complexes are pathogenic in SLE, though it remains unclear whether these are deposited preformed in the tissues or are formed *in situ*. The mechanisms that underlie lupus can be conceived in two ways. Firstly, there may be an initiating disturbance in immune regulation such that B lymphocytes (and presumably autoreactive T cells) escape the usual mechanisms that hold autoantibody production in check. A second hypothesis is that the autoimmune response arises through the aberrant presentation of autoantigen and that once this has occurred the normal mechanisms that eliminate immune complexes fail and there is then tissue deposition of immune complexes which causes tissue damage and hence further autoantigen presentation. The association of SLE with genetic complement deficiency favours the interpretation that impaired immune complex handling is of primary significance.

The second hypothesis of lupus pathogenesis predicts that the autoantibody response in lupus is antigen-driven. Recent studies looking at the antibody binding characteristics and comparing autoantibody mRNA and germline sequences have suggested that anti-DNA antibodies comprise two populations. One group, which also occur in normal subjects, are predominantly IgM, have a low affinity for DNA, and bear germline sequences. Pathogenic anti-DNA antibodies, in contrast, are IgG, have a high affinity for their target, and show evidence of somatic mutation in their variable regions as would be expected in an antigen-driven response[78,79].

By combining the hypothesis which suggests that autoantibodies in SLE are antigen-driven with the role of complement in immune complex metabolism a model for lupus pathogenesis can be constructed in which immune complex deposition and hypocomplementaemia can be viewed as one of a vicious cycle of aberrant handling and deposition[80]. Active SLE is associated with a decrease in the total erythrocyte CR1 number and the concentration of the classical complement components is often markedly reduced. The hypocomplementaemia is in part a consequence of complement activation by immune complexes; this may occur at sites of tissue damage where complexes are formed and/or deposited. The result of reduced C4, C2 and C1q together with CR1 is impaired immune complex transport and a tendency for inappropriate tissue deposition. Once localized in the tissues there is local complement activation producing damage and further complement consumption. In addition, it can be postulated that tissue damage itself may generate neoantigens or promote local antigen presentation so that further autoantibodies can be generated.

Experiments using radiolabelled, aggregated IgG or preformed immune complexes have allowed the visualization of immune complex handling *in vivo*. Following injection into normal subjects both aggregated IgG and preformed immune complexes are rapidly bound to erythrocytes and delivered to the liver within minutes. The rate of elimination is inversely related to the erythrocyte CR1 number[81]. When such studies are performed in patients with SLE preformed, large immune complexes are cleared more rapidly than in normal controls, and there is rapid but temporary hepatic uptake and reduced splenic uptake[82]. This may reflect rapid deposition throughout the vascular system (although the technique does permit direct visualization of this) rather than transport to the monocyte-macrophage system in the liver and spleen which appears defective in binding immune complexes.

Rheumatoid arthritis, immune complexes and complement

The relationship between complement, immune complexes and RA is complex. Active RA is usually associated with normal or elevated serum complement levels. The latter arise because many components such as C3, C4, C5 and factor B are acute phase proteins; an increase in their synthesis has been shown to occur in response to interleukin-1 and TNF stimulation[83].

Patients with rheumatoid arthritis who develop vasculitis tend to become hypocomplementaemic and sustain a reduction in erythrocyte CR1 numbers[84]. Such patients have high titres of RF in the serum. In patients with rheumatoid vasculitis there is evidence of systemic complement consumption which may reflect activation by RF/immunoglobulin complexes. In RA *sine* vasculitis there is evidence of complement activation, but this is confined to the synovium (to be discussed later). Serum from patients with rheumatoid vasculitis can be shown to be defective in the inhibition of immune precipitation[85]. Taken together the evidence suggests that deposition of circulating immune complexes may occur in rheumatoid vasculitis.

Complement may also play a subtle role in the pathogenesis of RA by its relationship to the generation of the immune response. The circulating IgG RFs in RA appear different from those found in other connective tissue diseases in that there is evidence that they arise by antigenic stimulation rather than as strict germline copies as do the monoclonal IgM RFs found in other inflammatory diseases. The RFs in RA are derived from all immunoglobulin isotypes[86], they are somatically hypermutated, and they may derive their light chain component from multiple light chain variable gene families[87]. This suggests that the autoantibodies are T cell dependent and that their production is maintained by continued antigen presentation, that is presentation of immunoglobulin within immune complexes. Complement can be activated by large circulating complexes of RF, this then favours their transport and localization to lymphoid germinal centres. Once there, the complexes bind to complement receptors on the surface of follicular dendritic cells (they express CR1, CR2, and CR3). This allows immune complex, and hence antigen retention[88]. This system has been demonstrated using immune complexes obtained from the serum of patients with RA. When these immune complexes were injected into mice the ability of the complexes to localize to the splenic germinal centres was seen to be optimal when the complexes were large, as occurs in RA with vasculitis and Felty's syndrome. Furthermore, efficient localization was related to the activation of the complement system via the classical pathway in the patient's serum[89].

COMPLEMENT IN DIAGNOSIS AND DISEASE MONITORING

The commonest assays of the complement system in the majority of clinical laboratories are the measurement of C3, C4 and CH50. Both C3 and C4 can be quantified immunochemically. The total haemolytic activity is measured by the CH50, that is the amount required to achieve 50% lysis of antibody coated red cells. These assays for complement protein concentrations and activity can be used as an aid to the differential diagnosis of connective tissue disease and as a means of monitoring disease activity.

Hypocomplementaemia is a feature of active SLE and rheumatoid vasculitis. Particularly in relation to SLE, low serum complement protein levels provide an early clue to the diagnosis enabling distinction from many of the other connective diseases such as rheumatoid arthritis, mixed connective tissue disease and scleroderma. In SLE and rheumatoid vasculitis it is predominantly the levels of the classical pathway proteins that are reduced, producing a low C4 and CH50 on routine analysis. The C3 concentration in the serum is often normal or only slightly depressed even in the presence of significant reduction in C4 concentration. This reflects the efficient regulation of classical pathway activation in the fluid phase which limits the conversion of C3. If C3 is substantially lowered this implies recruitment of the amplification loop of the alternative pathway activation. In SLE, low C3 concentrations are associated with severe disease[89]. In RA, hypocomplementaemia is associated with high titres of RF, vasculitis and extra-articular manifestations as outlined above in the discussion of immune complexes.

In an individual patient with SLE, sequential serum complement estimation can provide a valuable tool for disease monitoring since the classical pathway protein concentrations have an inverse relationship with disease activity[89]. This is not true for all lupus patients and it is difficult to demonstrate the reciprocal correlation between disease activity and complement protein levels in cohorts of patients[90]. It may well be that inter-individual variations in the synthetic rates of complement proteins account for the lack of a reproducible correlation. In fact, by using radiolabelled complement proteins in patients with SLE, such variability in synthetic rates has been shown to exist *in vivo*[91]. It is important to note that in pregnancy the concentration of complement proteins rises physiologically and hence pregnancy may mask the hypocomplementaemia of active lupus[92].

In patients with mixed essential cryoglobulinaemia the markedly low C4 values in the presence of pertinent clinical features such as Raynaud's/digital ischaemia, neuropathy and glomerulonephritis are a pointer to the diagnosis. Quantification of C4 may, together with an estimation of the amount of cryoglobulin, be useful in disease monitoring too.

Glomerulonephritis can be associated with hypocomplementaemia. The most characteristic circumstances are the particular lowering of C3 found with the nephritic factor in mesangiocapillary nephritis and the depression of C4 and C3 in post-streptococcal nephritis. Chronic infectious endocarditis can also give rise to an immune complex syndrome with glomerulonephritis and hypocomplementaemia.

Hypocomplementaemia also occurs in hypocomplementaemic urticarial vasculitis syndrome (HUVS) as described above. The relationship between this condition and SLE is close, as has been demonstrated by the anti-C1q antibody and the fact that a few cases of HUVS have progressed to SLE. Complement consumption can also be a feature of hypersensitivity vasculitis syndromes following infection or drug administration in which immune complexes are pathogenic.

In cases of SLE and lupus-like conditions in which there is profound and persistent hypocomplementaemia, the possibility of a hereditary complement deficiency should be considered. The commonest instance in the Caucasian population is that of C2 deficiency. In this case the CH50 is absent despite a preserved C3 and C4. Hereditary C3 deficiency can cause immune complex disease but it should be borne in mind that C3 deficiency may also occur as a result of factor I and factor H deficiency as well as with C3 nephritic factor.

COMPLEMENT AND INFLAMMATION

Complement is an important source of mediators for the inflammatory response. Activation of the complement cascade produces the anaphylatoxins C3a, C4a and C5a, which cause inflammatory mediators to be released from mast cells, monocytes and neutrophils. C5a is a potent chemotactic factor for neutrophils and macrophages, on whose surfaces it upregulates the expression of CR1 and CR3; the latter promotes leucocyte adhesion to endothelium. Of the anaphylatoxins, C5a is the most potent. Following binding to a specific C5a receptor on neutrophils, the cell is stimulated to degranulate, undergo a respiratory burst, and release prostanoid mediators, including leukotriene B4, itself a very potent chemotactic agent for neutrophils and monocytes.

The role of complement in the connective tissue diseases is most relevant to those in which the humoral autoimmune processes dominate pathogenesis. In any inflammatory process, whatever its aetiology, there may be evidence of local complement deposition although this may be a secondary event. Injured tissue releases various substances, such as nucleic acids, cardiolipin and anionic polymers, that have the capacity to activate complement[93]. In addition, other triggered enzyme cascades such as the kinin system, coagulation and fibrinolytic pathways, which are activated at inflammatory foci, have the facility to initiate the complement cascade[94].

The evidence for complement being pathogenic at the site of tissue damage comes in part from direct histological demonstration by immunofluorescence. However, such findings must be interpreted with caution because it can be shown in SLE that there is immunoglobulin and C3 present at the dermo-epidermal junction of clinically uninvolved skin – this forms the basis of the lupus band test for SLE. If the area is clinically affected then there is usually evidence of deposition of terminal complement components implying that the MAC is pathogenic in this circumstance[95]. However, recent studies have suggested that MAC localization does not prove a local pathogenic role for complement; some terminal complexes are bound to the inhibitory protein vitronectin, producing non-lytic complexes[96].

Complement and lupus nephritis

The nephritis of lupus has been well studied in relation to complement. In the kidney there are a number of histological patterns of lupus nephritis which probably represent different pathogenic mechanisms although complement deposition is a common feature. Immunofluorescent staining of lupus nephritis usually reveals IgG, IgM, IgA, C3, C4 and C1q. Immune complex deposition may be relevant in some cases, although whether these are locally formed or deposited from the circulation is unclear. There is some evidence that immune complexes in nephritis may involve anti-native DNA antibodies as they can be eluted from renal biopsy material from lupus patients[97]. An alternative mechanism is that complexes are formed *in situ* within the kidney as is believed to occur in membranous nephritis. In this case the complexes are localized subepithelially and the basement membrane acts as a barrier against cellular infiltrate. However, complement proteins can penetrate to the subepithelial region and in experimental animals it can be shown that development of the nephritis is critically dependent on the presence of the MAC[98]. In animal models in which immune complexes deposit in the subendothelium, experimental depletion of either leucocytes or complement ameliorates tissue damage, which suggests that both cells and complement are involved in pathogenesis. As mentioned above, the pathology of lupus nephritis is diverse and intraglomerular thrombosis is common when there is a diffuse proliferative nephritis. Complement, via its terminal pathway components, may interact with platelets to promote clotting. The MAC can insert into the platelet membrane and induce a rise in intracellular calcium levels. This releases procoagulant mediators such as: coagulation factors Va and Xa; and thromboxane A_2 (reviewed in [99]).

Rheumatoid arthritis

Although the cell mediated immune response is considered to play a dominant role in rheumatoid arthritis, there is evidence that complement activation takes place in rheumatoid joints. It is well known that the concentration of complement proteins in the active rheumatoid exudate (as found in the joint, pleural and pericardial cavities) is often low compared with the serum[100]. Various studies have demonstrated that this reflects activation of both classical and alternative pathways because of the presence of breakdown products such as C5a and Bb in synovial fluid[101]. This is probably triggered by local immune complex formation involving RF; indeed the main pathogenic potential of RF may lie in its ability to activate complement. Thus in rheumatoid arthritis, formation of immune complexes within the joint activates the complement system which propagates the synovitis. As well as being involved in rheumatoid exudative processes within the pleural and pericardial cavities, complement activation may well be pathogenic in other extra-articular manifestations. Terminal pathway components are deposited in rheumatoid nodules and in the skin in rheumatoid vasculitis[102].

Dermatomyositis

Another disease in which humoral mechanisms may be important is juvenile dermatomyositis. Histologically, there is perivascular inflammatory infiltrate and perifascicular atrophy in the affected muscle. Immunofluorescence shows that there is perivascular MAC deposition[103]. This is in contrast to adult polymyositis in which complement deposition is a less apparent feature and there is T lymphocyte infiltration in involved muscle.

LOCAL VERSUS SYSTEMIC SYNTHESIS OF COMPLEMENT PROTEINS

With the notable exceptions of C1q and factor D the bulk of the circulating complement proteins are manufactured in the liver. The main site of C1q synthesis remains controversial; C1q synthesis has been demonstrated in macrophages, fibroblasts and intestinal epithelial cells. Almost all of the circulating complement proteins are also synthesized by tissues outside the liver, particularly by monocytes/macrophages, polymorphs and fibroblasts[104]. These cells are usually capable of augmenting synthesis in response to cytokine stimulation[105]. Thus when there is local inflammation the predominant source of complement within that local environment is debatable. Is complement systemically derived because of locally increased vascular permeability, or locally produced by the ingress of inflammatory cells and/or by local cells such as fibroblasts responding to cytokines which stimulate them to produce complement proteins? There is good evidence that synovial tissue from both inflamed and degenerative joints is able to synthesize classical pathway proteins and factor B[106]. Using radiolabelled C3 it has been shown that in a synovial effusion from a patient with rheumatoid arthritis approximately one-half of the total intra-articular C3 was locally synthesized[107]. By performing *in situ* hybridization, synovial cells from rheumatoid joints have been demonstrated to express an increased amount of mRNA for C2 and C3 compared with synovial cells from osteoarthritic joints[108]. The exact cellular origin of complement within the joint is unsettled, possibilities include macrophages, B lymphocytes, endothelial cells and fibroblasts. The latter have been shown to synthesize complement components during *in vitro* culture[109].

THERAPEUTIC USE OF COMPLEMENT REGULATORS

Because of its role in the inflammatory response, complement inhibition has potential therapeutic uses in a wide range of diseases. In animal models of both immunological disease (e.g. myasthenia gravis) and ischaemic disease (e.g. coronary artery occlusion) the use of cobra venom factor to cause complement depletion has been shown to ameliorate the pathology[110]. A recombinant, soluble form of CR1 (sCR1) has been recently engineered[111]. The sCR1 contains all the extracellular domains of the parent molecule; the transmembrane and intracellular regions have been deleted. This molecule is a potent inhibitor of complement activation and on a molar basis is more efficacious than the naturally occurring complement inhibitory proteins of the fluid-phase – factor H and C4-binding protein. Beneficial effects have been described in non-immunological models, such as ischaemic reperfusion injury in the rat myocardium[112]; and in immunological models, e.g. after intra-alveolar and intradermal deposition of IgG immune complexes[113]; and in the rejection of xenografts and hyperacute rejection of allografts[114].

References

1. Law SK, Levine RP. Interaction between the third complement protein and cell-surface macromolecules. Proc Natl Acad Sci USA. 1977; 74: 2701–2705.
2. Panburn MK, Muller-Eberhard HJ. The C3 convertase of the alternative pathway of human complement. Enzymic properties of the bimolecular proteinase. Biochem J. 1986; 235: 723–730.
3. Burton DR, Boyd J, Brampton AD, Easterbrook-Smith ED, Emanuel EJ, Novotny J, Rademacher TW, van Schravendij MR, Sterberg MJ, Dwek RA. The C1q receptor site on immunoglobulin G. Nature. 1980; 288: 338–344.
4. Schumaker VN, Zavodsky P, Poon PH. Activation of the first component of complement. Ann Rev Immunol. 1987; 5: 21–42.
5. Law SK, Fearon DT, Levine RP. Action of the C3b-inactivator on cell bound C3b. J Immunol. 1979; 122: 7262–7265.
6. Muller-Eberhard HJ. Molecular organisation and function of the complement system. Ann Rev Biochem. 1988; 57: 321–347.
7. Lublin DM, Atkinson JP. Decay-acceleration factor: Biochemistry, molecular biology and function. Ann Rev Immunol. 1979; 7: 35–58.
8. Liszewski MK, Post TW, Atkinson JP. Membrane cofactor protein (MCP or CD46): newest member of the regulators of complement activation gene cluster. Ann Rev Immunol. 1991; 9: 431–455.
9. Ahearn JM, Fearon DT. Structure and function of the complement receptors, CR1 (CD35) and CR2 (CD21). Adv Immunol. 1989; 46: 183–219.
10. Nagaki K, Iida K, Inai S. The inactivator of the first component of human complement (C1INA). The complex formation with the activated first component of human complement (C1) or with its subcomponents. Int Arch Allergy Appl Immunol. 1974; 46: 935–948.
11. Podack ER, Muller-Eberhard HJ. Isolation of human S-protein, an inhibitor of the membrane attack complex of complement. J Biol Biochem. 1979; 254: 9908–9914.
12. Davies A, Simmons DL, Hale G, Harrison RA, Tighe H, Lachmann PJ, Waldmann H. CD 262, an Ly-6-like protein expressed in human lymphoid cells, regulates the action of the complement membrane attack complex on homologous cells. J Exp Med. 1989; 170: 637–654.
13. Schonermark S, Rauterberg EW, Shin ML, Loke S, Roelke D, Hansch GM. Homologous species restriction in lysis of human erythrocytes: a membrane derived protein with C8-binding capacity functions as an inhibitor. J Immunol. 1986; 136: 1772–1776.
14. Halperin JA, Nicholson-Weller A. Paroxysmal nocturnal haemoglobinuria. A complement-mediated disease. Complement Inflamm. 1989; 6: 65–72.
15. Reid KBM, Bentley DR, Campbell RD, Chung LP, Sim RB, Kristensen T, Tack BF. Complement system proteins which interact with C3b or C4b. Immunol Today. 1986; 7: 230–233.
16. Fearon DT. Cellular receptors for fragments of the third component of complement. Immunol Today. 1984; 5: 105–110.
17. Wong WW, Cahill JM, Rosen MD, Kennedy CA, Bonaccio ET, Morris MJ, Wilson JG, Klickstein LB, Fearon DT. Structure of the human CR1 gene. Molecular basis of the structural and quantitative polymorphisms and identification of a new CR1-like allele. J Exp Med. 1989; 169: 847–863.
18. Fingeroth JD, Weiss JJ, Tedder TF, Strominger JL, Biro PA, Fearon DT. Epstein-Barr virus receptor on human B lymphocytes is the C3d receptor, CR2. Proc Natl Acad Sci (USA). 1984; 81: 4510–4514.
19. Heyman B, Wiersma EJ, Kinoshita T. *In vivo* inhibition of the antibody response by a complement receptor specific monoclonal antibody. J Exp Med. 1990; 172: 665–668.
20. Papamichail M, Gutierrez C, Embling P, Johnson P, Holborow EJ, Pepys MB. Complement dependence of localisation of aggregated IgG in germinal centres. Scand J Immunol. 1975; 4: 343–347.
21. Klaus GGB, Humphrey JH. The generation of memory cells. The role of C3 in the generation of B memory cells. Immunology. 1977; 33: 31–40.
22. Ross GD, Medof ME. Membrane complement receptors specific for bound fragments of C3. Adv Immunol. 1985; 37: 217–267.

23. Doershuk CM, Winn RK, Coxson HO, Harlan JM. CD18-dependent and independent mechanisms of neutrophil emigration in the pulmonary and systemic microcirculation of rabbits. J Immunol. 1990; 144: 2327–2333.
24. Lachmann PJ, Walport MJ. Genetic deficiency diseases of the complement system. In: Ross GD, ed. Immunobiology of the Complement System. New York, Academic Press, 1986: 237–261.
25. Sellar GC, Cockburn D, Reid KBM. Localisation of the gene encoding the A chain, B chain and C chain of human C1q to 1p34.1 to 1p36.3. Immunogenetics. 1992; 35: 214–216.
26. Steinsson K, McClean RH, Merrow M, Rothfield NF, Weinstein A. Selective complete C1q deficiency associated with systemic lupus erythematosus. J Rheumatol. 1983; 10: 590–594.
27. Thompson RA, Haeney M, Reid KBM, Davies JG, White RHR, Cameron AH. A genetic defect of the C1q component of complement associated with childhood (immune complex) nephritis. N Engl J Med. 1980; 303: 22–24.
28. McAdam R, Groundis D, Reid KBM. A homozygous point mutation results in a stop codon in the B-chain of a C1q-deficient individual. Immunogenetics. 1988; 27: 259–264.
29. Tosi M, Duponche C, Meo T, Julier C. Complete cDNA sequence of human C1s and close physical linkage of the homologous genes C1s and C1r. Biochem. 1987; 26: 8516–8524.
30. Baur MP, Neugebauer M, Deppe H, Sigmund M, Luton T, Mayr WR, Albert ED. Population analysis on the basis of deduced phenotypes from random families. In: Albert ED, Baur MP, Mayr WR, eds. Histocompatibility Testing. Berlin, Heidelberg: Springer-Verlag; 1984: 333–341.
31. Dunckley H, Gatenby PA, Hawkins B, Naito S, Serjeantson SW. Deficiency of C4A is genetic determinant of systemic lupus erythematosus in three ethnic groups. J Immunogenetics. 1987; 14: 209–218.
32. Batchelor JR, Fielder AHL, Walport MJ, David J, Lord DK, Davey N, Dodi IA, Malesit ID, Wanachiwanin W, Bernstein R. Family study of the major histocompatibility complex in HLA DR3 negative patients with systemic lupus erythematosus. Clin Exp Immunol. 1987; 70: 364–371.
33. Schifferli JA, Steiger G, Paccaud J-P, Sjoholm AJ, Hauptmann G. Difference in the biological properties of the two forms of the fourth component of human complement. Clin Exp Immunol. 1986; 63: 473–477.
34. Christiansen FT, McCluskey J, Dawkins RL, Kay PH, Uko G, Zilko PJ. Complement allotyping in SLE: association with C4A null. Aust and NZ J Med. 1983; 13: 483–488.
35. Jacob CO, McDevitt HO. Tumour necrosis factor in murine autoimmune lupus nephritis. Nature. 1990; 331: 356–357.
36. Jacob CO, Fronek Z, Lewis GD, Koo M, Hansen JA, McDevitt HO. Heritable major histocompatibility complex class-II associated differences in the production of tumour necrosis factor α: relevance to genetic predisposition to systemic lupus erythematosus. Proc Natl Acad Sci USA. 1990; 87: 1233–1237.
37. Carroll MC, Palsdottir A, Belt KT, Porter RR. Deletion of complement C4 and steroid 21-hydroxylase genes in the HLA class III region. EMBO J. 1985; 4: 2547–2552.
38. Mauff G, Alper CA, Awdeh ZL, Batchelor JR, Bertrams J, Brunn-Petersen G, Dawkins RL, Demant P, Edwards J, Grosse-Wilde H, Hauptmann G, Klouda P, Lamm L, Mollenhaur E, Nerl E, Olaison B, O'Neil GJ, Rittner C, Roos M, Skanes V, Teisberg P, Wells L. Statement of the nomenclature of C4 allotypes. Immunobiology. 1983; 164: 184–191.
39. Hauptmann G, Tappeiner G, Schifferli JA. Inherited deficiency of the fourth component of human complement. Immunodef Rev. 1988; 1: 3–22.
40. Braun L, Schneider NL, Giles CM, Bertrams J, Rittner C. Null alleles of human complement C4: evidence for pseudogenes at the C4A locus and for gene conversion at the C4B locus. J Exp Med. 1990; 171: 129–140.
41. Agnello V. Complement deficiency states. Medicine. 1978; 57: 1–23.
42. Glass D, Baum D, Gibson D, Stillman JS, Schur PH. Inherited deficiency of the second component of complement. J Clin Invest. 1976; 58: 853–861.
43. Johnson CA, Densen P, Hurford RK, Colten HR, Westel RA. Type 1 human complement C2 deficiency – a 28 base pair gene deletion causes skipping of exon 6 during RNA splicing. J Biol Chem. 1992; 267: 9347–9353.
44. Agostini A. Inherited C1 inhibitor deficiency. Complement. 1989; 6: 112–118.
45. Massa MC, Connolly MD. An association between C1-esterase inhibitor deficiency and

lupus erythematosus. Report of two cases and review of the literature. J Am Acad Dermatol. 1982; 7: 255–264.

46. Botto M, Fong KY, So AK, Rudge A, Walport MJ. Molecular basis of hereditary C3 deficiency. J Clin Invest. 1990; 86: 1158–1163.

47. Botto M, Fong KY, So AK, Barlow R, Routier R, Morley BJ, Walport MJ. Homozygous hereditary C3 deficiency due to a partial gene deletion. Proc Natl Acad Sci USA. 1992; 89: 4957–4961.

48. Thompson RA, Winterborn MH. Hypocomplementaemia due to genetic deficiency of β1H globulin. Clin Exp Immunol. 1981; 46: 110–119.

49. Fijen CAP, Kuijper EJ, Hannema AJ, Sjoholm AG, van Putten JPM. Complement deficiencies in patients over ten years old with meningococcal disease with uncommon serotypes. Lancet. 1989; 2: 585–588.

50. Petersen BH, Lee TJ, Snyderman R, Brooks GF. Neisseria meningitidis and neisseria gonorrhoeae bacteraemia associated with C6, C7 and C8 deficiency. Ann Int Med. 1979; 90: 917–920.

51. Trapp RG, Mooney E, Coleman TH, Forristal J, Herman JH. Hereditary complement (C6) deficiency associated with systemic lupus erythematosus, Sjøgren's syndrome and hyperthyroidism. J Rheumatol. 1987; 14: 1030–1033.

52. Wilson JG, Wong W, Schur PH, Fearon DT. Mode of inheritance of decreased C3b receptors on erythrocytes of patients with systemic lupus erythematosus. N Engl J Med. 1982; 307: 981–986.

53. Wilson JG, Murphy EE, Wong WW, Klickstein LB, Weis JH, Fearon DT. Identification of a restriction fragment length polymorphism by CR1 cDNA that correlates with the number of CR1 on erythrocytes. J Exp Med. 1986; 164: 50–59.

54. Miykawa Y, Yamada A, Kosaka K, Tsuda F, Kosugie E, Mayumi M. Defective immune adherence (C3b) receptor on erythrocytes of patients with systemic lupus erythematosus. Lancet. 1981; 2: 493–497.

55. Walport MJ, Lachmann PJ. Erythrocyte complement receptor type 1, immune complexes and the rheumatic diseases. Arth Rheum. 1988; 31: 153–158.

56. Spitzer RE, Vallota EH, Forristal J, Sudora E, Stitzel A, Davis NC, West CD. Serum C'3 lytic system in patients with glomerulonephritis. Science. 1969; 164: 436–437.

57. Sissons JGP, West RJ, Fallows J, Williams DG, Boucher BJ, Amos N, Peters DK. The complement abnormalities of partial lipodystrophy. N Engl J Med. 1976; 294: 461–465.

58. Daha MR, Hazevoet HM, Van Es LA, Cats A. Stabilisation of the classical pathway C3 convertase C42 by a factor F-42, isolated from serum of patients with systemic lupus erythematosus. Immunology. 1980; 40: 417–424.

59. Agnello V, Koffler D, Eisenberg JW, Winchester RJ, Kunkel HG. C1q precipitins in the sera of patients with systemic lupus erythematosus and other hypocomplementaemic states: characterisation of high and low molecular weight types. J Exp Med. 1971; 134: 228S.

60. Wener MH, Uwatako S, Mannik M. Antibodies to the collagen-like region of C1q in sera of patients with rheumatic diseases. Arthritis Rheum. 1989; 32: 544–551.

61. Wisnieski JJ, Naff GB. Serum IgG antibodies to C1q in hypocomplementemic urticarial vasculitis syndrome. Arthritis Rheum. 1989; 32: 1119–27.

62. Siegert CE, Daha MR, Halma C, van der Voort EA, Breedveld FC. IgG and IgA autoantibodies to C1q in systemic and renal diseases. Clin Exp Rheumatol. 1992; 10: 19–23.

63. Schifferli JA, Ng YC, Peters DK. The role of complement and its receptor in the elimination of immune complexes. New Engl J Med. 1986; 315: 488–495.

64. Møller NPH. Fc-mediated immune precipitation. I. A new role of the Fc portion of IgG. Immunology. 1979; 38: 631–640.

65. Schifferli JA, Woo P, Peters DK. Complement-mediated inhibition of immune precipitation. I. Role of classical and alternative pathways. Clin Exp Immunol. 1982; 47: 555–562.

66. Siegel I, Liu TL, Gleicher N. The red-cell immune system. Lancet. 1981; 2: 556–559.

67. Cornacoff JB, Hebert LA, Smead WL, Vaneman LE, Birmingham DJ, Waxman FJ. Primate erythrocyte immune-complex clearing mechanism. J Clin Invest. 1983; 71: 236–247.

68. Waxman FJ, Hebert LA, Cornacoff JB, Vaneman ME, Smead WL, Kraut EH, Birmingham DJ, Taguiam JM. Complement depletion accelerates the clearance of immune complexes from the circulation of primates. J Clin Invest. 1984; 74: 1329–1340.

69. Schifferli JA, Ng YC, Paccaud JP, Walport MJ. The role of hypocomplementaemia and low erythrocyte complement receptor type 1 numbers in determining abnormal immune complex clearance in humans. Clin Exp Immunol. 1989; 75: 329–335.
70. Theofilopoulos AN, Dixon FJ. The biology and detection of immune complexes. Adv Immunol. 1979; 28: 89–220.
71. Uwatako S, Mannik M. Low molecular weight C1q-binding immunoglobulin G in patients with systemic lupus erythematosus consists of autoantibodies to the collagen-like region of C1q. J Clin Invest. 1988; 82: 816–824.
72. Aguado MT, Lambris JD, Tsokos GC, Burger R, Bitter-Suermann D, Tamerius JD, Dixon FJ, Theofilopoulos AN. Monoclonal antibodies against complement 3 neoantigens for detection of immune complexes and complement activation. Relationship between immune complex levels, state of C3, and numbers of receptors for C3b. J Clin Invest. 1985; 76: 1418–1426.
73. Meltzer M, Franklin EC, Elias K, McCluskey RT, Cooper N. Cryoglobulinaemia – a clinical and laboratory study. II. Cryoglobulins with rheumatoid factor activity. Am J Med. 1966; 40: 837–851.
74. Alpert E, Isselbacher KJ, Schur PH. The pathogenesis of arthritis associated with viral hepatitis. N Engl J Med. 1971; 285: 185–190.
75. Michalak T. Immune complexes of Hepatitis B surface antigen in the pathogenesis of polyarteritis nodosa. A study of seven necropsy cases. Am J Pathol. 1978; 90: 619–632.
76. Cohen R, Conn DL, Illstup DM. Clinical features, prognosis, and response to treatment in polyarteritis. Mayo Clin Proc. 1980; 55: 146–154.
77. Garcia-Fuentes M, Chantler C, Williams DG. Cryoglobulinaemia in Henoch-Schonlein purpura. Br Med J. 1977; 2: 163–169.
78. Shlomchik M, Mascelli M, Shan H, Radic MZ, Pisetsky D, Marshak-Rothstein A, Weigert A. Anti-DNA antibodies from autoimmune mice arise by clonal expression and somatic mutation. J Exp Med. 1990; 171: 265–297.
79. Van Es JH, Meyling FHJG, Van De Akker WRM, Aanstoot H, Derksen RHWM, Logtenberg T. Somatic mutations in the variable regions of a human IgG anti-double-stranded DNA autoantibody suggest a role for antigen in the introduction of systemic lupus erythematosus. J Exp Med. 1991; 173: 461–470.
80. Lachmann PJ, Walport MJ. Deficiency of the effector mechanisms of the immune response and autoimmunity. In: Whelan J, ed. Ciba Foundation Symposium 129: Autoimmunity and autoimmune diseases. Chichester: Wiley; 1987: 149–171.
81. Schifferli JA, Ng YC, Estreicher J, Walport MJ. The clearance of tetanus toxoid/anti-tetanus toxoid immune complexes from the circulation of humans. Complement and erythrocyte complement receptor 1-independent mechanisms. J Immunol. 1988; 140: 899–904.
82. Davies KA, Peters AM, Beynon HLC, Walport MJ. Immune complex processing in patients with systemic lupus erythematosus – *in vivo* imaging and clearance studies. J Clin Invest. 1992; 90: 2075–2083.
83. Perlmutter DH, Strunk RC, Goldberger G, Cole FS. Regulation of complement protein C2 and factor B by interleukin-1 and gamma interferon acting on transfected L cells. Mol Immunol. 1986; 23: 1263–1266.
84. Heurkens AH, Breedveld FC, Keur CV, Brand R, Daha MR. Degradation of aggregates of activated C3 (C3b) by monocytes of patients with rheumatoid arthritis is related to vasculitis. Clin Exp Immunol. 1990; 80: 177–180.
85. O'Sullivan MM, Amos N, Bedwell A, Williams BD. Complement mediated inhibition of immune precipitation in rheumatoid vasculitis. Rheumatol Int. 1990; 10: 159–163.
86. Natvig JB, Randen I, Thompson K. Probing of the rheumatoid factor (RF) gene repertoire in rheumatoid arthritis (RA) by hybridoma clones. Clin Exp Immunol. 1990; 8 (Suppl 5): 75–80.
87. Gause A, Kuppers R, Mierau I. A somatically mutated Vκ IV gene encoding a human rheumatoid factor light chain. Clin Exp Immunol. 1992; 88: 430–434.
88. Mageed RA, Kirwan JR, Holborow EJ. Localisation of circulating immune complexes from patients with rheumatoid arthritis in murine spleen germinal centres. Scand J Immunol. 1991; 34: 323–331.
89. Lloyd W, Schur PH. Immune complexes, complement, and anti-DNA in exacerbations of systemic lupus erythematosus (SLE). Medicine Baltimore. 1981; 60: 208–217.

90. Cameron JS, Lessof MH, Ogg CS, Williams BD, Williams DG. Disease activity in the nephritis of systemic lupus erythematosus in relation to serum complement concentrations. DNA-binding capacity and precipitating anti-DNA antibody. Clin Exp Immunol. 1976; 25: 418–427.
91. Alper CA, Rosen FS, Watson L. Studies of the *in vivo* behaviour of human C3 in normal subjects and patients. J Clin Invest. 1967; 46: 2021–2034.
92. Lockshin MD, Qamar T, Levy RA, Druzin ML. Pregnancy in systemic lupus erythematosus. Clin Exp Rheumatol. 1989; 7 (Suppl 3): S195–197.
93. Kovacsovics T, Tschopp J, Kress A, Isliker H. Antibody-independent activation of C1, the first component of complement by cardiolipin. J Immunol. 1985; 135: 2695–2700.
94. Hugli TE. Biochemistry and biology of anaphylatoxins. Complement. 1986; 3: 111–127.
95. Biesecker G, Lavin L, Ziskind M, Koffler D. Cutaneous localisation of the membrane attack complex in discoid and systemic lupus erythematosus. N Engl J Med. 1982; 306: 264–270.
96. Dahlback K, Lofberg H, Dahlback B. Vitronectin colocalises with Ig deposits and C9 neoantigen in discoid lupus erythematosus and dermatitis herpetiformis, but not in bullous pemphigoid. Br J Dermatol. 1989; 120: 725–733.
97. Krishnan C, Kaplan MH. Immunopathologic studies of systemic lupus erythematosus. II. Anti-nuclear reaction of gamma-globulin eluted from homogenates and isolated glomeruli of kidneys from patients with lupus nephritis. J Clin Invest. 1967; 46: 569–580.
98. Biesecker G, Katz S, Koffler D. Renal localisation of the membrane attack complex in systemic lupus erythematosus. J Exp Med. 1981; 154: 1779–1794.
99. Sims PJ, Wiedmer T. The response of human platelets to activated components of the complement system. Immunology Today. 1991; 12: 338–342.
100. Peltier AP, Vial MC, de Seze S. Etudes sur le méchanisme de la baisse du taux de complément dans le liquide synovial au cours de la polyarthrite rheumatoide. 1. Variations respectives des taux de C'1, C'2, et C'3 et du taux de complément total. Pathologie et Biologie. 1970; 18: 959–967.
101. Brodeur JP, Ruddy S, Schwartz LB, Mosley G. Synovial fluid levels of complement to SC5b-9 and fragment Bb are elevated in patients with rheumatoid arthritis. Arthritis Rheum. 1991; 34: 1531–1537.
102. Mellbye OJ, Førre O, Mollnes TE, Kvarnes L. Immunopathology of subcutaneous rheumatoid nodules. Ann Rheum Dis. 1991; 50: 909–912.
103. Kissel JT, Mendel JR, Rammahon KW. Microvascular deposits of complement membrane attack complex in dermatomyositis. N Engl J Med. 1986; 314: 329–334.
104. Colten HR. Biosynthesis of complement. Adv Immunol. 1976; 22: 67–118.
105. Colten HR, Strunk RC, Cole FS, Perlmutter DH. Regulation of complement protein biosynthesis in mononuclear phagocytes. In: Biochemistry of Macrophages. London: Pitman; 1986; 141–154.
106. Moffat BJ, Lappin D, Birnie GD, Whaley K. Complement biosynthesis in human synovial tissue. Clin Exp Immunol. 1989; 78: 54–60.
107. Ruddy S, Colten HR. Rheumatoid arthritis. Biosynthesis of complement proteins by synovial tissues. N Engl J Med. 1974; 290: 1284–1288.
108. Firestein GS, Paine MM, Littman BH. Gene expression (collagenase, tissue inhibitor of metalloproteinases, complement, and HLA-DR) in rheumatoid arthritis and osteoarthritis synovium. Quantitative analysis and effect of intraarticular corticosteroids. Arthritis Rheum. 1991; 34: 1094–1105.
109. Katz Y, Strunk RC. Synovial fibroblast-like cells synthesise seven proteins of the complement system. Arthritis Rheum. 1988; 31: 1365–1371.
110. Cochrane CGH, Muller-Eberhard HG, Aikon BS. Depletion of plasma complement in vivo by a protein of cobra venom: its effect on various immunologic reactions. J Immunol. 1970; 105: 55–64.
111. Klickstein LB, Barlow TJ, Miletic V, Robson LD, Smith JA, Fearon DT. Identification of distinct C3b and C4b recognition sites in the human C5b/C4b receptor (CR1, CD35) by deletion mutagenesis. J Exp Med. 1988; 168: 1699–1717.
112. Weisman HF, Barlow T, Leppo MK, Marsh HC, Carson GR, Concino MF, Boyle MP, Roux KH, Weisfeldt ML, Fearon DT. Soluble human complement receptor type 1: in vivo inhibitor of the complement suppressing post-ischaemic myocardial inflammation

and necrosis. Science. 1990; 249: 146–151.
113. Mulligan MS, Yeh CG, Rudolph AR, Ward PA. Protective effects of soluble CR1 in complement- and neutrophil-mediated tissue injury. J Immunol. 1992; 148: 1479–1485.
114. Pruitt SK, Baldwin WM, Marsh HC, Lin SS, Yeh CG, Bollinger RR. The effect of soluble complement receptor type 1 on hyperacute allograft rejection. Transplantation. 1991; 50: 868–873.

8
The Acute Phase Response

P. WOO

The acute phase response is the physiological systemic response to tissue injury and infection[1,2]. This occurs during the first few days following the insult to the organism and consists of a large number of systemic and metabolic changes. These events are generally considered to be protective in nature by containing or destroying infectious agents, removal of damaged tissue and foreign organisms, and tissue repair. Although the term 'acute phase' is usually used to describe these changes, they are also present in chronic inflammatory situations.

SYSTEMIC AND METABOLIC CHANGES

One of the earliest physiological changes to be recognized is fever. There is a rise in the number of granulocytes in the peripheral blood as a result of their increased release from bone marrow stores, and later from increased production of mature granulocytes and their precursors. There is also a rise in blood platelet count. A number of endocrine changes have been described in infected and trauma victims where there is an increased synthesis of a number of hormones including glucagon, insulin, ACTH, adrenal catecholamines, growth hormone, thyroxin related hormones, thyroxin, aldosterone and vasopressin.

Studies of total body metabolism in the acute phase have shown that plasma levels of phenylalanine and tryptophan are increased due largely to accelerated release of these amino acids from skeletal muscles. They reflect catabolism of muscle protein and inability of these amino acids to be utilized in skeletal muscle[3]. Plasma levels of triglycerides, free fatty acids, VLDL and other plasma lipids have been reported to be changed in the acute phase response[4]. In some instances, evidence of reduced lipoprotein lipase activity has been found. For example, patients with moderate burns show drastic falls in serum high density lipoprotein levels resulting in hypertriglyceridaemia, hypercholesterolaemia and hyperphospholipidaemia[5]. There are alterations in serum concentration of trace metal like copper, zinc and iron in the acute phase response, e.g. caeruloplasmin levels are increased resulting in higher copper levels but plasma zinc and iron levels are diminished.

The immune system is profoundly affected in the acute phase response. The reticuloendothelial function is transiently suppressed[6]. General activation of humoral and cellular response has been noted, but immuno-suppression has been observed following major surgical operations, trauma and burns. There is evidence of impaired cell mediating immunity by anergy to skin test antigens[7]. There is lymphocyte hypo-reactivity to stimuli such as phytohaemaglutinin *in vitro*[8]. Neutrophil bacteriocidal activity[9] and macrophage phagocytic activity[7] have been reported to diminish in some cases. On the other hand, the complement proteins C3 and Factor B, crucial to activation of complement both by the classical and by the alternative pathways, are elevated during the acute phase response[1].

The major event during the acute phase response occurs in the liver which increases considerably in size. There is increased synthesis of a range of proteins that are responsible for innate and adaptive immunity and tissue repair. These proteins are the 'acute phase proteins'. There are approximately 30 such proteins described so far and more are being found. Some of these proteins are useful indicators of the presence and extent of the inflammatory process.

THE LIVER AND PRODUCTION OF ACUTE PHASE PROTEINS

Studies of liver metabolism during the acute phase response have demonstrated increased formation of microtubules and Golgi complex. The endoplasmic reticulum is dilated and has increased amounts of smooth endoplasmic reticulum. There is increased synthesis of cholesterol and other lipids as well as acute phase proteins. A large number of enzymes have been found to be increased in the liver during the acute phase including hydroxymethyl-glutaryl-CoA reductase, which catalyses the first committed step in steroid synthesis, and the oxidative and catabolic enzymes, NADH-cytochrome C reductase. Enzymes that play a role in glycosylation of proteins are also increased as expected because of the increased synthesis of plasma-glycoproteins.

The synthesis of acute phase protein is probably the best studied of all the liver's metabolic alterations[2]. The rise in serum concentrations of these proteins ranges from 25% up to several hundred fold. Table 1 shows some of the acute phase proteins and their known and proposed functions in inflammation. They are varied in function and include proteins which mediate local inflammatory changes like complement proteins, carrier proteins, e.g. haptoglobin, ferritin and caeruloplasmin (which has also been shown to be a scavenger of oxygen derived free radicals), and key enzyme inhibitors like the alpha-1 proteinase inhibitors. C-reactive protein (CRP) and serum amyloid A protein (SAA) are distinctive in that their normal serum concentrations are practically undetectable, but can increase up to one thousand fold

Table 1 The acute phase proteins and their proposed functions

Protein	Magnitude of increase	Proposed functions in inflammation
Inflammatory mediators		
Complement components C3, C4	<2-fold	Opsonization, chemotaxis
C-reactive protein	<1000-fold	Opsonization via phosphorylcholine bonds, complement activation, cytokine induction
Plasminogen	<2-fold	Activation of complement, clotting and fibrinolysis
Fibrinogen	2–4 fold	Clotting
Kininogen	<2-fold	Vascular permeability
Scavengers		
Haptoglobin	2–4 fold	Scavenger of haemoglobin
C-reactive protein	<1000-fold	Scavenger of nuclear debris
Caeruloplasmin	<2-fold	Scavenger of free radicals
Serum amyloid A	<1000-fold	?? reverse cholesterol transport
Protease inhibitors		
α_1-antitrypsin	2–4 fold	Serine protease inhibitor, e.g. elastase
α_1-antichymotrypsin	2–4 fold	Cathepsin G inhibitor
Thiol protease inhibitor	2–4 fold	Cysteine protease inhibitor
Haptoglobin	2–4 fold	? Cathepsin B, H, L inhibitor
Antithrombin III C1 esterase inhibitor Factors I, H	<2-fold	Control of complement and coagulation pathways
Repair		
α_1-acid glycoprotein	2–4 fold	Fibroblast growth
Fibrinogen	2–4 fold	Formation of matrix
Cellular interactions		
α_1-acid glycoprotein	2–4 fold	Membrane protein of lymphocytes and monocytes
C-reactive protein	$\leqslant$1000 fold	Lymphocytes

or more within 24 hours of injury. The rate of increase in concentration, as well as the rate of decline vary among the acute phase proteins (Figure 1). In contrast, the concentrations of some proteins like albumin and transferrin have been found to fall during an acute phase: the so called 'negative acute phase reactants'. It is not clear whether this fall in plasma level is the result of reduced synthesis or increased catabolism.

There are significant species differences among the acute phase proteins. One notable example is alpha-2 macroglobulin which is a major acute phase protein in rats but is not in humans. Another example is C-reactive protein and its homologue serum amyloid-P protein (SAP). In man, CRP is an acute phase protein while SAP is very marginally raised, but the situation is reversed in mice.

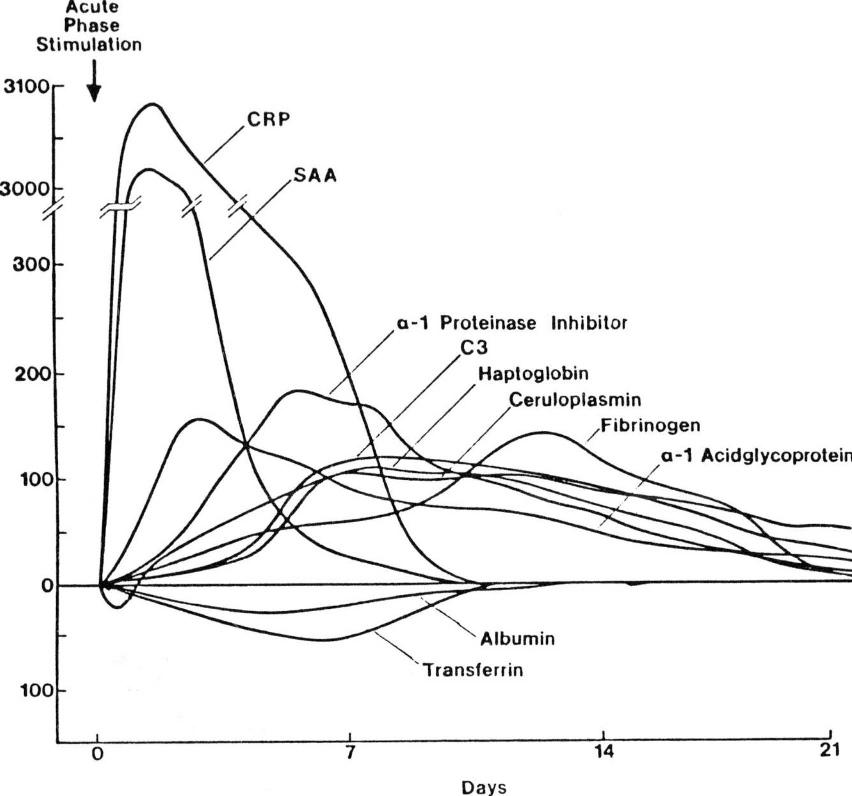

Figure 1 Rate of increase and decline among some acute phase proteins (after Gitlin and Colten)

INDUCER OF ACUTE PHASE PROTEIN SYNTHESIS

The inflammatory cytokines, in particular interleukin-6 (IL-6), interleukin-1 (IL-1), and tumour necrosis factor alpha (TNFα) have been shown to be important in the induction of acute phase protein synthesis. These cytokines are predominantly derived from activated macrophages at the site of injury although they can be produced by many other cell types such as fibroblasts and endothelial cells. In addition, they have been implicated in mediating other aspects of the acute phase response such as fever. In a sense, the production of these inflammatory cytokines can be included as part of the acute phase response. From experimental work involving primary hepatocyte cell lines from animals and humans, as well as cultured hepatoma cell lines, it is clear that the synthesis of some acute phase proteins is also regulated by the endocrine system, in particular the glucocorticoids[2]. Recently, other inducers of the hepatocyte acute phase protein response have been described, but none of them have the same degree of *in vitro* effects as the above three cytokines. A notable example is leukaemia inhibitory factor (LIF) which was

Table 2 Inducers of acute phase protein synthesis

Inducer	Acute phase protein
Crude activated macrophage supernatant	All
Class 1	
IL-1, IL-6, LIF, TNFα or combination	Serum amyloid A
	C-reactive protein
	Haptoglobin
	Complement FB
	Angiotensinogen
Class 2	
IL-6 and glucocorticoids	α_2-Macroglobulin
	α_1-Antichymotrypsin
	Fibrinogen
	Rat α_1-acid glycoprotein

IL-1 = interleukin 1
IL-6 = interleukin 6
LIF = leukaemia inhibitory factor
TNFα = tumour necrosis factor alpha

found to be the same as HSF3, first described by Baumann and colleagues. It has its own binding receptor which interacts with the membrane signalling protein for IL-6, gp130. Thus its spectrum of action is similar to IL-6, but weaker. Other related factors including ciliary neurotrophic factor (CNTF)[10], oncostatin M[11] and interleukin-11[12]; all of these belong to the α-helical cytokine family and utilize gp130 for intracellular signalling.

The cyokines that down-regulate IL-1 and TNFα synthesis may also have direct and indirect effects on acute phase protein synthesis. Preliminary results from *in vitro* experiments have shown that TGFβ may directly down-regulate SAA. The net result, therefore, depends on the interaction between the different cytokines and glucocorticoids on the gene in question.

Table 2 illustrates that subsets of acute phase proteins are induced by different cytokines. These observations are largely based on *in vitro* experiments involving hepatoma cell lines of different species. The most important regulations of these acute phase genes appear to be at the transcriptional level, for example C-reactive protein[13] and serum amyloid-A[14,15]. In addition, stabilization of messenger RNA (mRNA) by interleukin-1 has been described for IL-8[16] and increased secretory rate of C-reactive protein has also been attributed to IL-1 (MacIntyre, personal communication).

The intracellular signalling pathways that lead to gene activation are an active area of research currently and a number of transcription factors have been identified which mediate interleukin-1 and interleukin-6 action (see Table 3). The signalling receptor for IL-1 has been identified to be the 80 kD (type 1) and not the 65 kD (type 2) protein[17]. The IL-1 intercellular signal is a phosphorylation event which probably involves a novel kinase that activates the NFκB transcription factor complex[17], which migrates into the nucleus and binds to the SAA promoter to initiate gene transcription. The subunits of NFκB are homologous to the oncogene *rel* and the transcription

Table 3 Signal transduction by cytokines

Interleukin	Signalling receptor	Transcription factor
IL-1	Type 1 (80 kD)	AP 1 NFκB C/EBPβ or NFIL-6
IL-6 or LIF	gp130	C/EBPβ or NFIL-6 C/EBPδ or NFIL-6β APRF

IL-1 = interleukin 1
IL-6 = interleukin 6
LIF = leukaemia inhibitory factor

factor *dorsal* in drosophilia, and their inter-relationships are the subject of active research in major molecular biology laboratories (see review [18]). The signalling pathways for AP1 and NFIL-6 activation are likely to be different from the above. NFIL-6 and NFIL-6β have been cloned and shown to mediate transcription of acute phase genes responsive to IL-6[19,20]. IL-6 binds to its 80 kD receptor which then interacts with the signalling membrane protein gp130. The intracellular pathways that trigger the NFIL-6 factor to bind to DNA are less clear. Time course experiments using human hepatoma cell lines have shown that both APRF (a third factor induced by IL-6) and NFIL-6β are likely to be present in an inactive state intracellularly, and a post-translational event like phosphorylation has been shown to activate APRF binding to the α2-macroglobulin promoter[21]. Interestingly, the 80 kD IL-6 binding receptor is shed from hepatocytes and this soluble IL-6 receptor can also stimulate acute phase protein synthesis via gp130. From such studies another level of fine control which is tailor-made for each acute phase gene is emerging.

Synergy between cytokines is an important factor in the acute phase response. Synergistic action at the transcription level between IL-1 and IL-6 is most likely to be the physiological stimulus for the enormous increase in SAA serum levels[22]. As mentioned above, glucocorticoid is important in the synthesis of some acute phase proteins. For example, the synthesis of rat alpha$_1$-acid glycoprotein increases only under the dual stimulus of glucocorticoids and IL-6[2]. Female sex steroids too appear to act synergistically in the induction of human caeruloplasmin[23] and the acute phase female protein in Golden Syrian hamster[24].

It is clear that extra-hepatic tissue can also produce acute phase proteins. For example, cells of the monocyte-macrophage lineage can produce several complement components, alpha$_1$-antitrypsin and mouse SAA. The significance of this and the extent to which this normally occurs *in vivo*, particularly at the site of inflammation, could be important especially in relation to chronic inflammation.

A small group of proteins including albumin, prealbumin, retinol binding proteins, and transferrin decrease in serum concentration during inflammation. Relatively less experimental work has been done to elucidate the reason for lower serum levels of these proteins compared to the acute phase proteins.

THE ROLE OF ACUTE PHASE PROTEINS IN THE PATHOGENESIS OF RHEUMATIC DISEASES

There are marked differences in the acute phase response between different inflammatory diseases. During flares of SLE, several investigators have reported an absent or moderate rise in CRP in spite of pyrexia and a markedly increased erythrocyte sedimentation rate, in contrast to the brisk acute phase response in rheumatoid arthritis and juvenile chronic arthritis. Failure to mount an acute phase response can have deleterious effects. In view of the fact that one of the functions of CRP could be opsonization and clearance of damaged chromatin because of its high affinity binding to nuclear materials[25], the absence of CRP may predispose to development of nuclear antibodies, or the transcription of aberrant chromatin. Consumption of complement unmatched by an increased synthetic rate, as in SLE[26], results in low serum concentrations that reduce the opsonizing capacity of the serum. Insufficient supplies of protease inhibitors and repair proteins will also have an adverse effect. Scleroderma and dermatomyositis are other examples of inflammatory diseases that do not elicit a marked CRP response. The acute phase response may also be downregulated in chronic infection as illustrated by one study of recurrent attacks of iritis[27]. Therefore, studies to elucidate the mechanism of differential acute phase response and its regulation have exciting therapeutic possibilities.

LABORATORY MEASUREMENTS OF THE ACUTE PHASE RESPONSE IN RHEUMATIC DISEASES

The rate and extent in the increase in plasma concentration of any acute phase protein depends on the size of the protein, its intravascular versus extravascular distribution, its synthetic rate and also its catabolic rate. There are considerable kinetic differences seen between the various proteins during an episode of acute inflammation (see Figure 1). Thus the 'profile' of different acute phase proteins at any one point during acute inflammation as well as chronic inflammation would be different. Furthermore, if intravascular coagulation is a complication, levels of fibrinogen will be lower than would be expected and haptoglobin is lower if haemolysis is occurring.

The main acute phase proteins CRP and SAA have been used as indicators of disease activity in therapeutic studies in rheumatoid arthritis. It is important to note that although most of the time the levels of CRP and SAA are coincident, the two have been observed to be divergent in 40% of 185 RA patients[28]. This phenomenon has also been observed by others in chronic infectious states such as leprosy (MacAdam, personal communication). This may be related to the fact that CRP is transcriptionally responsive to IL-6 and SAA mainly to IL-1. There have been reports that SAA is a closer correlate of RA disease activity and may be more indicative of the production of IL-1 in this disease. It is interesting to speculate that this may have some bearing on the fact that erosive changes are one of the hallmarks of rheumatoid arthritis since IL-1 stimulates bone resorption. However, the relationship between the acute phase response and radiological progression is controversial at present.

The measurement of serum SAA is of particular importance in systemic reactive amyloidosis. The precursor protein of amyloid fibres is SAA. The effective lowering of SAA serum levels has led to the regression of amyloid as shown recently by a longitudinal study of amyloid patients using radioactive I^{123}-SAP scintigraphy[29]. Close monitoring of SAA and serum CRP levels has revealed that there are discrepancies between the two acute phase proteins. Therefore the measurement of SAA is of increasing importance in reactive amyloidosis. An acute phase SAA standard is currently being prepared with the aid of WHO, and ELISA measurement of SAA is now being refined in several laboratories.

MEASUREMENTS OF OTHER ACUTE PHASE PROTEINS IN RHEUMATIC DISEASES

The erythrocyte sedimentation rate (ESR) is still the most widely used index of the acute phase response. It measures the rate of sedimentation of the erythrocyte depending on the degree of aggregation as a result of the concentration of large asymmetrical proteins such as fibrinogen, alpha$_2$-macroglobulin and immunoglobulins. In addition, it is influenced by red cell number and red cell characteristics, age and sex, drugs and dietary lipids. Since the main influence of the ESR is fibrinogen, which is slow to increase and persists long after the inflammation has subsided as a result of its long half-life, it is a poor and insensitive measurement of the time course of the inflammation. In addition it is artificially low in anaemia and intravascular coagulation, and artificially high in vascular disease.

The plasma viscosity has been advocated increasingly to be used in place of ESR. However, this measurement is also dependent on the concentration of the same group of large molecule weight proteins like fibrinogen. Other acute phase proteins like haptoglobin, alpha$_1$-antitrypsin, complement proteins and caeruloplasmin are all acute phase proteins but too insensitive and slow to increase to be of use as markers of the acute phase response.

USE OF THE ACUTE PHASE RESPONSE MARKERS

In general, measurement of the acute phase proteins is important in assisting the rheumatologist to detect the presence of inflammatory disease, the extent of the disease activity, the monitoring of drugs therapy and also detection of infection in the case of systemic lupus erythematosus. For example, it has been proposed that the serum CRP level >60 mg/l is strongly indicative of an infection and CRP levels <30 mg/l shows that severe infection is unlikely to be present[30]. This rule has been shown to be useful only in the absence of serositis and arthritis.

A recent finding that the glycosylation status of several acute phase proteins is altered during active disease compared to inactive disease may be yet another important marker. Many serum glycoproteins exhibit microheterogeneity due to variations in their N-linked heteroglycan side chains. In patients with acute polymyalgia rheumatica for example, the glycan microheterogeneity of alpha$_1$-antichymotrypsin is altered, with a decrease in concanavalin A reactivity[31]. In this study, Hachulla and colleagues were able to discriminate between active and inactive disease with a sensitivity of 97% and a specificity of 91%. In another study by Mackiewicz et al.[32,33], glycosylation of alpha$_1$-acid glycoprotein in patients with ankylosing spondylitis and active RA is decreased in terms of concanavalin A reactivity compared with healthy controls.

SUMMARY

The acute phase protein response in acute infection, inflammation and tissue necrosis can be viewed as a beneficial response, and can be classified as part of our innate immunity. Failure to mount an acute phase response may have harmful sequelae, and a prolonged acute phase response can also be harmful, for example in reactive amyloidosis. Further research into the regulatory mechanisms of the acute phase protein response should yield insight into the pathogenesis of the diseases mentioned above and indicate novel therapeutic approaches.

References

1. Kushner I. The phenomenon of the acute phase response. Ann NY Acad Sci. 1982; 389: 39–48.
2. Baumann H, Prowse KR, Marinkovic S, Won A, Jahreis GP. Stimulation of hepatic acute phase response by cytokines and glucocorticoids. Ann NY Acad Sci. 1989; 557: 280–295.
3. Wannemacker RW. Key role of various individual amino acids in host response to injection. Am J Clin Nutr. 1977; 30: 1269–1280.
4. Blackburn GL. Lipid metabolism in infection. Am J Clin Nutr. 1977; 30: 1321–1332.
5. Coombes EJ, Shakespeare PG, Batstone GF. Lipoprotein changes after burn injury in man. J Trauma. 1980; 20: 971–975.
6. Saba TM, Jaffe E. Plasma fibronectin (opsonic glycoprotein): Its synthesis by vascular endothelial cells and role in cardiopulmonary integrity after trauma as related to reticulendothelial function. Am J Med. 1980; 68: 577–594.
7. Wang BS, Heacock, Wu AVO, Mannick JA. Generation of suppressor cells in mice after surgical trauma. J Clin Invest. 1980; 66: 200–209.
8. Constantian MB, Menzoian JO, Nimburg RB, Schmid K, Mannick JA. Association of a circulating immunosuppressive polypeptide with operative and accidental trauma. Ann Surg. 1977; 185: 73–79.
9. Alexander JW, Ogle CK, Stinnett JD, MacMillan BG. A sequential, prospective analysis of immunologic abnormalities and infection following severe thermal injury. Ann Surg. 1978; 188: 809–816.
10. Schooltink H, Stoyan T, Roeb E, Heinrich PC, Rose-John S. Ciliary neurotrophic factor induces acute phase protein expression in hepatocytes. FEBS Lett. (In press).

11. Richards CD, Brown TJ, Shoyib M, Baumann H, Gaeddie J. J Immunol. 1992; 148: 1731–1736.
12. Baumann H, Schendel P. Interleukin-11 regulates the hepatic expression of the same plasma protein genes as interleukin-6. J Biol Chem. 1991; 266: 20424–20427.
13. Ciliberto G, Arcone R, Wagner EF, Ruther U. Inducible and tissue-specific expression of human C-reactive protein in transgenic mice. EMBO J. 1987; 6: 4017–4022.
14. Lowell CA, Stearman RS, Morrow JF. Transcriptional regulation of serum amyloid A gene expression. J Biol Chem. 1986; 261: 8453–8461.
15. Edbrooke M, Burt D, Cheshire J, Woo P. Identification of cis-acting sequences responsible for phorbol tester induction of human serum amyloid A gene expression via a NFκB-like transcription factor. Mol Cell Biol. 1989; 9: 1908–1916.
16. Stoeckle MY. Post-transcriptional regulation of gro alpha, beta, gamma and IL-8 mRNAs by IL-1 beta. Nucl Acid Res. 1991; 19: 917–920.
17. Stylianou E, O'Neill AJ, Rawlinson L, Edbrooke M, Woo P, Saklatvala J. Interleukin 1 induces NFκB through its type I, but not its type II receptor in lymphocytes. J Biol Chem. 1992; 267: 15836–15841.
18. Blank V, Kourisky P, Israel A. NFκB and relation proteins: *Rel/dorsal* homologies meet ankyrin-like repeats. TIBS. 1992; 17: 135–140.
19. Akira S, Isshiki H, Sugita T, Tanabe O, Kinoshita S, Nishio Y, Nakajima T, Hirano T, Kishimoto T. A nuclear factor for IL-6 expression (NF-IL6) is a member of a C/EBP family. EMBO J. 1990; 9: 1897–1906.
20. Kinoshita S, Akira S, Kishimoto T. A member of the C/EBP family NF-IL6β, form a heterodimer and transcriptionally synergises with NF-IL6. Proc Nat Acad Sci USA. 1992; 89: 1473–1476.
21. Wegenka U, Buschmann J, Lutticken C, Heinrich P. A nuclear factor, APRF, binding to acute phase response elements, is rapidly activated by interleukin-6 at the post-translational level. Mol Cell Biol. (In press).
22. Betts JC, Cheshire JK, Akira S, Kishimoto T, Woo P. The role of NFκB and NFIL6 transactivating factors in the synergistic activation of human serum amyloid A gene expression by interleukin 1 and interleukin 6. (Submitted).
23. Weiner AL, Cousins RJ. Hormonally produced changes in caeruloplasmin synthesis and secretion in primary cultured rat hepatocytes. Biochem J. 1983; 212: 297–304.
24. Coe JE, Ross MJ. Hamster female protein: a divergent acute phase protein in male and female Syrian hamsters. J Exp Med. 1983; 157: 1421–1435.
25. Robey F, Jones KD, Tanaka T, Liu TY. Binding of C-reactive protein to chromatin and nucleosome core particles. J Biol Chem. 1984; 259: 7311–7316.
26. Sliwinski AJ, Zvaifler NJ. Decreased synthesis of the third component of complement (C3) in hypocomplementic systemic lupus erythematosus. Clin Exp Immunol. 1972; 11: 21–29.
27. Wicher JT. Interleukin 1 and acute phase proteins. Br J Rheumatol. 1985; 24(1): 21–24.
28. Chambers RE, MacFarlane DG, Wicher JT, Dieppe PA. Serum amyloid A protein concentration in rheumatoid arthritis and its role in monitoring disease activity. Ann Rheum Dis. 1983; 42: 665–667.
29. Hawkins PN, Richard S, Vigushin DM, David J, Kelsey CR, Gray RES, Hall MA, Woo P, Lavender JP, Pepys MB. Serum amyloid P component scintigraphy and turnover studies for diagnosis and quantitative monitoring of AA amyloidosis in juvenile rheumatoid arthritis. (Submitted).
30. Pepys MB, Lanham JG, De Beer FC. C-reactive protein in SLE. Clin Rheum Dis. 1982; 8: 91–103.
31. Hachulla E, Laine A, Hayem A. Microheterogeneity of α_1-antichymotrypsin in the management of giant cell arteritis and polymyalgia rheumatica. Clin Sci. 1990; 78: 557–564.
32. Mackiewicz A, Pawlowski T, Mackiewicz-Pawlowska A, Wiktorowicz K, Mackiewicz S. Microheterogeneity of α_1-acid glycoprotein as indicative of rheumatoid arthritis activity. Clinica Chimica Acta. 1987; 163: 185–190.
33. Mackiewicz A, Khan MA, Reynolds TL, Van der Linden S, Kushner I. Serum IgA, acute phase proteins, and glycosylation of α_1-acid glycoprotein in ankylosing spondylitis. Ann Rheum Dis. 1989; 48: 99–103.

9
Animal Models of Systemic Lupus Erythematosus

D. BUSKILA and Y. SHOENFELD

INTRODUCTION

Since the aetiology and pathogenesis of autoimmune diseases are not clear[1,2], it is evident that the pathogenesis of these diseases cannot readily be analysed without appropriate animal models. These models may help to define aetiology, determine pathogenesis, and design innovative therapies. Indeed, systemic lupus erythematosus (SLE), as well as other autoimmune diseases, has animal models. Not surprisingly, they vary considerably in the 'closeness of fit' to the human disease they are supposed to be mimicking. These models have been the subject of intense study for the last several years. Although our understanding of human autoimmune diseases has certainly been increased by insights gained from studies in animal models, it has become painfully clear that pathogenic mechanisms or therapeutic success observed in one strain may not operate and/or may fail in the others[3].

In recent years, therefore, investigators have performed experiments on several of the autoimmunity mice (spontaneous as well as induced SLE models), before arriving at generalized conclusions. In this chapter we review the classical animal models of SLE developing spontaneously, but concentrate in particular on the new models induced actively in animals which thus circumvent the genetic contribution to the development of the disease.

CLASSICAL MODELS OF SLE (see Table 1)

A number of animal models of human lupus have been described which tend to reflect different aspects of the disease as indicated in Table 1 (see also next section on clinical manifestations of autoimmunity).

The prototype murine model of spontaneous autoimmunity is the New

Table 1 Selected features of mouse models of systemic lupus erythematosus

Model	Immunopathology	Mean life span (months)	autoantibodies
NZB	Haemolyic anaemia, glomerulonephritis pulmonary infiltrates, lymphoid hyperplasia and lymphomas	15–18	Anti-DNA, antierythrocyte rheumatoid factor
(NZB x NZW)F$_1$*	Severe glomerulonephritis, pulmonary infiltrates	7–9	Anti-DNA, rheumatoid factor
MRL-lpr/lpr*	Glomerulonephritis, vasculitis, erosive arthritis lymphadenopathy myocardial infarcts	3–5	Anti-DNA, anti-Sm rheumatoid factor, cryoglobulins
(NZB x SWR)F$_1$*	Accelerated severe nephritis	13	Anti-DNA
BXSB**	Glomerulonephritis haemolytic anaemia, myocardial infarcts	4–6	Anti-DNA antierythrocyte
Moth-eaten	Pulmonary infiltrate, hair loss, mild glomerulonephritis	1	Anti-DNA antierythrocyte, rheumatoid factor
Palmerston-North	Vasculitis, glomerulonephritis	10–12	Anti-DNA
Swan	Mild glomerulonephritis	18	Anti-DNA

*female; **male

Zealand black (NZB) mouse, first derived 30 years ago by Marianne Bielschowsky and her colleagues at the University of Dunedin, New Zealand. It was selected for inbreeding on the basis of a solid black coat colour[3,4]. These animals are principally a model of autoimmune haemolytic anaemia which develops at the age of nine months; by 12 months, virtually all of the animals have the erythrocyte bound antibodies, detectable by a Coombs' test. In addition to the erythrocyte antibodies, a number of other autoantibodies can be detected, including anti-ss and ds-DNA. Kidney disease may develop in these animals, that have a 50% survival rate at 18 months and by this time will have developed splenomegaly, lymphoid hyperplasia and, invariably, detectable circulating immune complexes[3].

A hybrid strain derived from the NZB mouse is one produced by mating this strain with the New Zealand white mouse, the offspring being known as (NZB x NZW)F$_1$. This hybrid animal is in many respects an excellent model of human lupus. As with the human disease, it is the female which is most likely to get the disease, and in a more severe form[3].

Clinically, the symptoms become apparent around the age of 6 months and most animals are dead of immune complex nephritis by 9 months. In males, the disease becomes apparent after 10–12 months, with most of the animals dying at around 15 months[3]. Renal disease and also proteinuria may be detected as early as 3 months of age and this is often accompanied by the presence of ANA. Antibodies to ds and ss DNA and RNA, and a number of synthetic polynucleotides have all been described. In addition, an erythrocyte antibody and a positive Coombs' test are usually present. The class of antibody appears to be important in determining the development of the disease. In addition to autoantibody production, T cell abnormalities have also been described. The thymus involutes at an early age in both the NZB and the NZB/W mice and there is accompanying loss of thymic hormone production which may be partly responsible for an imbalance in the maturation of the various populations of thymus-derived cells.

Dysfunction in the Ly-1,2,3 post-thymic precursor cells, which are involved in feedback regulation, has also been noted[5]. The function of this population is to exert inhibitory effects after a signal from Ly-1 (helper) cells participating in a particular immune response. B lymphocytes have an independent defect as well. They spontaneously produce high levels of IgM even in neonatal animals and there is also an overproduction of IgG which increases throughout life and which cannot be regulated, at least *in vitro* by addition of healthy T cells to the culture system. The presence of such an abnormality long before T lymphocyte malfunction becomes evident is a very strong argument that the B lymphocyte is primarily responsible for the disease.

The MRL/lpr strain has been extensively studied since it was introduced in 1978 by Murphy and Roths[3]. This mouse strain is a model for an accelerated membranoproliferative glomerulonephritis associated with anti-DNA production[6,7]. Additional clinical features include lymphoproliferation, synovitis and vasculitis. These mice carry a single gene mutation, referred to as lymphoproliferation (lpr) which is characterized by abnormal proliferation of the T cell subset $CD3^+ CD4^- CD8^-$, resulting in lymphoid enlargement. MRL/lpr mice are further characterized by hypergamma globulinaemia and production of a wide array of autoantibodies[6,7].

Until recently, the function of lpr has been obscure. The identification of lpr as the *Fas* gene offers new insight into the mechanism of lpr autoimmunity[8]. The *Fas* gene, or APO-1, encodes a 48 kD transmembrane protein with homology to the receptors for nerve growth and tumour necrosis factor. Ligation of the Fas membrane protein has been shown to trigger apoptosis – the reverse effect of the bcl-2 protein (a mitochondrial membrane protein), which blocks apoptosis. The *Fas* gene may be involved in the clonal deletion of thymic T cells, and a defect in *Fas* has been linked to the marked accumulation of T cells in the autoimmune MRL-lpr/lpr mouse[8].

Another strain developed by Murphy and Roths, the BXSB mouse, is unusual in that the males develop autoimmunity quite early, dying at 5 to 7 months of age, whereas the female BXSB mice develop an indolent autoimmune syndrome that does not lead to death until well into the second year of life[7]. These mice are a recombinant inbred strain resulting from crossing of C57BL/6j females with SB/le males. The life span is approximately 5 months and they usually die of a severe exudative proliferative nephritis. As in the NZB/W mouse, the BXSB mice develop anti-DNA and anti-erythrocyte antibodies as well as hypocomplementaemia and immune complex disease.

Finally, the F_1 progeny (SNF_1) derived from crossing autoimmune NZB with normal SWR mice uniformly develop lethal glomerulonephritis in marked contrast to the NZB parents[9-11]. SWR mice, in contrast to NZB

Table 2 Clinical and pathological features
of autoimmunity in autoimmune mice

Glomerulonephritis
Heart disease (myocardial infarctions)
Arthritis
Vasculitis
Myositis
Central nervous system disease
Pneumonitis
Haemolytic anaemia
Skin disease
Sialadenitis
Lymphoid hyperplasia
Neoplasia

and ZNW strains, do not express retroviruses, and they develop neither autoimmune disease nor autoantibodies[10,11]. It was found that anti-DNA autoantibodies produced by the NZB x SWR crossing were qualitatively different from those made by the NZB parents with respect to their isotype, charge, and antigenic specificity patterns.

CLINICAL AND PATHOLOGIC MANIFESTATIONS OF AUTOIMMUNITY IN AUTOIMMUNE MICE (See Table 2)

Autoimmune mice develop a variety of clinical and pathological manifestations. The major cause of death in all lupus mice is *glomerulonephritis* which ranges from a chronic obliterative form in the NZB/W female to an exudative and proliferative acute form in the BXSB male and largely subacute proliferative form in the MRL/lpr male and female mice[3]. NZB/W mice develop an extensive membrano-proliferative glomerulonephritis leading to death between 8 and 10 months of age. The glomerular lesions are associated with the deposition of DNA/anti-DNA immune complexes and complement[12]. The obliterative lesion in the NZB/W female is accompanied by heavy mesangial and, at times, intravascular proteinaceous deposits, moderate proliferation of all glomerular cellular elements, and crescent formation[3]. Murine retroviral glycoprotein antigen, GP-70, and its specific antibody also have been eluted from glomerular lesions in NZB/W mice[13,14]. The relative nephritogenicity of these two antigen-antibody systems in murine lupus is still unclear. The MRL/lpr/lpr is a model for an accelerated membrano-proliferative glomerulonephritis associated with anti-DNA production[7]. The glomerular lesions involve the accumulation of monocytes and proliferation of both endothelial and mesangial cells with occasional crescent formation and basement membrane thickening[3]. Both male and female members of this strain die between 5 and 7 months of age.

Another strain of mouse, the BXSB, develops a rapidly progressive immune complex membrano-proliferative glomerulonephritis[7]. The incidence of glomerulonephritis in the NZB mice is approximately 1% at one year of age, but when they are crossed with the normal SWR mice almost 100% of the female F_1 (SNF$_1$) hybrids die from accelerated lupus nephritis[9]. Studies performed by Gavalchin et al.[10,11] in NZB x SWR model of lupus nephritis have suggested that selected families of nephritogenic idiotypes that are dormant in the autoimmune NZB and the normal SWR parents become expressed in the SNF$_1$ progeny due to genetic and immunoregulatory defects.

Ebling and Hahn[15] have observed that MRL/lpr and NZB/W mice contain a restricted number of DNA-binding bands, all of which focus at pH 8.0–9.0. This suggests that subpopulations of IgG-anti-DNA antibodies, i.e. those with an alkaline pH, are more pathogenic than others. Recently, studies by Kalunian et al.[16] and Shoenfeld et al.[17] suggested that certain pathogenic (common) anti-DNA antibody idiotypes (GN2, 16/6) may have a role in the pathogenesis of SLE nephritis. Furthermore, polyclonal anti-DNA from human sera and monoclonal anti-DNA from an NZB/NZW F_1 hybridoma directly bind to an isolated perfused rat kidney and initiate glomerulonephritis[18].

Fifteen to thirty per cent of each of the above types of mice have, at autopsy, old and/or acute *myocardial infarcts*[3]. Accinni and Dixon[19] demonstrated that medium and small coronary arteries and arterioles of such animals have focal degenerative lesions consisting of PAS positive or eosinophilic material deposited in the intima and media[19]. Recently, F_1 male mice (NZW x BXSB) have been reported to show a high incidence of coronary vascular disease and myocardial infarction[20]. Many of the mice had multiple small infarcts with whirloop configuration, which reflected the special anatomy of the intramural coronary arteries in the mice.

Another consistent feature of SLE pathology in all strains is severe *cortical thymic atrophy*[3,18]. Marked *splenic and lymph node hyperplasia* exist in all murine lupus strains. Lymphoid infiltrates may also occur in the lungs, kidneys, liver, salivary glands and bone marrow[3].

There is considerable variation in the reported incidence of lymphoid neoplasms in NZB mice ranging from 2–3% to a high of 50%[3,21]. This may reflect in part the problems in diagnosing lymphomas in face of profound lymphoid hyperplasia.

The MRL/lpr/lpr mouse is the only strain that develops a detectable synovitis in up to 75% of animals in addition to immune complex glomerulonephritis[7,22]. This feature has been used to promote the MRL/lpr/lpr mouse as a naturally occurring model of human rheumatoid arthritis as well as SLE. In no animal model are there significant neurological disorders, serositis, or skin involvement.

The studies describing the variety of features of autoimmune disease in autoimmune mice have shed little insight into the immunopathogenesis of autoimmune disease. An exception is what can be learned from immunohistochemical analysis of human autoimmune disease tissue. The analysis of the genetics that predispose to the development of autoimmune disease may clarify immunopathogenesis of these diseases. Indeed, breeding of MRL/lpr/lpr and C57BL/6-lpr/lpr mice dissociated the development of arteritis and glomerulonephritis as separate genetic traits in lpr/lpr mice[23]. Arthritis was observed in MRL/lpr/lpr mice but not in C57BL/6-lpr/lpr, C3H-lpr/lpr, or AKR-lpr/lpr mice. Production of IgM RF was elevated in MRL, C57BL/6 and C3H-lpr/lpr mice, suggesting that MRL background genes, and not RF production, are important in induction of arthritis[24].

NONMURINE MODELS OF LUPUS ERYTHEMATOSUS

A lupus-like disease has been reported not only in mice but also in rats, rabbits, guinea pigs, pigs, monkeys, dogs, cats, goats, hamsters, and Aleutian minks[25-29]. Nonmurine lupus animal studies have involved experiments with infusion of LE-positive plasma, attempts to induce positive LE preparations in animals, attempts to produce drug induced LE, transmissibility studies and treatment[25-29]. Canine lupus colonies have been set up and it appears that their clinical features and serological abnormalities do mirror those of human lupus. However, these colonies as well as those of other domestic pets are clearly more expensive to run and have therefore not proven as popular as lupus mouse colonies.

NEW MUTANT MICE OF AUTOIMMUNITY

Analysing a variety of animal models has led to a better understanding of the serological and histopathological characteristics of autoimmune disorders. However, the aetiologic mechanisms (including genetic factors) underlying mouse SLE are not well determined. Congenic strains bearing well-defined mutations would be extremely useful for isolating genes responsible for disease expression.

gld mutation

A newly discovered autosomal recessive mutation, generalized lymphoproliferative disease (gld) in the C3H/HeJ strain of mice, determines the development of severe lymphadenopathy, splenomegaly and autoimmune disease manifested by circulating anti-DNA antibodies and immune complex disease[30]. The interstitial pneumonitis in gld mice resembles the pathology in the human autoimmune disease[30].

Serologically, gld/gld mice develop ANA (including anti-ds DNA), thymocyte-binding autoantibodies, and hypergammaglobulinaemia with major increases in several immunoglobulin isotypes[30]. Mutant gld mice live only one-half as long as normal controls (12 and 23 months, respectively).

Only 14% of the autopsied mice had significant lupus-like nephritis. The pattern of early onset massive lymph node enlargement, hypergammaglobulinaemia, and production of ANA resembles the basic abnormal phenotype induced by the lpr mutation. gld is located between pep-3 and Lp on chromosome 1 and is apparently linked to the gene Dip-1[30]. Most of the large increase in lymph node size is due to the accumulation of Thy-1$^+$ and Thy-1$^-$ ('null') CD8$^-$ CD4$^-$ cells, although they lack both CD4 and CD8 T-cell surface proteins and express B-cell markers such as B-220[31,32].

The cells which accumulate in the peripheral lymphoid tissue of these mice are T cells which rearrange TCR genes and express surface alpha/beta TCR. The CD4$^-$ CD8$^-$ 'double-negative' T cells in gld mice also express aberrantly high levels of the *C-myb* proto-oncogene which is normally only expressed in immature thymocytes and cycling T cells[33].

CBA/KiJms-lpr^{cg}/lpr^{cg} mutation

Kimmura et al.[34] have recently described a new mutant mouse of autoimmunity (CBA/KiJms-lpr^{cg}/lpr^{cg}) that could link the *lpr* and *gld* genes. In this model, mice homozygous for both lpr^{cg} and mu (lpr^{cg}mu) were established by intercrossing (CBA-lpr^{cg} x DDD-mu)F$_1$ mice.

Lymphoproliferation and autoantibody formation were virtually absent in these mice. Furthermore, pregmu mice implanted with thymuses showed lymphoproliferation and autoantibody formation. This model is important in that a mutant gene causes a similar type of disease by the interaction with another gene on a different chromosome.

BXSB x MpJScr-ll/ll

Kofler et al.[35] have reported the generation and serological, cellular, histological and genetic characteristics of a BXSB/MpJScr-ll/ll that has lost early-life male lupus disease. Classic genetic analysis suggested that delayed disease expression results from the action of a single autosomal recessive gene. This putative gene, referred to as ll (long-lived), causes a significant delay in expression of autoimmune serology (total serum IgG and ANA levels), monocytosis, and immune complex-mediated histopathological changes such as glomerulonephritis, arteritis, and myocardial infarction. Presumably as a consequence of the delayed immunopathology, male BXSB/MpJScr-ll/ll mice live three to four times longer than regular BXSB/MpJScr. This strain might be useful for analysis of single genes responsible for severe autoimmune disease expression[35].

The BM12 mutation

Chiang et al.[36] have examined two inbred strains of mice in order to study the contribution of MHC-class II genes to the development of murine lupus. These new strains of mice, NZB.H-2^{bm12} and NZB.H-^{sbi}, were studied and compared in the tenth generation backcross. Inbreeding was followed by H-2 typing, responses to beef/porcine insulin, and presence of the B6Ig allotype, IgG2a^b. Interestingly, it was found that NZB.H-2, in contrast to^{bm12} NZB.H-2^b or NZB(H-2^d) mice develop high titres of autoantibodies to dsDNA. This result is unique because NZB(H-2^d) mice, unlike MZB x NZW or NSB x SWR hybrids, do not develop autoantibodies to dsDNA, even after immunization. NZB mice, in contrast, are characterized only by autoantibodies to ssDNA.

In summary, the new mutant mice described herein add further genetically well-defined models to the list of murine autoimmune disorders that may be exploited to gain a clearer understanding of immunoregulatory defects and to identify common pathogenic factors involved in systemic autoimmune diseases.

TRANSGENIC MICE AS MODELS OF AUTOIMMUNE DISEASE

Erikson et al.[37] have recently constructed transgenic mice using the rearranged heavy and light chains from a monoclonal antibody 3H9, which is an IgM anti-DNA antibody occurring naturally in MRL-lpr/lpr mice. Transgenic mice produce large numbers of B-cells expressing the VH 3H9/Vk8 antibody on their surface. These B-cells bind biotinylated ssDNA. In normal mice, there is no increased in secretion of VH-3H9/Vk8 anti-DNA antibody above that observed in nontransgenic mice. These results suggested that B cell tolerance to DNA is developed similarly to other experimental models of tolerance that have been described and that autoimmune disease likely results from a breakdown of regulation of autoantibody expression.

NEW EXPERIMENTAL MODELS FOR SYSTEMIC LUPUS ERYTHEMATOSUS

As was shown earlier, a number of animal models of human SLE have been described that tend to reflect different aspects of the disease, and that occur spontaneously in the individuals or strains that are predisposed genetically to develop the disease.

It would be of great interest to have models in which the disease could be induced, thus circumventing the genetic contribution toward the development of the disease.

Induction of systemic lupus erythematosus-like disease by a common anti-DNA idiotype (16/6 Id)

The 16/6 idiotype (Id) is a representative pathogenic idiotype of anti-DNA autoantibodies[2,38,39]. This antibody was initially identified as anti-single stranded (ss) DNA antibody, but subsequent analysis also demonstrated its ability to bind to other polynucleotides including nucleic acids, nucleoproteins, cell membranes and phospholipids[2,17]. The expression of this idiotype was probed by a rabbit anti-16/6 polyclonal antibody[2,17]. Titres of the common idiotype (16/6 Id) correlated with clinical activity in SLE patients, and its presence has been demonstrated in the dermal and kidney lesions of patients with SLE[17].

An SLE disease was induced in healthy C3H/SW female mice by immunization with the 16/6 Id antibody. The mice were immunized in the footpads with 1 μg of the human monoclonal antibody carrying the 16/6 idiotype followed by a booster injection after three weeks[2,40]. The mice had sustained high titres of both anti-16/6 idiotype antibodies and detectable 16/6 idiotype. In addition, the full panoply of antibodies associated with SLE was found, such as anti-ss DNA, anti-ds DNA, anti-Sm, anti-RNP, anti-Ro and anti-La autoantibodies[2,40]. The mice developed an increased erythrocyte sedimentation rate, leucopenia, and proteinuria. By immunohistochemistry, antibodies bearing the 16/6 idiotype (of mouse origin) were shown to be deposited in the kidney. Electron microscopy showed these antibodies to be in dense deposits of immune complexes in the mesangium. Mice immunized with human monoclonal anti-DNA antibodies lacking the 16/6 idiotype did not develop these lupus-like features[40]. The disease was induced in various mice strains including BALB/c and seemed not to be major histocompatibility complex (MHC)-restricted. The sex hormone effects in this experimental SLE model resemble those reported in spontaneous mouse SLE models[40,41]. A similar lupus-like syndrome was induced in BALB/c mice following immunization with the human IgM monoclonal antibody SA-1. SA-1 is a 16/6[+] hybridoma monoclonal antibody derived from the fusion of lymphocytes from a patient with active polymyositis[42]. It shows much stronger binding to native DNA than the original 16/6 antibody and the idiotype is located on the heavy chain variable region[42]. Immunization of BALB/c mice with SA-1 induced the above SLE model after three months of incubation. SA-2alpha parallel human monoclonal IgM generated from the same patient while in remission, which does not carry the 16/6 Id, does not bind to DNA, and failed to induce SLE. Similar studies were performed by the same group, confirming the importance of pathogenic 16/6 Id in the induction of the experimental SLE[42] as well as the anti-16/6 Id[43].

A group of investigators had failed to fully reproduce the 16/16 model of SLE in normal mice and have suggested the possible importance of environmental factors in the induction of this model[44]. But further series of experiments by the same group[45] show that what they have described is in fact a form of adjuvant arthritis (possibly because of the technique of injection of the antigen) and not an SLE model. Other recent studies had, however, provided additional support for the 16/16 model[46,47].

Rombach et al.[46] have shown that rabbits produce SLE-like anti-RNA polymerase I and anti-DNA autoantibodies in response to immunization with either human or murine SLE anti-DNA antibodies. Furthermore, Dang et al.[47] have demonstrated the induction of autoantibodies in normal BALB/c mice immunized with the UBU idiotype. This study has suggested that

(1) specific autoantibodies (anti-ss-DNA, anti-ds-DNA, anti-Sm) can be induced in a non-autoimmune mouse strain;
(2) this induction is related to the expression of the UBU idiotype;
(3) the idiotype network partially contributes to the induction of auto-immunity.

The role of T-cells in the experimental induction of SLE

Nude BALB/c mice, in contrast to normal BALB/c mice, did not develop either serological or clinical manifestations associated with SLE induced experimentally, which suggests that T-cells are essential for the experimental induction of SLE. Indeed, we have shown previously that SLE-like disease can be induced in naive mice by anti-DNA antibodies carrying the pathogenic 16/6 idiotype (Id)[40,42], as well as by the T-cell line specific for the 16/6 Id[48].

T-cell lines and clones specific to the 16/6 Id were established from C3H.SW and BALB/c mice. The proliferative responses of the lines were found to be specific only to 16/6 Id-bearing and H-2-restricted antibodies. Injection of naive mice with 5×10^6 cells of the above lines resulted in the serological and clinical manifestations typical of SLE, as was shown after immunization with the 16/6 antibody. The importance of the T cell lines that are specific for 16/6 Id was further established by another series of T cell lines and clones that reacted specifically with TB-68 (mouse monoclonal anti-DNA, anti-Tb glycolipid, and 16/6 Id$^+$), Tb-72 (mouse monoclonal anti-DNA, anti-Tb glycolipid, and 16/6 Id$^-$), and 4B4 (human monoclonal antibody anti-Sm, 16/6 Id$^+$)[49,50]. Only cell lines recognizing the 16/6 Id, induced the SLE-like disease. In order to elucidate the importance of 16/6 Id-specific lymphocytes in the pathogenesis of SLE, we established T-cell clones specific for several antibodies carrying the 16/6 Id[51]. T-cell clones were generated from BALB/c mice immunized with the human mAb anti-DNA antibody (SA-1) and the mouse monoclonal anti-tuberculous Ab (TB/68), both carrying the 16/6 Id. The T-cell clones proliferated only in the presence of either human or mouse mAb carrying the 16/6 Id. All the T-cell clones were found to be of the helper type (L3T4) and were H-2 restricted in their function.

The injection of the clones to BALB/c mice resulted in serological (e.g. anti-DNA, anti-Sm), clinical manifestations (e.g. proteinuria, low white blood cell counts, increased erythrocyte sedimentation rate), and renal insult typical of SLE disease.

This study[51] added more information to our previous one[43]. In the latter we generated helper cell lines only to the original human anti-DNA 16/6. In the present study[51] we expanded our research with several cell lines against diverse antibodies carrying the 16/6 Id. Our data support previous work showing the involvement of T-cells in SLE, as was demonstrated in MRL/lpr mice[3]. Our data also suggest that the cell line may supply helper activity to Id production independently of the source of the Id (mouse or human) or the position of the Id conformation.

The mechanisms by which the T-cell clones induce experimental SLE remain obscure. It is possible that activated 16/6 Id-specific T-cells are immunogenic enough to evoke antibody production directed against the antigen-specific receptor on the T-cells (anti-idiotypic antibodies), which later initiate a cascade of autoantibody production. This in turn results in the serology and clinical picture of SLE-like disease. Alternatively, as was demonstrated for the T/SA-1 16/6 Id-specific clone cells, the mechanism could be attributed to providing help to B-cells in producing anti-16/6-specific antibodies.

Systemic lupus erythematosus-like graft-versus-host disease

A model of SLE-like disease has been developed that uses a chronic graft versus host (GVHR) achieved by the transfer of parental helper T cell-enriched suppressor T cell depleted, spleen cells into nonirradiated F_1 hosts[52,53]. The optimal development of SLE-like diseases in mice with GVH requires three critical factors: the presence of $CD4^+$ T-cells in the donor inoculum, the presence of functional autoreactive B cells in the F_1 host, and a class II-MHC disparity (i.e. Ia) between donor and host[52,53]. In the most frequently studied model, DBA/2 (D2, H-2^d) spleen and lymph node cells, as a source of T-cells, are injected intravenously into unirradiated (C57BL/6 x DBA/2 F_1, H-2$^{b/d}$) recipients. The disease is characterized by production of autoantibodies to DNA, erythrocytes and thymocytes. Less frequently, antibodies to Sm and RNA are found. Immunoglobulin is deposited at the dermal/epidermal junction and immune-complex glomerulonephritis follows with proteinuria and ascites. In contrast to spontaneous SLE, SLE-like GVH disease does not involve exacerbations or remissions, and in contrast to the 16/6 Id-induced model, there are no sex predilections. The model has been used to clarify the relationship between T and B cells and autoantigens presented to them.

Portanova et al.[54] have shown that the production of autoantibodies in GVH-induced SLE is selective. The anti-histone antibodies that were generated reacted predominantly against histone regions accessible in chromatin, e.g. H_1 and H2B. The responses to H2A, H3 and H4 were only marginally elevated above pre-GVH disease levels. The predominant production of antibodies to histone regions that are exposed in nucleosomes raises the possibility that chromatin is an antigenic stimulus for histone-specific cells in this disease. Bruijn et al.[55] summarized the possibility of using murine GVH disease as a model for human lupus nephritis. As in human SLE, during GVH disease autoantibodies directed against nuclear antigens (e.g. anti-dsDNA) and autoantibodies against erythrocytes are elicited. Corresponding to human lupus nephritis, antinuclear antibodies are thought to play a pathogenic role in renal involvement. Twelve to 14 weeks after injection of 'parental' lymphocytes, light microscopy shows glomerular mesangial, segmental, and diffuse proliferative as well as membranous nephritis and in the most severe cases global glomerular sclerosis. These lesions are typical of human lupus nephritis and have been classified by the World Health Organization.

As in human SLE, the majority of the animals show a proliferative type of glomerular lesions. Deposits of immunoglobulin and complement are observed in a granular pattern along the glomerular capillary wall (mostly IgG) and in the mesangium (IgM). Electron microscopic examination reveals the presence of mesangial and subepithelial electron-dense deposits with varying degrees of spike formation and incorporation of electron-dense material in the glomerular basement membrane.

Similar to the 16/6 Id-induced SLE model, the GVH disease model has two advantages over other models of SLE: the disease can be induced experimentally and it develops relatively rapidly.

Animal models for the antiphospholipid syndrome

Serum antiphospholipid antibodies (aPL) are often found in patients with autoimmune disorders such as SLE and idiopathic thrombocytopenia[56,57].

These immunoglobulins, when associated with arterial and venous thrombosis, recurrent abortion, neurological disease and thrombocytopenia have been classified as the primary antiphospholipid syndrome, or the secondary antiphospholipid syndrome if they are associated with autoimmune diseases[58,59].

The 'lupus anticoagulant' is an acquired autoantibody that acts by inhibiting the generation of the prothrombin activator complex. A strong correlation has been demonstrated between the lupus anticoagulant and raised anti-cardiolipin levels[56-59]. It was found that antibodies directed against negatively charged phospholipids, cardiolipin in particular, could be demonstrated in sera from patients with positive lupus anticoagulant tests[56-59]. There appears to be a close, but not absolute correlation between both antibodies.

Whether the anti-phospholipid antibodies constitute 'markers' or epiphenomena seen in particular 'subsets' of patients with the associated clinical syndromes, or whether they are in themselves pathogenic is as yet unclear[60]. Indeed, a direct pathogenic role for aPL has not been demonstrated. Because the *in vivo* examination of human aPL regulatory mechanisms are complex, the availability of an animal model for the antiphospholipid syndrome would be valuable in unravelling the pathological mechanisms attributed to these antibodies. Only recently have several such animal models been presented.

Smith et al.[61] have demonstrated the presence of aPL, thrombocytopenia and thrombosis in MRL/lpr/lpr mice and established this strain as a suitable animal model for the human secondary anti-phospholipid syndrome. They revealed that old MRL/lpr/lpr mice have titres of both IgG and IgM anti-cardiolipin antibodies which are at least one thousandfold greater than control MRL$^+$/$^+$ and C3H/HeJ mice. They further established that these antibodies have characteristics similar to human anti-cardiolipin antibodies (aCL). By immunodiffusion, these murine aCL, like human aCL[62,63], displayed cross-reactivity with the negatively charged phospholipid, phosphatidyl serine, but not with cholesterol or phosphatidyl choline. Furthermore, histological evidence of central nervous system thrombosis as well as perivascular infiltrates of the choroid plexus was observed[61]. The high titres of serum aPL, thrombocytopenia and thrombosis establish this strain as an animal model for the secondary antiphospholipid syndrome.

Another study[64] determined whether purified immunoglobulin G from patients with antiphospholipid antibodies causes fetal loss in pregnant mice. Sera were obtained from nonpregnant parous women (group 1) and nonpregnant women with antiphospholipid antibodies and a history of fetal loss (group 2). Pregnant BALB/c mice were given an *intraperitoneal* injection of 15 mg of IgG on day 8 of pregnancy. Typically, mice treated with IgG from antiphospholipid antibodies aborted within 48 hours. When animals were sacrificed on day 9 to 15, the uterus of each animal was inspected for the presence of live, dead, or resorbing fetuses. In contrast to mice injected with control IgG or saline solution, each mouse injected with IgG from antiphospholipid antibodies aborted and no live fetuses were found. Histological examination of the uteroplacental interface showed decidual necrosis in the mice treated with IgG containing antiphospholipid antibodies, and immunofluorescent studies also showed prominent intravascular decidual IgG and fibrin deposition. These authors[64] concluded that IgG from antiphospholipid antibodies of women with fetal loss causes fetal loss in BALB/c mice. It appeared that the fetal loss was mediated by IgG binding in the maternal decidual vasculature.

We have evaluated the effect of passive transfer of anti-cardiolipin (aCL) antibodies to the *tail vein* of naive mice, on fecundity, fetal loss (fetal resorption) and the weight of embryos and placentae[65]. Two types of aCL antibodies were employed: (a) mouse monoclonal aCL antibodies derived from a BALB/c mouse in which experimental SLE was induced by a pathogenic idiotype (16/6) of anti-DNA antibodies, and (b) polyclonal IgG and IgM aCL antibodies derived from serum of a patient with primary antiphospholipid syndrome.

After infusion of either antibody ($10\,\mu$g per mouse), we could demonstrate lower fecundity rate, increased resorption index of embryos (equivalent to recurrent fetal loss), lower number of embryos per pregnancy, and lower mean weights of embryos and placentae in comparison to mice infused with appropriate control immunoglobulins. It was concluded that the aCL antibodies may have direct effects on fecundity and on the outcome of pregnancy.

We have also induced experimental SLE associated with antiphospholipid syndrome (APLS), following active immunization of mice with a new human monoclonal anti-DNA antibody (MIV-7), carrying the pathogenic anti-DNA idiotype 16/6, as well as induction of APLS with monoclonal anticardiolipin antibodies derived from the mouse with the induced syndromes[66]. MIV-7 is a human monoclonal antibody that binds to DNA and carries a pathogenic anti-DNA idiotype 16/6[66].

The antibody was generated by fusing peripheral blood lymphocytes of a healthy donor which were stimulated with an anti-idiotypic antibody to B11 (a human Mo Ab anti-mouse mammary tumor virus-MMTV). The MIV-7, in addition to being an anti-DNA, binds to MMTV glycoproteins. Following immunization of naive BALB/c mice with MIV-7 in the footpads, the mice developed SLE and APLS. The SLE was characterized by serological markers (e.g. anti-DNA), clinical manifestations (increased sedimentation rate and proteinuria) and histological findings (deposition of immune-complexes in the glomeruli).

The APLS was characterized by thrombocytopenia, the presence of anti-cardiolipin antibodies and lupus anticoagulant (prolonged APTT), by low fecundity rate, high resorption rate of fetuses and lower mean weights of the placentae and fetuses. Moreover, the existence of anti-cardiolipin antibodies that may induce the '*primary*' APLS were also confirmed: passive transfer of anti-cardiolipin MAbs (CAM, CAL) which were generated from the mice with the combined experimental SLE and APLS led to the generation of primary APLS[66] without the association of SLE manifestations. Similarly, active immunization of naive mice with a human IgM monoclonal aCl antibody induced generation by the mice of sustained (5 months) high levels of aCl antibodies. In these mice the characteristics of primary APLS were demonstrated[67].

Table 3 Factors recently associated with autoimmunity in lupus-prone mouse strains

Genetics:	MHC, T-cell receptor genes
Hormones:	Oestrogen, Prolactin
Cytokines:	IL-1, IL-2, IL-3-like, IL-4, IL-5, IL-6, TNF-alpha, INF-gamma
Immunologic disorders:	B-cell tolerance defects, Ly-1$^+$ B cells, T-cell tolerance defects
Oncogenes and retroviruses:	Increased expression of c-*myc*, c-*myb*, c-abl

The existence of these different experimental models of SLE with APLS may enable controlled studies of novel therapeutic methods.

FACTORS INVOLVED IN AUTOIMMUNITY IN ANIMAL MODELS (see Table 3)

The aetiology of human autoimmune conditions is multifactorial, entailing genetic, environmental, hormonal and immunological factors[2].

Accordingly, virtually all animal models of spontaneous autoimmune disease have been shown to rely on a polygenic basis and experimental autoimmunity can be induced in certain susceptible strains. Recent studies have been directed toward a more fundamental understanding of mechanisms of loss of self-tolerance leading to different autoimmune features. The various autoimmune mouse strains share a number of immunological defects leading to autoimmune diseases. One of these defects is a strain-specific, antigen-driven production of autoantibodies resulting in autoimmunity[68,69]. Indeed, Kleinman et al.[68] have analysed the B cell repertoire of old MRL/lpr/lpr mice and demonstrated (1) an age-dependent shift from production of IgM to IgG and (2) an age-dependent shift from polyclonal autoantibody production to production of antibodies against a limited number of auto-antigens.

Another type of defect observed in autoimmune mice is a deficiency in the maintenance of self-tolerance by B or T lymphocytes[70–72]. This is an intrinsic defect due to genetic abnormalities that presumably affect an early development signalling mechanism. The disruption of early B- and T-cell development leads to the appearance of lymphocytes that are predisposed to loss of tolerance. Although it is beyond the scope of this chapter to enumerate all the factors involved in autoimmunity in autoimmune mice, some of them are discussed here in more detail.

Antigen-driven production of autoantibodies

Although autoantibodies are a hallmark of autoimmune diseases, the mechanisms by which they are produced remain obscure. Studies in both human SLE and the murine GVH disease model of SLE have suggested the important role of antigen in the antibody response to the chromatin-related antigens. If chromatin were the putative antigen driving the production of autoantibody, then a close association should exist between antibodies to the chromatic components histone and DNA. However, it might be expected that antibodies to non-chromatin-related antigens such as Sm should occur independently of these chromatin-related antibodies. Cohen et al.[73], in their study carried out in the spontaneous mice SLE strain, MRL/lpr/lpr and MRL-+/+, found that the association between autoantibodies is not restricted to double-stranded DNA and histone and the association extends to Sm. Their findings support the notion that specific antigen-driven responses are not solely responsible for autoantibody production in murine SLE.

In contrast to DNA, which basically is not immunogenic and thus raises the possibility that anti-DNA in SLE was probably not found after antigen stimulation, evidence exists to the contrary in anti-Sm. The spontaneous occurrence of antibodies against the Sm nuclear antigen is a highly specific marker for the diagnosis of SLE. It has been previously shown that anti-Sm can be elicited by immunization of SLE-prone mice with purified Sm antigen. Recently, this autoantibody was induced in normal mice by a similar immunization protocol[74]. Anti-Sm produced by normal strains was predominantly of the IgG_1 subclass, which is similar to the isotype distribution in Sm-immunized MRL mice, but different from the IgG2 alpha-dominated response seen for spontaneous anti-Sm. Anti-Sm raised by immunization in most strains recognized epitopes not seen by spontaneous human and murine SLE anti-Sm of the 11 normal strains tested. Only C3H and AKR, strains from which MRL was partially derived, responded to these determinants.

Further, immunoblot analysis of anti-Sm generated by immunization of MRL and normal mice revealed that the same proteins, recognized by spontaneous human and murine anti-Sm, were also seen by these sera. This study shows that an autoantibody highly characteristic of SLE can be produced in normal and MRL mice after appropriate immunization and that the fine specificity of such experimentally induced antibody can be similar to that of spontaneous anti-Sm autoantibodies. The results imply a role for autoimmunization with Sm in the production of anti-Sm.

Another example of an antigen-driven, organ-specific autoantibody response is found in the mouse anti-red blood cell (MRBC) antibody in NZB mice. Polyclonal B cell activation may play a role in autoantibody production and autoimmune disease in NZB mice[75]. However, the MRBC response in NZB mice may be antigen driven, because transfer of bone marrow from old NZB donors to young NZB recipients resulted in a significant IgM anti-MRBC response in the absence of significant polyclonal activation[76].

In contrast to the antigen-driven theory for antinuclear antibody production stands the study by Brennan et al.[77]. In this work, spleen cells from MRL/lpr/lpr, CBA and BALB/c mice were cultured *in vitro* and assayed for production of antinuclear antibodies. It was demonstrated that anti-RNP and anti-dsDNA precursor B cells are part of the normal murine immune repertoire, thus suggesting that the spontaneous development of anti-RNP and anti-dsDNA antibodies is dependent on clonal stimulation and removal of suppressive influence.

Ly-1[+] B-cells in murine systemic lupus erythematosus

CD5[+] B-cells (Ly-1[+]B in mice, Leu1[+]B in humans) represent a distinct lineage intimately involved in autoantibody production. CD5 is a pan-T cell antigen that is also found on some B cells[78,79]. These B cells respond well to endogenous antigens but poorly to exogenous antigens[80]. One of the most interesting features of these cells is their presence in increased numbers in newborn infants and in patients with autoimmune states, all of whom display humoral immunoincompetence[81]. In addition, Leu-1[+] B cells have been found to be the malignant cell type in a high proportion of chronic lymphocytic leukaemias[82]. Normally Ly-1[+] B cells are the predominant B cell in fetal spleen but constitute less than 10% of the adult spleen.

Ly-1[+] B-cells constitute about 20% of the peritoneal cells. Ly-1[+] B cells produce much of the autoantibody and possibly may be involved in anti-idiotype production in normal mice. Mercolino et al.[83] have shown that peritoneal Ly-1[+] B cells from normal mice recognize phosphatidylcholine and are related to the cells secreting antibodies to autologous erythrocytes. In both humans and mice, Leu-1[+] and Ly-1[+] B-cells have been reported to be expanded in autoimmune states[82]. Manohar et al. first described high numbers of splenic CD5[+] B cells in NZB mice, i.e. 20%, as opposed to 10% of the B cells in normal mice, including NZW[84].

These findings were confirmed and elaborated on by Hayakawa et al.[85]. Comparable numbers of CD5[+] B cells were found in all strains tested (BALB/c being relatively high and SJL particularly low) except NZB-related strains where elevated levels were detected from neonatal life onward. Interestingly the depletion of CD5[+] B cells due to total lymphoid irradiation of B/W mice was associated with a decrease in autoantibody production, although the return of CD5[+] B cells to pre-irradiation levels did not give rise to a relapse of the disease[86]. In contrast, CD5[+] B cells were found to be normal in MRL/lpr/lpr mice.

It has, however, been demonstrated that some hybridomas obtained from these mice also have messenger RNA transcripts detectable with the CD5 probe[87]. In reality, CD5[+] B cells constitute a major lymphoid subpopulation in the murine peritoneal cavity[88]. In general, B cells account for up to 60% of the harvested peritoneal cells, of which approximately one-half express CD5. This proportion is markedly augmented in lupus mice. Mice homozygous for either the allelic autosomal recessive moth-eaten *mev*[89] or viable moth-eaten *mev*[90] develop high levels of polyclonal and autoreactive Ig, and die at average ages of 3 and 9 weeks, respectively. Numerous abnormalities have been described in these mice, including an extreme overrepresentation of the CD5[+] B cell population[91].

Other strains of mice display an immunodeficiency syndrome. For example, CBA/N mouse is a mutant strain derived from CBA, with an X-linked recessive immune defect (termed Xid) at the B cell level[92]. These animals are unable to raise antibodies to a group of thymus-independent antigens, and to develop a spontaneous antibody response to bromelain treated mouse erythrocytes (Br-ME) following *in vitro* polyclonal B cell activation. This is consistent with the lack of a subset of B lymphocytes characterized by

Lyb-3 and Lyb-5 differentiation markers, since a low frequency of peritoneal CD5[+] B cells has been detected, which fall largely in the Lyb-5 compartment[93]. It is interesting that the CBA/N X-linked B cell defect may be fully expressed in (CBA/N x NZB) F_1 mice[94]. Despite not being expressed, the genetic synthesis of natural autoantibodies does exist in these mice[95], and they may develop CD5[+] B cells, if reconstituted with autologous bone marrow after treatment with cyclosporin A[96].

The immunodeficiency of R111 S/J mice is also characterized by a low anti-Br-ME splenic plaque-forming cell response, and associated with a reduced frequency of peritoneal CD5[+] B cells[97]. The inability to produce a response to Br-ME has also been found in the SJL mice. They are without CD5[+] B cells[98], but also unable to respond normally to lipopolysaccharide[99].

Many autoantibodies ascribed to Ly-1+ B cells are so-called 'natural autoantibodies'. These autoantibodies, found in normal as well as in autoimmune mice, bind to a variety of self-antigens with relatively low affinity, and cross-react with bacterial determinants. The contribution of Ly-1 B cells to the pathogenic antibodies precipitating in glomerulonephritis and haemolytic anaemia in autoimmune mice should be further investigated. Ly-1[+] B cells may be an important regulator of other B cells: the finding that the immune suppression observed in patients with multiple myelomas is mediated by CD5[+] B cells suggested that CD5[+] B cells (and Ly-1[+] B cells in mice) may be involved in the regulation of conventional B cell function. The effect of exogenous Ly-1[+] B cells on recipient lymphoid subpopulations was analysed by Raveche et al.[100] by injecting spleen cells possessing hyperdiploid NZB Ly-1[+] B cells into unirradiated (NZB x DBA/2) F_1 mice. The lymphoid subpopulations in the recipient mice were assayed by flow cytometric techniques. The study by Raveche et al.[100] suggests that hyperdiploid Ly-1[+] B cells are different from typical peritoneal Ly-1[+] B cells both in the lymphoid organs in which they home and in their proliferative capacity. NZB hyperdiploid Ly-1+ B cells, which may arise as a natural consequence of hyperactive Ly-1+ B cells, may play an immunoregulative role in the spleen.

T cells in autoimmune mice

One of the most striking features of lpr mice is the marked accumulation of abnormal lymphocytes in lymph nodes, and, to a lesser extent, in the spleen. The expanded population appears to be of T-cell lineage, since the cells bear T cell receptors[101,102] and have a germ line immunoglobulin gene configuration[102].

The major population of cells accumulating in the lymphoid tissue is the unique subset of Thy-1[+], L3T4, Lyt-2[−], B220[+] and Pgp-1[+][103,104]. They seem to belong to a T cell lineage in consideration for expression of TCR-alpha/beta[101], albeit at low density, lack of Ig gene rearrangements[103] and generation of thymus[101]. In lpr mouse, neonatal thymectomy completely prevents the disease at least during the first 15 months of life at which time observations were terminated[105–106]. Neonatal thymectomy followed by thymic grafting of the lpr mouse showed that an lpr thymus was not essential to the development of the characteristic early disease in this mouse, since transplantation of an MRL/n thymus following thymectomy resulted in a disease indistinguishable from that seen in an intact MRL/l mouse[107]. Transplantation of normal bone marrow into lpr mice prevents the development of the disease[108,109]. These phenomena suggest an importance of the existence of the thymus for development of the disease and an intrinsic abnormality in lpr stem cells.

A defect in clonal deletion and anergy induction by lpr T cells was demonstrated by transfer of bone marow cells from MI_sb MRL-lpr/lpr mice into H-2-compatible MI_sa AKR-lpr/lpr[110]. Transfer of bone marrow cells from MRL-lpr ($H-2^k$, MI_sb, Thy 1.2) mice resulted in decreased $CD4^+CD8^+$ T cells and increased mature thymocytes compared to transfer of bone marrow cells from MRL-+/+ mice.

A second defect was a failure to delete self-reactive T cells expressing V beta 6 in AKR recipients of lpr/lpr bone marrow compared with AKR recipients of +/+ bone marrow.

In contrast to lpr mice, the participation of the thymus in the SLE disease in other mice strains is not always essential. Neonatal thymectomy of BXSB mice of either sex does not detectably alter the course of the disease[111].

T-cell lines capable of augmenting the production of pathogenic anti-DNA autoantibodies were analyzed in (SWR x NZB) F_1 mice[112]. Four of 16 anti-DNA autoantibody-inducing T helper lines were $CD4^-CD8^-$. Two clones expressed V beta 6 and one expressed V beta 8.1. These clones are self-reactive in (SWR x NZB) F_1 mice because they are directed against the MI_{sa} antigen.

A similar failure of clonal deletion of autoreactive T cells was found by flow cytometry analysis of spleen cells, with an increase in V beta 17 alpha (I-E reactive) T cells. These results suggest that a defect in clonal deletion of autoreactive T cells in autoimmune mice can lead to increased autoantibody production. Magilavy et al.[113] reported recently that abnormal suppressor activity was found in T cells from the liver of MRL/lpr/lpr mice. The concordance of this increased suppressor activity with disease onset at 9 weeks of age suggested that this suppressor activity might be a compensatory response to the autoimmune disease.

Genetic factors

Among the factors involved in autoimmune disease, genetics has a major role. The most studied genes in this regard are the polymorphic class II major histocompatibility complex genes, some of which confer an increased risk of developing certain autoimmune diseases or different clinical manifestations of autoimmunity. Nephritis in (NZB x SWR) F_1 is linked to I-Aq beta chain locus of the SWR mouse. Antibodies to class II molecules ameliorate disease in (NZB x NZW)F_1 mice, indicating that the H-2-linked genes in the NZW mouse accelerate autoimmune disease. Polymorphism of the second exon of the first domain of I-A alpha, I-A beta, I-E alpha, and

I-E beta of NZB mice was investigated by sequence analysis. A single base pair and amino acid (arginine for threonine) change was found at amino acid position 72 in the NZWI-E beta chain[114]. Three-dimensional analysis revealed that this is in a position to interact with the T cell receptor/antigen complex and affect immune response.

The T cell receptor genes may be another set of candidate genes important for disease susceptibility. In the last few years, some studies have been reported that analyse the structure, genomic organization, and expression of T-cell receptor on mice with SLE. In MRL/lpr mice, an increase of the V beta 8 family of the T-cell receptor was identified.

This enhanced representation may indicate modification in thymic selection/maturation processing in these mice which may have relevance to the lpr gene-associated autoimmunity[115].

Another study using sodium dodecyl sulphate-polyacrylamide gel electrophoresis analysis has demonstrated a difference between MRL/lpr mice T-cell receptor and MRL/+ +[116]. These differences in T-cell receptor structure may be related to the autoimmune tendency of MRL/lpr[116]. Davignon et al.[117] have also shown relationships between the hyporesponsiveness of T-cells in MRL/lpr mice and the T cell structure.

Cytokines in murine systemic lupus erythematosus

Autoimmune diseases are characterized by decreased production of and/or response to IL2[118,119]. The CD4⁻CD8⁻ T cells of lpr/lpr autoimmune mice have a decreased response to IL2. The high affinity T cell receptor for IL2 is composed of the recently identified signal-transducing p75 chain and a p55 chain that can be detected by several antibodies. The CD4⁻CD8⁻ T-cells of lpr/lpr mice have decreased expression of the p55 chain. Expression of the p75 chain in B220⁻ T cells of lpr/lpr has been found to be expressed weakly by one investigation[120] and constitutively by another[121]. Preliminary results showed that the production of IL2 in the mice with induced SLE was reduced[2]. This led us to treat mice with experimentally induced SLE with the synthetic immunomodulator Aa-101 (ammonium trichlorotellurate)[122].

This immunomodulator has the ability to increase the production of IL2, and colony-stimulating factor *in vivo* and *in vitro*. The immunomodulating action on mice of AS-101 was not followed by improvement, showing that the decreased secretion of IL2 is a result, not the cause of SLE in these mice.

Interleukin-1 (IL1) is elevated in plasma and synovial fluid of patients with rheumatoid arthritis[123]. IL1 alpha accelerated the arthritis in 3-month-old MRL/lpr/lpr mice[124], but not glomerulonephritis or lymphadenopathy.

Interleukin-3 (IL/3) can induce the release of inflammatory mediators by mononuclear cells[125]. Two types of antibodies can mimic IL-3 effects in MRL/lpr/lpr[126] and C3H/gld/gld mice. One type of antibody binds to the IL-3 receptor, and the second type can support the growth of IL-3 dependent cell lines by binding to the IgG Fc receptor. Both antibodies can induce production of IL3 by cell lines. It is possible that antibodies that mimic IL3 increase monocyte activity in lpr/lpr and gld/gld mice.

Twenty-five per cent of resting B cells from both BALB/c controls as well as autoimmune MRL/lpr/lpr and (NZB x NZW) F_1 mice secreted IgG_1 after *in vitro* stimulation with interleukin 4 (IL4). Nearly all resting B cells in NZB mice were IgM^+IgG^-, and IL4 did not induce IgG_1 production in B cells from these mice[127]. Interleukin-5 was shown to promote immunoglobulin and anti-DNA production in (NZB x NZW) F_1 mice[128]. In yet another study[129], interleukin-6 induced production of IgM and IgG anti-DNA from freshly isolated B cells from thymectomized and nonthymectomized (NZB x NZW) F_1 mice. Anti-interleukin-6 blocked the production of interleukin-6 induced production of anti-DNA *in vitro*.

Interferon gamma-treated NZB/NZW mice developed accelerated renal disease whereas treatment with a monoclonal antibody to interferon-gamma delayed disease[130]. High levels of interferon-gamma and tumour necrosis factor (TNF) alpha RNA have been found in peripheral lymph nodes of old MRL/lpr/lpr mice[131]. Because TNF synergizes with interferon-gamma in a number of activities, the *in vivo* effects of TNF-alpha have been tested in this murine model[127]. This study showed that lupus nephritis in NZB/NZW may be due to a lack of the genes producing TNF. Treatment with TNF prevented nephritis and prolonged the life of treated mice[132].

On the other hand, Boswell et al.[133] found that over-expression of mRNA of TNF and interleukin-1 and oversecretion of the lymphokine were associated with nephritis in MRL/lpr mice. To complicate the issue of the contrasting effects of TNF *in vivo*, Kettelhurt and Goldberg[134] have shown that TNF treatment in rats can induce fever without producing the catabolic state commonly noted when TNF secretion is induced by endotoxin.

These studies point to the need for further investigations in the field to clarify the role cytokines play in autoimmunity.

Oncogenes and retroviruses

Proto-oncogenes encode for normal cellular proteins involved in regulation of growth and differentiation, and altered expression reflects differences in these processes in autoimmune disease. Increased expression of c-*myc*, c-*myb*, c-*abl*, and other oncogenes has been reported in B-cells, T-cells and autoimmune disease tissue. The most striking association between cellular oncogene expression and generalized autoimmunity is the 30- to 60-fold increase in c-*myb* RNA in the lymph nodes of MRL/lpr/lpr mice compared to MRL-+/+ mice[135]. The lpr/lpr genotype is implicated because this degree of c-*myb* expression is also found in the lymph nodes of AKR/lpr/lpr, C3H/lpr/lpr, and C57BL/6-lpr/lpr mice but not in congenic +/+ strains[136]. The high c-*myb* expression is associated with the $CD4^-CD8^-$ T cells, which markedly expand in the lpr/lpr lymph nodes[103,137]. High c-*myb* expression is found in precursor cells for all of the other haemotopoietic lineages[138,139].

Mountz and Steinberg[140] have shown recently that nuclear extract from lymph nodes of MRL/lpr/lpr mice binds specifically to the 5^1 genomic region of the c-*myb* oncogene and correlates with high expression of c-*myb* messenger RNA.

Elevated expression of proto-oncogenes in synovial tissue in autoimmune disease is sometimes interpreted as evidence that tissues may be undergoing a process similar to malignant transformation[141], but there is no direct evidence to support this claim.

The genomes of most vertebrates contains numerous retroviral sequences, the great majority of which are non-infectious. The endogenous retroviral sequences are transcribed and translated in many host tissues, and are induced by mitogens. Endogenous type C retroviral proteins and RNA are expressed in the lymphoid tissues of all studied mouse strains[142,143]. This expression is rapidly induced by T or B-cell mitogens[144,145].

The consequences of this inducible expression have been unclear inasmuch as direct effects of endogenous retroviral proteins on the host immune system have been elusive. A possible role of endogenous type C retrovirus in autoimmune mice was analysed using specific antisense oligonucleotides complementary to the gag-pol initiation site as well as other sites[146]. This resulted in increased spleen cell RNA synthesis and increased Ia and immunoglobulin expression. These data[146] suggest that an endogenous retrovirus can encode for gene products that exert a negative feedback circuit after immune stimulation.

Retrovirus infection has often been suggested as the aetiology for autoimmune diseases (rheumatoid arthritis and SLE), but without experimental support. There are many immunopathological similarities between these diseases and those caused by lentiviruses in animals[147]. So far, however, most attempts to detect retrovirus infections in patients with rheumatoid arthritis and SLE have given negative results. Neither antibodies to HIV nor those to human T-cell leukaemia virus type I (HTLV-I) were found in patients with SLE by Boumpas et al.[148]. These antibodies were also undetectable in patients with rheumatoid arthritis and SLE studied by Pelton et al.[149]. In contrast, Olsen et al.[150] reported that the sera of 12 African patients with SLE contained antibodies to HTLV-1 in titres ranging from 1:20 to 1:80.

Recently, Gavalchin et al.[151] found that 26% of 53 SLE sera had titres of antibody to HTLV-I compared to only 5% in normal controls. Ziegler et al.[152] demonstrated antigenic sequences recognized by monoclonal antibodies to p19 and p24 of HTLV-I in cells of the proliferating synovium in rheumatoid arthritis. These findings, although intriguing, still do not constitute proof as to the involvement of the virus in the pathogenesis of autoimmune diseases.

Hormones and autoimmunity

Sex hormones strongly influence the development of autoimmune disease in NZB/W mice. Oestrogen administration decreased survival and increased autoantibody production, whereas testosterone had the opposite effect[153]. In another study[154], testosterone inhibited delayed-type hypersensitivity and antibody production in MRL/lpr/lpr and C57BL/6-lpr/lpr mice, while oestrogen suppressed delayed-type hypersensitivity but enhanced antibody production.

The immunomodulatory effects of sex hormones varied in other strains of mice. Ahmed et al.[155] have shown that prenatal exposure of C57BL/6J mice to oestrogen resulted in increased numbers of antibody plaque-forming cells to bromelain-treated mouse erythrocytes and development of lesions indistinguishable from Sjøgren's syndrome. These results suggest that oestrogen acts directly on B cells as well as on T-cells.

Sex hormones were found to influence antihistone antibody production in MRL/lpr/lpr and (NZB x NZW)F$_1$ mice[156]. Antihistone antibodies are associated with drug-induced systemic lupus erythematosus in humans. These antibodies increase in number with age, and this increase occurs earlier in females. Oestrogen increased and testosterone decreased antihistone antibody levels in both (NZB x NZW) F$_1$ and MRL/lpr/lpr mice. Aside from this common influence by hormones, different autoimmune mouse strains tend to produce different antihistone antibodies. Thus, MRL/lpr/lpr mice produce antibodies reactive with histone component H1, whereas (NZB x NZW)F$_1$ mice tend to produce antibodies reactive with histone components H2b and H3.

The effects of sex hormones were shown in several experiments with our model of experimental SLE[157]. Females treated with oestrogen before immunization with 16/6 Id showed an accelerated experimental SLE induction when compared with control females immunized only with 16/6 Id. Testosterone treatment of mice before 16/6 Id immunization (females and orchidectomized males) resulted in a milder disease on serological (autoantibody production) and clinical levels (increased ESR, proteinuria, and leucopenia). Histological findings indicate that testosterone administered to immunized, orchidectomized males could prevent kidney damage, whereas oestrogen administration led to an earlier onset of and more pronounced kidney damage[157]. Recent studies support a link between prolactin (PRL), the immune system and autoimmune diseases[158,159]. McMurray et al.[160] have demonstrated that hyperprolactinaemia accelerates disease activity in the male NZB/W mouse model of SLE. In this study, hyperprolactinaemia was associated with elevated anti-DNA, IgM and IgG levels, and accelerated mortality in male B/W mice when compared to normoprolactinaemic male B/W controls.

NEW TREATMENT MODALITIES OF AUTOIMMUNE DISEASE IN MICE (see Table 4)

One advantage of each of the mouse models is their availability for studies of therapeutic interventions. Many such interventions have been studied including modification of the environment or hormone status, immuno-suppressive drugs, antiviral agents, and total lymphoid irradiation[3,39,70]. More recently, newer therapeutic modalities of autoimmunity in animal models have been introduced.

Table 4 Therapeutic modalities that suppress murine SLE

Drugs	Glucocorticoids
	Immunosuppressive reagents
	(azathioprine, cyclophosphamide)
	Cyclosporin A
Dietary manipulation	Low calorie diet
	Low protein diet
	Diet rich in saturated fat
	High eicosapentanoic acid in diet
	Low zinc
Hormones	Androgens
	Anti-oestrogens
Total lymphoid irradiation	
Anti-lymphocyte reagents	
Treatment with idiotypes and anti-idiotypes	

Cyclosporin A

It has been previously shown that various organ-specific autoimmune diseases such as gastritis, oophoritis, thyroiditis or insulitis develop in mice by depleting Lyt T-cells, including L3T4 (CD4$^+$) T-cells as well as Lyt-2$^+$ (CD8$^+$) T-cells, leaving Thy-1, Lyt- T-cells in the immune system. Cyclosporin A (CsA) is a fungal metabolite and a potent immunosuppressant that has a specific effect on T-cells. Cyclosporin A can selectively abrogate L3T4$^+$ T-cells and Lyt-2$^+$ T-cells in the murine thymus. Sakaguchi and Sakaguchi[161] have shown an induction of gastritis, oopheritis and insulitis in athymic *nu/nu* mice after engrafting the thymus from euthymic *mu/+* mice treated with CsA. Their controlled study demonstrated that cyclosporin A appears to interfere selectively with the thymic production of certain suppressor T-cells controlling self-reactive (autoimmune) T-cells, allowing the latter to expand and cause autoimmune disease.

In a recent study, we attempted to examine the role of CsA on the development of SLE in a model of experimental SLE described earlier. The immunosuppressive agent was injected into naive mice at an early stage of the disease (two months after immunization) and at four months after immunization, when clinical parameters had already been observed. Cyclosporin A was found to have a suppressive effect on antibody production as well as on the appearance of clinical manifestations in the 16/6 lupus model[162]. The most prominent effect of the drug was noted when the mice were treated at an early stage of the disease. This was reflected in the dramatic decrease to normal levels of autoantibody titres to DNA, histones, cardiolipin, Sm, RNP, SS-A (Ro), SS-B(La) and 16/6 idiotype. A similar effect was noted on erythrocyte sedimentation rate, white blood cell count and proteinuria. These data were supported by the electron micrographs of the CsA treated SLE kidneys, as well as by analysis of *in vitro* helper activity to anti-16/6 Id production by lymph node cells from the above animals.

The study demonstrates that, similar to other autoimmune conditions (e.g.

insulin dependent diabetes mellitus), the early administration of CsA in SLE may be more beneficial than when given at later stages. Our study also supports previously described data suggesting that CsA induced a decrease in anti-DNA antibody producing B cells in NZB/NZW (F_1) mice[163,164]. Similarly, it has been reported that CsA affected the production of autoantibody against thyroid antigens in insulin-dependent diabetic patients[165]. Previously, we also showed that CsA treatment in patients with uveitis leads to a significant decrease in the titres of antibodies to DNA, cardiolipin, histones, Sm/RNP and SS-A (Ro). The effect was selective on autoantibody production without affecting the total immunoglobulin levels[166].

All these studies are in agreement with a recent report on successful treatment of SLE patients with CsA[167]. These facts may raise the question of initiating treatment with CsA in SLE in early stages of the disease rather than in very late ones.

Fish oil

Fish oils contain long chain, highly polyunsaturated, omega-3 (ω-3) fatty acids, particularly eicosapentaenoic (20:5 omega-3) and docosahexaenoic (22:6 omega-3) acid of the linolenic or omega-3 class, unlike linoleic acid (18:2 omega-6) which is the predominant polyunsaturated fatty acid in a Western diet.

The rationale behind the treatment is that high dietary levels of essential fatty acids would increase the levels of prostaglandins of the three series which are less inflammatory than prostaglandins of the two series derived from arachidonic acid. Indeed, Prickett et al.[168] showed that the incidence of glomerulonephritis in the (NZB x NZW) F_1 mouse lupus model was decreased in animals fed with a diet rich in eicosapentaenoic acid (EPA)[168]. This was accompanied by a decrease in overall mortality. Suppression of autoimmune lupus in MRL-lpr mouse model as measured by decreased lymphoid hyperplasia and delay in onset of renal disease by diets rich in fish oil have also been noted[169].

Diets high in ω-3 fatty acids have also been shown to decrease the incidence of collagen induced arthritis in susceptible mouse strains[170] and to retard the formation of experimental amyloid in azocasein treated mice[171].

Ito et al.[172] have examined the impact of fish oil on rats and found it had a significant effect on serum lipid eicosanoid production and fibrinolysis, and even protected the renal function. Fish oil also had an effect on the kidney morphology in rats in which nephrotic syndrome was induced by doxorubicin. Therefore, the authors recommended fish oil, rich in ω-3 fatty acids, as an adjunct to other therapeutic measures in autoimmune conditions associated with kidney involvement.

The detrimental effect of ultraviolet light on SLE is well-established. The mechanism by which ultraviolet light induces this disease remains uncertain. In part, it is believed that DNA becomes more immunogenic due to defects in DNA repairs.

Licastro et al.[173] have suggested that the beneficial results of dietary restriction in autoimmunity are explained by its effect on DNA repair. The authors analysed DNA repair following ultraviolet irradiation in mice. Two mouse cohorts received restricted amounts of purified hypocaloric diets: one was minimally restricted (75%), and the other was severely restricted (50%). An inverse correlation between age and DNA repair was present in the two cohorts. However, the regression lines in the two cohorts showed different slopes: dietary restriction appeared to decelerate the age-associated decline of DNA repair capacity. This delay might account in part for the improved immune function shown by old mice on dietary restriction.

Total lymphoid irradiation (TLI)

Total lymphoid irradiation (TLI) is a technique in which high doses of radiation (more than the LD50 for man) are delivered to lymphoid tissues while other tissues are shielded. X-rays are targeted to cervical, axillary, mediastinal, para-aortic and inguinal lymph nodes, as well as to the thymus and spleen. TLI is now a routine treatment for human lymphoid malignancies, e.g. Hodgkin's disease.

TLI produces many alterations in the immune functions. It induces a marked lymphopenia, but the lymphocyte count gradually returns to normal, 1–2 years after treatment[174]. However, after the lymphocyte count returns to its pretreatment level, there is a reversal of the B to T cell ratio in the peripheral blood, and a long-lasting T lymphopenia and B lymphocytosis. There are also changes in the T cell subsets[175]. In addition, it was noted that there is a marked decrease in the spontaneous secretion of IL-1 by synovial biopsy specimens[175]. TLI also suppresses cellular immunity as judged by its ability to eliminate the mixed leucocyte reaction, depresses the response of peripheral blood lymphocytes to phytohaemagglutinin, and induces the disappearance of the delayed hypersensitivity skin reaction to dinitrochlorbenzene[176].

Studies performed in mice have shown that cells from the spleen of an animal given TLI non-specifically suppressed the T cell-dependent antibody response. Furthermore, after treatment with TLI, there is a transient appearance of antigen-nonspecific suppressor cells of the mixed lymphocyte reaction[177]. These cells prevent responder cells from any strain of mice from reacting to stimulation by cells of any other strain.

Another important effect of TLI is the induction of a state of tolerance which is mediated by antigen-specific suppressor T cells. For example, BALB/c mice given TLI and injected with bovine serum albumin (BSA) developed a state of tolerance and made no anti-DNP antibody response when challenged with DNP-BSA. This tolerance was antigen-specific, and when the same mice were challenged with DNP-BCG, they made a normal anti-DNP response[178].

Most of the trials of TLI have been in experimental models of human autoimmune diseases. Kotzin and Strober[179] demonstrated that TLI given to (NZB/NZW)F$_1$ mice early in the course of the disease reversed the proteinuria, decreased the titres of anti-DNA antibodies, and markedly prolonged the life of the animals relative to the controls. TLI also prolonged the survival of mice with advanced disease, unlike most other immunosuppressive methods which prevent the disease from developing only if administered before mice became ill.

The mechanism of action of TLI in these mice might be through non-specific suppression of the antibody response found after TLI. It is well known that (NZB/NZW)F$_1$ mice have deficiencies of suppressor T-cells and TLI may exhibit its effects by swinging the balance back in the direction of tolerance to self by favoring suppressor cells.

TLI given to MRL/n and MRL/l mice induced a marked decrease in proteinuria and doubling of their life span. Histopathological examination of TLI-treated mice revealed normal kidneys, while the controls showed generalized glomerular lesions by light microscopy and large electron dense deposits[179].

Few trials of TLI in human autoimmune diseases have been performed. The results are encouraging but a major obstacle involves the serious complications involved in such a treatment.

Anti-lymphocyte reagents

Monoclonal antibodies (mAb) to T-helper (Th) cells have been used successfully to treat murine models for several human autoimmune diseases[180–182]. In these studies, the anti-Th cell mAb used have been directed against the L3T4 molecule. L3T4, which is homologous to human CD4, is selectively expressed on mouse T 'helper/inducer' cells. In these studies[180–182], successful treatment with anti-L3T4 has been associated with profound depletion of L3T4+ cells which could account for immune suppression. However, in a recent study[183], treatment of NZB/NZW F$_1$ (B/W) mice with F (ab^l)2 anti-CD4 resulted in decreased anti-DNA antibody production, improved renal function and prolonged survival without the depletion of CD4$^+$ T cells observed after treatment with the intact anti-CD4 antibody. The inhibitory effect was postulated to result from the blocking of CD4-mediated signal transduction normally associated with interaction of the CD4 molecule with Ia on antigen-presenting cells. Treatment of mice with the intact anti-CD4 antibody was associated with tolerance induction to the rat anti-CD4, whereas treatment with the F (ab^l)2 anti-CD4 was complicated by the development of a host immune response to the rat monoclonal antibody fragments. However, mice could be made tolerant to the F(ab^l)2 fragment by pretreating with a single high dose of intact rat anti-CD4. Similar treatment strategies for tolerance induction by monoclonal antibodies may be applicable to human autoimmune disease therapies.

The contribution of the abnormal CD4$^-$CD8$^-$B220$^+$ T cells to auto-immunity in MRL/lpr/lpr mice is unknown. Administration of the anti-B220 antibody to MRL/lpr/lpr mice reduced autoantibodies production and lymphadenopathy[184]. The authors proposed that the effect might be mediated through B220$^+$, CD4$^+$ T cells[101]. Mel-14 is a peripheral lymph node homing receptor found on T cells. Treatment of MRL/lpr/lpr mice with anti-Mel-14 mAb resulted in reduction (10 to 20 fold) in lymphadenopathy[185].

Manipulation of anti-DNA idiotypes

The realization that the expression of idiotype-bearing antibodies is regulated by anti-idiotypes has led to a new approach to the treatment of autoimmune diseases via manipulations of the idiotype–anti-idiotype interactions[186].

The rationale for such treatment is the evidence that there are certain pathogenic idiotypes (cross-reactive) that are directly involved in the pathogenesis of autoimmune diseases and that manipulation of such idiotypes may result in down-regulation of pathogenic autoantibodies and beneficial effect of patients with autoimmune disease[186]. Certainly, encouraging results have been reported in experimental autoimmune diseases. These studies[187–189] involved *in vitro* manipulation of the idiotype network (animal and human studies) as well as *in vivo* modulation of idiotypes (animal studies)[189].

Three distinct methods were used to manipulate the idiotype network: (a) passive administration of anti-Id; (b) syngeneic immunization with idiotypes; (c) injection of anti-idiotype conjugated to a cytotoxic agent whereby the anti-idiotype targets antibody-producing cells and the toxin specifically destroys them[38,186].

Kim et al.[190] have demonstrated that anti-DNA production by anti-DNA secreting hybridomas can be inhibited by the addition of anti-idiotypes to anti-DNA. Hahn and Ebling[191] have shown that in lupus-prone mice, anti-idiotype administration suppressed both production of anti-DNA antibodies and nephritis. The effect was transient, however, and anti-DNA antibodies appeared which did not bear the injected idiotype[191].

Zouali et al.[192] inoculated mice with syngeneic anti-DNA IgG together with muramyl dipeptide and found that anti-DNA antibody levels were suppressed and that anti-idiotype specific for the injected IgG appeared[192]. Conjugation of anti-idiotype to a cytotoxic agent has been shown by Sasaki et al.[193] to eliminate anti-DNA antibody producing cells *in vivo*. Still another approach introduced recently by Shoenfeld et al.[194] utilizes T suppressor cells specific to pathogenic idiotypes. These authors have shown that treatment of BALB/c mice, in which SLE was induced experimentally, with T suppressor cells specific to the pathogenic idiotype 16/6 resulted in a decline in the titres of the autoantibodies and in the clinical manifestations[189].

SUMMARY

The clinical, serological and pathogenetic characteristics of a number of different strains of mice that spontaneously develop an autoimmune disease are described herein. All these models have in common the production of characteristic autoantibodies leading to immune complex mediated injury. In addition, newer experimental models of SLE induced in mice are discussed. These models of SLE-like disease induced experimentally have the advantage of circumventing the genetic contribution toward the development of the disease. The factors involved in the pathogenesis of autoimmunity in these mice are also discussed.

More studies in animal models of SLE are needed to yield information regarding basic common mechanisms relevant to our understanding and treatment of lupus in humans.

References

1. Shoenfeld Y. Autoimmune diseases: multiple factors involved in the etiology. Isr J Med Sci. 1988; 24: 351–352.
2. Shoenfeld Y, Mozes E. Pathogenic idiotypes of autoantibodies in autoimmunity: lesson from new experimental models of SLE. FASEB J. 1990; 4: 2646–2651.
3. Theofilopoulos AN, Dixon FJ. Murine models of systemic lupus erythematosus. Adv Immunol. 1985; 37: 269–390.
4. Bielschowsky M, Helyer BJ, Howie JB. Spontaneous anemia in mice of the NAB/Bl strain. Proc Unit Otago Med School. 1959; 37: 9–11.
5. Cantor H, McVay-Boudreau L, Hugenberger J, Naidorf J, Shen FW, Gershon RK. Immunoregulatory circuits among T-cell sets. II. Physiologic role of feedback inhibition in vivo absence in NZB mice. J Exp Med. 1978; 147: 1116–1125.
6. Gutierrez-Ramos JC, Andreu JL, Moreno De Alboran I, et al. Insights into autoimmunity: from classical models to current perspectives. Immunol Reviews. 1990; 118: 73–101.
7. Andrews BS, Eisenberg RS, Theofilopoulos AN, et al. Spontaneous murine lupus-like syndromes. Clinical and immunopathological manifestations in several strains. J Exp Med. 1978; 148: 1198–1215.
8. Cohen PL, Eisenberg RA. The lpr and gld genes in systemic autoimmunity: life and death in the Fas lane. Immunol Today. 1992; 13: 427–428.
9. Manny N, Datta SK, Schwartz RS. Synthesis of IgM by cells of NZB and SWR mice and their crosses. J Immunol. 1979; 122: 1220–1222.
10. Gavalchin J, Seder RA, Datta SK. The NZB x SWR model of lupus nephritis. I. Cross-reactive idiotypes of monoclonal anti-DNA antibodies in relation to antigen specificity, charge, and allotype. Identification of interconnected idiotype families inherited from the normal SWR and the autoimmune NZB parents. J Immunol. 1987; 138: 128–137.
11. Gavalchin J, Datta SK. The NZB x SWR model of lupus nephritis. II. Autoantibodies deposited in renal lesions show a distinctive and restricted idiotypic diversity. J Immunol. 1987; 138: 138–148.
12. Lambert PH, Dixon FJ. Pathogenesis of glomerulonephritis of NZB/W mice. J Exp Med. 1968; 127: 507–522.
13. Izui S, McConahey PJ, Clark JP, Hang LM, Hara I, Dixon FJ. Retroviral gp70 immune complexes in NZB x NZW F1 mice with murine lupus nephritis. J Exp Med. 1981; 54: 517–528.
14. Izui S, McConahey PJ, Theofilopoulos AN, Dixon FJ. Association of circulating retroviral gp-70 anti-gp70 immune complexes with murine systemic lupus erythematosus. J Exp Med. 1979; 149: 1099–1116.
15. Ebling F, Hahn BH. Restricted subpopulations of DNA antibodies in kidneys of mice with systemic lupus. Arthritis Rheum. 1980; 23: 392–403.
16. Kalunian K, Panosian-Sahakian N, Ebling FM, Cohen AH, Louie JS, Kaine J, Hahn BH. Idiotypic characteristics of immunoglobulins associated with systemic lupus erythematosus: studies of antibodies deposited in glomeruli of humans. Arthritis Rheum. 1989; 32: 513–522.
17. Shoenfeld Y, Amital-Teplizki H, Mendlovic S, Blank M, Mozes E, Isenberg DA. The role of the human anti-DNA idiotype 16/6 in autoimmunity. Clin Immunol Immunopathol. 1989; 51: 313–325.
18. Raz E, Brezis M, Rosenmann E, Eilat D. Anti-DNA antibodies bind directly to renal antigens and induce kidney dysfunction in the isolated perfused rat kidney. J Immunol. 1989; 142: 3076–3082.
19. Accinni L, Dixon FJ. Degenerative vascular disease and myocardial infarction in mice with lupus-like syndrome. Am J Pathol. 1979; 96: 477–486.
20. Yoshida H, Fujiwara H, Fujiwara T, Ikehara S, Hamashima Y. Quantitative analysis of myocardial infarction in (NZW x BXSB) F_1 hybrid mice with systemic lupus erythematosus and small coronary artery disease. Am J Pathol. 1987; 129: 477–485.

21. Howie JB, Helyer FJ. The immunology and pathology in NZB mice. Adv Immunol. 1968; 9: 215–225.
22. Hang L, Theofilopoulos AN, Dixon FJ. A spontaneous rheumatoid arthritis-like disease in MRL/1 mice. J Exp Med. 1982; 155: 1690–1701.
23. Nose M, Nishimura M, Kyogoku M. Analysis of granulomatous arteritis in MRL/Mp autoimmune disease mice bearing lymphoproliferative genes: the use of the mouse genetics to dissociate the development of arteritis and glomerulonephritis. Am J Pathol. 1989; 135: 271–280.
24. Gilkeson GS, Ruiz P, Grudier JP, Kurlander RJ, Pisetsky DS. Genetic control of inflammatory arthritis in congenic lpr mice. Clin Immunol Immunopathol. 1989; 53: 460–474.
25. Akhnazarova VD, Vasil'eva EG. Aleutian mink disease as an experimental model of systemic lupus erythematosus. Voprosy Revmatizma. 1981; 1: 46–52.
26. Monier JC. Lupus in the dog for a better understanding of human lupus. Pathologie Biologie. (Paris) 1981; 10: 255–258.
27. Steinberg AD, Reinertsen JL. Lupus in New Zealand mice and in dogs. Bull Rheum Dis. 1978; 28: 940–945.
28. Lewis RM, Schwartz RS. Canine systemic lupus erythematosus. Genetic analysis of an established breeding colony. J Exp Med. 1971; 134: 417–420.
29. Lewis RM, Schwartz RS, Gilmore CE. Autoimmune diseases in domestic animals. Part 1. Ann NY Acad Sci. 1965; 124: 178–200.
30. Roths JB, Murphy ED, Eichner EM. A new mutation, gld, that produces lymphoproliferation and autoimmunity in C3H/HeJ mice. J Exp Med. 1984; 159: 1–20.
31. Hashimoto Y, Yui K, Littman D, Greene MI. T-cell receptor genes in autoimmune mice: T-cell subsets have unexpected T-cell receptor gene programs. Proc Natl Acad Sci USA. 1987; 84: 5883–5887.
32. Yui K, Hashimoto Y, Greene MI. T cell receptors of autoimmune mice: Functional and molecular analysis of novel T cell subsets in C3H-gld/gld mice. Immunol Res. 1988; 7: 173–188.
33. Mountz JD, Mushinski JF, Steinberg AD. Differential gene expression in autoimmune mice. Surv Immunol Res. 1985; 4: 48–64.
34. Kimura M, Ogata Y, Shimada K, Moriyama T, Matsuzawa A. New mutant mice of autoimmunity, CBA/KIJms-lpr^{cg}/lpr^{cg}, that could link the lpr and gld genes. Autoimmunity. 1991; 9: 359–361.
35. Kofler R, McConahey PJ, Duchosal MA, Balderas RS, Theofilopoulos AN, Dixon FJ. An autosomal recessive gene that delays expression of lupus in BXSB mice. J Immunol. 1991; 146: 1375–1379.
36. Chiang BL, Bearer E, Ansari A, Dorshkind K, Gershwin ME. The BM12 mutation and autoantibodies to dsDNA in NZB.H-2^{bm12} mice. J Immunol. 1990; 145: 94–101.
37. Erikson J, Radic MZ, Campe SA, Hardy RR, Carmack C, Weigaert M. Expression of anti-DNA immunoglobulin transgenes in non-autoimmune mice. Nature. 1991; 349: 331–334.
38. Buskila D, Shoenfeld Y. Anti-DNA idiotypes: their pathogenic role in autoimmunity. In: Cruse JM, Lewis RE, jr., eds. Clinical and Molecular Aspects of Autoimmune Diseases. Concepts Immunopathol. Vol 8. Basel: Karger; 1992: 85–113.
39. Shoenfeld Y, Isenberg DA. The Mosaic of Autoimmunity. Amsterdam: Elsevier; 1989: 1–540.
40. Mendlovic S, Brocke S, Shoenfeld Y, Ben-Bassat M, Meshorer A, Bakimer R, Mozes E. Induction of a SLE-like disease in mice by a common anti-DNA idiotype. Proc Natl Acad Sci USA. 1988; 85: 2260–2264.
41. Mozes E, Shoenfeld Y, Brocke S, Mendlovic S. Induction of experimental systemic lupus erythematosus in mice. Isr J Med Sci. 1988; 24: 741–744.
42. Blank M, Mendlovic S, Mozes E, Shoenfeld Y. Induction of SLE-like disease in naive mice with a monoclonal anti-DNA antibody derived from a patient with polymyositis carrying the 16/6 Id. J Autoimmun. 1988; 1: 683–691.
43. Mendlovic S, Fricke H, Shoenfeld Y, Mozes E. The role of anti-idiotype antibodies in the induction of experimental SLE. Eur J Immunol. 1989; 19: 729–735.
44. Isenberg DA, Katz DR, Le Page S. Independent analysis of the 16/6 idiotype lupus model: a role for an environmental factor? J Immunol. 1991; 147: 4172–4177.
45. Knight B, Katz DR, Isenberg DA, Ibrahim MA, Le Page S, Hutchings P, Schwartz RS,

Cooke A. Induction of adjuvent arthritis in mice. Clin Exp Immunol. 1992; 90: 459–465.

46. Rombach E, Stetler DA, Brown JC. Rabbits produce SLE-like anti-RNA polymerase I and anti-DNA autoantibodies in response to immunization with either human or murine SLE anti-DNA antibodies. Autoimmunity. 1992; 13: 291–302.

47. Dang H, Laridis K, Talar N. Induction of autoantibodies in normal BALB/C mice by perturbation of the idiotype network. Arthritis Rheum. 1992; 35 (suppl): S155.

48. Fricke H, Mendlovic S, Blank M, Shoenfeld Y, Ben-Bassat M, Mozes E. Idiotype specific T cell lines inducing experimental SLE in mice. Immunology. 1991; 73: 421–427.

49. Shoenfeld Y, Wilner Y, Coates AR, Rauch J, Lavie G, Pinkhas J. Infection and autoimmunity: monoclonal anti-tuberculosis antibodies react with DNA autoantibodies bound to myco-bacterial derived glycolipids. Clin Exp Immunol. 1986; 66: 255–261.

50. Blank M, Fricke H, Mozes E, Talal N, Coates ARM, Shoenfeld Y. The importance of the pathogenic 16/6 idiotype of anti-DNA antibodies in the induction of SLE in naive mice. Scand J Immunol. 1990; 31: 45–52.

51. Blank M, Mendlovic S, Mozes E, Coates ARM, Shoenfeld Y. Induction of systemic lupus erythematosus in naive mice with T-cell lines specific for human anti-DNA antibody SA-1 (16/6 Id$^+$) and for mouse tuberculosis antibody TB-68 (16/6 Id$^+$). Clin Immunol Immuno-pathol. (In press).

52. Elson CJ. Autoantibodies typical of SLE and graft-vs-host reactions. Immunol Today. 1982; 3: 181–182.

53. Gleichmann E, Van Elven EH, Vanden Veen JPW. A systemic lupus erythematosus (SLE)-like disease in mice induced by abnormal T-B cell cooperation. Preferential formation of autoantibodies characteristic of SLE. Eur J Immunol. 1982; 12: 152–159.

54. Portanova JP, Arndt RE, Lotzin BL. Selective production of autoantibodies in graft-vs-host-induced and spontaneous murine lupus: predominant reactivity with histone regions accessible in chromatin. J Immunol. 1988; 140: 755–759.

55. Bruijn JA, Van Elven EH, Hogendoom PCW, Corver WE, Hoedemarker PJ, Fleuren GJ. Murine chronic graft-vs-host disease as a model for lupus nephritis. Am J Pathol. 1988; 130: 639.

56. Harris EN, Gharavi AE, Boey ML, Patel S, Mackworth-Young CG, Loizon S, Hughes GRV. Anticardiolipin antibodies: detection by radioimmuno-assay and association with thrombosis in systemic lupus erythematosus. Lancet. 1983; 2: 1211–1214.

57. Harris EN, Gharavi AE, Hegde U, et al. Anticardiolipin antibodies in autoimmune thrombocytopenia purpura. Br J Haematol. 1985; 59: 231–234.

58. Hughes GRV, Harris EN, Gharavi AE. The anticardiolipin syndrome. J Rheumatol. 1986; 13: 486–489.

59. Harris EN, Gharavi AE, Hughes GRV. Anti-phospholipid antibodies. Clin Rheum Dis. 1985; 11: 591–609.

60. Alarcon-Segovia D, Sanchez-Guerrero J. Primary antiphospholipid syndrome. J Rheumatol. 1989; 16: 482–485.

61. Smith HR, Hansen CL, Rose R, Canoso RT. Autoimmune MRL-lpr/lpr mice are an animal model for the secondary antiphospholipid syndrome. J Rheumatol. 1990; 17: 911–915.

62. Branch DW, Rote NS, Dostal DA, Scott JR. Association of lupus anticoagulant with antibody against phosphatidyl serine. Clin Immunol Immunopathol. 1987; 42: 63–75.

63. Thiagarajan P, Shapiro SS, De Marco L. Monoclonal immunoglobulin M coagulation anticoagulant with phospholipid specificity. J Clin Invest. 1980; 66: 396–405.

64. Branch WD, Dudley DJ, Creighton KA, Abbott TM, Hammond EH, Daynes RA. Immunoglobulin G fractions from patients with antiphospholipid antibodies causes fetal death in BALB/c mice: A model for autoimmune fetal loss. Am J Obstet Gynecol. 1990; 163: 210–216.

65. Blank M, Cohen J, Toder V, Shoenfeld Y. Induction of anti-phospholipid syndrome in naive mice with mouse lupus monoclonal and human polyclonal anticardiolipin antibodies. Proc Natl Acad Sci USA. 1991; 88: 3069–3073.

66. Blank M, Krause I, Ben-Bassat M, Shoenfeld Y. Induction of experimental SLE associated with anti-phospholipid syndrome following immunization with human monoclonal patho-genic anti-DNA idiotype. J Autoimmunity. (In press).

67. Bakimer R, Fishman P, Blank M, Sredni B, Shoenfeld Y. Induction of primary anti-phospholipid syndrome following immunization with human anti-cardiolipin (H-3). J Clin

Invest. 1992; 89: 1558–1562.
68. Kleinman DM, Eisenberg RA, Steinberg AD. Development of the autoimmune B cell repertoire in MRL-lpr/lpr mice. J Immunol. 1990; 144: 506–511.
69. Caulfield MJ, Stanko D, Calkins C. Characterization of the spontaneous autoimmune (anti-erythrocyte) response in NZB mice using a pathogenic monoclonal autoantibody and its anti-idiotype. Immunology. 1989; 66: 233–237.
70. Shoenfeld Y. Experimental and induced animal models of systemic lupus erythematosus and Sjøgren's syndrome. Current Opinion Rheumatol. 1989; 1: 360–368.
71. Mountz J. Animal models of systemic lupus erythematosus and Sjøgren's syndrome. Current Opinion Rheumatol. 1990; 2: 740–748.
72. Mountz JD, Gause WC, Jonsson R. Murine models for systemic lupus erythematosus and Sjøgren's syndrome. Current Opinion Rheumatol. 1991; 3: 738–756.
73. Cohen MG, Pollard KM, Schreiber L. Relationship of age and sex to autoantibody expression in MRL-+/+ and MRL-lpr/lpr mice: demonstration of an association between the expression of antibodies to histones, denatured DNA and Sm in MRL-+/+. Clin Exp Immunol. 1988; 72: 50–54.
74. Shorer EW, Pisetsky DS, Grudier J, Eisenberg RA, Cohen PL. Immunization with the Sm nuclear antigen induces anti-Sm antibodies in normal and MRL mice. Immunology. 1988; 65: 473–478.
75. Kastner DL, Steinberg AD. Determinants of B-cell hyperactivity in murine lupus. Concepts Immunopathol. 1988; 6: 22–88.
76. Reininger L, Shibata T, Schurmans S, Merino R, Fossati L, Lacour M, Izui S. Spontaneous production of anti-mouse red blood cell antibodies is independent of the polyclonal activation in NZB mice. Eur J Immunol. 1990; 20: 2405–2410.
77. Brennan FM, Andrew EM, Williams DG, Maini RN. Anti-n RNP anti-nuclear antibody-secreting cells are represented in the lymphocyte-B repertoire of normal and MRL/Mp-lpr/lpr lupus mice. Immunology. 1988; 63: 213–218.
78. Casali P, Notkins A. CD5+ B polyreactive antibodies and the human B cell repertoire. Immunol Today. 1989; 10: 364–368.
79. Raveche ES. Possible immunoregulatory role for CD5+ B cells. Clin Immunol Immuno-pathol. 1990; 56: 135–150.
80. Kocks C, Rajewsky K. Stable expression and somatic hypermutation of antibody regions in B-cell developmental pathways. Ann Rev Immunol. 1989; 7: 537–559.
81. Buskila D, Mackenzie L, Shoenfeld Y, Youinou P, Lydyard P. The biology of CD5+ cells. In: Shoenfeld Y, Isenberg DA, eds. Natural Autoantibodies: Their Physiological Role and Regulatory Significance. CRC Press Inc; 1992: 125–142.
82. Youinou P, Buskila D, Mackenzie I, Shoenfeld Y, Lydyard P. CD5-positive B-cells and diseases. In: Shoenfeld Y, Isenberg DA, eds. Natural Autoantibodies: Their Physiological Role and Regulatory Significance. CRC Press Inc; 1992: 143–145.
83. Mercolino TJ, Arnold LW, Hawkins LA, Haughton G. Normal mouse peritoneum contains a large population of Ly1+ (CD5) B-cells that recognize phosphatidyl choline: relationship to cells that secrete hemolytic antibody specific for autologous erythrocytes. J Exp Med. 1988; 168: 687–698.
84. Manohar V, Brown E, Leiserson WM, Chused TM. Expression of Lyt-1 by a subset of B lymphocytes. J Immunol. 1982; 129: 532–538.
85. Hayakawa K, Hardy RR, Parks DR, Herzenberg LA. The Ly-1 B cell subpopulation in normal, immunodefective and autoimmune mice. J Exp Med. 1983; 157: 202–218.
86. Carmen M, Stall AM, Solovera JJ, Tarlington DM, Herzenberg LA, Strober S. Ly-1 B cells and disease activity in (NZB x NZW)F$_1$ mice. Effect of total lymphoid irradiation. Arthritis Rheum. 1990; 33: 553–561.
87. Bailey NC, Fidanza V, Mayer R, Mazza G, Fougereau M, Bona C. Activation of clones producing self reactive antibodies by foreign antigens and anti-idiotype antibody carrying the internal image of the antigen. J Clin Invest. 1989; 84: 744–756.
88. Hayakawa K, Hardy RR, Herzenberg LA. Peritoneal Ly-1 B-cells. Genetic control, autoantibody production, increased lambda light chain expression. Eur J Immunol. 1986; 16: 450–456.
89. Green MC, Shultz LD. Motheaten, an immunodeficient mutant of the mouse. I-Genetic and pathology. J Hered. 1975; 66: 250–258.

90. Schultz LD, Coman DL, Bailey CL, Beamer WG, Sidman CL. Viable motheaten, a new allele at the motheaten locus. Am J Pathol. 1984; 116: 179–192.
91. Sidman CL, Shultz LD, Hardy RR, Hayakawa K, Herzenberg LA. Production of immunoglobulin isotypes by Ly-1$^+$ B cells in viable motheaten and normal mice. Science. 1985; 232: 1423–1425.
92. Scher I. The CBA/N mouse strain. An experimental model illustrating the influence of the X chromosome on immunity. Adv Immunol. 1982; 33: 2–31.
93. Smith HR, Yaffe LJ, Chused TM, Reveche ES, Steinberg AD. Analysis of B cell subpopulations. I, Relationships among splenic Xid Ly1$^+$ and Lyb5$^+$ cells. Cell Immunol. 1985; 92: 190–196.
94. Taurog JP, Moutsopoulos HM, Rosenberg J, Chused TM, Steinberg AD. CBA/N X-linked B cell defect prevents NZB B cell hyperactivity in F_1 mice. J Exp Med. 1979; 150: 31–43.
95. Dighiero G, Poncet P, Rouyre S, Mazie JC. Newborn Xid mice carry the genetic information for the production of natural autoantibodies against DNA, cytoskeletal proteins and TNP. J Immunol. 1986; 136: 4000–4005.
96. De La Hera A, Marcos MA, Toribio ML, Marquez C, Caspar ML, Martinez C. Development of Ly-1$^+$ B cells in immunodeficient CBA/N mice. J Exp Med. 1987; 166: 804–808.
97. Hiernaux JR, Goidl EA, Martin McEvoy SJ, Stashak PW, Baker PJ, Holmes KL. Characterization of the immunodeficiency of R111 S/J mice. I. Association with the CD5 B cell lineage. J Immunol. 1989; 142: 1813–1817.
98. Poncet P, Kocher HP, Pages J, Jaton JC, Bussard AE. Monoclonal autoantibodies against mouse red blood cells. A family of structurally restricted molecules. Molec Immunol. 1985; 22: 541–544.
99. Hutchings PR, Varey AM, Cooke A. Immunological defects in SJL mice. Immunology. 1986; 59: 445–450.
100. Raveche ES, Lalor P, Stall A, Conroy J. In vivo effects of hyperdiploid Ly1+ B cells of NZB origin. J Immunol. 1988; 141: 4133–4139.
101. Nenazee DA, Studer S, Steinmetz M, Dembic Z, Kiefer M. The lymphoproliferating cells of MRL-lpr/lpr mice are a polyclonal population that bear the T lymphocyte receptor for antigen. Eur J Immunol. 1985; 15: 760–764.
102. Davidson WF, Dumont FJ, Bedigian HG, Fowlkes BJ, Morse HC III. Phenotypic, functional and molecular genetic comparisons of the abnormal lymphoid cells of C3H-lpr/lpr and C3H-gld/gld mice. J Immunol. 1986; 136: 4075–4078.
103. Morse HC III, Davidson WF, Yetter RA, Murphy ED, Roths JB, Coffman RB. Abnormalities induced by the mutant gene lpr: expansion of a unique lymphocyte subset. J Immunol. 1982; 129: 2612–2615.
104. Wofsy D, Hardy RR, Seanan WE. The proliferating cells in autoimmune MRL/lpr mice lack L3T4 antigen on helper T cells that is involved in the response to class II major histocompatibility antigens. J Immunol. 1984; 132: 2686–2690.
105. Steinberg AD, Roths AD, Murphy ED, Steinberg RT, Raveche ES. Effects of thymectomy or androgen administration upon the autoimmune disease of MRL-lpr/lpr mice. J Immunol. 1980; 125: 871–874.
106. Hang L, Theofilopoulos AN, Balderas RS, Francis SJ, Dixon FJ. The effect of thymectomy on lupus-prone mice. J Immunol. 1984; 132: 1809–1812.
107. Theofilopoulos AN, Balderas RS, Shawler DL, Lee S, Dixon FJ. Influence of thymic genotype on the systemic lupus erythematosus-like disease and T cell proliferation of MRL/Mp-lpr/lpr mice. J Exp Med. 1981; 153: 1405–1410.
108. Theofilopoulos AN. Role of the thymus in murine lupus and cellular transfer of the disease. Arthritis Rheum. 1982; 25: 726–729.
109. Ikehara S, Good RA, Nakamura T, Sekita K, Inoue S, Oo M, Muso E, Ogawa K, Hamashima Y. Rationale for bone marrow transplantation in the treatment of autoimmune disease. Proc Natl Acad Sci USA. 1985; 82: 2483–2485.
110. Matsumoto K, Yoshikai Y, Asano T, Himeno K, Iwasaki A, Nomoto K. Defect in negative selection in lpr donor-derived T cells differentiating in non-lpr host thymus. J Exp Med. 1991; 173: 127–136.
111. Dixon FJ. Basic elements of murine systemic lupus erythematosus. J Rheumatol. 1987; 14

(suppl 13): 3–10.

112. Adams S, Zordan T, Sainis K, Datta SK. T cell receptor V beta genes expressed by IgG anti-DNA autoantibody inducing T cells in lupus nephritis: forbidden receptors and double negative T cells. Eur J Immunol. 1990; 20: 1435–1443.

113. Magilavy DB, Rowley DA, Davis M. The liver of MRL/lpr mice contains defective accessory cells and a population of immunosuppressive lymphocytes. Cell Immunol. 1990; 125: 469–479.

114. Schiffenbauer J, McCarthy DM, Nygard NR, Woulfe SI, Didier DK, Schwartz BD. A unique sequence of the NZW I-E beta chain and its possible contribution to autoimmunity in the (NZB x NZW) F_1 mouse. J Exp Med. 1989; 170: 971–984.

115. Theofilopoulos AN, Kofler R, Singer PA, Noonan DJ, Dixon FJ. Genomic organization and expression of B and T cell antigen receptor genes in murine lupus. Rheum Dis Clin North Am. 1987; 13: 511–530.

116. Dang H, Talal N. T-cell antigen receptor studies in mice expressing the lpr genetic defect. Cell Immunol. 1988; 115: 393–402.

117. Davignon JL, Cohen PL, Eisenberg RA. Rapid T-cell receptor modulation accompanies lack of in vitro mitogenic responsiveness of double negative T cells to anti-CD3 monoclonal antibody in MRL/Mp-lpr/lpr mice. J Immunol. 1988; 141: 1848–1854.

118. Alcocer-Varela G, Alarcon-Segovia D. Decreased production of and response to IL-2 by cultured lymphocytes from patients with SLE. J Clin Invest. 1982; 63: 1388–1392.

119. Chathely G, Amor B, Fournier C. Defective IL-2 production in active rheumatoid arthritis regulation by radio sensitive suppressor cells. Clin Rheumatol. 1986; 5: 482–492.

120. Rosenberg YJ, Nurse F, Begley CG. IL-2 receptor expression in autoimmune MRL-lpr/lpr. The expanded L3T4$^-$, Lyt2$^-$ population does not express p^{75} and cannot generate functional high-affinity IL-2 receptors. J Immunol. 1989; 143: 2216–2222.

121. Gutierrez-Ramos JC, Pezzi I, Palacios R, Martinez AC. Expression of the p^{75} interleukin 2-binding protein on CD3$^+$4-8-TAC$^-$ cells from autoimmune MRL-lpr/lpr mice. Eur J Immunol. 1980; 19: 201–204.

122. Blank M, Sredni B, Albeck N, Mozes E, Shoenfeld Y. The effect of the immunomodulator AS-101 on IL-2 production in SLE disease induced in mice by a pathogenic anti-DNA idiotype. Clin Exp Immunol. 1990; 49: 443–447.

123. Arend WP, Dayer JM. Cytokines and cytokine inhibitors or antagonists in rheumatoid arthritis. Arthritis Rheum. 1990; 33: 305–315.

124. Hom JT, Cole H, Bendele AM. Interleukin 1 enhances the development of spontaneous arthritis in MRL/lpr mice. Clin Immunol Immunopathol. 1990; 55: 109–119.

125. Sakihama T, Akasu F, Iwamoto M, Shirakura-Shibata Y, Okada Y, Nakahma Y, Tasaka K. Polyclonal and monoclonal IgGs from MRL/Mp-lpr/lpr mice induce an interleukin 3-dependent cell line to produce interleukin-3 through an Fc gamma-receptor-mediated mechanism. Cell Immunol. 1990; 125: 160–170.

126. Iwamoto M, Akasu F, Sakihama T, Onaya T, Nakajima Y, Tasaka K. Serum IgG from an autoimmune prone mouse C3H/HeJ-gld/gld supports the interleukin-3-dependent cell line through an autocrine mechanism. Cell Immunol. 1990; 125: 151–159.

127. Klinman DM. IgG$_1$ and IgG$_{2a}$ production by autoimmune B cells treated in vitro with IL-4 and IFN-gamma. J Immunol. 1990; 144: 2529–2534.

128. Umland SP, Go NF, Cupp JE, Howard M. Responses of B cells from autoimmune mice to IL-5. J Immunol. 1989; 142: 1528–1535.

129. Mihara M, Fukui H, Koishihara Y, Saito M, Ohsugi Y. Immunologic abnormality in NZB/W F_1 mice: thymus-independent expansion of B cells responding to interleukin 6. Clin Exp Immunol. 1990; 82: 533–537.

130. Jacobs CO, Van Der Meide PH, McDevitt HO. In vivo treatment of (NZB x NZW) F_1 lupus-like nephritis with monoclonal antibody to gamma interferon. J Exp Med. 1987; 166: 798–803.

131. Murray L, Martens C. The abnormal T lymphocytes in lpr mice transcribe interferon-gamma and tumor necrosis factor-alpha genes spontaneously in vivo. Eur J Immunol. 1989; 19: 563–565.

132. Jacob CO, McDevitt HO. Tumor necrosis factor alpha in murine autoimmune 'lupus' nephritis. Nature. 1988; 335: 356–358.

133. Boswell JM, Yui MA, Burt DW, Kelley VE. Increased tumor necrosis factor and IL-1

beta gene expression in the kidneys of mice with lupus nephritis. J Immunol. 1988; 141: 3050–3053.

134. Kettelhurt TC, Goldberg AL. Tumor necrosis factor can induce fever in rats without activating protein breakdown in muscle or lipolysis in adipose tissue. J Clin Invest. 1988; 188: 1384–1389.

135. Mountz JD, Steinberg AD, Klinman DM, Smith HR, Mushinski JF. Autoimmunity and increased c-myb transcription. Science. 1984; 226: 1087–1090.

136. Mountz JD, Mushinski JF, Mark GE, Steinberg AD. Oncogene expression in autoimmune mice. J Mol Cell Immunol. 1985; 2: 121–122.

137. Murphy ED, Roths JB. A single gene model for massive lymphoproliferation with autoimmunity in new mouse strain MRL. Fed Proc. 1977; 36: 1246–1249.

138. Thompson CB, Challoner PB, Neiman PE, Groudine M. Expression of the c-myb proto-oncogene during cellular proliferation. Nature. 1986; 319: 374–378.

139. Westin EH, Gallo RL, Arya SK, Eva A, Souza LM, Baluda JA, Aaronson A, Wong-Staal F. Differential expression of the amv gene in human hematopoietic cells. Proc Natl Acad Sci USA. 1982; 79: 2194–2198.

140. Mountz JD, Steinberg AD. Studies of c-myb gene regulation in MRL-lpr/lpr mice: Identification of a 5^1c-myb nuclear protein binding site and high levels of binding factors in nuclear extracts of lpr/lpr lymph node cells. J Immunol. 1989; 142: 328–335.

141. Lafyatis R, Renmers EF, Roberts AB, Yocum DR, Sporn MB, Wieder RL. Anchorage-dependent growth of synoviocytes from arthritic and normal joints. Stimulation by exogenous platelet-derived growth factor and inhibition by transforming growth factor-beta and retinoids. J Clin Invest. 1989; 83: 1267–1276.

142. Morse HC III, Chused TM, Boehm-Truitt M, Mathieson BJ, Sharrow SO, Hartley JW, Xen CSA. Cell surface antigens related to the major glycoproteins (gp70) of xenotropic murine leukemia viruses. J Immunol. 1979; 122: 443–446.

143. Krieg AM, Khan AS, Steinberg AD. Expression of an endogenous retroviral transcript is associated with murine lupus. Arthritis Rheum. 1989; 32: 322–326.

144. Greenberger JS, Phillips SM, Stephenson JR, Aaronson SA. Induction of mouse type-C RNA virus by lipopolysaccharide. J Immunol. 1975; 115: 317–320.

145. Krieg AM, Khan AS, Steinberg AD. Multiple endogenous xenotropic and mink cell focus-forming murine leukemia virus-related transcripts are induced by polyclonal immune activators. J Virol. 1988; 62: 3545–3548.

146. Krieg AM, Gause WC, Gourley MF, Steinberg AD. A role for endogenous retroviral sequences in the regulation of lymphocyte activation. J Immunol. 1989; 143: 2448–2451.

147. Phillips PE. Infectious agents in the pathogenesis of rheumatoid arthritis. Semin Arthritis Rheum. 1986; 16: 1–10.

148. Boumpas DT, Popovic M, Mann DL, Balow JE, Tsokos GC. Type C retroviruses of the human T cell leukemia family are not evident in patients with systemic lupus erythematosus. Arthritis Rheum. 1986; 29: 185–188.

149. Pelton BK, North M, Palmer RG, Hylton W, Smith-Burchnell C, Sinclair AL, Malkovsky M, Dalgleish AG, Denman AM. A search for retrovirus infection in systemic lupus erythematosus and rheumatoid arthritis. Ann Rheum Dis. 1988; 47: 206–209.

150. Olsen RG, Tarr MJ, Mathes LE, Whisler R, Du Plessis D, Schulz EJ, Blakeslee JR. Serological and virological evidence of human T lymphotropic virus in systemic lupus erythematosus. Med Microbiol Immunol. 1987; 176: 53–64.

151. Gavalchin J, Phillips PE, Ginzler EM, Froehlich CJ, Poiesz BJ. Antibody to human T lymphotropic virus type I (HTLV-I) in systemic lupus erythematosus. Arthritis Rheum. 1987; 30 (suppl 4): S 121.

152. Ziegler B, Huang G, Cay RE, Fassbender HG, Gay S. Immunohistological demonstration of retroviral sequences in rheumatoid synovium utilizing monoclonal anti-HTLV-I p19 and anti-HTLV-I p24 antibodies. Arthritis Rheum. 1988; 31 (suppl 4): S35.

153. Matsunaga A, Miller BC, Cottam GL. Dehydroisoandrosterone prevention of autoimmune disease in NZB/W F_1 mice: Lack of an effect on associated immunological abnormalities. Biochim Biophys Acta. 1988; 992: 265–271.

154. Carlsten H, Holmdahl R, Tarkowski A, Nilsson LA. Oestradiol- and testosterone-mediated effects on the immune system in normal and autoimmune mice are genetically linked and inherited as dominant traits. Immunology. 1989; 68: 209–214.

155. Ahmed SA, Aufdemorte TB, Chen JR, Montoya AI, Olive D, Talal N. Estrogen induces the development of autoantibodies and promotes salivary gland lymphoid infiltrates in normal mice. J Autoimmun. 1989; 2: 543–552.

156. Brick JE, Ong SH, Bathon JM, Walker SE, O'Sullivan FX, Di Bartolomeo AG. Anti-histone antibodies in the serum of autoimmune MRL and (NZB/NZW) F_1 mice. Clin Immunol Immunopathol. 1990; 54: 372–381.

157. Blank M, Mendlovic S, Fricke H, Mozes E, Talal N, Shoenfeld Y. Sex hormone involvement in induction of experimental SLE by a pathogenic anti-DNA idiotype in naive mice. J Rheumatol. 1990; 69: 228–236.

158. Jara LJ, Lavalle C, Fraga A, et al. Prolactin, immunoregulation and autoimmune diseases. Seminars Arthritis Rheum. 1991; 20: 273–284.

159. Buskila D, Sukenik S, Shoenfeld Y. The possible role of prolactin in autoimmunity. Amer J Reprod. Immunol. 1991; 26: 118–123.

160. McMurray RW, Keisler D, Walker SE. Hyperprolactinemia accelerates disease activity in the male NZB/W mouse model of SLE. American College of Rheumatology, 55th annual meeting 1991; C 182.

161. Sakaguchi S, Sakaguchi N. Thymus and autoimmunity: transplantation of the thymus from cyclosporine-treated mice causes organ-specific autoimmune disease in athymic nude mice. J Exp Med. 1988; 167: 1479–1485.

162. Blank M, Ben-Bassat M, Shoenfeld Y. The effect of cyclosporine A on early and late stages of experimental SLE induction in mice. Arthritis Rheum. (In press).

163. Jones MG, Harris G. Prolongation of life in female NZB/NZW (F_1) hybrid mice by cyclosporin A. Clin Exp Immunol. 1985; 59: 1–9.

164. Israel-Biet DI, Noel LH, Bach MA. Marked reduction of DNA antibody production and glomerulopathy in thymulin (FTS-Zn) or cyclosporin A treated (NZB x NZW) F_1 mice. Clin Exp Immunol. 1983; 54: 359–365.

165. Boitard C, Fentren G, Castano L, Debray-Sachs M, Assan R, Hors J, Back JF. Effect of cyclosporin A treatment on the production of antibody in insulin-dependent (Type 1) diabetic patients. J Clin Invest. 1987; 80: 1607–1612.

166. Blank M, Palestine A, Nussenblatt R, Shoenfeld Y. Down regulation of autoantibody levels by cyclosporine treatment in patients with uveitis. Clin Immunol Immunopathol. 1990; 4: 87–89.

167. Miescher PA, Favre H, Zubler R, Huang VP. The place of cyclosporin in the treatment of SLE. Proceeding of the 2nd International Conference of SLE. Nov. Singapore. 1989; 133–139.

168. Prickett JD, Robinson DR, Steinberg AD. Dietary enrichment with the polyunsaturated fatty acid eicosapentaenoic acid prevents proteinuria and prolongs survival in NZB x NZW F_1 mice. J Clin Invest. 1981; 68: 556–559.

169. Kelley VE, Ferreeti A, Izu S, Strom TB. A fish oil diet rich in eicosapentaenoic acid reduces cyclooxygenase metabolites, and suppresses lupus in MRL-lpr mice. J Immunol. 1985; 134: 1914–1919.

170. Leslie CA, Gonnerman WA, Ullman MD, Hayes KC, Franzblace C, Cathcart ES. Dietary fish oil modulates fatty acids and decreases arthritis susceptibility in mice. J Exp Med. 1985; 162: 1336–1349.

171. Cathcart ES, Leslie CA, Meydani SN, Hayes KC. A fish oil diet retards experimental amyloidosis modulates lymphocyte function and decreases macrophage arachidonate metabolism in mice. J Immunol. 1987; 139: 1850–1854.

172. Ito Y, Barceli U, Yamashita W, Weiss M, Glasgreenwalt P, Pollak VE. Fish oil has beneficial effects on lipids and renal disease of nephrotic rats. Metabolism. 1988; 37: 352–357.

173. Licastro F, Weindroch R, Davis IJ, Walford RI. Effect of dietary restriction on the age-associated decline of lymphocyte DNA repair activity in mice. Age Aging. 1988; 11: 48–53.

174. Trentham DE, Belli JA, Anderson RJ. Clinical and immunologic effects of fractionated total lymphoid irradiation in refractory rheumatoid arthritis. N Engl J Med. 1981; 305: 976–982.

175. Gaston JSH, Strober S, Solovera JJ. Dissection of the mechanism of immune injury in RA using TLI. Arthritis Rheum. 1988; 31: 21–30.

176. Strober S. Overview: effect of total lymphoid irradiation on autoimmune disease and transplantation immunity. J Immunol. 1984; 132: 968–970.
177. Oseroff A, Okada S, Strober S. Natural suppressor cells found in the spleen of neonatal mice and of adult mice given total lymphoid irradiation (TLI) express null surface phenotype. J Immunol. 1984; 132: 101–110.
178. Zan-Bar I, Slavin S, Strober S. Induction and mechanism of tolerance to bovine serum albumin in mice given total lymphoid irradiation (TLI). J Immunol. 1978; 121: 1400–1404.
179. Andrews BS, Eisenberg RA, Theofilopoulos A. Spontaneous murine lupus-like syndromes: clinical and immunopathological manifestations in several strains. J Exp Med. 1978; 148: 1198–1218.
180. Wofsy D, Seaman WE. Successful treatment of autoimmunity in NZB/NZW F_1 mice with monoclonal antibody to L3T4. J Exp Med. 1985; 161: 378–391.
181. Ranges GE, Sriram S, Cooper SM. Prevention of type II collagen-induced arthritis by in vivo treatment with anti-L3T4. J Exp Med. 1985; 162: 1105–1110.
182. Wofsy D. Administration of monoclonal anti-T cell antibodies retards murine lupus in BXSB mice. J Immunol. 1986; 136: 4554–4560.
183. Carteron NL, Schimenti CL, Wofsy D. Treatment of murine lupus with $F(ab^1)_2$ fragments of monoclonal antibody to L3T4: suppression of autoimmunity does not depend on T helper cell depletion. J Immunol. 1989; 142: 1470–1475.
184. Asensi V, Kimeno K, Kawamura I, Sakumoto M, Nomoto K. Treatment of autoimmune MRL-lpr mice with anti-B220 monoclonal antibody reduces the level of anti-DNA antibodies and lymphadenopathy. Immunology. 1989; 68: 204–208.
185. Mountz JD, Gause WC, Finkelman FS, Steinberg AD. Prevention of lymphadenopathy in MRL-lpr/lpr mice by blocking peripheral lymph node homing with Mel-14 in vivo. J Immunol. 1988; 2943–2949.
186. Buskila D, Shoenfeld Y. Manipulation of anti-DNA idiotypes: a possible treatment approach to autoimmune diseases. In: Cruse JM, Lewis RE, Jr., eds. Clinical and Molecular Aspects of Autoimmune Diseases. Concepts Immunopathol. Vol 8, Basle: Karger; 1992: 114–128.
187 Hahn BH, Ando D, Ebling FM, Panosian-Sahakian N, Tsao B, Kalunian K. T cell up-regulation of B cells via their idiotypes contributing to the development of systemic lupus erythematosus. Am J Med. 1988; 85 (suppl 6A): 32–34.
188. Paul E, Manheimer-Lort A, Livneh A, et al. Pathogenic anti-DNA antibodies in SLE: idiotypic families and genetic origins. Int Rev Immunol. 1990; 5: 295–313.
189. Zouali M, Diamond B. Idiotype mediated intervention in systemic lupus erythematosus. J Autoimmun. 1990; 3: 381–388.
190. Kim YT, Puntillo E, DeBlasio T, Weksler ME, Siskind GW. Regulation of antibody production by hybridoma cultures. I. Anti-idiotype antibody-mediated down-regulation of anti-DNA antibody production by hybridoma cells. Cell Immunol. 1987; 105: 65–74.
191. Hahn B, Ebling F. Suppression of NZB/NZW mice murine nephritis by administration of a syngeneic monoclonal antibody to DNA: possible role of anti-idiotypic antibodies. J Clin Invest. 1983; 71: 728–736.
192. Zouali M, Jolivet M, Leclerc C. Suppression of murine lupus autoantibodies to DNA by administration of muramyl d peptide and syngeneic anti-DNA IgG. J Immunol. 1985; 135: 1091–1096.
193. Sasaski T, Muryoi T, Takai O, et al. Selective elimination of anti-DNA antibody producing cells by anti-idiotypic antibody conjugated with neocarzinostatin. J Clin Invest. 1986; 77: 1382–1386.
194. Blank M, Ben-Bassat N, Shoenfeld Y. Modulation of SLE induction in naive mice by specific T cells with suppressor activity to pathogenic anti-DNA antibody idiotype. Cell Immunol. 1991; 137: 474–486.

10
Animal Models of Arthritis

L. J. CROFFORD and R. L. WILDER

INTRODUCTION

Inflammatory polyarthritis has multiple potential aetiologic agents and complex pathogenetic mechanisms. Both acute and chronic inflammatory processes are modulated by the immune, endocrine and nervous systems. Animal models are essential to study the influence of these interrelated systems on the development and course of inflammatory arthritis. Additionally, animal models contribute to our understanding of the genetic influences on susceptibility to inflammatory diseases. This chapter will discuss the use of animal models to understand the aetiology and pathogenesis of inflammatory polyarthritis, with particular focus on new observations that contribute to the understanding of inflammatory arthritides, such as rheumatoid arthritis, in humans. The chapter will also discuss the use of transgenic technology in developing new models of arthritis.

SPONTANEOUS MODELS OF INFLAMMATORY ARTHRITIS

MRL.lpr/lpr mice

MRL.lpr/lpr mice, a strain that develops a lupus-like autoimmune syndrome and a lymphoproliferative disorder, spontaneously develop inflammatory arthritis with clinical and histological features similar to RA. Histopathological features over time have been described in detail, but there are discrepancies in the literature. Hang and colleagues[1] found that 45% of 3–4 month old mice had synovial pathology characterized by thickening of the synovia and subsynovial mononuclear inflammatory infiltration. They also described coexistent periarticular vasculitis and/or arteritis, and early articular erosion. By 5–6 months of age, 75% of mice had significant joint pathology with synoviocyte proliferation and subsynovial infiltration of lymphocytes and plasma cells. In a later study by O'Sullivan and colleagues[2], the earliest histopathological changes developed at 13–14 weeks of age in most animals and were characterized by synovial cell proliferation in the joint recesses with marginal erosion of cartilage. They, as well as others, noted a conspicuous lack of lymphocytic infiltrates[2,3]. However, there was a distinctive morphology of the proliferating synovial fibroblast-like cells reminiscent of transformed cells, in that there are plentiful cytoplasm, large nuclei, and multiple nucleoli. By 16–19 weeks of age, MRL.lpr/lpr mice developed an aggressive destructive arthritis, again with a scarcity of inflammatory cells. These proliferating synovial cells were closely associated with destructive lesions of cartilage and subchondral bone. At 21–25 weeks, extensive destructive joint changes were seen, with the formation of fibrous scar tissue and fibrocartilage in areas of extensive destruction.

MRL.lpr/lpr mice are one of few animal models that have IgG and IgM rheumatoid factors, and the level of IgM rheumatoid factors correlates with arthritis[1]. These mice have also been reported by some authors to develop antibodies against types I, II, III, IV and V collagen, as well as fibronectin[4,5]. Much smaller amounts of antibodies against proteoglycan, type IV collagen, and laminin have been found[4]. The pathogenicity of these extracellular matrix antibodies is controversial, and injection of MRL.lpr/lpr mice with mouse type II collagen leads to a humoral response, which does not influence the course of arthritis[6].

The background strain for MRL.*lpr/lpr* mice, MRL.+/+, are also genetically autoimmune-prone. The recessive *lpr* mutation, however, leads to the massive lymphadenopathy and earlier-onset autoimmune disease. It has recently been shown that the *lpr* locus codes for the mouse Fas cell-surface glycoprotein, which mediates apoptosis, or programmed cell death, of lymphocytes[7]. The lack of expression of Fas on lymphocytes provides an explanation for the phenotypes of *lpr* mice. Other genes of the MRL.+/+ strain must also play a role in autoimmunity. These other genes may also be important for the development of spontaneous inflammatory arthritis.

Canine arthritis

Dogs develop inflammatory joint disease that is similar to RA, with diagnostic criteria for canine RA being essentially the same as for the human disease. Canine RA is a symmetrical polyarthritis of the peripheral joints, which show swelling and pain. Similar to humans, dogs also develop joint stiffness after rest. Canine RA is progressive and may lead to severe joint destruction with characteristic deformities. Radiographic and histological findings are also similar to human RA. IgM rheumatoid factors, immune complexes, and antibodies to type II collagen are elevated in the sera and synovial fluids of dogs with RA, but they are also elevated in dogs with osteoarthritis, infectious arthritis, and traumatic joint injury[8,9]. This suggests that in canine arthritides, rheumatoid factors, immune complexes and anti-type II collagen antibodies may be a response to injury rather than an aetiologic factor.

The aetiology of canine RA is unknown, but, as in human RA, infectious agents are one potential cause. Recently, elevated levels of antibodies in canine distemper virus (CDV) have been found in dogs diagnosed with canine RA. CDV antigens were also found in the serum and, to a greater extent, the joint fluids from dogs with RA, but not dogs with osteoarthritis, infectious arthritis, or traumatic injury[10]. Most dogs are exposed to this paramyxovirus either by becoming infected or by being vaccinated. The role of this agent in the development of canine RA in susceptible dogs is under investigation.

EXPERIMENTAL MODELS OF INFLAMMATORY ARTHRITIS

SCW- and other bacterial cell wall-induced arthritis

Cell wall fragments from Group A streptococci (SCW), as well as from many other gram positive bacteria, produce acute and chronic polyarthritis in susceptible rats when injected intraperitoneally in aqueous suspension. These fragments are composed of peptidoglycan and group-specific polysaccharide. The clinical course of SCW-induced arthritis in rats is highly reproducible. Acute arthritis, which reflects synovial microvascular injury, appears within 24 hours and reaches maximum severity at about three days after injection. Then 14–28 days after injection, there is a recrudescence of proliferative synovitis that may persist for months, and leads to destruction of cartilage and bone in the affected joints. The arthritis is characterized by swelling and erythema of peripheral joints, particularly the carpus, tarsus, metacarpo- and tarso-phalangeal joints, and interphalangeal joints. The acute phase of SCW arthritis is T lymphocyte independent, but development of chronic arthritis is dependent on the presence of thymus-derived cells. This has been demonstrated by athymic nude LEW.rnu/rnu rats that develop acute arthritis, but do not go on to develop chronic disease[11]. Additionally, chronic arthritis may be passively transferred to a naive recipient by sensitized T cells[12]. Treatment studies have provided further evidence of T cell mediation of the chronic arthritis since cyclosporin A effectively treats the disease[13], and the demonstration that monoclonal antibodies directed against the T cell receptor $\alpha\beta$[14] or monoclonal anti-CD4 antibodies[15] prevent the development of chronic arthritis.

Studies in SCW-induced arthritis have demonstrated phenotypic characteristics of proliferative and locally invasive synovial tissue, most of which are also displayed by human rheumatoid arthritic synovia. There is up-regulation of class II major histocompatibility complex antigens in the acute phase of SCW-induced arthritis[16]. The proto-oncogenes c-*fos* and c-*myc*, markers of mitotically activated cells, are also up-regulated in SCW-arthritic synovium[17,18]. Phosphotyrosine, a component of activated growth factor receptors and other proteins, is markedly up-regulated early in the course of CSW-induced arthritis and is localized in proximity to cells expressing increased fibroblast growth factor-1 (FGF-1; also called heparin binding growth factor-1 and acidic fibroblast growth factor) and platelet-derived growth factor (PDGF). FGF-1, a major stimulus to angiogenesis, and PDGF, a mitogen for synovial fibroblast-like cells, could contribute to the massive proliferation of synovial tissue in inflammatory arthritis[18,19]. There is also increased expression of cyclooxygenase, an enzyme in the prostaglandin pathway that could lead to increases in pro-inflammatory prostaglandins[20]. Other cytokines, such as transforming growth factor-β, a multi-functional cytokine that stimulates deposition of extracellular matrix and modulates cells of the immune system, are also present in synovial tissue[21]. Inflamed synovial tissue also expresses peptides thought of as neuropeptides, such as substance P and corticotropin-releasing hormone, that may modulate the inflammatory process[22]. Transin/stromelysin is a connective tissue-degrading enzyme active against proteoglycan, type IV collagen, and denatured type I collagen, and activates collagenase. Transin/stromelysin is expressed in acute, as well as chronic SCW-induced arthritis, indicating that enzymes which destroy bone and cartilage are up-regulated very early in the pathogenesis of inflammatory arthritis[17]. All of these molecules may play important roles in the pathogenesis of SCW-induced arthritis and other inflammatory arthritides.

SCW-induced arthritis exhibits considerable variability in severity depending on the inbred rat strain utilized. This suggests that considerable genetic influences are involved in the expression of inflammatory arthritis. Lewis rats are susceptible to severe SCW-induced arthritis[16,23], as well as many other experimental inflammatory diseases, such as experimental autoimmune encephalomyelitis[24] and experimental autoimmune uveitis[25], while Fischer rats are resistant to these diseases. While the major histocompatibility complex (MHC) may be important for susceptibility to these experimental arthritides, genetic analysis shows that genetic loci other than the MHC are responsible for the differences between Lewis and Fischer rats[26]. Lewis and Fischer rats exhibit other differences that may be important in their differing susceptibility to inflammatory arthritis. Activation of the hypothalamic–pituitary–adrenal (HPA) axis is a major counter-regulatory response to stress, including inflammation. Stimulation of the HPA axis leads to increased glucocorticoid production that exerts anti-inflammatory effects primarily through suppression of inflammatory cell recruitment, decreased cytokine production, and suppression of the arachidonic acid/prostaglandin pathway. Lewis rats have a blunted HPA axis response to SCW and other inflammatory mediators, such as interleukin-1. Fischer rats have a vigorous HPA axis response to the same stimuli[27,28]. This could contribute to the differing susceptibility of Lewis and Fischer rats to inflammatory diseases.

There are also differences in the T-cell responses between Lewis and Fischer rats, which may be influenced by exposure to bacterial antigens[29]. Fischer rats raised in a germ-free environment are susceptible to SCW- and adjuvant-induced arthritis[30,31]. Recent experiments utilizing bone marrow chimeras between Lewis and Fischer rats implicate bone marrow-derived cells as the genetic factor responsible for determining severity of SCW- and adjuvant-induced arthritis[31]. Ultimately, genetic mapping of the loci responsible for the differences in susceptibility to severe autoimmune and inflammatory diseases in Lewis and Fischer rats may clarify some of the factors important in human susceptibility to similar autoimmune and inflammatory diseases.

As previously noted, cell walls from numerous bacteria are arthritogenic when administered to a genetically susceptible host. Of interest, common intestinal bacterial flora are among those organisms that induce arthritis[32–36]. Arthritis induced by the cell walls of these organisms is similar in course and histological appearance to SCW-induced arthritis, suggesting common pathogenetic mechanisms.

The minimal arthritogenic constituent of the bacterial cell wall is the peptidoglycan subunit, muramyl dipeptide. Muramyl dipeptide induces acute polyarthritis after a single aqueous injection; however, chronic arthritis does not develop. The pro-inflammatory properties of muramyl dipeptide include activation of macrophages and endothelial cells[37]. Induction of chronic arthritis seems to require both the peptidoglycan and polysaccharide components of the cell wall. Arthritogenic strains of bacteria share common properties in their constituent polysaccharides, including resistance to lysozyme degradation and, commonly, high rhamnose content[34,36,38]. These properties of the polysaccharide side-chains influence the persistence of the cell wall fragments in tissues, including synovium, bone marrow, liver, and spleen. There is evidence from the SCW model that persistence in tissues is important in the development of chronic arthritis[39].

Bacteria have been linked to many types of inflammatory arthritis in humans, including post-streptococcal arthritis[40], Reiter's syndrome[41–43], and the arthritis of infectious bowel diseases[44–46]. Nevertheless, the relationship between bacterial cell wall-induced arthritis in animals and human inflammatory polyarthritides requires further study. For example, the streptococcal M protein is a major determinate of virulence. M protein specific antibodies from patients with acute rheumatic fever cross-react with joint tissues, including vimentin[47]. However, M protein is not necessary for the induction of SCW-induced arthritis in rats[48].

Adjuvant-induced arthritis

Chronic, erosive polyarthritis develops in genetically-susceptible rat strains injected intradermally with Freund's complete adjuvant, an oil vehicle containing *Mycobacteria tuberculosis*, *M. butyricum*, or *M. phlei*. Adjuvant-induced arthritis is highly species specific, and develops only in certain strains of rats. After injection, there is a latent period of 10–12 days followed by the abrupt onset of inflammation in distal joints. The arthritis increases in intensity until 20–28 days after injection, then the inflammation slowly resolves. Histologically, an initial perivascular mononuclear cell infiltration and oedema are prominent. As the disease progresses, more intense cellular infiltration, fibrin deposition, and proliferation of synovial fibroblasts and periosteal osteoblasts are noted. Pannus begins to invade the subchondral bone and occasionally the surface of the articular cartilage. Severe involvement can lead to joint destruction and fibrous and bony ankylosis[49].

Adjuvant-induced arthritis is clearly T-lymphocyte dependent. A T-cell line, A2b, derived from adjuvant-arthritic rats induces arthritis when injected into naive recipient animals[50]. It is of considerable interest that the A2b cell line proliferates in response to the mycobacterial 65 kD heat shock protein (HSP)[51]. The epitope of the 65 kD HSP recognized by this cell line shares homology with a mammalian cartilage proteoglycan link protein, which can also stimulate the A2b cell line to proliferate[52,53]. While injection of the 65 kD HSP does not itself induce arthritis, it protects naive animals from adjuvant-induced arthritis[53,54]. This resistance can be overcome by injection of arthritogenic T-cells, suggesting that the resistance may be due to prevention of clonal proliferation of autoreactive T-lymphocytes[53]. These observations support the idea that molecular mimicry between bacterial proteins and components of mammalian joint tissues is operative in the development of adjuvant-induced arthritis, and perhaps in the etiopathogenesis of other chronic inflammatory polyarthritides. This hypothesis is made more attractive in the light of observations that animals can also be rendered resistant to the development of SCW-induced arthritis by injection of 65 kD HSP[55], and T-lymphocytes isolated from some patients with rheumatoid arthritis and reactive arthritis proliferate in response to the 65 kD HSP shared epitope[56-58].

Collagen-induced arthritis

Intradermal injection of type II collagen (CII) in complete or incomplete Freund's adjuvant induces chronic inflammatory polyarthritis in susceptible strains of mice, rats, and monkeys. Collagen-induced arthritis may be produced with heterologous or homologous CII, but the immune responses may differ depending on which type of collagen is utilized to generate arthritis[59,60]. Although the native triple-helical composition of collagen was initially felt to be critical to the development of arthritis, the arthritogenic determinant resides in one cyanogen bromide fragment of CII, the CB-11 peptide. This fragment is capable of producing arthritis, but with a lower incidence and severity than that of native collagen[61]. In both mice and rats, there is a latent period followed by the onset of polyarthritis, especially in the distal hind extremities[60].

Collagen-induced arthritis differs from both SCW- and adjuvant-induced arthritis in that the disease involves a humoral response to a normal cartilage protein. Transient arthritis can be induced by injecting naive recipient animals with purified anti-collagen antibodies[62]. However, cellular immunity is also operative, and the disease can be transferred to naive recipients by T-cells[63]. Genetic susceptibility to collagen-induced arthritis is polygenic, but involves the MHC in both rats and mice[64,65]. Another genetic locus that appears to be important to the development of collagen-induced arthritis in mice is complement component 5, an important mediator of inflammation[66].

Antigen-induced arthritis

Chronic arthritis is induced by intra-articular injection of antigen into previously immunized rats, mice, and rabbits. Several hours after intra-articular injection, severe, acute joints swelling develops. The swelling usually decreases over 2 weeks, but a recrudescence of disease characterized by invasive pannus and cartilage erosions occurs after 4 to 6 weeks. The acute synovitis is dependent on high titres of precipitating IgG antibodies. However, the chronic disease is dependent on both humoral and cellular immune mechanisms. Flare-up reactions triggered by very small amounts of antigen are dependent on T-lymphocytes retained in the joint[67].

TRANSGENIC MODELS OF ARTHRITIS

Transgenic animals are generated in the laboratory by the introduction of a foreign gene, or transgene, into the germline[68,69]. This may be accomplished by microinjection of the foreign gene into the pronucleus of a fertilized ovum, retrovirus infection of embryos, or manipulation of embryonic stem cells. Microinjection usually leads to integration of multiple copies of the transgene and may lead to abnormalities of host DNA sequences at the insertion site. The microinjected transgene is present in all cells, including the germ line, and is stably transmitted to progeny in a Mendelian fashion. Retroviruses mediate integration of a single copy of proviral sequences at a single host site, usually without significant alteration of the host chromosome. Embryonic stem cells are explanted blastocysts manipulated *in vitro*, then re-injected into an intact blastocyst. This procedure results in a chimeric animal that, in some instances, carries the transgene in the germline and transmits the transgene to its progeny. The expression of the transgene-encoded protein is determined by the promoter/enhancer sequences used to construct the transgene, the site of integration, and, in certain situations, the number of copies of the transgene. Transgenic models provide a means to test hypotheses as to possible aetiologies and contributing factors for the development of arthritis.

HLA-B27 transgenic model for spondyloarthropathies

Transgenic technology has been applied to the study of spondyloarthropathies by developing transgenic LEW/N and F344/N rats that express human HLA-B27 and β_2-microglobulin on the surface of lymphocytes[70,71]. One LEW/N and one F344/N transgenic rat line developed clinical and histological features resembling human spondyloarthropathies. The most consistent finding is diarrhoea associated with chronic inflammation of the gastrointestinal tract. Inflammatory synovitis of peripheral and axial joints occurs most frequently in LEW/N males (>90%), but also in 50% of LEW/N females and F344/N males, and <25% of F344/N females. Severe psoriasiform changes of the tail skin with hyperkeratosis and dystrophy of the nails occur in 30–50% of LEW/N males and females, but is rare in the F344/N transgenic line. The clinical and histological appearance of these lesions bears a striking resemblance to psoriasis vulgaris. Male transgenic rats also develop orchitis and epididymitis. Inflammation of the aortic valve and myocardium also occurred in 45% of the hearts examined in the LEW/N rat line that was similar to cardiac involvement in ankylosing spondylitis. Further evaluation of these transgenic animals may elucidate the molecular mechanisms behind the association of HLA-B27 and the spondyloarthropathies.

HTLV-1 transgenic mice

Transgenic mice containing the genome of the HTLV-1 retrovirus develop polyarticular synovitis that occurs earlier in females (2–3 months) than in males (5–10 months)[72]. Histologically, synovial tissue shows proliferation of fibroblast-like cells and new blood vessel formation, with infiltration of inflammatory cells and erosion of cartilage and bone. Low level rheumatoid factor and antibodies to double- and single-stranded DNA are very rarely seen. Additionally, the thymuses of these HTLV-1 transgenic mice are frequently atrophied and they have a decreased proliferative response to concavalin A. This study provides further evidence to support retroviruses as one possible aetiology of chronic inflammatory arthritis.

Transgenic mice expressing TNF-α

Pro-inflammatory cytokines, such as tumour necrosis factor-α (TNF-α), interleukin-1 and interleukin-6, are thought to play a role in the inflammatory process. These cytokines are found in the synovial fluid of RA patients and have effects on synovial cells *in vitro*. Transgenic mice carrying a human TNF-α transgene truncated at the 3′ end, important for post-transcriptional regulation of TNF-α expression, develop chronic inflammatory poly-arthritis[73]. This arthritis was inherited with 100% incidence and was clinically evident by 3–4 weeks of age. These animals also developed weight loss, a known biological effect of TNF-α. Additionally, the arthritis could be prevented by injections of anti-TNF-α antibody given intra-peritoneally twice weekly starting at birth. Transgenic animals containing the full-length human TNF-α gene did not develop arthritis. The reason for the phenotypic difference between the truncated and full-length TNF-α transgenic animals may be related to the regulation of the transgene. For example, the truncated TNF-α transgene is also expressed constitutively at low levels in many tissues, but there is no expression in peritoneal macrophages and no regulation by endotoxin. However, the full human TNF-α transgene is expressed at low levels in many tissues, including peritoneal macrophages, and there is a large increase in mRNA expression in peritoneal macrophages in response to lipopolysaccharide treatment similar to the endogenous murine TNF-α gene. These transgenic animal studies can potentially be utilized to evaluate the regulated expression and biological function of TNF-α *in vivo*.

Transgenic animal models will undoubtedly become increasingly important in the study of aetiologies and pathogenic mechanisms of inflammatory arthritis.

References

1. Hang L, Theofilopoulos AN, Dixon FJ. A spontaneous rheumatoid arthritis-like disease in MRL/1 mice. J Exp Med. 1982; 155: 1690–1701.
2. O'Sullivan FX, Fassbender H-G, Gay S, Koopman WJ. Etiopathogenesis of the rheumatoid arthritis-like disease in MRL/1 mice. Arthritis Rheum. 1985; 28: 529–536.
3. Tarkowski A, Jonsson R, Holmdahl R, Klareskog L. Immunohistochemical characterization of synovial cells in arthritic MRL-lpr/lpr mice. Arthritis Rheum. 1987; 30: 75–82.
4. Ratkay LG, Tonzetich J, Waterfield JD. Antibodies to extracellular matrix proteins in the sera of MRL-*lpr* mice. Clin Immunol Immunopathol. 1991; 59: 236–245.
5. Phadke K, Fouts R, Parrish J, Baker RS. Autoreactivity to collagen in a murine lupus model. Arthritis Rheum. 1984; 27: 313–319.
6. Boissier M-C, Texier B, Carlioz A, Fournier C. Polyarthritis in MRL-lpr/lpr mice: Mouse type II collagen is antigenic but not arthritogenic. Autoimmunity. 1989; 4: 31–41.
7. Watanabe-Fukunaga R, Brannan CI, Copeland NG, Jenkins NA, Nagata S. Lymphoproliferation disorder in mice explained by defects in Fas antigen that mediates apoptosis. Nature. 1992; 356: 314–317.
8. Carter SD, Bell SC, Bari ASM, Bennett D. Immune complexes and rheumatoid factors in canine arthritides. Ann Rheum Dis. 1989; 48: 986–991.
9. Bari ASM, Carter SD, Bell SC, Morgan K, Bennett D. Anti-type II collagen antibody in naturally occurring canine joint diseases. Br J Rheum. 1989; 28: 480–486.
10. Bell SC, Carter SD, Bennett D. Canine distemper viral antigens and antibodies in dogs with rheumatoid arthritis. Res Vet Sci. 1991; 50: 64–68.
11. Allen JB, Malone DG, Wahl SM, Calandra GB, Wilder RL. Role of the thymus in streptococcal cell wall-induced arthritis and hepatic granuloma formation. J Clin Invest. 1985; 76: 1042–1056.
12. DeJoy SQ, Ferguson KM, Sapp TM, Zabriskie JB, Oronsky AL, Kerwar SS. Streptococcal cell wall arthritis. Passive transfer of disease with a T cell line and crossreactivity of streptococcal cell wall antigens with *Mycobacterium tuberculosis*. J Exp Med. 1989; 170: 369–382.
13. Yocum DE, Allen JB, Wahl SM, Calandra GB, Wilder RL. Inhibition by cyclosporin A of streptococcal cell wall-induced arthritis and hepatic granulomas in rats. Arthritis Rheum. 1986; 29: 262–273.
14. Yoshino S, Cleland LG, Mayrhoger FG, Brown RR, Schwab JH. Prevention of chronic erosive streptococcal cell wall-induced arthritis in rats by treatment with a monoclonal antibody against the T cell antigen receptor $\alpha\beta$. J Immunol. 1991; 146: 4187–4189.
15. van den Broek MF, van de Langerijt LGM, van Bruggen MCJ, Billingham MEJ, van den Berg WB. Treatment of rats with monoclonal anti-CD4 induces long-term resistance to streptococcal cell wall-induced arthritis. Eur J Immunol. 1992; 22: 57–61.
16. Wilder RL, Allen JB, Hansen C. Thymus-dependent and -independent regulation of Ia antigen expression in situ by cells in synovium of rats with streptococcal cell wall-induced arthritis. Differences in site and intensity of expression in euthymic, athymic, and cyclosporin A-treated LEW and F344 rats. J Clin Invest. 1987; 79: 1160–1171.
17. Case JP, Sano H, Lafyatis R, Remmers EF, Kumkumian GK, Wilder RL. Transin/stromelysin expression in the synovium of rats with experimental erosive arthritis. In situ localization and kinetics of expression of the transformation-associated metalloproteinase in euthymic and athymic Lewis rats. J Clin Invest. 1989; 84: 1731–1740.
18. Sano H, Forough R, Maier JA, Case JP, Jackson A, Engleka K, Maciag T, Wilder RL. Detection of high levels of heparin binding growth factor-1 (acidic fibroblast growth factor) in inflammatory arthritic joints. J Cell Biol. 1990; 110: 1417–1426.
19. Sano H, Engleka K, Mathern P, Hla T, Crofford LJ, Remmers EF, Jelsema C, Maciag T, Wilder RL. Co-expression of tyrosine phosphoproteins, PDGF-B and FGF-1 *in situ* in the synovial tissues of patients with rheumatoid arthritis and rats with adjuvant and streptococcal cell wall arthritis. J Clin Invest. 1993; 91: 553–565.
20. Sano H, Hla T, Maier JAM, Crofford LJ, Case JP, Maciag T, Wilder RL. *In vivo* cyclooxygenase expression in synovial tissues of patients with rheumatoid arthritis and osteoarthritis and rats with adjuvant and streptococcal cell wall arthritis. J Clin Invest. 1992; 89: 97–108.

21. Lafyatis R, Thompson NL, Remmers EF, Flanders KC, Roche NS, Kim SJ, Case JP, Sporn MB, Roberts AB, Wilder RL. Transforming growth factor-beta production by synovial tissues from rheumatoid patients and streptococcal cell wall arthritic rats. Studies on secretion by synovial fibroblast-like cells and immunohistologic localization. J Immunol. 1989; 143: 1142–1148.

22. Crofford LJ, Sano H, Karalis K, Webster EL, Goldmuntz EA, Chrousos GP, Wilder RL. Local secretion of corticotropin-releasing hormone in the joints of Lewis rats with inflammatory arthritis and patients with rheumatoid arthritis. Submitted.

23. Wilder RL, Calandra GB, Garvin AJ, Wright KD, Hansen CT. Strain and sex variation in the susceptibility to streptococcal cell wall-induced polyarthritis in the rat. Arthritis Rheum. 1982; 25: 1064–1072.

24. Patterson PY. Experimental autoimmune (allergic) encephalomyelitis: Induction, pathogenesis, and suppression. In: Miescher PA, Muller-Eberhard HS, ed Textbook of Immunopathology. New York: Grune and Stratton; 1976; 179–213.

25. Caspi R, Wilder R, Roberge F, Chan C, Leake W, CT H, Nussenblatt R. Studies of EAU induction in different rat strains compatible in RT1 (abstract). Invest Ophthalmol Vis Sci. 1989; 30 (Suppl): 81.

26. Crofford LJ, Remmers EF, Misiewicz-Poltorak B, Sano H, Goldmuntz EA, Cash JM, Sternberg EM, Hansen CT, Wilder RL. Genetic control of acute inflammatory arthritis severity in Lewis and Fischer rats is not linked to the MHC (abstract). Arthritis Rheum. 1991; 34: s68.

27. Sternberg EM, Young III WS, Bernardini R, Calogero AE, Chrousos GP, Gold PW, Wilder RL. A central nervous system defect in biosynthesis of corticotropin-releasing hormone is associated with susceptibility to streptococcal cell wall-induced arthritis in Lewis rats. Proc Natl Acad Sci USA. 1989; 86: 4771–4775.

28. Sternberg EM, Hill JM, Chrousos GP, Kamilaris T, Listwak SJ, Gold PW, Wilder RL. Inflammatory mediator-induced hypothalamic-pituitary-adrenal axis activation is defective in streptococcal cell wall arthritis-susceptible Lewis rats. Proc Natl Acad Sci USA. 1989; 86: 2374–2378.

29. van den Broek MF, van Bruggen MC, van de Putte LB, van den Berg WB. T cell responses to streptococcal antigens in rats: relation to susceptibility to streptococcal cell wall-induced arthritis. Cell Immunol. 1988; 116: 216–229.

30. Kohashi O, Kohashi Y, Takahashi T, Ozawa A, Shigematsu N. Suppressive effect of *Escherichia coli* on adjuvant-induced arthritis in germ-free rats. Arthritis Rheum. 1986; 29: 547–553.

31. van Bruggen MCJ, van den Broek MF, van den Berg WB. Streptococcal cell wall-induced arthritis and adjuvant arthritis in F344–Lewis and in Lewis–F344 bone marrow chimeras. Cellular Immunol. 1991; 136: 278–290.

32. Lehman TJA, Allen JB, Plotz PH, Wilder RL. Polyarthritis in rats following the systemic injection of *Lactobacillus casei* cell walls in aqueous suspension. Arthritis Rheum. 1983; 26: 1259–1265.

33. Lehman TJA, Allen JB, Plotz PH, Wilder RL. *Lactobacillus casei* cell wall-induced arthritis in rats: Cell wall fragment distribution and persistence in chronic arthritis-susceptible LEW/N and resistant F344/N rats. Arthritis Rheum. 1984; 27: 939–942.

34. Severijnen A, van Kleef R, Hazenberg MP, van de Merwe JP. Cell wall fragments from major residents of the human intestinal flora induce chronic arthritis in rats. J Rheumatol. 1989; 16: 1601–1608.

35. Severijinen AJ, van Kleef R, Hazenberg MP, van de Merwe JP. Chronic arthritis induced in rats by cell wall fragments of Eubacterium species from the human intestinal flora. Infect Immun. 1990; 58: 523–528.

36. Stimpson SA, Brown RR, Anderle SK, Klapper DG, Clark RL, Cromartie WJ, Schwab JH. Arthropathic properties of cell wall polymers from normal flora bacteria. Infect Immun. 1986; 55: 240–249.

37. Wilder RL. Proinflammatory microbial products as etiologic agents of inflammatory arthritis. Rheum Dis Clin North Am. 1987; 13: 293–306.

38. Lehman TJA, Allen JB, Plotz PH, Wilder RL. Bacterial cell wall composition, lysozyme resistance and the induction of chronic arthritis in rats. Rheumatol Int. 1985; 5: 163–167.

39. Eisenberg R, Fox A, Greenblatt JJ, Anderle SK, Cromartie WJ, Schwab JH. Measurement

of bacterial cell wall in tissues by solid phase radioimmunoassay: Correlation of distribution and persistence with experimental arthritis in rats. Infect Immun. 1982; 38: 127–135.

40. Gibofsky A, Zabriskie JB. Acute rheumatic fever: Clinical and immunopathologic aspects. In: Espinoza L, Goldenberg D, Arnett F, Alarcon G, eds. Infections in the Rheumatic Diseases. New York: Grune & Stratton, Inc.; 1988: 367–373.
41. Keat A. Reactive arthritis, Reiter's syndrome, and genitourinary infections. In: Espinoza L, Goldenberg D, Arnett F, Alarcon D, eds. Infections in the Rheumatic Diseases. New York: Grune & Stratton, Inc.; 1988: 281–286.
42. Inman RD. Reactive arthritis, Reiter's syndrome, and enteric pathogens. In: Espinoza L, Goldenberg D, Arnett F, Alarcon G, eds. Infections in the Rheumatic Diseases. New York: Grune & Stratton, Inc.; 1988: 273–279.
43. Keat A, Rowe I. Reiter's syndrome and associated arthritides. Rheum Dis Clin North Am. 1991; 17: 25–42.
44. Utsinger PD, Spalding DM, Weiner SR, Clarke J. Intestinal immunology and rheumatic diseases: inflammatory bowel disease and intestinal bypass arthropathies. In: Espinoza L, Goldenberg D, Arnett F, Alarcon G, eds. Infections in the Rheumatic Diseases. New York: Grune & Stratton, Inc.; 1988: 317–341.
45. Granfors K, Jalkanen S, von Essen R, Lahesmaa-Rantala R, Isomaki O, Pekklow-Heino K, Merilahti-Palo R, Saario R, Isomaki H, Toivanen A. Yersinia antigens in synovial fluid cells from patients with reactive arthritis. N Engl J Med. 1989; 320: 216–221.
46. Granfors K, Jalkanen S, Lindberg AA, Maki-Ikola O, von Essen R, Isomaki H, Saario R, Arnold WJ, Toivanen A. Salmonella lipopolysaccharide in synovial cells from patients with reactive arthritis. Lancet. 1990; 335: 685–688.
47. Baird RW, Bronze MS, Kraus W, Hill HR, Veasey LG, Dale JB. Epitopes of group A streptococcal M protein shared with antigens of articular cartilage and synovium. J Immunol. 1991; 146: 3132–3137.
48. DeJoy SQ, Ferguson-Chanowitz KM, Sapp TM, Oronsky AL, Lapierre LA, Zabriskie JB, Kerwar SS. M protein deficient streptococcal cell walls can induce acute and chronic arthritis in rats. Cell Immunol. 1990; 125: 526–534.
49. Pearson CM, Wood FD. Studies of polyarthritis and other lesions induced in rats by injection of mycobacterial adjuvant. I. General clinical and pathological characteristics and some modifying factors. Arthritis Rheum. 1959; 2: 440–459.
50. Holoshitz J, Naparstek Y, Ben-Nun A, Cohen I. Lines of T-lymphocytes induce or vaccinate against autoimmune arthritis. Science. 1983; 217: 56–58.
51. Cohen IR, Holoshitz J, van Eden W, Frenkel A. T-lymphocyte clones illuminate pathogenesis and affect therapy of experimental arthritis. Arthritis Rheum. 1985; 28: 841–845.
52. van Eden W, Holoshitz J, Nevo A, Frenkel A, Klajman A, Cohen IR. Arthritis induced by a T-lymphocyte clone that responds to *Mycobacterium tuberculosis* and to cartilage proteoglycans. Proc Natl Acad Sci USA. 1985; 82: 5117–5120.
53. van Eden W, Thole JER, van der Zee R, Noordzij A, van Embden JD, Hensen EJ, Cohen IR. Cloning of the mycobacterial epitope recognised by T-lymphocytes in adjuvant arthritis. Nature. 1988; 331: 171–173.
54. Billingham MEJ, Carney S, Butler R, Colston MJ. A mycobacterial 65-Kd heat shock protein induces antigen-specific suppression of adjuvant arthritis, but is not itself arthritogenic. J Exp Med. 1990; 171: 339–344.
55. van den Broek MF, Hogervorst EJ, van Bruggen MC, van Eden W, van der Zee R, van den Berg WB. Protection against streptococcal cell wall-induced arthritis by pretreatment with the 65-kD mycobacterial heat shock protein. J Exp Med. 1989; 170: 449–466.
56. Res PCM, Schaar CG, Breedveld RC, van Eden W, van Embden JDA, Cohen IR, de Vries RR. Synovial fluid T cell reactivity against 65 kD heat shock protein of mycobacteria in early chronic arthritis. Lancet. 1988; 2: 478–480.
57. Gaston JS, Life PF, Bailey LC, Bacon PA. In vitro responses to a 65-kilodalton mycobacterial protein by synovial T cells from inflammatory arthritis patients. J Immunol. 1989; 15: 2494–2495.
58. Gaston JS, Life PF, Jenner PJ, Colston MJ, Bacon PA. Recognition of a mycobacteria-specific epitope in the 65-kD heat-shock protein by synovial fluid-derived T cell clones. J Exp Med. 1990; 171: 831–841.
59. Holmdahl R, Jansson L, Larsson E, Rubin K, Klareskog L. Homologous type II collagen

induces chronic and progressive arthritis in mice. Arthritis Rheum. 1986; 29: 106–113.
60. Cremer M. Type II collagen-induced arthritis in rats. In: Greenwald RA, Diamond HS, eds. CRC Handbook of Animal Models for the Rheumatic Diseases, Vol. I. Boca Raton: CRC Press, Inc. 1988; 17–27.
61. Terato K, Hasty KA, Cremer MA, Stuart JM, Townes AS, Kang AH. Collagen-induced arthritis in mice. Localization of an arthritogenic determinant to a fragment of the type II collagen molecule. J Exp Med. 1985; 162: 637–646.
62. Stuart JM, Cremer MA, Townes AS, Kang AH. Type II collagen-induced arthritis in rats: passive transfer with serum and evidence that IgG anticollagen antibodies can cause arthritis. J Exp Med. 1982; 155: 1–16.
63. Holmdahl R, Klareskog L, Rubin K, Larrson E, Wigzell H. T-cells in collagen-induced arthritis in mice: Characterization of arthritogenic collagen II specific T-lymphocyte lines and clones that can transfer arthritis. Scand J Immunol. 1986; 22: 295–301.
64. Watson WC, Townes AS. Genetic susceptibility to murine collagen II autoimmune arthritis. Proposed relationship to the IgG2 autoantibody subclass response, complement C5, major histocompatibility complex (MHC) and non-MHC loci. J Exp Med. 1985; 162: 1878–1891.
65. Watson WC, Thompson JP, Terato K, Cremer MA, Kang AH. Human HLA-DRb gene hypervariable region homology in the biobreeding BB rat: Selection of the diabetic-resistant subline as a rheumatoid arthritis research tool to characterize the immunopathologic response to human type II collagen. J Exp Med. 1990; 172: 1331–1339.
66. Spinella DG, Jeffers JR, Reife RA, Stuart JM. The role of C5 and the T-cell receptor Vb genes in susceptibility to collagen-induced arthritis. Immunogenetics. 1991; 34: 23–27.
67. Cooke TDV. Antigen-induced arthritis, polyarthritis, and tenosynovitis. In: Greenwald RA, Diamond HS, eds. CRC Handbook of Animal Models for the Rheumatic Diseases, Vol. I. Boca Raton: CRC Press, Inc.; 1988: 53–81.
68. Jaenisch R. Transgenic Animals. Science. 1988; 240: 1468–1474.
69. Westphal H. Molecular genetics of development studied in the transgenic mouse. Annu Rev Cell Biol. 1989; 5: 181–196.
70. Hammer R, Maika SD, Richardson JA, Tang J-P, Taurog JD. Spontaneous inflammatory disease in transgenic rats expressing HLA-B27 and human B_2m: An animal model of HLA-B27-associated human disorders. Cell. 1990; 63: 1099–1112.
71. Taurog JD, Maika SD, Hlavaty JL, Simmons WA, Hastings BA, Richardson JA, Breban M, Hammer RE. Inflammatory disease in HLA-B27 transgenic rats is accompanied by a dramatic rise in B27 expression (abstract). Arthritis Rheum. 1991; 34: s33.
72. Iwakura Y, Tosu M, Yoshida E, Takiguchi M, Sato K, Kitajima I, Nishioka K, Yamamoto K, Takeda T, Hatanaka M, Yamamoto H, Sekigichi T. Induction of inflammatory arthropathy resembling rheumatoid arthritis in mice transgenic for HTLV-1. Science. 1991; 253: 1026–1028.
73. Keffer J, Probert L, Cazlaris H, Georgopoulos S, Kaslaris E, Kioussis D, Kollias G. Transgenic mice expressing human tumour necrosis factor: a predictive genetic model of arthritis. EMBO J. 1991; 10: 4025–4031.

11
Lyme Arthritis: Pathogenetic Principles Emerging from Studies in Man and Mouse

M. M. SIMON, M. D. KRAMER, R. WALLICH and U. E. SCHAIBLE

HISTORY AND AETIOLOGY OF LYME DISEASE

Lyme arthritis was originally discovered in 1977 by Allen Steere and co-workers in Old Lyme (Connecticut, USA) in a population of young children and initially misdiagnosed as juvenile arthritis[1]. Extensive epidemiological studies revealed that the disease is a vector-borne infection transmitted to humans primarily by ixodic ticks[2]. In 1982, the aetiological agent was isolated from the midgut of ticks and identified as a Gram-negative spirochaete, later termed *Borrelia burgdorferi*[3,4].

Like other spirochaetes, *B. burgdorferi* organisms consist of an outer cell membrane, underlying periplasmic flagella and a protoplasmic cylinder complex[5] (Figure 1). From more than 100 spirochaete-associated proteins seen after electrophoretic separation, a variety of structures including two plasmid-encoded outer surface proteins A and B (OspA, OspB)[6] as well as the chromosome encoded structures HSP60[7], HSP70[8], and the flagella-associated 41 kDa protein, flagellin[9], have been defined by antibodies[9-12] (Figure 1) and their genes have been cloned and sequenced[13-18,25].

In humans, *B. burgdorferi* causes a complex disease affecting mainly the skin, joints, nervous system and heart[19]. Some of the manifestations have been known since the turn of the century but had not been ascribed to one clinical entity[20-22].

CLINICAL MANIFESTATIONS OF LYME DISEASE

The clinical course of *B. burgdorferi* infection, also termed Lyme Borreliosis or Lyme disease, can be divided into early and late infection with three

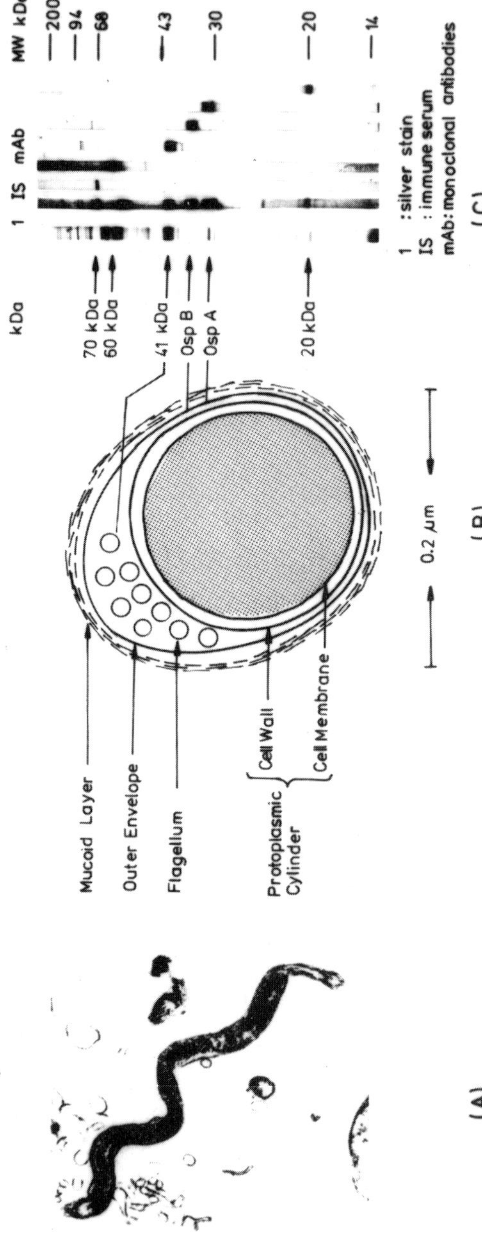

Figure 1a Electron micrograph of *Borrelia burgdorferi* (Magnification 1:32 000; reproduced with kind permission from [119]). *B. burgdorferi* is grouped together with *Treponema* and *Spirochaeta* into the family of spirochaetaceae. It is a Gram-negative microaerophilic bacterium with a length of around 20–30 μm, and width of the helices is approximately 0.2–0.3 μm. It can be grown in artificial culture medium (Barbour-Stoenner-Kelly medium), but only with a low generation time (12–40h).
b Schematic drawing of a cross-section of *B. burgdorferi*, showing the outer cell membrane surrounded by a mucoid layer, multiple flagella and the protoplasmic cylinder complex. The localization of immunologically important structures is indicated.
c Analysis of *B. burgdorferi* proteins. Electrophoretically separated whole cell lysates of *B. burgdorferi* visualized by silver staining[1] and by Western blotting using a *B. burgdorferi* specific mouse immune serum (IS), or monoclonal antibodies specific for spirochaetal proteins of molecular masses of approximately 70 kDa, 60 kDa, 41 kDa, 34 kDa, 31 kDa and 20 kDa

stages (Table 1). This is analogous to syphilis, another spirochaetal infection[23]. The different stages of the disease are usually characterized by distinct clinical manifestations which may develop independently of each other or may occur in different combinations[19] (Table 1).

Early infection is defined as stage 1 and is a local infection of the skin at the site of the tick bite. The clinical picture is termed erythema (chronicum) migrans (EM)[20,24,25]. At this stage, there is no involvement of the musculo-skeletal system. Stage 2 corresponds to disseminated infection and can develop within days or weeks after haematogenous spread of the spirochaetes. This stage is characterized by intermittent organ involvement, particularly of joints (musculo-skeletal pain, arthritic attacks[26]), nervous system (meningo-polyneuritis[27]), and heart (carditis[28]). Nonspecific symptoms such as fatigue, headache, fever, arthralgia and lymphadenitis may accompany the specific ones[19]. Stage 3 usually begins only months after infection and is characterized by persistent organ involvement presenting as chronic arthritis[26], encephalo-myelitis[19,29], carditis[30] and/or a localized scleroderma-like lesion, acrodermatitis chronica atrophicans[31].

CLINICAL FEATURES OF LYME ARTHRITIS

The best information on the natural history of Lyme arthritis available to date is provided by an extensive study performed on 55 infected patients in the eastern part of the USA, who did not receive antibiotic therapy[26]. As reported in this survey, 18% of the infected individuals began to experience brief episodes of periarticular or musculo-skeletal pain within 6 years of observation. 51% of all patients had at least one episode of arthritis; only a few had polyarticular involvement. The knee was most frequently involved. Chronic erosive joint lesions developed in approximately 10% of the patients. These findings suggest that arthritis, whether intermittent or chronic, is a major clinical feature of *B. burgdorferi* infection, at least in North America. Although still a matter of debate, the prevalence of arthritides in Europe in patients with Lyme disease appears to be lower[32]. The reason for this difference is not known, but strain variability of *B. burgdorferi* may play a role. In fact, genotypic/phenotypic variations have been shown to be much less pronounced in spirochaetal isolates from North America than from Europe[11,33–35]. However, association of the different variants with distinct clinical symptoms has not been established.

X-ray examinations of joints afflicted with Lyme arthritis show early changes in joint fluid, and/or synovial proliferation, and diffuse soft tissue swelling[36]. Later, thickening of joints, calcification, in particular of articular cartilage or meniscus, or ossification may be observed. Patients with chronic arthritis show both inflammatory and degenerative changes. The latter include articular or periarticular erosions, osteoporosis, subarticular cysts and sclerosis, proliferative osteophyte formation and cartilage loss.

Table 1

System	Early infection Stage 1 Local infection Skin manifestation	Late infection	
		Stage 2 Generalized infection Early organ manifestation	Stage 3 Generalized infection Chronic organ manifestation
Skin	Erythema migrans	Polytopic erythemata	Acrodermatitis chronica atrophicans
Nervous system		Meningo-polyneuritis Peripheral neuritis	Encephalomyelitis
Heart		Myocarditis Pancarditis	Chronic carditis
Musculo-skeletal system		**Intermittent arthritic attacks**	**Chronic arthritis**

This summary is not meant to be comprehensive: it serves to place joint involvement into the time course of *B. burgdorferi* infection. For more detailed information reference [19] is recommended

HISTOPATHOLOGY OF LYME ARTHRITIS

Histopathological findings in synovial lesions of Lyme arthritis are reminiscent of those found in other chronic inflammatory arthritides, including rheumatoid arthritis: villus hypertrophy of the synovium, vascular proliferation, and the presence of macrophages, T cells and plasma cells are observed[37,38]. Sometimes, the lymphocytic infiltrations are organized as follicle-like structures, the significance of which, however, is not understood. Numerous mast cells may be observed and in only a few cases neutrophils are the predominant inflammatory cells. Early hypertrophy of synovial lining cells is frequently accompanied by focal necrosis, deposition of fibrin, and sometimes microvascular lesions resembling those of obliterative endarteritis[37]. Chronically inflamed adherent synovium ('pannus') is often associated with erosion of the underlying cartilage. In addition, periarticular tissues such as tendons and ligaments can be affected, and both noninflammatory myositis with muscle-fibre necrosis[39] and inflammatory myositis[40,41] have been observed.

Only in a few cases have *B. burgdorferi* organisms been identified in tissues, either within the walls of thickened vessels and in the loose tissue of the vascular bed[37,42,43] or isolated from synovial fluid[44]. The difficulty in detecting and isolating spirochaetes from clinical specimens may be due to their low frequency in tissues or to inadequacy of the methods used. As shown recently, molecular genetic techniques, in particular the polymerase chain reaction (PCR), offer a more sensitive and reliable way by which to determine unequivocally the presence or absence of *B. burgdorferi* in joints and other affected tissues during different disease stages[45–47].

The scarcity of spirochaetes in synovial lesions of afflicted joints is reminiscent of tertiary syphilis, where only small numbers of organisms persist and maintain inflammation[48]. At present, little is known about the factors targeting spirochaetes to the joints or other tissues and allowing their survival. The recent finding that cartilage proteoglycans are able to bind to *B. burgdorferi* suggests that these structures may focus spirochaetes to synovial tissue thereby providing the stimulus for chronic synovial inflammation[49]. The underlying pathological processes may then be initiated by the spirochaete itself as indicated by its ability to readily induce inflammatory mediators, such as interleukin 1 (IL-1) and tumour necrosis factor alpha (TNFα) *in vitro* and *in vivo*[50,51].

TREATMENT OF LYME ARTHRITIS

Patients with Lyme arthritis mostly respond to oral or parenteral antibiotic treatment, indicating that arthritis and possibly also other disease manifestations are the result of spirochaete persistence[52]. On the other hand, some patients only seem to react to prolonged or multiple anti-microbial regimens or do not respond at all[52,53]. The lack of, or reduced, susceptibility of spirochaetes to antibiotics may be due to (i) suboptimal concentrations of antibiotics in tissues, (ii) development of resistant strains *in vivo*, (iii) their ability to sequester themselves from therapeutic drugs in extra- or intracellular compartments, as suggested recently[54], or (iv) involvement of immunological and spirochaete-independent processes in the pathogenesis of arthritis.

INVOLVEMENT OF B AND T CELLS AND OTHER HOST FACTORS IN LYME ARTHRITIS

B. burgdorferi infection in humans is usually accompanied by both B and T cell responses in the late phase of stage 1 and in stages 2 and 3 of the disease[55-58]. In many cases, however, these immune reactions are not able to protect against disease. On the other hand, the analysis of specific antibody production during infection is valuable for the serodiagnosis of Lyme disease[56]. However, because of the limited specificity and sensitivity of the currently available tests they can only be used to support a clinical diagnosis of Lyme arthritis but not to prove it[59,60].

The spectrum of specific antibodies to *B. burgdorferi* antigens generated in patients with Lyme disease increases with time. Antibodies include those to flagellin, p39, HSP60, HSP70, 80 kD–100 kD antigens and occasionally also to the two outer surface proteins A and B (OspA, OspB[19,55,56,61]). Oligoclonal anti-*B. burgdorferi* IgG antibodies have been found in the paired joint fluid and serum samples during *B. burgdorferi* infection but no qualitative differences were observed[62]. The proposed association of joint symptoms and the presence of antibodies to a particular polypeptide is questionable. The mere demonstration of an increased level of antibodies to recombinant OspA in patients with Lyme arthritis cannot be taken as evidence that these proteins induce an arthritogenic immune response[63]. It may rather reflect the generation of anti-OspA antibodies later during disease as pointed out by a number of independent studies[55,56,64].

Several reports have demonstrated that patients with Lyme disease have an increased level of polyclonal IgM in serum and a high proportion of constitutively activated B cells[65,66]. These antibody responses may be attributed to a recently described *B. burgdorferi*-associated B cell mitogen[67,68,120]. It remains to be established whether the elevated serum IgM levels and/or the presence of cryoprecipitating and circulating immune complexes contribute to the development of arthritis[19,69].

The idea that the T cell response to *B. burgdorferi* antigens may play a role in joint destruction of Lyme arthritis has derived from the observations that inflammatory cells of synovial lesions consist of T cells in addition to macrophages and B cells as well as plasma cells[38]. *B. burgdorferi*-specific T cells have been isolated at various stages of the disease from blood and joint fluid of patients with Lyme arthritis[70,71]. Further analyses showed that the overall T cell response to *B. burgdorferi*, both in synovial fluid and in blood, is polyclonal, as reflected by the heterogeneous antigen specificities recognized by unselected T cells or T cell clones, their utilization of T cell receptor (TCR) variable region gene segments, and the multiple HLA class II alleles involved in the recognition process[71,72]. Finally, the fact that all *B. burgdorferi*-specific T cell clones isolated so far from Lyme arthritis patients produce cytokines such as TNFα, granulocyte-macrophage colony stimulating factor (GM-CSF) and interferon gamma (IFNγ) in response to antigen, suggests that one subset of human CD4$^+$ T cells, in particular Th1, can contribute to the development and/or progression of inflammatory processes in the joint[73].

The increased expression of HLA-DR and HLA-DQ antigens within the synovial lesions[38] and the observation that the *duration* rather than the *induction* of Lyme arthritis is associated most frequently with HLA-DR4 and less so with HLA-DR2, at least in North American populations[74], suggest that an immunogenic trait may be involved in the chronicity of the disease. It is possible that infection in genetically predisposed individuals preferentially leads to the induction of spirochaete-specific T cells mediating inflammatory processes or that some of the T cells sensitized to *B. burgdorferi* are also reactive with structures of the affected tissue. When exposed to the relevant antigen(s) *in situ*, these T cells may secrete cytokines thereby inducing and/or perpetuating an inflammation in the presence or absence of spirochaetes.

Although the aetiology of Lyme disease is firmly linked to *B. burgdorferi*, the process(es) leading to induction and chronicity of Lyme arthritis is far from being clear; it may be initiated by direct interaction of intact spirochaetes or their products with either resident or inflammatory cells at the local tissue, such as fibroblasts, macrophages and granulocytes, respectively, or by specific T and B cells sensitized during infection, or by both. The fact that classical proinflammatory cytokines such as IL-1[75], TNFα[51], other mediators such as chemotactic factors for neutrophils[76] and prostaglandin E2 as well as collagenase[77] are found in joint fluids of patients with Lyme arthritis and that *B. burgdorferi*-associated structures such as peptidoglycans and glycolipids[78,79] can trigger adherent monocytes to produce those cytokines *in vitro* suggests that these and possibly other as yet undefined mediators may account for the synovial pathology. However, the processes which lead to the generation of these factors *in vivo* and their mode of action during the initial and later phases of Lyme arthritis remain elusive.

THE MOUSE MODEL FOR LYME ARTHRITIS

In an effort to obtain more information on the immunological and pathogenetic processes underlying Lyme disease in general and Lyme arthritis in particular, various laboratory models for *B. burgdorferi* infection have been established. The most prominent finding common to rat[80,81], hamster[82,83] and mouse[84–88] models is that, upon experimental inoculation with viable *B. burgdorferi* organisms, all three species can develop arthritic lesions which are morphologically similar to those of patients with Lyme arthritis. The fact that pathological responses are much more pronounced in immunocompromised than in normal animals supports the idea of an immunological control of the disease in these species[80,82,84]. In the following sections we will mainly focus on the pathology of Lyme arthritis and the immune response to *B. burgdorferi* in mice and we will refer to other animal models only where appropriate. This review is not meant to be comprehensive and the reader is referred to the cited literature for further information.

PATHOGENESIS OF *B. BURGDORFERI* INFECTION IN IMMUNODEFICIENT MICE

Recent studies have shown that many immunocompetent inbred[84–88] and outbred[89] mice do not or only marginally develop clinical signs of arthritis upon experimental inoculation with *B. burgdorferi*. One explanation for resistance to the disease in these animals might be the development of an effective immune response. If this assumption is correct, then mice with a compromised immune system can be expected to develop disease. We have therefore exploited the severe combined immunodeficient (SCID) mouse, which lacks functional B and T cells[90], to study the course of infection with *B. burgdorferi*. Upon subcutaneous inoculation with live but not with either UV-treated or sonicated spirochaetes, SCID mice develop a persistent spirochaetaemia leading to a multisystem disease with the preponderance of chronic arthritis, myositis, carditis and hepatitis[84,85,91]. As few as ten spirochaetes are sufficient to induce chronic arthritis[92,121]. Clinical symptoms are observed between days 7 and 22 post-inoculation in both tibiotarsal joints depending on the numbers of spirochaetes transferred[92,121]. Later on in the disease, additional joints, i.e. ulnacarpal and metatarsal, show similar clinical manifestations[85].

Natural infection of SCID mice via tick bites also leads to clinical arthritis with a time course similar to that of mice experimentally inoculated with 10 to 1000 spirochaetes[92,121]. This indicates that not more than 1000 spirochaetes are transmitted during a tick's blood meal on SCID mice and most probably also on humans (see below).

The arthritis in SCID mice is characterized by early inflammatory lesions around large joints and their subsequent expansion into surrounding connective tissue and synovium, proliferation of synovial lining cells ('pannus' formation) and erosion of cartilage and bone (Figure 2a–e).[85] However, inflammation of periarticular tissues, such as ligaments, tendons, fascia and skeletal muscle with perivascular and interfibrillar lesions, represents additional key manifestations of the disease (Figure 2d,e). Similar histopathological changes of joint tissues have also been described for other immunocompromised animals after experimental inoculation with live spirochaetes, in particular the young C3H/HeJ mouse[86,87], neonatal rat[80,81] and irradiated hamster[82,83].

The inflamed tissue of the joint of infected SCID mice is characterized by intense vascularization. Inflammatory infiltrates in this and other affected organs consist mostly of Mac-1$^+$ cells of the macrophage/monocyte cell lineage as well as some polymorphonuclear leucocytes (Figure 3)[85,91,93,94]. Neither B nor T lymphocytes are detectable. These data show that inflammatory processes observed in joints and other tissues can proceed in the absence of immunological pathways.

Inflammation of joints, tendons and striated muscles in experimentally

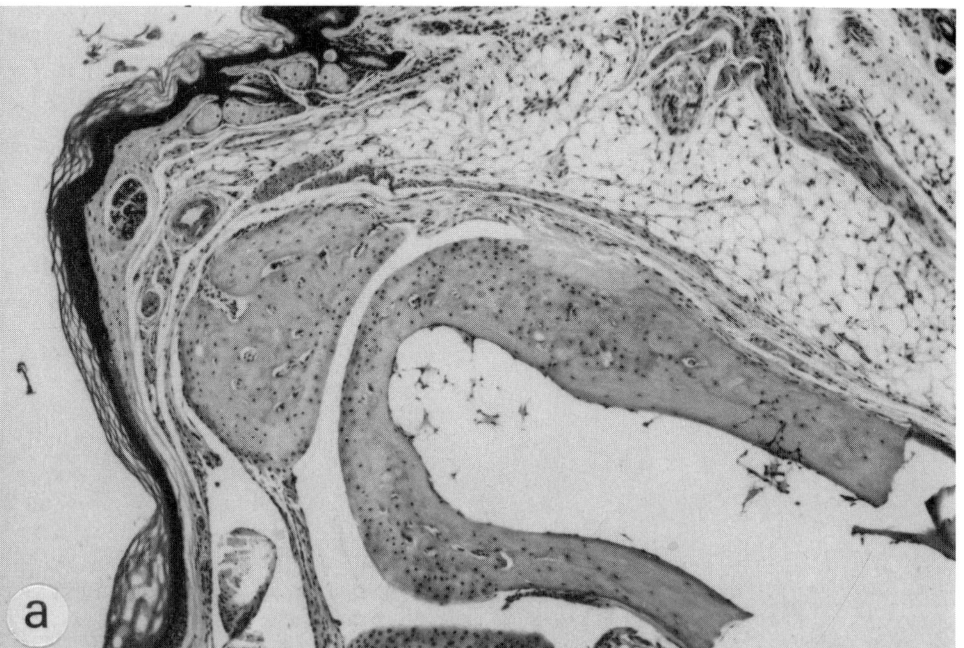

Figure 2a Tibiotarsal joint from a non-infected SCID mouse (magnification 100 ×; H&E).
b Meta-tarsal joint of a SCID mouse at day 36 post-inoculation with 10^8 spirochetes showing infiltrations with polymorpho- and mononuclear leucocytes (200 ×; H&E)
c Higher magnification (435 ×) of (b) reveals inflammatory mononuclear cells, hyperplastic synovial lining cells associated with erosion of cartilage (H&E).
d, e Tibiotarsal joint of a SCID mouse at day 36 post-inoculation with 10^8 spirochetes showing cellular intra- and periarticular infiltration (200 ×; H&E)

inoculated SCID mice was shown to coincide with the presence of spirochaetes in connective tissues of the joint (Figure 4), skeletal muscle, heart and kidney as well as in synovial fluid and blood. In a number of independent studies on *B. burgdorferi* infection in SCID and normal mice, the pathogen was identified either by silver staining[87], immunohistology (Figure 3)[85], *in situ* hybridization[87], reisolation and cultivation *in vitro*[84,85,87,89] or by PCR analysis[87,122]. In infected normal mice, spirochaetes were predominantly associated with collagen fibres[87]. When studied by electron microscopy, *B. burgdorferi* organisms were shown to be localized mostly extracellularly in the pericapillary space and were only occasionally found intracellularly[94].

The finding that only viable, low-passage organisms are able to induce the disease in SCID mice is in agreement with other recent reports in normal mice[86–88], rats[80] and hamsters[82] and indicates that motility of spirochaetes *per se* is an important component in the pathogenesis of Lyme arthritis. In fact, viable *B. burgdorferi* organisms have been shown to bind to and penetrate through vascular endothelial cells *in vitro*[95,96] and to cross the blood–brain barrier shortly after intravenous inoculation of rats[97]. It is therefore most likely that after their tissue colonization the spirochaetes

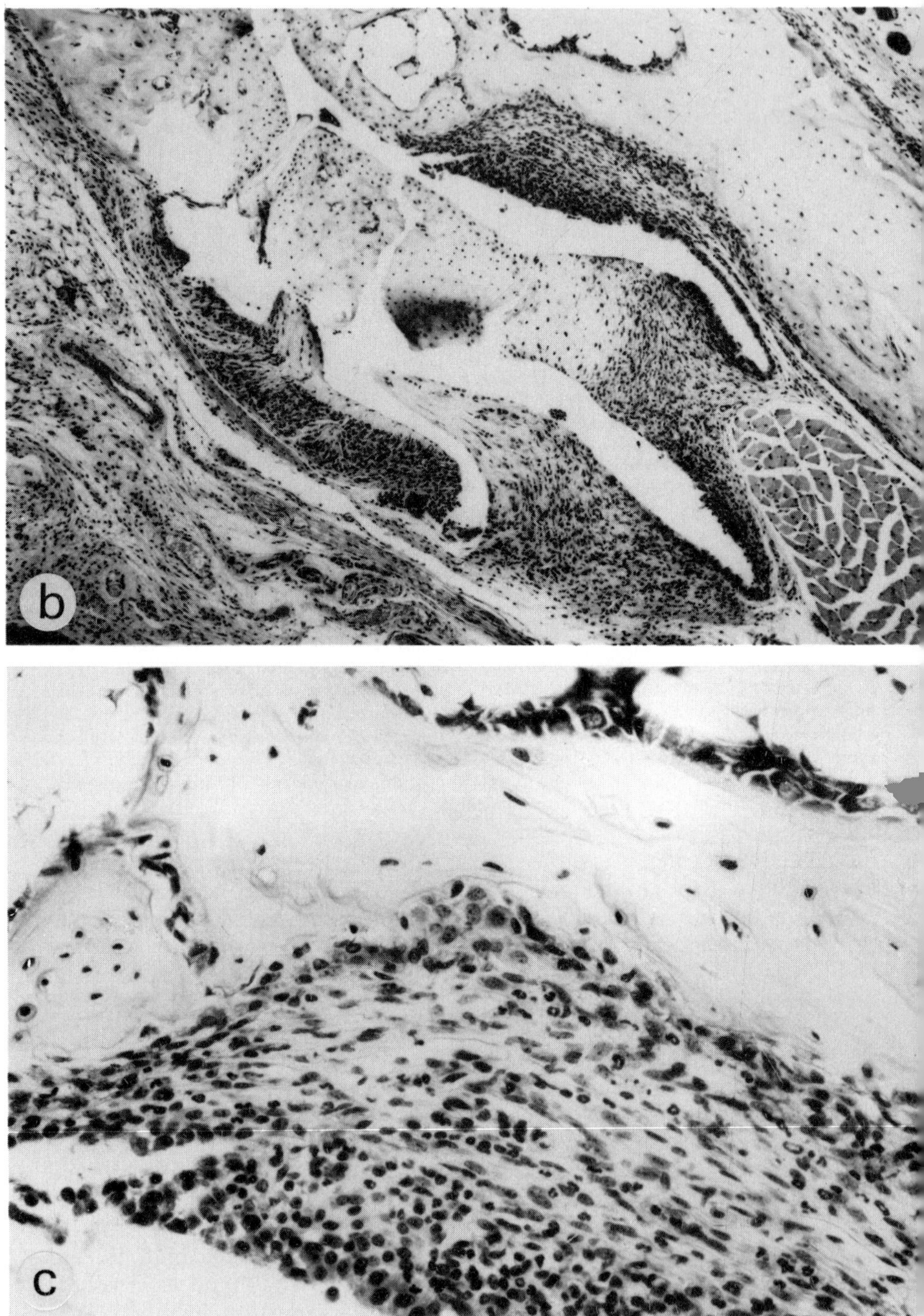

Figure 2b–c

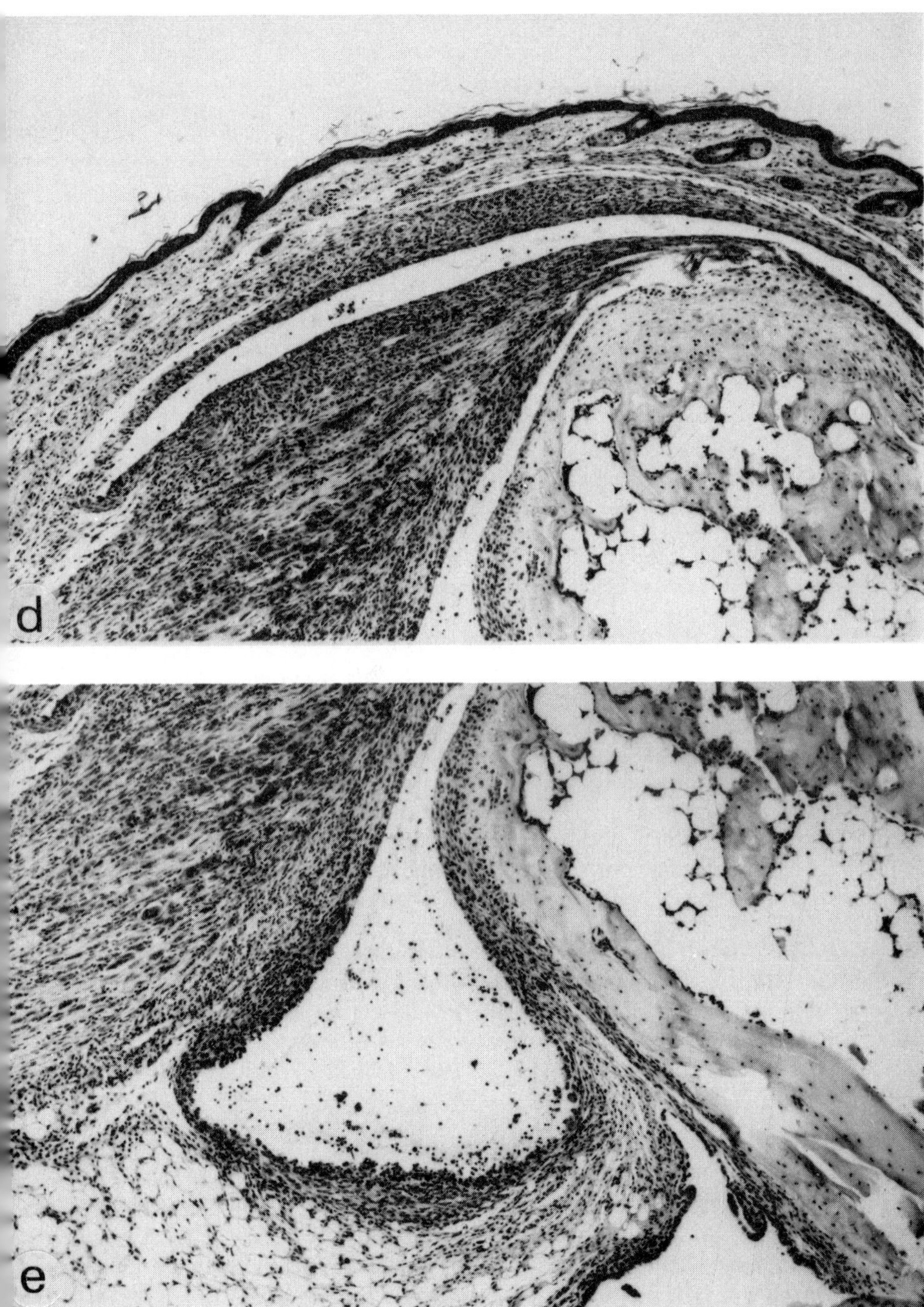

Figure 2d–e

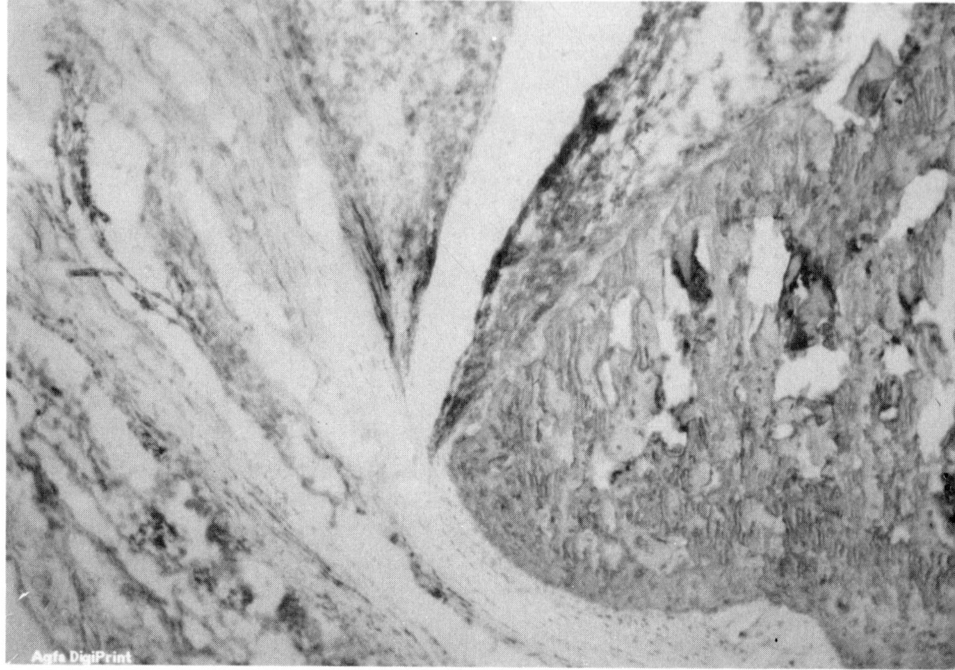

Figure 3 Immunohistological staining of the tibiotarsal joint of a SCID mouse at day 21 post-inoculation using a mAb specific for the macrophage/monocyte marker Mac-1; most of the infiltrating cells stain positive for Mac-1 (Magnification 100×)

themselves and/or their resulting degradation products initiate the various inflammatory reactions in immunocompromised and probably also normal recipients (see below).

PATHOGENESIS AND IMMUNE RESPONSE OF *B. BURGDORFERI* INFECTION IN IMMUNOCOMPETENT MICE

The analysis for clinical and microscopical arthritis in immunocompetent mice experimentally inoculated with viable *B. burgdorferi* organisms revealed three distinct patterns[88]: (i) C.B-17 mice (H-2^d), the coisogenic partner of SCID mice as well as other recipients of the H-2^d haplotype irrespective of their background genes or Igh allotypes (BALB/c, DBA/2, C.B-17, B10.D2, Cal.20) develop, if at all, only marginal signs of a self-limiting clinical arthritis; (ii) mice of H-2 haplotypes H-2^b (C57BL/6), H-2^j (B10.WB), H-2^r (B10.R111) and H-2^s (B10.S) develop arthritis of variable duration and intensity which is not progressive; and (iii) mice of the H-2^k haplotype, in particular AKR/N and C3H/HeJ, develop a chronic progressive arthritis of their tibiotarsal joints (Figure 4a–c). The appearance of clinical arthritis in AKR/J[88] and C3H/HeJ[86] mice, which may be seen with as few as 10 spirochaetes[121] is

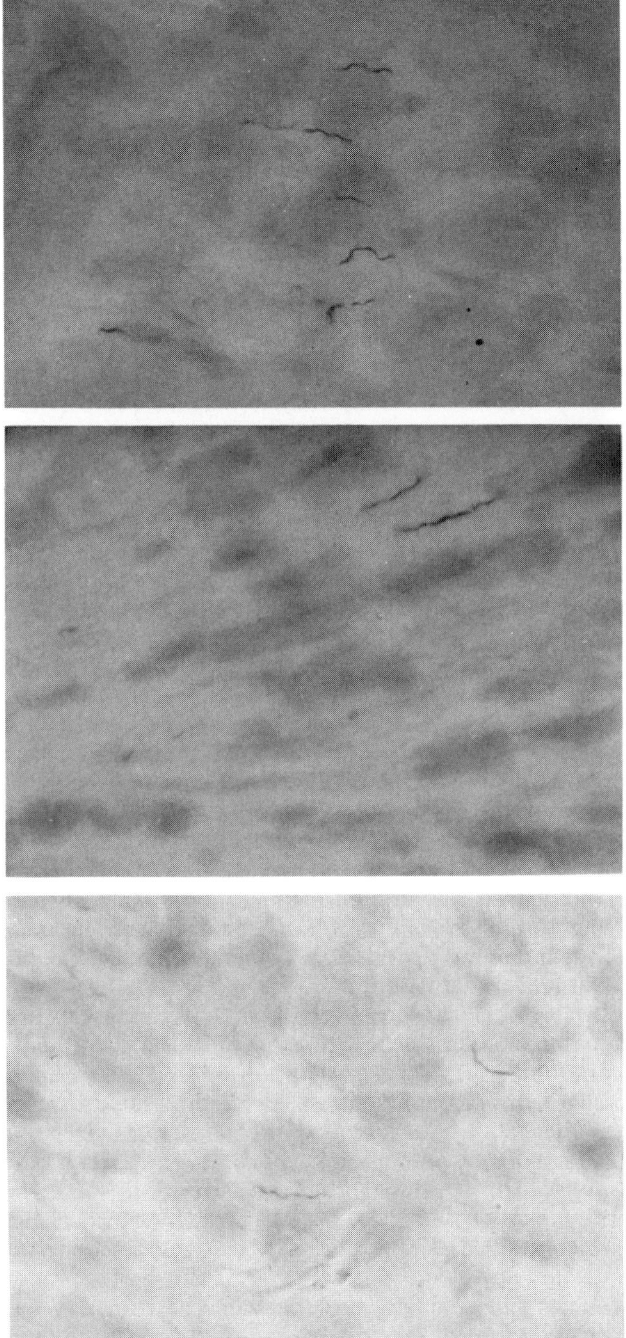

Figure 4 Detection of *B. burgdorferi* in the inflamed tibiotarsal joint of a SCID mouse at day 96 post-inoculation by immunohistological staining using a peroxidase labelled mAb to flagellin (Magnification 400 ×)

always delayed compared to SCID mice. Most notably, however, the morphology of the resulting inflammatory lesions is similar in all three recipients[88,94]. The cellular infiltrations in the joints of AKR/N and C57BL/6 mice mainly consist of macrophages and granulocytes (Mac1[+] cells; Figure 5a) with only a few scattered T but not B cells, even in the late stage of infection[94] (Figure 5b). These experiments yield two important pieces of information. First, they indicate that even in the presence of the immune system, inflammatory processes are initiated by non-immune processes, as in SCID mice, but that lymphocytes may also participate in the pathogenic events. Second, they suggest a H-2 linkage with either resistance or susceptibility to developing arthritis and indicate that in normal mice both protection and pathogenesis are controlled, at least in part, by the immune system. This is also supported by the finding that the highly susceptible H-2^k mouse strains, AKR/N and C3H/He, develop arthritic lesions in spite of an early protective antibody response: transfer of sera from these donors and from resistant animals protect SCID mice similarly against infection (see also below, and [94]).

Most notably, no correlation was seen between the quality and quantity of spirochaete-specific antibodies generated in mice and susceptibility or resistance to clinical arthritis. It is likely that in genetically predisposed mice some of the *B. burgdorferi*-specific T cells raised during infection contribute to the development of disease by virtue of their autoreactivity and/or their pathogenic potential. Alternatively, exacerbation of Lyme arthritis may be indirectly controlled by costimulatory factors for the activation of T cells, which are induced by microbial structures, such as LPS, on B cells[98]. Lastly, genetic traits in the development of arthritis in mice may also be related to non-immune cell types.

Experimental inoculation of immuno-competent mice with *B. burgdorferi* leads to the development of specific cellular and humoral immune responses in all inbred and outbred strains tested[84,86–89,92,94,99,100]. Together with the fact that SCID mice cannot clear *B. burgdorferi* infection, these results suggested that specific B and/or T cells are necessary to eliminate spirochaetes and to control the disease. Subsequent reconstitution experiments in SCID mice with the component parts of the immune system derived from coisogenic donors showed that presensitized mixtures of B and T cells but not T cells alone[101] as well as *B. burgdorferi*-specific immune sera derived from various inbred strains of mice[88,102] can protect against challenge with spirochaetes.

One major characteristic of *B. burgdorferi* infection in mice is the development of early and strong antibody responses to OspA and OspB[86–89]. This is in sharp contrast to patients with Lyme disease who do not seem to generate antibodies with these specificities in the early stages of infection and rarely (if at all) as the disease progresses[55,56,64]. The differential patterns of antibody responses and development of disease in both species suggested that anti-OspA and anti-OspB antibodies can clear the spirochaetes. It was subsequently shown in the SCID[102–104] and C3H/HeJ[105,106] mouse models that monoclonal and polyclonal antibody preparations specific for OspA and OspB can prevent or mitigate spirochaetemia and the development of the disease. Protection was also achieved in normal mice following active immunization with recombinant OspA and OspB[105,106].

Most importantly, optimal protection against the development of Lyme arthritis is only achieved when anti-OspA/OspB antibodies are present at the time or before the spirochaetal inoculation. This corroborates earlier studies in hamsters[107] and emphasizes the necessity for the presence of protective antibodies early during infection to reduce the spirochaetal load and to prevent disease. Whether this response is also sufficient to eradicate the spirochaetes from the host, is questionable. This is indicated by the fact that spirochaetes are occasionally found in peripheral blood of experimentally inoculated immunocompetent mice, and are readily isolated from spleen and urinary bladder triturates (30%) of similarly infected but otherwise symptomless white-footed mice[108]. These wild mice represent the primary reservoir for *B. burgdorferi* and the primary host for infecting larvae and nymphal ticks in the Northern Midwest and North Eastern United States[89]. Most probably, *B. burgdorferi* organisms escape immune surveillance due to (i) a delayed immune response, (ii) their ability to migrate to immunoprivileged sites, i.e. interstitial spaces within muscular and synovial tissues[87], or (iii) their capacity to survive intracellularly[54,96,97].

If antibodies to OspA and OspB are the protective elements against *B. burgdorferi* infection why are they not produced in patients with Lyme disease? A possible explanation comes from recent observations that only experimentally but not naturally infected dogs develop anti-OspA and anti-OspB antibodies[109]. Furthermore, experimental inoculation of laboratory mice with a range of 10 to 10^8 spirochetes and natural infection using infected ticks result in comparable levels of *B. burgdorferi*-specific antibodies[92]. However, anti-OspA or anti-OspB antibodies are *not* generated in mice inoculated with low numbers of spirochaetes, i.e. 10–1000, or in tick-infected recipients[92,121]. These findings suggest that the load of spirochaetes rather than the infection route has an important bearing on the quality of the immune response.

CONCLUSIONS FROM THE MOUSE MODEL OF LYME ARTHRITIS

The major findings derived from studies of *B. burgdorferi* infection in mice are that (i) viable infective low-passage spirochaetes are required for the development of arthritis and other clinical symptoms, (ii) chronic arthritis and persistent spirochaetemia can develop in the absence and presence of immune responses and (iii) anti-OspA and anti-OspB antibodies convey protection against development of disease.

The presence of viable spirochaetes within synovial tissue indicates a direct effect of the pathogenic agent rather than an indirect effect of spirochaetal products on the permeability of vessel walls or the underlying tissue. The findings that *B. burgdorferi* organisms are able to directly induce inflammatory cytokines such as IL-1 (interleukin 1)[50], TNFα[51], IL-6[110] and IL-8[111] as well as oxygen radicals and nitric oxide[123] in various target cells *in vitro* and that the composition of cellular infiltrates in inflammatory foci were quite

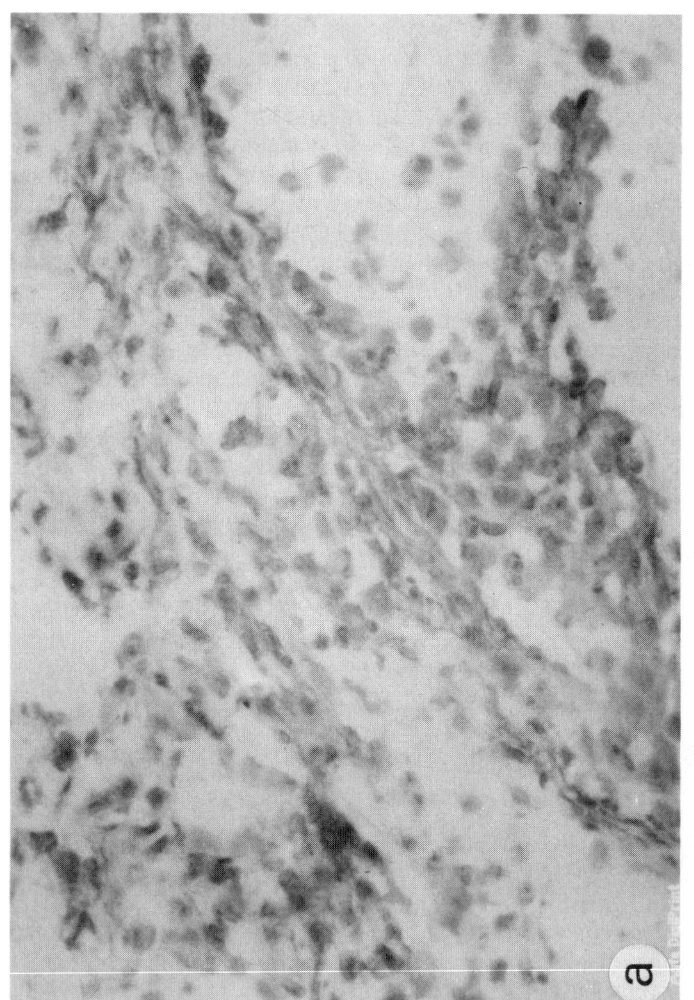

Figure 5a Immunohistological staining of the periarticular infiltration with inflammatory cells in the tibio-tarsal joint of an AKR/N mouse at day 148 post-inoculation using a mAb specific for the macrophage/monocyte marker Mac-1; most of the infiltrating cells stain positive for Mac-1 (Magnification 200 ×)

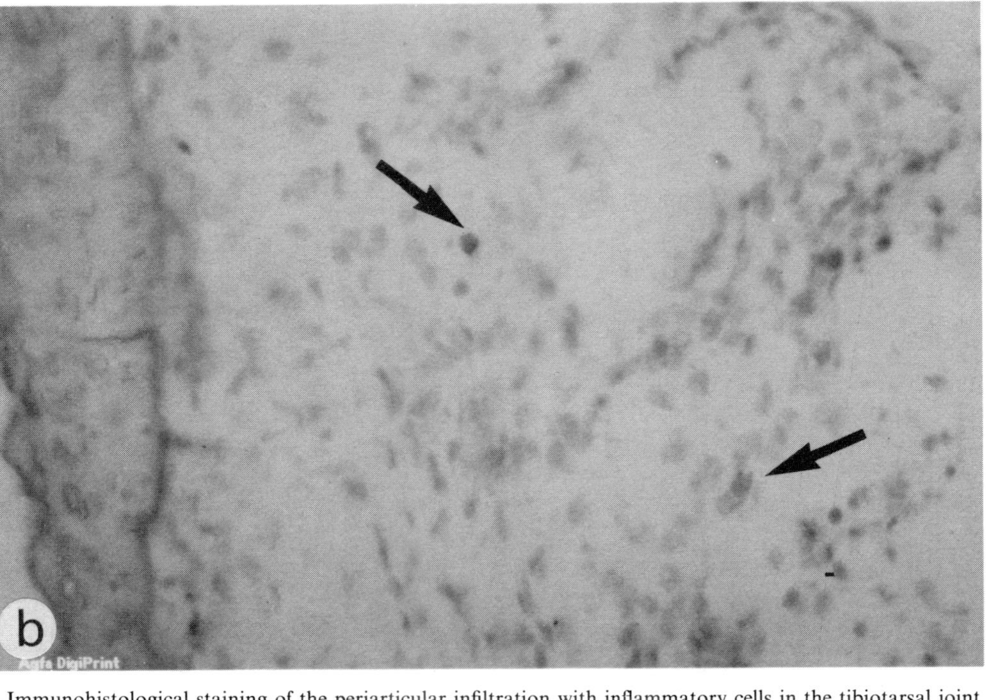

b Immunohistological staining of the periarticular infiltration with inflammatory cells in the tibiotarsal joint of an AKR/N mouse at day 148 post-inoculation using a mAb specific for the mouse T cell surface molecule CD3; only two cells (arrows) can be identified as T cells using this marker (Magnification 200×)

similar in infected SCID and normal mice[94] further emphasize their potential to initiate tissue destruction by non-immunological processes.

The predisposition of normal mice with certain H-2 haplotypes to develop chronic Lyme arthritis, even in the presence of protective antibodies, indicates the involvement of immunogenetic traits and suggests that pathogenic processes leading to joint destruction in immunocompetent mice may be independent of *B. burgdorferi* organisms and are probably controlled by T cells and/or other as yet unknown factors.

One major problem in preventing arthritis in humans and mice seems to be concerned with the ability of spirochaetes to evade protective host immune responses early during infection and to sequester in immunoprivileged sites where they exert their pathogenic potential irrespective of the host's defence mechanisms. The presence of relevant anti-spirochaetal antibodies at the time or shortly after exposure to the pathogen is therefore a prerequisite to achieving sterile immunity and full protection against disease.

Hopefully, the mouse model for Lyme arthritis will not only help to elucidate some of the underlying molecular processes but also further our understanding of the pathological processes which are involved in other chronic arthritides of unknown aetiology including rheumatoid arthritis.

WORKING HYPOTHESIS

From available evidence in humans with Lyme arthritis and in mouse models for *B. burgdorferi* infection and from current concepts of inflammatory processes, it is possible to formulate a hypothesis about non-immunological and immunological processes leading to chronic arthritis. The hypothesis is meant to provide a framework for future research rather than a definitive explanation of Lyme disease.

Intradermal injection of spirochaetes by ticks induces a local skin lesion at the site of inoculation. As long as the spirochaetes remain localized in the skin, the inflammatory process(es), i.e. perivascular and interstitial cellular infiltration and production of soluble mediators, do(es) not affect distant organs such as joints. Only after haematogenous spread do *B. burgdorferi* organisms colonize joints and other tissues by engaging their surface-bound adhesins with receptors on endothelial cells (EC) or with structures of basement membranes and extracellular matrices. This is supported by the following findings: spirochaetes attach to and penetrate EC monolayers *in vitro*, through intercellular tight junctions and through the cytoplasma of EC[95,96], and these processes are inhibitable by antibodies to OspB[112] or to fibronectin[96]. It is possible that differential recognition of *B. burgdorferi* adhesins by organ-specific EC receptors accounts for the tissue tropism of the pathogen. Invasion may be initiated by the spirochaetes themselves or by secondary host reactions. The fact that *Treponema pallidum* induces expression of ICAM-1 in EC[113] and that microbial structures are able to induce IL-1 production in EC[114] suggests similar activities for *B. burgdorferi*. Thus, spirochaetes would induce EC to secrete IL-1 which in turn would elicit the production of various other cytokines including IL-1, IL-6 or those with chemotactic activities (IL-8, monocyte chemotactic protein 1;[115]), the release of factors involved in vasodilatation, and the expression of adhesion structures such as ICAM-1[113] and ELAM[115]. If this is correct, the first encounter of spirochaetes with EC of the capillaries within the subsynovial tissue and the subsequent recruitment and activation of leukocytes would lead to the disruption of the integrity of the vessel wall and of underlying tissue. These processes appear to be the key events in the induction of joint pathology. This is indicated by the demonstration of perivascular cuffing and infiltrations of neutrophils and leukocytes into subsynovial tissue as the first histopathological alteration in infected mice[85,87,89].

Once present in the tissue, spirochaetes may induce infiltrating cells, i.e. monocytes/macrophages and polymorphonuclear leukocytes, to produce an array of inflammatory cytokines, such as IL-1, TNFα and IL-6, which can then stimulate the production of secondary mediators such as proteolytic enzymes and prostaglandins[116,117]. It is also possible that *B. burgdorferi* organisms can interact with and activate resident synovial lining cells, either directly or indirectly, to secrete IL-1, IL-6 and IL-8, hydrolytic enzymes and other molecules contributing to joint pathology[118]. The finding of hyperplastic synovial lining cells at sites of cartilage and/or bone destruction in infected SCID mice[85] and the fact that IL-1 induces collagenase production in chondrocytes[114] support this concept. If not successfully treated with antibiotics or eliminated by protective antibodies, inflammation then becomes chronic and does not resolve.

Activation of the immune system and, in particular, the early generation of protective anti-OspA and anti-OspB antibodies during *B. burgdorferi* infection would prevent or mitigate the development of chronic arthritis. Obviously, most of the spirochaetes are eliminated by antibody-mediated processes during their haematogenous spread or within the inflammatory lesions, and under optimal conditions this may lead to sterile immunity. On the other hand, some spirochaetes may escape the immune reaction by migrating into immunoprivileged sites or by their ability to gain entrance into and to survive intracellularly in EC[95,96] or fibroblasts[54]. In this case, spirochaetes would persist, even in the presence of optimal protective immune responses or of antibiotics and would create a permanent threat for induction of arthritis in the host.

Activation of the immune system by spirochaetes may also have deleterious effects on the host, as indicated particularly by the genetic linkage of chronic Lyme arthritis to genes of the MHC complex[74,88]. Thus, *B. burgdorferi*-specific T cells with pathogenic properties or autoreactive T cells generated during infection would invade, together with other cells, joint tissues and would participate either directly or indirectly in the pathological processes. Under these conditions, chronic arthritis could develop even after eradication of spirochaetes and would be insensitive both to protective antibodies and to antibiotic therapy.

For an optimal protection of the host against the development of arthritis it is therefore mandatory that protective antibodies are present at the time of exposure. Most probably the only way by which this could be achieved is by prophylactic immunization with an appropriate vaccine. In the case of infection of non-vaccinated individuals, simultaneous passive administration of protective antibodies may prevent the disease.

Acknowledgments

We are indebted to Drs S. Gay, L. Gern, Ch. Eckerskorn, N. Honarvar, S. Moter, M. Modolell, H. Mossman, C. Museteanu and M. Rittig for their collaboration in many of the experiments reported here. The expert technical assistance of G. Nerz, I. Neuman, M. Prestner U, Schirmer, T. Stehle and T. Tran is gratefully acknowledged. The authors wish to thank Drs U. Hurtenbach and J. Langhorne for their valuable suggestions and critical reviews of this manuscript. Work from the authors' laboratories described here was supported by grants from the BMFT (01 KI 8909/8, 01 KI 9001), from the Boehringer Ingelheim Fund and from SmithKline Beecham Biologicals.

References

1. Steere AC, Malawista SE, Snydman DR, et al. Lyme arthritis: An epidemic of oligoarthriticular arthritis in children and adults in three Connecticut communities. Arthritis Rheum. 1977; 20: 7–17.
2. Steere AC, Broderick TF, Malawista SW. Erythema chronicum migrans and Lyme disease: Epidemiologic evidence for a tick vector. Am J Epidemiol. 1978; 108: 312–321.
3. Burgdorfer W, Barbour AG, Hayes SF, Benach JL, Grunwaldt E, Davis JP. Lyme disease – A tick-borne spirochetosis? Science. 1982; 216: 1317–1319.
4. Barbour AG, Burgdorfer W, Hayes SF, Peter O, Aeschlimann A. Isolation of a cultivable spirochete from *Ixodes ricinus* ticks. Curr Microbiol. 1983; 8: 123–126.
5. Barbour AG, Hayes SF. Biology of Borrelia species. Ref Infect Dis. 1986; 50: 381–400.
6. Howe TR, Mayer LW, Barbour AG. A single recombinant plasmid expressing two major outer surface proteins of the Lyme disease spirochete. Science. 1985; 227: 645–646.
7. Hansen K, Bangsborg JM, Fjordvang H, Pedersen NS, Hindersson P. Immunochemical characterization of and isolation of the gene for a Borrelia burgdorferi immunodominant 60-kilodalton antigen common to a wide range of bacteria. Infect Immun. 1988; 56: 2047–2053.
8. Luft BJ, Gorevic PD, Jiang W, Munoz P, Dattwyler RJ. Immunologic and structural characterization of the dominant 66- to 73-kDa antigens of *Borrelia burgdorferi*. J Immunol. 1991; 146: 2776–2782.
9. Barbour AG, Tessier SL, Todd WJ. Lyme disease spirochetes and Ixodid tick spirochetes share a common surface antigenic determinant defined by a monoclonal antibody. Infect Immun. 1983; 41: 795–804.
10. Barbour AG, Hayes SF, Heiland RA, Schrumpf ME, Tessier SL. A Borrelia-specific monoclonal antibody binds to a flagellar protein. Infect Immun. 1986; 52: 549–554.
11. Barbour AG, Heiland RA, Howe TR. Heterogeneity of major proteins in Lyme disease borreliae: A molecular analysis of North American and European isolates. J Infect Dis. 1985; 152: 478–484.
12. Kramer MD, Schaible UE, Wallich R, Moter S, Petzoldt D, Simon MM. Characterization of Borrelia burgdorferi associated antigens by monoclonal antibodies. Immunobiology. 1990; 181: 357–360.
13. Bergström S, Bundoc VG, Barbour AG. Molecular analysis of linear plasmid-encoded major surface proteins, OspA and OspB, of the Lyme disease spirochate Borrelia burgdorferi. Mol Microbiol. 1989; 3: 479–486.
14. Wallich R, Schaible UE, Simon MM, Heiberger A, Kramer MD. Cloning and sequencing of the gene encoding the outer surface protein A (OspA) of a European *Borrelia burgdorferi*

isolate. Nucleic Acids Res. 1989; 17: 8864.
15. Gassmann GS, Kramer M, Göbel UB, Wallich R. Nucleotide sequence of a gene encoding the Borrelia burgdorferi flagellin. Nucl Acid Res. 1989; 17: 1590-
16. Wallich R, Moter SE, Simon MM, Ebnet K, Heiberger A, Kramer MD. The *Borrelia burgdorferi* flagellum-associated 41-kilodalton antigen (flagellin): Molecular cloning, expression, and amplification of the gene. Infect Immun. 1990; 58: 1711–1719.
17. Gassmann GS, Jacobs ES, Deutzmann R, Göbel UB. Analysis of the *Borrelia burgdorferi* GeHo *fla* gene and antigenic characterization of its gene product. J Bacteriol. 1991; 173: 1452–1459.
18. Shanafelt M-C, Hindersson P, Soderberg C, et al. T cell and antibody reactivity with the *Borrelia burgdorferi* 60-kDa heat shock protein in Lyme arthritis. J Immunol. 1991; 146: 3985–3992.
19. Steere AC. Lyme disease. N Engl J Med. 1989; 321: 586–596.
20. Afzelius A. Erythema chronicum migrans. Arch Dermatol et Venereol. 1921; 2: 120–125.
21. Herxheimer K, Hartmann K. Ueber Acrodermatitis chronica atrophicans. Arch Dermatol Syph. 1902; 61: 57–76.
22. Bannwarth A. Zur Klinik und Pathogenese der 'chronischen lymphozytären Meningitis'. Arch Psychiatr Nervenkr. 1944; 117: 161–185.
23. Asbrink E, Hovmark A. Early and late manifestations in Ixodes-borne borreliosis (Erythema migrans borreliosis, Lyme Borreliosis). Ann NY Acad Sci. 1988; 539: 4–15.
24. Weber K, Puzik A, Becker T. Erythema-migrans-Krankheit. Dtsch Med Wschr. 1983; 108: 1182–1190.
25. Ackermann R, Kabatzki J, Boisten HP, et al. Spirochäten-Ätiologie der Erythema-chronicum-migrans-Krankheit. Dtsch Med Wschr. 1984; 109: 92–97.
26. Steere AC, Schoen RT, Taylor E. The clinical evolution of Lyme arthritis. Ann Intern Med. 1987; 107: 725–731.
27. Pachner AR, Steere AC. The triad of neurologic abnormalities of Lyme disease. Neurol. 1985; 35: 47–53.
28. Marcus LC, Steere AC, Duray PH, Anderson AE, Mahoney EB. Fatal pancarditis in a patient with coexistent Lyme disease and Babesiosis. Ann Intern Med. 1985; 103: 374–376.
29. Ackermann R, Gellmer E, Rehse-Küpper B. Progressive Borrelien-Enzephalomyelitis. Chronische Manifestation der Erythema-chronicum-migrans Krankheit am Nervensystem. Dtsch Med Wschr. 1985; 110: 1039–1042.
30. Steere AC, Batsford WP, Weinberg M, et al. Lyme carditis: Cardiac abnormalities of Lyme disease. Ann Intern Med. 1980; 93: 8–16.
31. Ackermann R, Boisten HP, Kabatzki J, Runne U, Krüger K, Herrmann WP. Serumanti-körper gegen die Ixodes-ricinus-Spirochäte bei Acrodermatitis chronica atrophicans (Herxheimer). Dtsch Med Wschr. 1984; 109: 6–10.
32. Herzer P, Wilske B, Preac-Mursic V, Schierz G, Schattenkirchner M, Zöllner N. Lyme arthritis: Clinical features, serological, and radiographic findings of cases in Germany. Klin Wschr. 1986; 64: 206–215.
33. Wilske B, Preac-Mursic V, Schierz G, Kühbeck R, Barbour AG, Kramer M. Antigenic variability of Borrelia burgdorferi. Ann NY Acad Sci. 1988; 539: 126–143.
34. Wilske B, Barbour AG, Bergström S, Soutschek E, Wallich R. Antigenic variation among strains of B. burgdorferi (Antigenic heterogeneity). 1992; Summary of the Annecy Meeting on 'Molecular Biology of Spirochaetes'.
35. Wallich R, Helmes C, Schaible UE, et al. Evaluation of genetic divergence among Borrelia burgdorferi isolates using OspA, fla, HSP60 and HSP70 gene probes. Infect Immunol. 1992; 60: 4856–4866.
36. Lawson JP, Rahn DW. Lyme disease and radiologic findings in Lyme arthritis. Am J Roentgenol. 1992; 158: 1065–1069.
37. Johnston YE, Duray PH, Steere AC. Lyme arthritis. Spirochetes found in synovial microangiopathic lesions. Am J Pathol. 1985; 118: 26–34.
38. Steere AC, Duray PH, Butcher EC. Spirochetal antigens and lymphoid cell surface markers in Lyme. Arthritis Rheum. 1988; 31: 487–495.
39. Schoenen J, Sianardgainko J, Carpentier M, Reznik M. Myositis during *Borrelia-burgdorferi* infection (Lyme disease). J Neurol Neurosurg Psychiatry. 1989; 52: 1002–1005.
40. Reimers CD, Pongratz DE, Neubert U, et al. Myositis caused by Borrelia burgdorferi:

report of four cases. J Neurol Sci. 1990; 91: 215–226.

41. Atlas E, Novak SN, Duray PH, Steere AC. Lyme myositis: Muscle invasion by Borrelia burgdorferi. Ann Intern Med. 1988; 109: 245–246.

42. Duray PH, Steere AC. Clinical pathology correlation of Lyme disease by stage. Ann NY Acad Sci. 1988; 539: 65–79.

43. deKoning J, Hoogkamp-Korstanje AA, Van Der Linde MR, Crijna HJGM. Demonstration of spirochetes in cardiac biopsies in patients with Lyme disease. J Infect Dis. 1989; 1: 150–153.

44. Schmidli J, Hunziker T, Moesli P, Schaad UB. Cultivation of *Borrelia burgdorferi* from joint fluid three months after treatment of facial palsy due to Lyme borreliosis. J Infect Dis. 1988; 158: 1905–1906.

45. Debue M, Gautier P, Hackel C, et al. Detection of *Borrelia burgdorferi* in biological samples using the polymerase chain reaction assay. Res Microbiol. 1991; 142: 565–572.

46. Moter SE, Wallich R, Simon MM, Petzoldt D, Kramer MD. Die Polymerase-Kettenreaktion zum Nachweis von Borrelia burgdorferi. Ärztl Lab. 1991; 37: 88–94.

47. Moter SE, Wallich R, Simon MM, Kramer MD. Nachweis von B. burgdorferi DNS mit der Polymerase-Ketten-Reaktion (PCR) in läsionaler Haut von Erythema chronicum migrans und Acrodermatitis chronica atrophicans. In Massler D, ed. Infection, Fortschrifte der Infektiologie: Lyme Borreliose. München: MMV Medizin Verlag; 1992: 58–70.

48. Steere AC. Pathogenesis of Lyme arthritis: Indications for rheumatic disease. Ann NY Acad Sci. 1988; 539: 87–92.

49. Switalski LM, Butcher WG, Barker JR, Hook M, Piesman J, Johnson BJB. Interactions of Borrelia burgdorferi with cartilage proteoglycan (PGC). V Int Conf Lyme Borreliosis 1992; 160.

50. Habicht GS, Beck G, Benach JL, Coleman JL, Leichtling KD. Lyme disease spirochetes induce human and murine interleukin 1. J Immunol. 1985; 134: 3147–3154.

51. Defosse DL, Johnson RC. In vitro and in vivo induction of tumor necrosis factor alpha by *Borrelia burgdorferi*. Infect Immun. 1992; 60: 1109–1113.

52. Dattwyler RJ, Halperin JJ. Failure of tetracycline therapy in early Lyme disease. Arthritis Rheum. 1987; 30: 448–450.

53. Preac-Mursic V, Weber K, Pfister HW, et al. Survival of Borrelia burgdorferi in antibiotically treated patients with Lyme borreliosis. Infection. 1989; 17: 355–359.

54. Georgilis K, Peacocke M, Klempner MS. Fibroblast protect the Lyme disease spirochete, Borrelia burgdorferi, from ceftriaxone *in vitro*. J Infect Dis. 1992; 166: 440–444.

55. Barbour AG, Burgdorfer W, Grunwaldt E, Steere AC. Antibodies of patients with Lyme disease to components of the Ixodes dammini spirochete. J Clin Invest. 1983; 72: 504–515.

56. Craft JE, Grodzicki RL, Steere AC. Antibody response in Lyme disease: Evaluation of diagnostic tests. J Infect Dis. 1984; 149: 789–795.

57. Dattwyler RJ, Volkman DJ, Halperin JJ, Luft BJ, Thomas J, Golightly MG. Specific immune response in Lyme borreliosis: Characterization of T cell and B cell responses to Borrelia burgdorferi. Ann NY Acad Sci. 1988; 539: 93–102.

58. Dattwyler RJ. Seronegative Lyme disease: Dissociation of specific T- and B-lymphocyte responses to Borrelia burgdorferi. N Engl J Med. 1991; 319: 1441–1446.

59. Magnarelli LA, Anderson JF, Johnson RC. Cross-reactivity in serological tests for Lyme disease and other spirochetal infections. J Infect Dis. 1987; 156: 183–188.

60. Olsson I, Von Stedingk L-V, Hanson H-S, Von Stedingk M, Åsbrink E, Hovmark A. Comparison of four different serological methods for detection of antibodies to *Borrelia burgdorferi* in erythema migrans. Acta Derm Venereol (Stockh). 1991; 71: 127–133.

61. Simpson WJ, Schrumpf ME, Schwan TG. Reactivity of human Lyme borreliosis sera with a 39-kilodalton antigen specific to *Borrelia burgdorferi*. J Clin Microbiol. 1990; 28: 1329–1337.

62. Cruz M, Hansen K, Ernerudh J, Steere AC, Link H. Lyme arthritis: Oligoclonal anti-*Borrelia burgdorferi* IgG antibodies occur in joint fluid and serum. Scand J Immunol. 1991; 33: 61–71.

63. Kalish RA, Leong JM, Steere AC. Evidence for a deleterious immune response to the Osp proteins of Borrelia burgdorferi in chronic Lyme arthritis. V Int Conf Lyme Borreliosis. 1992; 147.

64. Nadal D, Taverna C, Hitzig WH. Immunoblot analysis of antibody binding to polypeptides

of Borrelia burgdorferi in children with different clinical manifestations. Pediatr Res. 1989; 26: 377–382.

65. Sigal LH, Steere AC, Dwyer JM. In vivo and in vitro evidence of B cell hyperactivity during Lyme disease. J Rheumatol. 1988; 15: 648–654.

66. Zoschke DC, Skemp AA, Defosse DL. Lymphoproliferative responses to *Borrelia burgdorferi* in Lyme disease. Ann Intern Med. 1991; 114: 285–289.

67. Schoenfeld R, Araneo B, Ma Y, Yang L, Weis JJ. Demonstration of a B-lymphocyte mitogen produced by the Lyme disease pathogen, *Borrelia burgdorferi*. Infect Immun. 1992; 60: 455–464.

68. De Souza MS, Fikrig E, Smith AL, Flavell RA, Barthold DW. Nonspecific proliferative responses of murine lymphocytes to *Borrelia burgdorferi* antigens. J Infect Dis. 1992; 165: 471–478.

69. Hardin JA, Walker LC, Steere AC, Malawista SE. Immune complexes and the evolution of Lyme arthritis: Dissemination and localization of abnormal C1q binding activity. N Engl J Med. 1979; 301: 1358–1363.

70. Neumann A, Schlesier M, Schneider H, Vogt A, Peter HH. Frequencies of Borrelia burgdorferi-reactive T lymphocytes in Lyme arthritis. Rheumatol Int. 1989; 9: 237–241.

71. Yoshinari NH, Reinhardt BN, Steere AC. T cell responses to polypeptide fractions of *Borrelia burgdorferi* in patients with Lyme arthritis. Arthritis Rheum. 1991; 34: 707–713.

72. Yssel H, Nakamoto T, Schneider P, et al. Analysis of T lymphocytes cloned from the synovial fluid and blood of a patient with Lyme arthritis. Int Immunol. 1990; 2: 1081–1089.

73. Yssel H, Shanafelt M-C, Soderberg C, Schneider PV, Anzola J, Peltz G. *Borrelia burgdorferi* activates a T helper type 1-like T cell subset in Lyme arthritis. J Exp Med. 1991; 174: 593–601.

74. Steere AC, Dwyer E, Winchester R. Association of chronic Lyme arthritis with HLA-DR4 and HLA-DR2 alleles. N Engl J Med. 1990; 323: 219–223.

75. Beck G, Benach JL, Habicht GS. Isolation of interleukin 1 from joint fluids of patients with Lyme disease. J Rheumatol. 1989; 16: 800–806.

76. Georgilis K, Noring R, Steere AC, Klempner MS. Neutrophil chemotactic factors in synovial fluids of patients with Lyme disease. Arthritis Rheum. 1991; 34: 770–775.

77. Steere AC, Brinckerhoff CE, Miller DJ, Drinker H, Harris ED, Malawista SE. Elevated levels of collagenase and prostaglandin E2 from synovium associated with erosion of cartilage and bone in a patient with chronic Lyme arthritis. Arthritis Rheum. 1980; 23: 591–599.

78. Beck G, Benach JL, Habicht GS. Isolation, preliminary chemical characterization, and biological activity of *Borrelia burgdorferi* peptidoglycan. Biochem Biophys Res Commun. 1990; 167: 89–95.

79. Beck G, Habicht GS, Benach JL, Coleman JL. Chemical and biologic characterization of a lipopolysaccharide extracted from the Lyme disease spirochete (Borrelia burgdorferi). J Infect Dis. 1985; 152: 108–117.

80. Barthold SW, Moody KD, Terwilliger GA, Jacoby RO, Steere AC. An animal model for Lyme arthritis. Ann NY Acad Sci. 1988; 539: 264–273.

81. Moody KD, Barthold SW, Terwilliger GA, Beck DS, Hansen GM, Jacoby RO. Experimental chronic Lyme Borreliosis in Lewis rats. Am J Trop Med Hyg. 1990; 42: 165–174.

82. Schmitz JL, Schell RF, Hejka A. Induction of Lyme arthritis in LSH hamsters. Infection and Immunity. 1988; 56: 2336–2342.

83. Hejka A, Schmitz JL, England DM, Callister SM, Schell RF. Histopathology of Lyme arthritis in LSH hamsters. Am J Pathol. 1989; 134: 1113–1123.

84. Schaible UE, Kramer MD, Museteanu C, Zimmer G, Mossmann H, Simon MM. The severe combined immunodeficiency (*scid*) mouse. A laboratory model for the analysis of Lyme arthritis and carditis. J Exp Med. 1989; 170: 1427–1432.

85. Schaible UE, Gay S, Museteanu C, Kramer MD, Zimmer G, Eichmann K, Museteanu U, Simon MM. Lyme Borreliosis in the severe combined immunodeficiency (*scid*) mouse manifests predominantly in the joints, heart, and liver. Am J Pathol. 1990; 137: 811–820.

86. Barthold SW, Beck DS, Hansen GM, Terwilliger GA, Moody KD. Lyme Borreliosis in selected strains and ages of laboratory mice. J Infect Dis. 1990; 162: 133–138.

87. Barthold SW, Persing DH, Armstrong AL, Peeples RA. Kinetics of *Borrelia burgdorferi* dissemination and evolution of disease after intradermal inoculation of mice. Am J Pathol.

1991; 139: 263–273.

88. Schaible UE, Kramer MD, Wallich R, Tran T, Simon MM. Experimental *Borrelia burgdorferi* infection in inbred mouse strains: Antibody response and association of H-2 genes with resistance and susceptibility to development of arthritis. Eur J Immunol. 1991; 21: 2397–2405.

89. Schwan TG, Kime KK, Schrumpf ME, Coe JE, Simpson WJ. Antibody response in white-footed mice (Peromyscus leucopus) experimentally infected with the Lyme disease spirochete (Borrelia burgdorferi). Infection and Immunity. 1989; 57: 3445–3451.

90. Bosma GC, Custer RP, Bosma MJ. A severe combined immunodeficiency mutation in the mouse. Nature. 1983; 301: 527–530.

91. Museteanu C, Schaible UE, Stehle T, Kramer MD, Simon MM. Myositis in mice inoculated with *Borrelia burgdorferi*. Am J Pathol. 1991; 139: 1267–1271.

92. Gern L, Schaible UE, Simon MM. Mode of inoculation of the Lyme disease agent Borrelia burgdorferi influences infection and immune responses in inbred strains of mice. J Infect Dis. 1993; 167: 971–975.

93. Zimmer G, Schaible UE, Kramer MD, Mall G, Museteanu C, Simon MM. Lyme carditis in immunodeficient mice during experimental infection of *Borrelia burgdorferi*. Virchows Arch [A]. 1990; 417: 129–135.

94. Schaible UE, Wallich R, Kramer MD, et al. The immune response in Lyme disease: Lessons from the mouse model. In: Curr Commun Cell Mol Biol. 1992; 6: 243–262.

95. Comstock LE, Thomas DD. Penetration of endothelial cell monolayers by Borrelia burgdorferi. Infection and Immunity. 1989; 57: 1626–1628.

96. Szcepanski A, Furie MB, Benach JL, Lane BP, Fleit HB. Interaction between Borrelia burgdorferi and endothelium in vitro. J Clin Invest. 1990; 85: 1637–1647.

97. Garcia-Monco JC, Villar BF, Alen JC, Benach JL. *Borrelia burgdorferi* in the central nervous system: Experimental and clinical evidence for early invasion. J Infect Dis. 1990; 161: 1187–1193.

98. Liu Y, Janeway CJ. Microbial induction of costimulatory activity for CD4 T-cell growth. Int Immunol. 1991; 3: 323–332.

99. Schaible UE, Kramer MD, Justus CWE, Museteanu C, Simon MM. Demonstration of antigen-specific T cells and histopathological alterations in mice experimentally inoculated with Borrelia burgdorferi. Infect Immun. 1989; 57: 41–47.

100. Benach JL, Coleman JL, Garcia-Monco JC, Deponte PC. Biological activity of Borrelia burgdorferi antigens. Ann NY Acad Sci. 1988; 539: 115–125.

101. Schaible UE, Wallich R, Kramer MD, Museteanu C, Simon MM. Protection against Borrelia burgdorferi infection in SCID mice is conferred by presensitized spleen- as well as B cells but not by T cells alone. 1993; submitted.

102. Schaible UE, Kramer MD, Eichmann K, Modolell M, Museteanu C, Simon MM. Monoclonal antibodies specific for the outer surface protein A (OspA) of Borrelia burgdorferi prevent Lyme Borreliosis in severe combined immunodeficiency (scid) mice. Proc Natl Acad Sci USA. 1990; 87: 3768–3772.

103. Simon MM, Schaible UE, Kramer MD, Müller-Hermelink HK, Wallich R. Recombinant outer surface protein A of Borrelia burgdorferi induces antibodies protective against spirochetal infection in mice. J Infect Dis. 1991; 164: 1230–1232.

104. Simon MM, Schaible UE, Wallich R, Kramer MD. A mouse model for *Borrelia burgdorferi* infection: Approach to a vaccine against Lyme disease. Immunol Today. 1991; 12: 11–16.

105. Fikrig E, Barthold SW, Kantor FS, Flavell RA. Protection of mice against the Lyme disease agent by immunizing with recombinant OspA. Science. 1990; 250: 553–556.

106. Fikrig E, Barthold SW, Marcantonio N, Deponte K, Kantor FS, Flavell RA. Roles of OspA, OspB, and flagellin in protective immunity to Lyme Borreliosis in laboratory mice. Infect Immun. 1992; 60: 657–661.

107. Johnson RC, Kodner C, Russel M. Passive immunization of hamsters against infection with the Lyme disease spirochete. Infect Immun. 1986; 53: 713–714.

108. Schwan TG, Burgdorfer W, Schrumpf ME, Karstens RH. The urinary bladder, a consistent source of Borrelia burgdorferi in experimentally infected white-footed mice (*Peromysetes Leucoptes*). J Clin Microbiol. 1988; 26: 893–895.

109. Greene RT, Walker RL, Nicholson WL, et al. Immunoblot analysis of immunoglobulin G response to the Lyme disease agent (Borrelia burgdorferi) in experimentally and naturally

infected dogs. J Clin Microbiol. 1988; 26: 648–653.

110. Habicht GS, Katona LI, Benach JL. Cytokines and pathogenesis of neuroborreliosis: *Borrelia burgdorferi* induces glioma cells to secrete interleukin-6. J Infect Dis. 1991; 164: 568–574.

111. Porat R, Poutsiaka DD, Miller LC, Granowitz EV, Dinarello CA. Interleukin-1 (IL-1) receptor blockade reduces endotoxin and *Borrelia burgdorferi*-stimulated IL-8 synthesis in human mononuclear cells. FASEB J. 1992; 6: 2482–2486.

112. Thomas DD, Comstock LE. Interaction of Lyme disease spirochetes with cultured eucaryotic cells. Infect Immun. 1989; 57: 1324–1326.

113. Riley BS, Oppenheimer-Marks N, Hansen EJ, Radolf JD, Norgard MV. Virulent *Treponema pallidum* activates human vascular endothelial cells. J Infect Dis. 1992; 165: 484–493.

114. Oppenheim JJ, Kovacs EJ, Matsushima K, Durum SK. There is more than one interleukin 1. Immun Today. 1986; 7: 45–56.

115. Mantovani A, Dejana E. Cytokines as communication signals between leukocytes and endothelial cells. Immunol Today. 1989; 10: 370–375.

116. Wevers MD. Cytokines and macrophages. In: Kunkel SC and Remick GR, eds. Cytokines in Health and Disease. NY, Basel, Hong Kong: Marcel Dekker Inc.; 1992: 327–352.

117. Dayer JM, deRochemoteix B, Burrus B, Dembczik S, Dinarello C. Human recombinant Interleukin-1 stimulates collagenase and prostaglandin E2 production by synovial cells. J Clin Invest. 1986; 77: 645–648.

118. Karmiol S, Phan SK. Fibroblasts and cytokines. In: Kunkel SC and Remick GR, eds. Cytokines in Health and Disease. NY, Basel, Hong Kong: Marcel Dekkar Inc.; 1992: 271–296.

119. Putzker M, Walscheid R. Die Diagnostik von Infektionen mit Borrelia burgdorferi. II. Diagnostik und epidemiologische Aspekte der Lyme-Erkrankung. Wehrmed Wschr. 1988; 32: 257–266.

120. Honarvar N, Böggameyer E, Galanos C. et al. Borelia burgdorferei infection in mice: aspects of inflammation and immune reponse. Proceeding of the 2nd European Symposium on Lyme Borreliosis. New York: Plenum. 1993; in press.

121. Schaible UE, Gern L, Wallich R, Kramer MD, Prester M, Simon MM. Distinct pattern of protective antibodies are generated against Borrelia burgdorferei in mice experimentally inoculated with high and low doses of antigen. Immunol Lett. 1993; 36: 219–226.

122. Moter SE. Nachweis und Charakterisierung das Ervagers aber Lyme Borreliose, Borrelia burgdorferei, mit der Polymerase-Kettenreaktion (PCR). Dissertation; 1993, Darmstadt, Germany.

123. Modolell M, Schaible UE, Gooralita I, Riley M, Simon MM. The role of macrophages in experimental Lyme borreliosis. Patholbiologie. 1992; 60/1: 23.

12
Retroviral Arthritis in Animals and Man

G. D. HARKISS

INTRODUCTION

Retroviruses are classified into three families: oncoviruses, which cause cancer, lentiviruses, which cause 'slow virus disease'; and spumaviruses, which are generally thought not to cause disease. The lentiviruses, which include ovine maedi–visna virus (MVV), caprine arthritis–encephalitis virus (CAEV) and the human and simian immunodeficiency viruses (HIV and SIV), cause chronic inflammatory and degenerative disease of the lungs, brain, joints, mammary glands and lymphoid tissue characterized by insidious onset, slow progression, and variable clinical course[1,2]. CAEV was the first lentivirus to be associated with naturally occurring chronic arthritis, and was shown to cause a similar inflammatory joint disease when inoculated experimentally into newborn goats[3]. Subsequently, it was found that sheep naturally or experimentally infected with MVV also developed chronic inflammatory arthritis[4,5]. More recently, it has become clear that HIV infection is associated with a variety of joint problems[6], and that SIV can induce chronic inflammatory joint disease in both natural and experimental infections in monkeys[7,8]. The association with joint disease is not restricted to lentiviruses, but is also found in patients infected with the oncovirus human T-cell leukaemia virus 1 (HTLV-I)[9].

The pattern and extent of clinical disease caused by MVV and CAEV varies within and between infected individuals, but chronic inflammatory disease is common to all affected tissues and the animals become progressively cachectic. Organ-specific changes such as cartilage degradation in joints, demyelination in brain and spinal cord, and interstitial disease in lungs may accompany or follow the inflammatory changes. Infected individuals vary in which organ system is primarily affected and rarely have clinical disease at all sites. However, subclinical disease at these other sites is common, indicating that infected animals have a widespread multiorgan disease in which one or more target tissues become clinically diseased with time. The most salient feature of the disease syndromes caused by MVV, CAEV and other lentiviruses is that the virus infection persists for life. The consequences of this persistence on immune cell activation and dysregulation of normal intracellular function are likely to underlie much of the pathology observed with these infections. The focus of this article will be mainly on joint disease caused by MVV and CAEV, though available data on HIV and HTLV-I will be included for comparison.

CLINICAL DISEASE AND JOINT PATHOLOGY

Ovine and caprine lentiviruses

The arthritic disease caused by MVV and CAEV has been the subject of several recent reviews[10-14]. The prevalence of clinical arthritis in CAEV-infected goats has been estimated to be between 20–30% of animals[15-17]. However, in a flock of MVV-infected sheep studied by the author, less than 5% of MVV-infected animals were clinically arthritic, although a substantially higher proportion had subclinical joint disease. The clinical signs include lameness or stiffness accompanied by unilateral or bilateral swelling of the carpal joints due to soft tissue swelling and increased amounts of synovial fluid (SF). Radiography often shows discrete deposits due to mineralization[16,18-20]. The joint changes described in naturally- and experimentally-infected sheep and goats appear to be identical[5,20], and cross-infection studies have shown that the caprine and ovine viruses can induce arthritis in sheep and goats respectively[21]. The carpal joints are affected most frequently, followed by the tarsal, stifle and occasionally the atlanto-occipital joints. Both viruses initiate an inflammatory process involving joints, tendon sheaths, bursae and capsular tissue[3,4,16,18]. The process in natural infections usually has an insidious onset, which may be followed by a rapidly progressive arthritis or more usually by a slow chronic course interspersed by acute inflammatory episodes[3,15,20]. In animals infected experimentally via the joint, the disease starts as a proliferative synovitis which progresses to marked synovial proliferation, hyperplasia, hyperaemia, and villous hypertrophy[3,18,22,23]. The synovial lining layer is variably thickened depending on the severity of the inflammatory changes, and vessels often show marked smooth muscle hyperplasia[24].

The synovium is infiltrated to varying degrees by lymphocytes, macrophages (Mϕ) and plasma cells. In early disease, the inflammatory infiltrate is present just beneath the synovial lining layer and around blood vessels. The infiltrate aggregates into follicular- and germinal centre-like structures resembling organized lymphoid tissue in advanced disease[4,18,21]. In a proportion of cases, pannus formation and cartilage erosion occur[18,19]. Rarely, severe cartilage erosion and destruction of bone occur giving rise to joint deformities.

Phenotypic analysis of the inflammatory infiltrate in the synovial membrane (SM) and SF of MVV-infected sheep showed that increased numbers of all major subsets of T cells were present[24-26]. The CD8 + T cell subset tended to predominate over CD4 + and $\gamma\delta$ T cells, although in some SF and SM $\gamma\delta$ T cells were the main subset[24,25]. However, although normal SF and SM had very few total lymphocytes, a similar predominance of CD8 + over CD4 + T cells was noted. Thus the T cell subset ratios in MVV-infected animals appears to represent an exaggerated version of the normal trafficking pattern of these cells through joints. CD8 + T cells tended to be found just under the synovial lining layer. CD4 + T cells were also found at this site but in much lower numbers[24]. Both of these T cell subsets were observed in a perivascular distribution in approximately equal numbers. In contrast, $\gamma\delta$ T cells were distributed randomly throughout the synovium. B cells were few in number in both SF and SM, although plasma cells could be distinguished in SM by histology[24]. At present, no information is available on the specificity or function or these infiltrating lymphocytes.

In SF and SM from normal sheep, cells with the morphological characteristics of macrophages (Mϕ) or dendritic cells (DC) are present. These cells stain with monoclonal antibodies that recognize ovine alveolar and mammary Mϕ[24,25]. In addition, some of these Mϕ/DC react with monoclonals to sheep CD1[24,25], a marker found on sheep afferent lymph DC and skin Langerhan's cells (LC)[27] which may act as a restriction element for $\gamma\delta$ T cells. In addition to staining with anti-Mϕ monoclonals, some of the lining layer cells stain with anti-CD1 antibodies, suggesting that they might have similar functions to DC. In MVV-infected sheep, increased staining for CD1 was observed in both SF and SM, including the lining layer[24,25]. In adult sheep, as in man, the lining layer normally expresses Class II molecules of the Major Histocompatibility Complex (MHC). However, staining for Class II molecules was greatly increased in MVV-infected animals over normal on Mϕ/DC in the subsynovium, lining layer and SF[24,25]. The upregulation of MHC Class II was not confined to the Mϕ/DC, but was observed by sequential sectioning on the CD8 + and CD4 + T cells residing just below the lining layer and in a perivascular distribution.

The arthritis induced by CAEV and MVV is thus characterized by the presence of both activated Mϕ/DC and lymphocytes and increased expression of MHC Class II and CD1 molecules, and is consistent with a disease process driven by chronic antigen presentation and lymphoproliferation.

Joint disease associated with HIV and SIV

Although joint disease was not reported in the early descriptions of HIV infection, it has become clear from recent studies that HIV infection is associated with the development of a variety of arthritic conditions. Several reviews on this subject are available[6,28-30]. The commonest joint problem encountered in HIV patients resembles that found in Reiter's syndrome or psoriatic arthritis[31-34]. The prevalence of Reiter's syndrome in HIV-infected individuals is about 5%, which represents about a 100-fold increase over that in normal populations. The arthritis is persistent and more painful in many patients than that occurring in non-HIV-associated Reiter's syndrome. It has been estimated that approximately one-third of HIV-associated Reiter's cases are due to coinfection by micro-organisms known to precipitate reactive arthritis (e.g. *Salmonella*, *Shigella*, *Yersinia* and *Campylobacter*), while a further third may involve infection by organisms that do not usually induce reactive arthritis (e.g. *Mycobacterium avium intracellulare*, *Giardia lamblia*, and *Borrelia burgdorferi*)[30]. The lack of any obvious inciting enteric, urogenital or other opportunistic infection in the remainder of cases has raised the suggestion that HIV itself may be arthritogenic. It was noted in early studies that HIV-associated Reiter's syndrome could occur in patients with marked deficiencies in circulating CD4+ T cell levels[31]. Some patients had an absolute increase in the numbers of CD8+ T cells in blood. Although blood T cell counts may not reflect joint changes, the observations suggested a possible role for CD8+ T cells in the arthritic disease rather than the CD4+ T cells usually found in the synovium of Reiter's syndrome patients. A study of synovial tissue from HIV-infected individuals with arthritis indeed showed a predominance of CD8+ T cells, lending support to this suggestion[35]. The joint disease in these patients thus shows some resemblance to CAEV- and MVV-induced arthritis.

In addition to reactive or psoriatic arthritis, several other joint problems have been described in HIV-infected patients. Rosenberg and colleagues[36] described an acute symmetric polyarthritis which resembled rheumatoid arthritis (RA) in some respects, including marginal erosions and joint deviations and deformities. Another inflammatory arthropathy was described consisting of painful but short-lived (1–6 weeks) synovitis which responded to therapy[6]. The synovium contained a mononuclear inflammatory infiltrate indicating an ongoing chronic process. HIV was isolated from the SF of one patient, suggesting that this 'AIDS-associated arthritis' may be due directly to the lentivirus infection. Septic arthritis has also been reported[37,38], though the incidence is lower than might be expected from the number of opportunistic infections associated with the development of AIDS. A post mortem study of patients with AIDS showed extensive synovial fibrosis and hyperplasia of arterial vessel walls[39].

The question of whether HIV can cause arthritis itself remains uncertain. However, SIV, a closely related primate lentivirus, can induce chronic inflammatory synovitis experimentally in monkeys[8]. The inflammatory infiltrate consisted of lymphocytes and macrophages in a perivascular distribution. In advanced cases, there was a tendency to form syncytia in both the lining layer and the subsynovium, and viral antigen was detected in the syncytial structures. These results suggest that lentiviruses including HIV may have a general propensity to cause joint disease in susceptible hosts.

HTLV-I-associated arthritis

Recent studies have indicated that HTLV-I may cause inflammatory synovitis and erosive joint disease[9,40–43]. The disease is characterized by synovitis, villous proliferation and synovial cell hyperplasia, with infiltration of the synovium by leukaemic lymphocytes but without germinal centre formation[42]. Erosions in cartilage and bone and swan-neck deformities were observed in some patients[9], while in one case a severe osteolytic disease was present[41]. A role for HTLV-I in the joint disease is suggested by the observations that the virus was detected by immunostaining in the synovium in some patients, and that antibody to the virus core proteins p19, p24 and p28 was present in the synovial fluid.

The mechanisms underlying the development of chronic inflammatory arthritis induced by lentiviruses and HTLV-I are not understood. However, studies of lentiviral pathogenesis have indicated that the virus/host cell interaction at the subcellular level and the host's immune response to viral antigens play a crucial role in the disease process. In the following sections, these aspects will be discussed in more detail with reference mainly to CAEV and MVV, but also to HIV and HTLV-I where appropriate.

RETROVIRUS STRUCTURE AND FUNCTION

The genomic arrangement of retroviruses consists of three groups of genes encoding the viral structural proteins, i.e. core proteins (*gag*), reverse transcriptase (*pol*), and the surface glycoproteins (*env*), flanked at either end by the long terminal repeat (LTR) sequences containing the viral promoters and enhancers. In addition, the lentiviruses contain several non-structural regulatory genes which control the rate and extent of viral replication[2,44]. In MVV and CAEV these include genes for the transactivating proteins tat and rev, and a protein, Q, which shows sequence homology with the HIV protein, vif, involved in enhancing viral infectivity[2,45]. HTLV-I possesses regulatory genes encoding proteins analogous to tat and rev called P40^{tax} and rex respectively[46].

The HIV and MVV tat proteins act on an RNA response element named TAR in the viral LTR to increase the amounts of steady state viral RNA[44,47]. The degree of upregulation by MVV and CAEV tat on the LTR *in vitro* is modest compared to HIV-1 tat's effect on the HIV LTR[55–58]. This is presumably due to these proteins operating through different mechanisms. In the case of HIV, the tat protein binds either directly or indirectly through cellular proteins to the TAR region on viral RNA via a highly ordered stem-loop secondary structure and requires the cellular factor NFκB for full activation[44]. In contrast, MVV tat appears to act on LTR sequences which resemble sites for the cellular enhancer factors AP1 and AP4[47].

The P40^{tax} transactivating protein of HTLV-I is thought to mediate its effect indirectly through the interaction of host cell transcription factors with a cyclic AMP-responsive element in the viral LTR[48]. In addition to functioning intracellularly as transactivating proteins, P40^{tax} and HIV tat can act extracellularly to upregulate viral transcription *in vitro*[49]. However, it is not known if this occurs *in vivo*, or if MVV or CAEV tat can mediate transactivation in this way.

The lentiviral rev proteins are thought to function as posttranscriptional regulators that are critical in determining whether the viral structural proteins are expressed or not[50,51]. In HIV, MVV and CAEV, rev functions by binding to the rev responsive element (RRE) target sequence on mRNA transcripts which is incorporated within the sequences encoding the transmembrane component of the envelope glycoprotein[51,52]. It is thought that once rev concentrations reach a critical level it binds to the RRE and inhibits splicing of the transcripts, thereby enabling the larger mRNA molecules encoding the viral structural proteins to be exported to the cytoplasm for translation[53]. The MVV and CAEV Q proteins, like vif, are produced late in the replication cycle and are found exclusively in the cytoplasm[54].

LENTIVIRUS LIFE CYCLE

Life cycle *in vitro*

The life cycle of lentiviruses *in vitro* begins with the virus binding via its surface envelope glycoprotein to a receptor on the host cell membrane[2,44]. In the case of HIV, the main receptor is the CD4 molecule expressed on T cells and at lower levels on Mϕ and other cell types[44]. The receptor for MVV or CAEV is not known, but recent work has shown that MHC class II molecules bind MVV *in vitro* suggesting that they may act as components of the MVV receptor[55], while another study found proteins of 15, 30 and 50 kD to be involved[56]. Following internalization via receptor-mediated endocytosis or fusion with the cell membrane, the virus uncoats and the viral RNA is transcribed into proviral DNA by the enzyme reverse transcriptase which is carried as part of the intact virion. Upon entering the nucleus, some of the proviral DNA may integrate into the host genome while the rest remains as linear molecules. When the host cell becomes activated the proviral DNA is transcribed to produce genomic RNA and several messenger RNA species which become translated in the cytosol into viral structural proteins. The genomic RNA, reverse transcriptase and structural proteins are assembled into new virions just below the plasma membrane or in cytoplasmic vacuoles[57]. Dissemination of the infection takes place either by viral particles budding from the cell membrane, causing membrane fusion between adjacent cells, or by lysis, depending on the cell type. The infection in tissue culture cells usually results in a syncytial cytopathic effect with complete destruction of the cell monolayer within a few days depending on the amount of input virus.

Replication *in vivo*

Viral replication *in vivo* appears to be greatly restricted compared to the generally permissive state of cells in tissue culture. Infectious MVV or CAEV can be isolated from blood monocytes by cocultivation with permissive cells such as synovial fibroblasts or choroid plexus cells. However, using virus titrations, *in situ* hybridization, or immunohistology techniques it has been shown that very few cells are productively infected *in vivo*, and that the numbers of viral DNA positive cells greatly exceed the numbers of viral antigen-positive cells[1,58,59]. In joints, CAEV has been found in the synovium using *in situ* hybridization[60]. In one study, 1/400 SF cells of a clinically arthritic sheep harboured MVV by infectious centre assay[26]. CAEV, however, could be isolated more frequently at early rather than later time points following experimental infection[18,61]. The low rate of productive infection *in vivo* is paradoxical given the extent of inflammation in target tissues and the evidence supporting a major role for anti-viral responses in the disease process (see later).

Possible mechanisms of virus restriction

The reasons for this relative lack of live virus or viral antigens *in vivo* are not known. However, several lines of evidence suggest that (1) cell tropism, (2) restricted replication, or (3) anti-viral cytokines may be important.

Cell tropism

Lentiviruses are tropic for cells of the monocyte/Mϕ lineage, with HIV and SIV additionally infecting CD4 + T cells and DC[2,57,62]. A recent report provided evidence that MVV also infects DC[63]. Quantitative analysis of HIV has shown that the number of virions released by Mϕ into culture fluids was one or two orders of magnitude less than by T cells, despite the former having a five-fold greater amount of HIV RNA[57]. This was thought to be due to the infection in T cells being lytic in nature, compared to Mϕ where new virions budded internally into cytoplasmic vacuoles and were retained within the cell. Given the very low frequency of infection in T cells and that Mϕ appear to be the predominant cell type infected *in vivo*, the restricted release of virions except via cell fusion might explain in part the low number of HIV antigen-positive cells in target tissues. MVV and CAEV infected Mϕ probably retain their virions in a similar way.

Restricted replication

In addition to the narrow set of target cells infected *in vivo*, mechanisms exist which slow the rate of viral replication. HIV, MVV and CAEV exist in one of three replicative states *in vivo*: latent, restricted or productive. There is likely to be a mixture of these states at any one time and the relative balance may differ within and between animals and target tissues depending on genetic, environmental or other factors. The emergence from latency of MVV and CAEV depends on the normal maturation of infected monocytes to mature Mϕ following tissue localization. In sheep and goats, the bone marrow is thought to act as a central reservoir for latently-infected promonocytes, with approximately 2% of cells in infected foci expressing viral RNA[58]. After release from the bone marrow and circulation as monocytes these cells move into tissues and differentiate into adult Mϕ. At this point the cells are capable of supporting a degree of viral replication, but only after the cells are activated. In mice transgenic for the MVV LTR, Mϕ harbouring the LTR transgene had to be activated by phorbol esters *in vitro* before the LTR would direct reporter gene expression[64]. Viral replication probably requires activated mature Mϕ because of a requirement for certain developmentally regulated host cell proteins to act as cofactors in the replication process. In the restricted state, some mRNA transcripts and a small amount of viral protein can be found, though the mechanisms responsible for this restriction are not understood. It is likely that the latent or restricted replication states represent the norm in otherwise quiescent joints and other target tissues.

Cytokines

Previous work with MVV and CAEV demonstrated that T cells responding to virus-infected Mϕ *in vitro* released one or more cytokines which possessed anti-viral effects and the ability to upregulate MHC class II expression[65,66]. Although not characterized at the molecular level, the cytokines had biological features in common with interferons (IFN) and were produced by T cells rather than the Mϕ. These cytokines also had the property of inhibiting maturation and proliferation of monocytes[67], an effect which could result in slowing the development of the relevant permissive cells *in vivo*. SF taken from a clinically arthritic sheep infected with MVV was shown to possess an anti-viral effect, indicating that a similar factor(s) may be produced *in vivo*[26]. These studies show that cytokines which possess opposing effects may be generated in MVV/CAEV infection. On the one hand they have anti-viral and anti-proliferative effects, and on the other they result in cell activation as judged by induction of MHC class II expression which would enhance viral replication. The activation effects of CAEV were demonstrated in an *in vivo* study which showed that allergic (antigen) arthritis in goats was augmented by concurrent infection with CAEV[68]. In this study, antigen-induced arthritis in CAEV-infected and noninfected goats was generated by first priming the animals with methylated human serum albumin (mHSA) in Freund's Complete Adjuvant, then injecting mHSA into the left carpal joint. In noninfected goats, a typical acute inflammatory arthritis consisting of joint swelling and infiltration by neutrophils was observed which lasted about 3 weeks. In the CAEV-infected goats, however, the joint swelling persisted and increased with time and was accompanied by infiltration of the synovium with lymphocytes and macrophages and other chronic inflammatory changes. Although CAEV titres in the joints receiving antigen were elevated, the increases were slight, suggesting that enhanced production of CAEV was not the main factor involved. Also, in contrast to the inhibiting effects of the IFNs induced by MVV/CAEV described above, CAEV infection has been shown to enhance proliferation of Mϕ *in vitro*[69]. Thus, it is possible that shifts in a balance between the down-regulating effects of viral-induced IFNs and CAEV-induced Mϕ-activation may play a role in determining the course of the arthritic process.

Patients infected with HIV also produce IFNs including an αIFN which belongs to an unusual subclass characterized by lability at low pH[70-73]. B cells and monocytes have been implicated as sources of this acid-labile αIFN[74], and a high serum level of this cytokine is a poor prognostic indicator that predicts the onset of opportunistic infection[75]. Recombinant IFNs of all three classes appear to inhibit HIV replication at concentrations attainable *in vivo*[76]. Gendelman and colleagues[77] reported that monocytes stimulated with granulocyte-colony stimulating factor (G-CSF) and infected with HIV had a highly selective defect in their ability to produce IFNα in response to known IFN inducers. This result suggested that the diminished capacity of HIV-infected monocytes to make IFNα might enable the virus to survive and persist in these cells. This effect, however, is specific for G-CSF treated monocytes, as HIV infection of unstimulated monocytes has recently been shown to induce both acid-stable and acid-labile IFNα molecules[78]. These results indicate that IFNα production by HIV-infected monocytes is greatly influenced by the differentiation or activation state of the cells. It is also clear that while IFNs may exert an anti-viral effect, other cytokines upregulate HIV replication *in vitro*. These include granulocyte macrophage-colony stimulating factor (GM-CSF), TNFα and β, IL-1β, and IL-6, but not IFNγ, IL-4 or platelet-derived growth factor[79,80]. Activation of T cells via the antigen receptor is also known to induce HIV replication. Again, it is likely that the balance between these opposing effects will determine the disease course.

IMMUNE RESPONSES TO CAEV AND MVV

Anti-viral immune responses and disease

Immune responses to viral proteins are thought to play a major role in initiating and perpetuating the disease process in all target organs. The evidence supporting this comes from studies which show that the lesions in MVV infection can be abrogated by immunosuppressive treatment[81] and that T and B cell responses to MVV or CAEV could be detected in and correlated with tissue lesions.

Humoral responses

The involvement of anti-viral antibodies in CAEV-induced joint disease was suggested in studies showing that polyclonal IgG subclass 1 (IgG₁) levels in SF were elevated 2–5 fold over serum[82], and that the SF contained IgG antibodies to viral glycoproteins in high titre[83]. These increased SF antibody levels were found to correlate with the degree of subluminal plasma cell infiltration. These results provided evidence for local synthesis of anti-viral antibodies in joints. A more general activation of the B cell component of the immune response was indicated by the adenopathy of lymph nodes draining inflammatory sites[84]. The mediastinal lymph node draining the lungs was increased several fold in size, and while enlargement of both B and T cell areas was found, the increase occurred mainly in the follicular and germinal centre areas.

The involvement of anti-viral antibodies in the arthritic process was further suggested in experiments where goats vaccinated with inactivated CAEV then challenged intra-articularly with live CAEV developed a more rapid and severe arthritis than non-vaccinated animals[85]. Similarly, goats with persistent CAEV infection developed an acute arthritis after live CAEV was injected into carpal joints[85]. The inflammatory infiltrate consisted of both neutrophils and mononuclear cells. These results indicated that excess viral antigen introduced into joints containing anti-viral antibodies caused an acute arthritis resembling the well established allergic arthritis model, where immune complex formation and complement activation cause acute inflammation and lead to chronic inflammatory changes such as lining cell and villous hyperplasia, lymphoid infiltration, follicle formation, pannus and erosion of cartilage and bone[86]. Consistent with this model of inflammation are studies showing correlations between the severity of lesions and the frequency of CAEV isolation from joints[61,87]. Indeed, it has been shown that the severity of arthritis not only correlates with, but is predicted by, the antibody response to the CAEV gp135 glycoprotein[88]. In the latter study, anti-gp135 titres in SF gave a much better correlation with disease severity than either anti-p28 antibody titres in SF or anti-gp135 antibody titres in blood, possibly because local antibody responses appear to be directed preferentially against gp135[83]. Antibodies to gp90 and gp120, which are oligomeric forms of the transmembrane glycoprotein gp38, were found to be predominant in the serum of goats with CAEV-induced arthritis[89]. Why the local humoral response in joints should be focused in this manner is not known. One possible explanation is that gp135 is released into the extracellular fluid at a high rate, whereas gag proteins are retained within infected cells[90]. Preferential shedding of gp135 by infected cells in joints could result in stimulation of B cells locally to produce antibodies. However, whether the allergic arthritis model forms the basis of the chronic arthritis seen in naturally infected animals remains to be determined.

Although animals infected with MVV or CAEV make neutralizing antibodies[91,92], they do not clear these viruses and they remain persistently infected. One reason for this might be the relatively low affinity and slow association kinetics of the antibodies for viral epitopes compared with virus binding to receptors on $M\phi$[93]. Another possible reason could relate to the existence of two modes of viral uptake, one via a cell receptor and a second through a membrane fusion site[94]. These two functions appear to be mediated via different epitopes on MVV envelope proteins, and antibodies to one site would not affect the other site. Jolly and coworkers[95] provided evidence for enhanced binding, internalization, and uncoating of virus mediated by non-neutralizing antibody, possibly by an Fc receptor, but found the effect resulted in delayed appearance rather than increased replication of the virus. This result differs from the enhanced replication of HIV following uptake via Fc receptors[96].

Cell-mediated responses

Animals infected experimentally produce a primary cellular immune response of normal magnitude and kinetics[91,97,98]. In persistently infected animals, the blood T cell responses to MVV or CAEV were noted to be transient and/or irregular[99-101], suggesting intermittent and irregular production of virus. These results were consistent with the virus isolation data showing that virus was reliably detectable only in the first few weeks following infection[91,99] and thereafter was intermittent[99-101]. Adams and coworkers[99], though, found that while fluctuant, the proliferative T cell responses to CAEV increased in magnitude with time. A recent report also found T cell responses to be continuously present in MVV-infected sheep using live MVV or recombinant MVV gag as antigen[102]. The latter report also showed that the proliferative responses were due mainly to CD4+ T cells, though some proliferation was noted in CD8+ T cells obtained by depletion of CD4+ T cells. Less information is available concerning cell-mediated anti-viral immune responses in target tissues. One study showed that T cells in SF from CAEV-infected goats proliferated in response to CAEV antigens *in vitro*, but the stimulation indices were modest and responses obtained from only some joint fluids[68]. The phenotype of the *in vitro* responding T cells was not determined. However, the preponderance of CD8+ T cells in joints in infected animals[24-26] suggests that this subset is preferentially activated *in vivo*. Recently, cytotoxic CD8+ lymphoblasts have been demonstrated in the efferent lymph from persistently infected sheep following culture *in vitro*[103]. These results suggest that the CD8+ T cells in the joints of MVV-infected sheep might show anti-viral cytotoxic activity.

Role of antigenic variation

Like all lentiviruses, MVV and CAEV undergo point mutations during replication which result in antigenic drift. Molecular analysis of MVV escape mutants showed that a small number of nucleotide changes can markedly affect the gp135 neutralizing epitopes[104]. Early studies suggested that antigenic variation could result in virus escaping from neutralization and thereby persisting. However, it was found that while viral variants arose, they did so in only 25% of MVV-infected animals[105], and did not replace the infecting parental strain[106]. Antigenic variation was thus thought to play no role in virus persistence, and that the principal mechanisms maintaining persistence of MVV and CAEV were cell-to-cell transmission and restricted viral replication resulting in infected cells forming a suboptimal target for immune elimination[1]. A recent report, though, showed that the presence of neutralization-resistant variants of CAEV was associated with the development of severe progressive arthritis[87]. Individual variants appeared to be clonally expanded within joints, suggesting that these variants were responsible for the recurrent antigenic stimulation involved in disease progression. It is possible that antigenic variation may alter cell or tissue tropism, thereby enhancing the disease process in a tissue-specific manner.

IMMUNE RESPONSES TO HIV

In HIV infections, no specific information is available relating to the immune response in arthritic joints. However, information obtained from analysis of blood and target tissues may be relevant to the joint disease. Polyclonal B cell activation and hypergammaglobulinaemia have been well documented[107], with anti-gp160 and anti-p24 antibodies constituting a high proportion of the elevated immunoglobulin levels[108]. A cytokine-driven mechanism has been proposed for the polyclonal B cell activation, since blood IL-6 levels are elevated in HIV-infected individuals[109], and HIV gp120 and gp160 envelope proteins have been shown to induce IL-6 in CD4+ T cell clones[110]. It can be envisaged that increased levels of anti-viral antibodies in joints harbouring productively infected cells could result in acute and/or chronic inflammatory arthritic processes analogous to the experimental studies described earlier with CAEV in goats[85].

Neutralizing antibodies and antibody-dependent cell-mediated cytotoxicity have been described in HIV-infected individuals[111], although their role in controlling the spread of HIV and the course of disease progression *in vivo* is unclear. Like MVV and CAEV, HIV undergoes antigenic drift which results in the generation of escape mutants *in vivo*[112,113], which could play a role in evasion of host immune responses. However, persistence of the parental virus gp120 sequences was noted in some cases[113] suggesting, like MVV and CAEV, that antigenic variation of B cell epitopes may contribute to recurrent immune stimulation rather than being an important determinant of HIV persistence.

The well established role of cytotoxic T cells (CTLs) in controlling viral infections suggests that cell-mediated immune responses are more likely to be able to control HIV infections. Infected individuals respond in T cell proliferation assays to HIV antigens, and MHC Class I-restricted cytotoxic T cell responses can be demonstrated in blood and target tissues such as the lungs, lymph nodes and CSF[114]. It is generally thought that the CTL activity is mainly beneficial in HIV disease, since CD8+ CTLs inhibit viral replication *in vitro* and anti-HIV-specific CTL activity declines with disease progression[114]. The demonstration of anti-HIV gag-specific CTL escape mutants in HIV-infected individuals[115] lends further support to the view that CTLs are important in controlling the viral infection. The role played by cell-mediated immune responses in HIV-associated joint disease is not known, but involvement of anti-viral T cell immune responses in joint inflammation is plausible given the CD8+ T cell predominance in some patients[35].

Studies by Patterson and colleagues[116] have shown a high proportion of DC in blood are infected in HIV seropositive individuals. Several reports also document the presence of HIV-infected DC in the joints of patients with arthritis[33,117,118]. Studies of HIV-infected non-lymphoid DC from blood have shown that they are defective functionally[62]. Normally, DC function as potent antigen-presenting cells in both primary and secondary immune responses. However, these cells are unable to present third party antigens when infected with HIV[62]. Thus, while HIV-infected DC may be unable to induce T cell responses *de novo* to third party infections, their ability to present HIV antigens remains undiminished. Therefore, it is likely that HIV-infected DC in joints will present viral antigen preferentially and contribute to the inflammatory response through stimulation of viral-specific T and B cells.

AUTOIMMUNE REACTIVITY

Autoimmune responses to normal host antigens

The joint disease observed in CAEV and MVV infected animals shows some resemblance to human RA, a disease of presumed autoimmune aetiology characterized by the presence of high titre IgM and IgG rheumatoid factors (RF) and other autoantibodies in blood and SF[119]. The question, therefore, arises as to whether CAEV and MVV infections are associated with autoimmune-like reactivities. However, no RFs have been found in goats with CAEV-induced chronic arthritis using latex agglutination or other unspecified methods[13,120]. In contrast, recent work has shown that sheep, naturally or experimentally infected with MVV for months or years and exhibiting mainly subclinical synovitis, had elevated serum titres of a variety of autoantibodies[121]. These included IgM and IgG antibodies to single-stranded DNA (ssDNA), histones and cardiolipin, as well as antiglobulins and RFs reactive with immobilized rabbit IgG and purified sheep Fc fragments. IgM autoantibodies, except for those reactive with histones, appeared transiently in blood 3 weeks after experimental infection with MVV. After a period of months the autoantibodies reappeared. The results indicated that MVV either directly or indirectly induced these autoreactivities. However, in SF from these sheep, antiglobulin titres were raised only slightly, and the other specificities were absent. This may have reflected the subclinical nature of the joint disease.

Autoimmune-like phenomena have also been described in HTLV-I and HIV-1 infections. In HTLV-I infections, autoantibodies reactive with actin, vimentin or brain endothelial cells have been documented[122]. In the case of HIV-1 infection, a plethora of autoantibody reactivities have been reported, including RFs and antibodies reactive with nuclear antigens, DNA, cardiolipin and other phospholipids, collagen, intermediate filaments, vimentin, and smooth muscle, as well as antibodies to lymphocytes, granulocytes and erythrocytes[28]. These autoreactivities tend to appear in the early asymptomatic stages of HIV-1 infection, suggesting that they are induced by the lentivirus itself rather than by opportunistic infections which occur later.

The significance of the autoreactivities found in MVV, HIV-1 and HTLV-I to the diseases caused by these retroviruses remains speculative, as it is with other viral infections[123]. They could contribute to the inflammation by forming immune complexes with antigens released from damaged cells. In HIV-1 infection, polyclonal B cell activation and raised immunoglobulin levels may provide an explanation for the elevated levels of autoantibodies. However, evidence has accumulated in recent years that RF and anti-DNA responses in autoimmune mice are antigen driven[124,125]. The observations that RF-producing B cells take up antigens in the form of immune complexes in antibody excess and present the processed antigen to T cells[126], suggests a mechanism whereby viral antigen could drive the RF response. It is also possible that viral nucleic acid-binding proteins, such as tat and rev, may provide new helper T cell epitopes on DNA/histone complexes or other subcellular particles[127] thereby providing help for B cells encoding DNA or histone autoreactivities.

Autoimmune responses to stress proteins

Heat shock proteins (HSP) are another class of antigens that have been implicated in arthritis and autoimmune disease[128]. It has been shown that blood and SF T and B cell responses to mycobacterial HSP65 are elevated in a variety of human arthritic conditions including RA, juvenile chronic arthritis, and reactive arthritis[128]. Recently, the author has examined MVV infected sheep to determine if similar responses were present in peripheral blood. The results showed that the sheep had elevated IgM but not IgG antibodies reactive with HSP65 from *M. leprae* and *M. bovis*, and responded in bulk T cell proliferation assays to HSP65 free of endotoxin (G.D.H. – unpublished observations). It is not known if the CD4+ or CD8+ T cells infiltrating the joints of these sheep will respond to HSP65 as yet. It is also not clear whether these blood T cell responses represent an elevated response to mycobacteria due to infection by the latter, or autoreactivity to an endogenous ovine HSP65 analogue which cross-reacts with mycobacterial HSP65. Consistent with either of these notions is the observation that the monoclonal antibody ML30, which recognizes an epitope common to both mycobacterial and human HSP65 molecules, also reacts with sections of inflamed lung and synovium from MVV-infected sheep (Watt, N.J. and G.D.H. – unpublished observations). Elevated responses to mycobacterial HSP65 could conceivably arise if MVV infection induced some defect in the ability of macrophages to kill mycobacteria. Increased susceptibility to mycobacterial infection is a well recognized early complication of HIV infection[129]. However, mycobacterial infection has not been documented in MVV or CAEV infected animals, although defects in the ability of CAEV infected Mϕ to kill intracellular Listeria organisms have been reported[130]. Another possible explanation is that MVV infection induces a stress response in infected tissues which results in increased ovine HSP65 expression and immune responses to it. Although the significance of elevated anti-HSP65 immune responses in CAEV- or MVV-induced arthritis is unknown, the above observations suggest further investigation is warranted.

DISEASE SUSCEPTIBILITY

All ages and breeds of sheep and goats are infectable experimentally with MVV and CAEV respectively and probably under natural conditions as well given the appropriate contact. However, only a small proportion of animals develop clinical disease, suggesting that the host genotype plays a significant role in determining disease progression. This notion is supported by the inability of the Icelandic MVV strain 1514 to produce in North American sheep the neurological disease found both naturally and experimentally in Icelandic sheep[131]. In addition, the Icelandic outbreaks of encephalitic disease (visna) and lung disease (maedi) were caused by the introduction of infected Karakul rams from Europe into the Icelandic stock which had been isolated from outside contact for many years. Thus disease was caused by the introduction of a virus from one genetic background into another. However, no breed susceptibilities to CAEV arthritic disease in goats have been found.

The nature of the disease susceptibility to CAEV or MVV infection is unknown. Studies of the genomic organization of the MHC in these species are at an early stage. In joint tissues of MVV infected sheep no preferential expression of DR or DQ by infiltrating macrophages or lymphocytes has been observed[24,25]. In Saanen goats, it has been shown that resistance to CAEV-induced chronic arthritis is associated with an MHC allele[132], and that MHC Class I disease susceptibility associations exist. At present, it is not known if these associations are due directly to a Class I gene or to linkage disequilibrium between genes conveying CAEV resistance/susceptibility and MHC genes.

In HIV infection, some studies have indicated there may be a genetic susceptibility related to the MHC in the development of AIDS. In particular, HLA-A1 and B8 were found to be associated with the development and progression of HIV-related symptoms[133]. Brancato and colleagues[134] found that HLA-B27 was present in 71% of Caucasians with HIV-associated Reiter's syndrome. This frequency is similar to that found in Reiter's patients without HIV infection, and compares with a B27 frequency of 6–8% in the normal population. In Zimbabweans, where B27 is a rare allele, HIV-associated Reiter's syndrome is B27 negative[135], indicating that other HLA determinants may confer susceptibility in African populations. In patients with HIV-associated psoriatic arthritis preliminary evidence suggests that the B27 frequency may be elevated[34], but further studies are required to confirm this association. The results suggest that certain HLA alleles may predispose HIV-infected patients towards developing AIDS-like symptoms, but the presence of HLA B27 will result in a chronic type of reactive arthritis in a large proportion of patients.

VIRUS GENOTYPE

While some of the variations in disease patterns and severity that occur in animals infected with MVV or CAEV can be attributed to the host, it is clear that genetic differences in virus strains also contribute to this diversity. It has been proposed that these virus strains can be divided into pneumo-encephalitic or pneumoarthritic groups, with CAEV strains tending towards the latter and MVV strains having the properties of either group[136]. Some strains of MVV have been selected progressively for increased neurovirulence in sheep[137]. Although sequence comparisons have been made between CAEV strain Co and two strains of MVV[52], it is not possible, as yet, to ascribe any of the differences with an arthritogenic function.

In a study by Cheevers and colleagues[138], two biologically cloned strains of CAEV (G63/75 and Co) were compared for their arthritogenic properties in Saanen goats. The results clearly showed that the G63/75 strain caused chronic joint disease more frequently and of greater severity than the Co strain. No differences were noted in seroconversion or virus isolation rates. Thus disease expression was at least partly determined by the relative pathogenicity of the two virus strains. Sequence analysis of the surface and transmembrane glycoproteins of the two strains revealed some differences[139], though it is not known which, if any, of these confer arthritogenic potential. The availability of completely sequenced infectious molecular clones of CAEV[52] should facilitate identification of genetic features important in joint disease.

DIRECT EFFECTS OF VIRAL PRODUCTS

Induction of cellular genes

Although anti-viral immune responses are thought to play a major role in the disease process induced by lentiviruses, it remains possible that retroviral infection itself results in some dysregulation of host cell or tissue function. For example, the transactivating proteins, tat and P40^{tax} may exert direct effects on cells and tissues. In HTLV-I infections, P40^{tax} is known to transactivate a variety of host genes including those for IL-2, IL-2 receptor, IL-6, GM-CSF, γIFN, TNFβ, and c-*fos*[140–143]. The ability of P40^{tax} to transactivate such a large number of cellular genes is probably due to it functioning via the transcription factor NFκB, since many cellular promoters contain recognition sites for this factor. Extracellular p40^{tax} also stimulates proliferation of lymphocytes[144] presumably by transactivating the IL-2 and IL-2R genes. It additionally induces TGFβ1[145], a cytokine known to be involved in angiogenesis and fibrosis and which could potentially be involved in HTLV-I disease in joints, muscles, and brain tissues. TNFβ may have important cytolytic effects and contribute to bone resorption and hypercalcaemia[146]. Since TNFα and TNFβ act on the same receptors, TNFβ is likely to have similar metalloproteinase induction and cartilage degradative effects as TNFα.

In contrast, HIV-1 tat appears to be much more fastidious than p40^{tax} in the promoters it will transactivate, and is not thought to transactivate cellular genes. One reason for this is the apparent necessity of the RNA TAR region in the HIV LTR adopting a complex stem-loop structure for tat in conjunction with cellular proteins to bind[44]. Although HIV tat inhibits rather than stimulates lymphocyte proliferation *in vitro*[44], it has been found that HIV-infected cells secrete increased levels of IL-1, IL-6 and TNFα *in vitro*, and that these cytokines can be induced via interaction of HIV gp120 with

CD4[147,148]. MVV-infected Mϕ also release increased amounts of TNFα (I. Green and D.R. Sargan – unpublished observations), though the mechanism of induction is not known. Since MVV tat operates largely through binding to AP1 sites[47] it might be expected that cellular genes containing AP1 elements in their promoters, such as c-*fos*, collagenase, and TNFα, would be transactivated by MVV tat.

These observations may provide important clues as to the mechanisms of disease induction by these viruses in joints, particularly since mice transgenic for a TNFα gene lacking a post-transcriptional 3' control element developed cachexia and a chronic inflammatory joint disease characterized by joint swelling and lameness[149]. Histologically, the mice showed synovial lining layer thickening, pannus formation, cartilage destruction and massive fibrosis. The source of the TNFα appeared not to be Mϕ, but may have been produced by chondrocytes. The well recognized effects of TNFα in activating endothelia and recruiting lymphocytes and monocytes to sites of infection or inflammation, may play a significant part not only in the joint disease in these mice, but also in the induction and maintenance of synovitis, pneumonitis, encephalitis, and cachexia in MVV, CAEV and HIV infections.

In the examples cited above, the viruses by their actions on host genes are proposed to cause abnormal synthesis and release of cytokines which have potent modulatory effects on immune cells and resident cells of the target tissues. The recent description of mice transgenic for the entire coding sequence of HTLV-I further illustrates this point[150]. The transgenic mice were judged to be tolerant to HTLV-I antigens, but nevertheless developed a chronic inflammatory arthritis which was similar to that described for HTLV-I infections in humans[9], consisting of proliferative synovitis, pannus formation, and cartilage and bone destruction. Thus, the viral infection induced a chronic inflammatory disease involving cells of the immune system but which apparently did not involve any anti-viral immune responses. Although the pathogenesis of this disease in transgenic mice is not understood, the authors suggested a mechanism involving transactivation of cellular genes by P40[tax]. Such a mechanism is unlikely to operate with HIV tat due to the requirement for the highly structured TAR response element. However, since AP1 sites are ubiquitous in cellular genes, it is possible that MVV and CAEV tat could mediate such effects.

Co-infections and heterologous transactivation

In the initial outbreaks of MVV in sheep in Iceland in the 1950s, co-infection with MVV and a type D retrovirus which induces lung tumours resulted in a more severe cancer and more rapidly spreading MVV infection[151]. Similarly, co-infections with other infectious agents such as herpesviruses and mycoplasmas and non-specific immune activation by other pathogens have been suggested as important cofactors in individuals with HIV. The ability of herpesviruses and other viruses to transactivate the HIV LTR may provide a partial explanation for the disease enhancement observed[44]. These observations indicate the potential for interaction between lentiviruses and other infectious agents, though their role in modulating retroviral-induced arthritis remains speculative at present.

SUMMARY

The principal feature of lentiviruses is their ability to persist in the face of an apparently normal immune response, giving rise to chronic inflammation which leads eventually to degenerative changes in tissues. Though many gaps in our knowledge exist and the exact mechanisms operating are conjectural, the sequence of events thought to occur in MVV and CAEV infections leading to joint disease can be summarized as follows. Virus-infected Mϕ are transferred to offspring via ingestion of colostrum or milk or through respiratory contact. The infection spreads following release of newly synthesized virions to lymph nodes, bone marrow and other lymphoid tissues, and uptake into cells occurs via specific cellular receptors or by membrane fusion with uninfected Mϕ. Following an initial round of replication, anti-viral and possibly autoimmune T and B cell immune responses are induced and the infection becomes latent or restricted in character with the bone marrow in particular forming a reservoir of infection. Some proviruses will integrate into the Mϕ genome. With time, latently infected promonocytes will enter the blood stream as monocytes and seed to joints and other tissues where they will differentiate into adult Mϕ capable of supporting productive infection. However, some activational events probably involving traumatic, infective, immunological or merely housekeeping stimuli will result in the production of either newly synthesized infectious virions or a restricted number and amount of viral proteins. Local anti-viral immune responses ensue. On the one hand these serve to initiate and amplify the joint inflammation by activating cells involved in the immune response and by recruiting others to this end by inducing MHC Class II expression, and on the other hand to dampen down viral replication through the effects of IFNα/β. Some viral proteins may contribute to the tissue damage by inducing inflammatory cytokines and growth factors via transactivation or through interaction with cell surface molecules. Restricted replication and the mainly cell-to-cell mode of virus spread in established infection allows the virus to escape the effects of humoral responses including neutralizing antibodies. With time, escape mutants develop which may allow the virus to evade anti-viral cytotoxic T cell responses as well as neutralizing antibodies. By failing to eliminate the viral infection, the immune system is continuously stimulated by low levels of viral antigen presented by infected Mϕ and DC. Such chronic antigen presentation results in turn in the typical effects of chronic inflammation – connective tissue proliferation, angiogenesis, fibrosis and degenerative changes.

References

1. Haase AT. Pathogenesis of lentivirus infections. Nature. 1986; 322: 130–136.
2. Narayan O, Clements JE. Biology and pathogenesis of lentiviruses. J Gen Virol. 1989; 70:

1617–1639.
3. Crawford TB, Adams DS, Cheevers WP, Cork LC. Chronic arthritis in goats caused by a retrovirus. Science. 1980; 207: 997–999.
4. Oliver RE, Gorham JR, Parish SF et al. Ovine progressive pneumonia: Pathologic and virologic studies on the naturally occurring disease. Am J Vet Res. 1982; 42: 1554–1559.
5. Oliver RE, Gorham JR, Perryman LE, Spencer GR (1982). Ovine progressive pneumonia: Experimental intrathoracic, intracerebral, and intra-articular infections. Am J Vet Res. 1982; 42: 1560–1564.
6. Rynes RI. Painful rheumatic syndromes associated with immunodeficiency virus infection. Rheum Dis Clin North Am. 1991; 17: 79–87.
7. Hendrickson RV, Maul DH, Lerche NW et al. Clinical features of simian acquired immunodeficiency syndrome (SAIDS) in rhesus monkeys. Lab Animal Sci. 1984; 34: 140–145.
8. Roberts ED, Martin LN. Arthritis in rhesus monkeys experimentally infected with simian immunodeficiency virus (SIV/DELTA). Lab Invest. 1991; 65: 637–643.
9. Kitajima I, Maruyama I, Maruyama Y et al. Polyarthritis in human T lymphotropic virus type I-associated myelopathy. Arthritis Rheum. 1989; 32: 1342–1344.
10. Cheevers WP, McGuire TC. The lentiviruses: maedi/visna, caprine arthritis-encephalitis, and equine infectious anaemia. Adv Virus Res. 1988; 34: 189–215.
11. McGuire TC, O'Rourke KI, Knowles DP, Cheevers WP. Caprine arthritis encephalitis lentivirus transmission and disease. Curr Top Micro Immunol. 1990; 160: 61–75.
12. Narayan O, Cork LC. Lentiviral diseases of sheep and goats: chronic pneumonia leuko-encephalomyelitis and arthritis. Rev Infect Dis. 1985; 7: 89–98.
13. Kennedy-Stoskopf S, Zink MC, Jolly PE, Narayan O. Lentivirus-induced arthritis. Chronic disease caused by a covert pathogen. Rheum Dis Clin North Am. 1987; 13: 235–247.
14. Narayan O, Zink MC, Gorrell M et al. Lentivirus induced arthritis in animals. J Rheumatol. 1992; 19 (Suppl 32): 25–32.
15. Crawford TB, Adams DS. Caprine arthritis-encephalitis: Clinical features and presence of antibody in selected goat populations. J Am Vet Med Assoc. 1981; 178: 713–719.
16. Woodard JC, Gaskin JM, Poulos PW et al. Caprine arthritis encephalitis: Clinicopathologic study. Am J Vet Res. 1982; 43: 2085–2096.
17. East NE, Rowe JD, Madewell BR, Floyd K. Serologic prevalence of caprine arthritis-encephalitis virus in California goat dairies. J Am Vet Med Assoc. 1987; 190: 182–186.
18. Adams DS, Crawford TB, Klevjer-Anderson P. A pathogenetic study of the early connective tissue lesions of viral caprine arthritis-encephalitis. Am J Pathol. 1980; 99: 257–278.
19. Cutlip RC, Lehmkuhl HD, Wood RL, Brogden KA. Arthritis associated with ovine progressive pneumonia. Am J Vet Res. 1985; 46: 65–68.
20. Crawford TB, Adams DS, Sande RD et al. The connective tissue component of the caprine arthritis-encephalitis syndrome. Am J Pathol. 1989; 100: 443–450.
21. Banks KL, Adams DS, McGuire TC, Carlson J. Experimental infection of sheep by caprine arthritis-encephalitis virus and goats by progressive pneumonia virus. Am J Vet Res. 1983; 44: 2307–2311.
22. Cork LC, Narayan O. The pathogenesis of viral leukoencephalomyelitis-arthritis of goats. I. Persistent viral infection with progressive pathologic changes. Lab Invest. 1980; 42: 596–602.
23. Ellis T, Robinson W, Wilcox G. Characterization, experimental infection and serological response to caprine retrovirus. Aust Vet J. 1983; 60: 321–326.
24. Anderson A, Harkiss GD, Watt NJ. Quantitative analysis of immunohistological changes in synovial membrane of sheep infected with maedi-visna virus. 1993; (Submitted for publication).
25. Harkiss GD, Watt NJ, King TJ et al. Retroviral arthritis: Phenotypic analysis of cells in the synovial fluid of sheep with inflammatory synovitis associated with visna virus infection. Clin Immunol Immunopathol. 1991; 60: 106–117.
26. Kennedy-Stoskopf S, Zink C, Narayan O. Pathogenesis of ovine lentivirus-induced arthritis: phenotypic evaluation of T lymphocytes in synovial fluid, synovium, and peripheral circulation. Clin Immunol Immunopathol. 1989; 52: 323–330.
27. Harkiss GD, Hopkins J, McConnell I. Uptake of antigen by afferent lymph dendritic cells mediated by antibody. Eur J Immunol. 1990; 20: 2367–2373.

28. Buskila D, Gladman D. Musculoskeletal manifestations of infection with human immunodeficiency virus. Rev Infect Dis. 1990; 12: 223–235.
29. Rowe IF. Arthritis in the acquired immunodeficiency syndrome and other viral infections. Curr Opin Rheum. 1991; 3: 621–627.
30. Soloman G, Brancato L, Winchester R. An approach to the human immunodeficiency virus-positive patient with a spondyloarthropathy. Rheum Dis Clin North Am. 1991; 17: 43–58.
31. Winchester R, Bernstein H, Fischer H et al. The co-occurrence of Reiter's syndrome and acquired immunodeficiency. Ann Int Med. 1987; 106: 19–26.
32. Espinosa LR, Berman A, Vasey FB et al. Psoriatic arthritis and acquired immunodeficiency syndrome. Arthritis Rheum. 1988; 31: 1034–1040.
33. Forster SM, Seifert MH, Keat AC et al. Inflammatory joint disease and human immunodeficiency virus infection. Br Med J. 1988; 296: 1625–1627.
34. Reveille JD, Conant MA, Duvic M. Human immunodeficiency virus-associated psoriasis, psoriatic arthritis, and Reiter's syndrome: a disease continuum? Arthritis Rheum. 1990; 33: 1574–1578.
35. Espinosa LR, Aguilar JL, Espinosa CG et al. HIV antigen demonstration in the synovial membrane. J Rheumatol. 1990; 17: 1195–1201.
36. Rosenberg ZS, Norman A, Soloman G. Arthritis associated with HIV infection: radiographic manifestations. Radiol. 1989; 173: 171–176.
37. Ragni MV, Hanley EN. Septic arthritis in hemophiliac patients and infection with human immunodeficiency virus (HIV). Ann Int Med. 1989; 110: 168–169.
38. Hughes RA, Rowe IF, Shanson D et al. Septic bone, joint and muscle lesions associated with human immunodeficiency virus infection. Br J Rheumatol. 1992; 31: 381–388.
39. Dalton ADA, Harcourt-Webster JN, Keat ACS. Synovium in AIDS: a post-mortem study. Br Med J. 1990; 300: 1239–1240.
40. Harden EA, Moore JO, Haynes BF. Leukemia-associated arthritis: identification of leukemic cells in synovial fluid using monoclonal and polyclonal antibodies. Arthritis Rheum. 1984; 27: 1306–1308.
41. Yufu Y, Nonaka S, Nobunaga M. Adult T cell leukemia-lymphoma mimicking rheumatic disease. Arthritis Rheum. 1987; 30: 599–600.
42. Taniguchi A, Takenaka Y, Noda Y et al. Adult T cell leukemia presenting with proliferative synovitis. Arthritis Rheum. 1988; 31: 1076–1077.
43. Nishioka K, Maruyama I, Sato K et al. Chronic inflammatory arthropathy associated with HTLV-I. Lancet. 1989; 1: 441.
44. Vaishnav YN, Wong-Staal F. The biochemistry of AIDS. Ann Rev Biochem. 1991; 60: 577–630.
45. Tiley LS, Brown PH, Le S-J et al. Visna virus encodes a post-transcriptional regulator of viral structural gene expression. Proc Natl Acad Sci USA. 1990; 87: 7497–7501.
46. Yoshida M, Seiki M. Recent advances in the molecular biology of HTLV-1: transactivation of viral and cellular genes. Ann Rev Immunol. 1987; 5: 541–559.
47. Gabuzda DH, Hess JL, Small JA, Clements JE. Regulation of the visna long terminal repeat in macrophages involves cellular factors that bind sequences containing AP-1 sites. Moll Cell Biol. 1989; 9: 2728–2733.
48. Jeang K-T, Boros I, Brady J et al. Characterization of cellular factors that interact with the human T-cell leukemia virus type I p40^x-responsive 21-base-pair sequence. J Virol. 1988; 62: 4499–4509.
49. Steffy K, Wong-Staal F. Genetic regulation of human immunodeficiency virus. Microbiol Rev. 1991; 55: 193–205.
50. Rosen CA, Pavlakis GN. Tat and Rev: positive regulators of HIV gene expression. AIDS. 1990; 4: 499–509.
51. Tiley LS, Cullen BR. Structural and functional analysis of the visna virus rev-responsive element. J Virol. 1992; 66: 3609–3615.
52. Saltarelli M, Querat G, Konings DAM et al. Nucleotide sequence and transcriptional analysis of molecular clones of CAEV which generate infectious virus. Virol. 1990; 179: 347–364.
53. Pomerantz RJ, Seshamma T, Trono D. Efficient replication of human immunodeficiency virus type 1 requires a threshold level of Rev: Potential implications for latency. J Virol.

1992; 66: 1809–1813.
54. Audoly G, Sauze N, Harkiss G et al. Identification and subcellular localization of the Q gene product of visna virus. Virol. 1992; 189: 734–739.
55. Dalzeil RG, Hopkins J, Watt NJ et al. Identification of a putative cellular receptor for the lentivirus visna virus. J Gen Virol. 1991; 72: 1905–1911.
56. Crane SE, Buz J, Clements JE. Identification of cell membrane proteins that bind visna virus. J Virol. 1991; 65: 6137–6143.
57. Meltzer MS, Skillman DR, Gomatos PJ et al. Role of mononuclear phagocytes in the pathogenesis of human immunodeficiency virus infection. Ann Rev Immunol. 1990; 8: 169–194.
58. Gendelman HE, Narayan O, Molineaux S et al. Slow, persistent replication of lentiviruses: Role of tissue macrophages and macrophage precursors in bone marrow. Proc Natl Acad Sci USA. 1985; 82: 7086–7090.
59. Gendelman HE, Narayan O, Kennedy-Stoskopf S et al. Tropism of sheep lentiviruses for monocytes: susceptibility to infection and virus gene expression increase during maturation of monocytes to macrophages. J Virol. 1986; 58: 67–74.
60. Zink MC, Yager JA, Mayers JD. Pathogenesis of caprine arthritis encephalitis. Cellular localization of viral transcripts in tissues of infected goats. Am J Pathol. 1990; 136: 843–854.
61. Klevjer-Anderson P, Adams DS, Anderson LW et al. A sequential study of virus expression in retrovirus-induced arthritis in goats. J Gen Virol. 1984; 65: 1519–1525.
62. Knight SC, Macatonia SE, Bedford PA, Patterson S. Dendritic cells and HIV infection. In: Racz P, Dijkstra CD, Gluckman JC, eds. Accessory Cells in HIV and Other Retroviral Infections. Basel: Karger; 1991: 145–154.
63. Gorrell MD, Brandon MR, Sheffer D et al. Ovine lentivirus is macrophagetropic and does not replicate productively in T lymphocytes. J Virol. 1992; 66: 2679–2688.
64. Small JA, Bieberich C, Ghotbi Z et al. The visna virus long terminal repeat directs expression of a reporter gene in activated macrophages, lymphocytes, and the central nervous systems of transgenic mice. J Virol. 1989; 63: 1891–1896.
65. Narayan O, Sheffer D, Clements JE, Tennenkoon G. Restricted replication of lentiviruses. Visna viruses induce a unique interferon during interaction between lymphocytes and infected macrophages. J Exp Med. 1985; 162: 1954–1969.
66. Kennedy PGE, Narayan O, Ghotbi Z et al. Persistent expression of Ia antigen and viral genome in visna-maedi virus-induced inflammatory cells. J Exp Med. 1985; 162: 1970–1982.
67. Zink MC, Narayan O. Lentivirus-induced interferon inhibits maturation and proliferation of monocytes and restricts the replication of caprine arthritis-encephalitis virus. J Virol. 1989; 63: 2578–2584.
68. Banks KL, Jacobs CA, Michaels FH, Cheevers WP. Lentivirus infection augments antigen-induced arthritis. Arthritis Rheum. 1987; 30: 1046–1053.
69. Jutila MA, Banks KL. Increased macrophage division in the synovial fluid of goats infected with caprine arthritis-encephalitis virus. J Infect Dis. 1988; 157: 1193–1202.
70. Rossol S, Voth S, Laubenstein HP, Muller WEG et al. Interferon production in patients infected with HIV-1. J Infect Dis. 1989; 159: 815–821.
71. Pomerantz RJ, Hirsch MS. Interferon and human immunodeficiency virus infection. Interferon. 1987; 9: 114–127.
72. Minagawa T, Mizuno K, Hirano S et al. Detection of high levels of immunoreactive human beta-1 interferon in sera from HIV-infected patients. Life Sci. 1989; 45: iii–vii.
73. Preble OT, Rook AH, Quinnan GV et al. Role of interferon in AIDS. Ann NY Acad Sci. 1984; 437: 65–75.
74. Copobianchanchi MR, De Marco F, Di Marco P, Dianzani F. Acid-labile human interferon alpha production by peripheral blood mononuclear cells stimulated by HIV-infected cells. Arch Virol. 1988; 99: 9–19.
75. Vadhan-Raj S, Wong G, Gnecco C et al. Immunological variables as predictors of prognosis in patients with Kaposi's sarcoma and the acquired immunodeficiency syndrome. Cancer Res. 1986; 46: 417–425.
76. Wells DE, Chatterjee S, Mulligan MJ, Compans RW. Inhibition of human immunodeficiency virus type 1-induced cell fusion by recombinant human interferons. J Virol. 1991; 65: 6325–6330.

77. Gendelman HE, Friedman RM, Joe S et al. A selective defect of interferon α production in human immunodeficiency virus-infected monocytes. J Exp Med. 1990; 172: 1433–1442.

78. Szebeni J, Dieffenbach C, Wahl SM et al. Induction of alpha interferon by human immunodeficiency virus type 1 in human monocyte-macrophage cultures. J Virol. 1991; 65: 6362–6364.

79. Rosenberg ZF, Fauci AS. Immunopathogenic mechanisms of HIV infection: cytokine induction of HIV expression. Immunol Tod. 1990; 11: 176–180.

80. Tornatore C, Nath A, Amemiya K, Major EO. Persistent human immunodeficiency virus type 1 infection in human fetal glial cells reactivated by T-cell factor(s) or by the cytokines tumor necrosis factor alpha and interleukin-1 beta. J Virol. 1991; 65: 6094–6100.

81. Nathanson J, Panitch H, Palsson PA et al. Pathogenesis of visna. II. Effect of immunosuppression upon early central nervous system lesions. Lab Invest. 1976; 35: 444–451.

82. Johnstone GC, Adams DS, McGuire TC. Pronounced production of polyclonal immunoglobulin G1 in the synovial fluid of goats with caprine arthritis-encephalitis virus infection. Infect Immun. 1983; 41: 805–815.

83. Johnston GC, Barbet AF, Klevjer-Anderson P, McGuire TC. Preferential immune response to virion surface glycoproteins by caprine arthritis-encephalitis virus-infected goats. Infect Immun. 1983; 41: 657–665.

84. Ellis JA, DeMartini JC. Immunomorphologic and morphometric changes in pulmonary lymph nodes of sheep with progressive pneumonia. Vet Pathol. 1985; 22: 32–41.

85. McGuire TC, Adams DS, Johnson GC et al. Acute arthritis in caprine arthritis-encephalitis virus challenge exposure of vaccinated or persistently infected goats. Am J Vet Res. 1986; 47: 537–540.

86. Dumonde DC, Jones EH, Kelly RH et al. Experimental models of rheumatoid inflammation. In: Glynn LE, Schlumberger HD, eds. Experimental Models of Chronic Inflammatory Diseases. Berlin, Heidelberg, New York: Springer; 1977: 4–27.

87. Cheevers WP, Knowles DP Jr, Norton LK. Neutralization-resistant antigenic variants of caprine arthritis-encephalitis lentivirus associated with progressive arthritis. J Infect Dis. 1991; 164: 679–685.

88. Knowles D Jr, Cheevers W, McGuire T et al. Severity of arthritis is predicted by antibody response to gp135 in chronic infection with caprine arthritis-encephalitis virus. J Virol. 1990; 64: 2396–2398.

89. McGuire TC, Knowles DP Jr, Davis WC et al. Transmembrane protein oligomers of caprine arthritis-encephalitis lentivirus are immunodominant in goats with progressive arthritis. J Virol. 1992; 66: 3247–3250.

90. Vigne R, Phillipi P, Querat G et al. Precursor polypeptides to structural proteins of visna virus. J Virol. 1982; 42: 1046–1056.

91. Griffen DE, Narayan O, Adams RJ. Early immune responses in visna, a slow viral disease of sheep. J Infect Dis. 1978; 138: 340–350.

92. McGuire TC, Norton LK, O'Rourke KI, Cheevers WP. Antigenic variation of neutralization-sensitive epitopes of caprine arthritis-encephalitis lentivirus during persistent arthritis. J Virol. 1988; 62: 3488–3492.

93. Kennedy-Stoskopf S, Narayan O. Neutralizing antibodies to visna lentivirus: Mechanism of action and possible role in virus persistence. J Virol. 1986; 59: 37–44.

94. Crane SF, Clements JE, Narayan O. Separate epitopes in the envelope of visna virus are responsible for fusion and neutralization: Biological implications for anti-fusion antibodies in limiting virus replication. J Virol. 1988; 62: 2680–2685.

95. Jolly PE, Huso D, Hart G, Narayan O. Modulation of lentivirus replication by antibodies. Non-neutralizing antibodies to caprine arthritis-encephalitis virus enhance early stages of infection in macrophages, but do not cause increased production of virions. J Gen Virol. 1989; 70: 2221–2226.

96. Takeda A, Tuazon CU, Ennis FA. Antibody-enhanced infection by HIV-1 via Fc receptor mediated entry. Science. 1988; 242: 580–583.

97. Larsen HJ. Experimental maedi virus infection in sheep: Early cellular and humoral immune response following parenteral inoculation. Am J Vet Res. 1982; 43: 379–383.

98. Sihvonen L. Early immune responses in experimental maedi. Res Vet Sci. 1981; 30: 217–222.

99. Adams DS, Crawford TB, Banks KL et al. Immune responses of goats persistently

infected with caprine arthritis-encephalitis virus. Infect Immun. 1980; 28: 421–427.
100. Larsen HJ, Hyllseth B, Krogsrud J. Experimental maedi virus infection in sheep: Cellular and humoral immune response during three years following intranasal inoculation. Am J Vet Res. 1982; 43: 384–389.
101. Sihvoven L. Late immune responses in experimental maedi. Vet Microbiol. 1984; 9: 205–213.
102. Reyburn HT, Roy DJ, Blacklaws BA et al. Characteristics of the T cell mediated immune response to maedi-visna virus. J Virol Meth. 1992; 37: 305–320.
103. Blacklaws et al. (Manuscript in preparation)
104. Clements JE, Gdovin SL, Montelaro RC et al. Antigenic variation in lentiviral diseases. Ann Rev Immunol. 1988; 6: 139–159.
105. Thormar H, Barshatzky MR, Andersen K, Kozlowski PB. The emergence of antigenic variants is a rare event in long-term visna virus infection *in vivo*. J Gen Virol. 1983; 64: 1427–1432.
106. Lutley R, Petursson G, Palsson PA et al. Antigenic drift in visna: virus variation during long-term infection of Icelandic sheep. J Gen Virol. 1983; 64: 1433–1440.
107. Zolla-Pazner S. B cells in the pathogenesis of AIDS. Immunol Tod. 1984; 5: 289–291.
108. Shirai A, Cosentino M, Leitman-Klinman SF, Klinman DM. Human immunodeficiency virus infection induces both polyclonal and virus-specific B cell activation. J Clin Invest. 1992; 89: 561–566.
109. Breen EC, Rezai AR, Nakajima K et al. Infection with HIV is associated with elevated IL-6 levels and production. J Immunol. 1990; 144: 480–484.
110. Oyaizu N, Chirmule N, Ohnishi Y et al. Human immunodeficiency virus type 1 envelope glycoproteins gp120 and gp160 induce interleukin-6 production in CD4+ T cell clones. J Virol. 1991; 65: 6277–6282.
111. Weiss RA, Clapham PR, Weber JN et al. Variable and conserved neutralization antigens of human immunodeficiency virus. Nature. 1986; 324: 572–575.
112. Albert J, Abrahamsson B, Nagy K et al. Rapid development of isolate-specific neutralizing antibodies after primary HIV-1 infection and consequent emergence of virus variants which resist neutralization. AIDS. 1990; 4: 107–112.
113. Simmonds P, Zhang LQ, McOmish F et al. Discontinuous sequence change of human immunodeficiency virus (HIV) type 1 env sequences in plasma viral and lymphocyte-associated proviral populations in vivo: Implications for models of HIV pathogenesis. J Virol. 1991; 65: 6266–6276.
114. Nixon DF. The cytotoxic T cell response to HIV. In: Bird AG, ed. Immunology of HIV Infection, Dordrecht: Kluwer 1992: 59–74.
115. Phillips EE, Rowland-Jones S, Nixon DF et al. Human immunodeficiency genetic variation that can escape cytotoxic T cell recognition. Nature. 1991; 354: 453–459.
116. Patterson S, Gross J, Bedford P, Knight SC. Morphology and phenotype of dendritic cells from peripheral blood and their productive and non-productive infection with human immunodeficiency virus type. Immunol. 1991; 72: 361–367.
117. Withrington RH, Cornes P, Harris JRW et al. Isolation of human immunodeficiency virus from synovial fluid of a patient with reactive arthritis. Br Med J. 1987; 294: 484.
118. Hughes RA, Macatonia SF, Rowe IF et al. The detection of human immunodeficency virus DNA in dendritic cells from the joints of patients with aseptic arthritis. Br J Rheumatol. 1990; 29: 166–170.
119. Zvaifler NJ. The immunopathology of joint inflammation in rheumatoid arthritis. Adv Immunol. 1973; 16: 265–336.
120. Zwahlen R, Spath PJ, Stucki M. Histological and immunopathological investigation in goats with carpitis/pericarpitis. In: Sharp JM, Hoff-Jorgensen R, eds. Slow Viruses in Sheep, Goats and Cattle. Proceedings of a C.E.C. Workshop on slow viruses. C.E.C., Luxembourg: Office for Official Publications of the European Communities; 1985: 239–248.
121. Harkiss GD, Veitch D, Dickson L, Watt NJ. Autoimmune reactivity in sheep induced by the visna retrovirus. J Autoimmun. 1993; 1: 63–75.
122. Tsukeda N, Tanaka Y, Yanagisawa N. Autoantibodies to brain endothelial cells in the sera of patients with human T-lymphotropic virus type I associated myelopathy and other demyelinating disorders. J Neurol Sci. 1989; 90: 33–42.

123. Schattner A, Rager-Zisman B. Virus-induced autoimmunity. Rev Infect Dis. 1990; 12: 204–222.
124. Schlomchik MJ, Marshak-Rothstein A, Wolfwicz CB et al. The role of clonal selection and somatic mutation in autoimmunity. Nature. 1987; 328; 805–811.
125. Schlomchik MJ, Mascelli M, Shan H et al. Anti-DNA antibodies from autoimmune mice arise by clonal expansion and somatic mutation. J Exp Med. 1990; 171: 265–292.
126. Roosnek E, Lanzaveccia A. Efficient and selective presentation of antigen-antibody complexes by rheumatoid factor B cells. J Exp Med. 1991; 173: 487–489.
127. Tan EM. Autoantibodies in pathology and cell biology. Cell. 1991; 67: 841–842.
128. Van Eden W. Heat-shock proteins as immunogenic bacterial antigens with the potential to induce and regulate autoimmune arthritis. Immunol Rev. 1991; 121: 5–28.
129. Kumararatne DS, Pithie A, Bassi EOE, Bartlett R. Mycobacterial immunity and mycobacterial disease in relation to HIV infection. In: Bird AG, ed. Immunology and Medicine, Vol. 17: Immunology of HIV infection. London: Kluwer Acad Pub.; 1992: 113–154.
130. Michaels FH, Banks KL, Reitz MS. Lessons from caprine and ovine retrovirus infections. Rheum Dis Clin North Am. 1991; 17: 5–23.
131. Georgsson G, Petursson G, Palsson PA et al. Experimental visna in fetal Icelandic sheep. J Comp Pathol. 1978; 88: 599–605.
132. Ruff G, Lazary S. Evidence for linkage between the caprine leucocyte antigen (CLA) system and susceptibility to CAE virus-induced arthritis in goats. Immunogen. 1988; 28: 303–309.
133. Steel CM, Ludlam CA, Beatson D et al. HLA haplotype A1 B8 DR3 as a risk factor for HIV-related disease. Lancet. 1990; 1: 1185–1188.
134. Brancato L, Itescu S, Skovron ML et al. Aspects of the spectrum, prevalence and disease susceptibility determinants of Reiter's syndrome and related disorders associated with HIV infection. Rheum Int. 1989; 9: 137–141.
135. Davis P, Stein M, Latif A et al. Acute arthritis in Zimbabwean patients: Possible relationship to human immunodeficiency virus infection. J Rheumatol. 1986; 16: 346–348.
136. Narayan O, Zink MC, Sheffer D et al. Lentiviruses of animals are biological models of the human immunodeficiency viruses. Microb Pathogen. 1988; 5: 149–157.
137. Georgsson G, Houwers DJ, Palsson PA, Petursson G. Expression of viral antigens in the central nervous system of visna-infected sheep: an immunohistochemical study on experimental visna induced by visna strains of increased neurovirulence. Acta Neuropathol. 1989; 77: 299–306.
138. Cheevers WP, Knowles DP Jr, McGuire TC et al. Chronic disease in goats orally infected with two isolates of the caprine arthritis-encephalitis lentivirus. Lab Invest. 1988; 58: 510–517.
139. Knowles DP Jr, Cheevers WP, McGuire TC et al. Structure and genetic variability of envelope glycoproteins of two antigenic variants of caprine arthritis-encephalitis lentivirus. J Virol. 1991; 65: 5744–5750.
140. Greene WC, Leonard WJ, Wano Y et al. Trans-activator gene of HTLV-II induces IL-2 receptor and IL-2 cellular gene expression. Science. 1986; 232: 877–880
141. Miyatake S, Seiki M, Yoshida N, Arai K-I. T-cell activation signals and human T-cell leukemia virus type I-encoded p40^x protein activate the mouse granulocyte-macrophage colony-stimulating factor gene through a common DNA element. Mol Cell Biol. 1988; 8: 5581–5587.
142. Joshi JB, Dave HPG. Transactivation of the proencephalin gene promoter by the Tax$_1$ protein of human T-cell lymphotropic virus type I. Proc Natl Acad Sci USA. 1992; 89: 1006–1010.
143. Fuji M, Sassone-Corsi P, Verma IM. c-fos promoter transactivation by the tax$_1$ protein of human T-cell leukemia virus type I. Proc Natl Acad Sci USA. 1988: 85: 8526–8530.
144. Marriott S, Lindholm P, Reid R, Brady J. Soluble HTLV-I Tax protein stimulates proliferation of human peripheral blood lymphocytes. New Biol. 1991; 3: 1–9.
145. Lindholm PF, Reid RL, Brady JN. Extracellular Tax$_1$ protein stimulates tumor necrosis factor-β and immunoglobulin kappa light chain expression in lymphoid cells. J Virol. 1992; 66: 1294–1302.
146. Thomson BM, Mundy GR, Chambers TJ. Tumor necrosis factors α and β induce osteoclastic cells to stimulate osteoclastic bone resorption. J Immunol. 1987; 138: 775–779.

147. Merrill JE, Koyanagi Y, Chen ISY. Interleukin 1 and tumour necrosis factor α can be induced from mononuclear phagocytes by HIV-1 binding to the CD4 receptor. J Virol. 1989; 63: 4404–4408.
148. Nakajima K, Martinez-Maza O, Hirano T et al. Induction of IL-6 (B cell stimulatory factor-2/IFN-β_2) production by HIV. J Immunol. 1989; 142: 531–536.
149. Keffer J, Probert L, Cazlaris H et al. Transgenic mice expressing human tumour necrosis factor: a predictive genetic model of arthritis. EMBO J. 1991; 10: 4025–4031.
150. Iwakura Y, Tosu M, Yoshida E et al. Induction of inflammatory arthropathy resembling rheumatoid arthritis in mice transgenic for HTLV-I. Science. 1991; 253: 1026–1028.
151. Dawson M, Done SH, Venebles C, Jenkins CE. Maedi-visna and sheep pulmonary adenomatosis: a study of concurrent infection. Br Vet J. 1990; 146: 531–538.

13
Autoantibodies Against DNA

N. A. STAINES

INTRODUCTION

The autoimmune connective tissue diseases are characterized by autoantibodies against a diverse range of antigens on and in cells, and associated with the extracellular matrix. For long, the idiosyncratic patterns of autoantibody production have been held to reflect the immunopathological processes that characterize the respective diseases. Although antibodies of a given specificity may appear commonly elsewhere, it is their associations with each other that may define characteristic disease patterns[1-4]. In many cases it is not known what their precise contribution is to the actual pathology, so their importance may be defined more by faith than fact. The issue of whether a particular antibody specificity is associated with a particular disease is of great importance in disease assessment, and such clinical associations are routinely sought in rheumatic diseases. However, there is no case of an *absolutely* complete and inclusive association between an antibody and a rheumatic disease: in general the associations are incomplete in that the antibody is found in a proportion of patients and often, but not always, in some individuals with other diseases or without diagnosed disease. This is a compeling parallel with the associations seen between HLA and disease, and indeed the similarity may have more than a passing significance. With HLA, the Class II genes clearly dictate T cell help for antibody production, so it appears that HLA type relates directly to production of autoantibodies of particular specificities.

The fact that some antibodies are found only in a proportion of patients with a particular disease could be interpreted to mean that they may have no significant role in pathology. On the other hand, they may define a subset of disease patients with variant pathology dictated by the antibodies. For example, antibodies against double stranded (ds) DNA are found almost uniquely in systemic lupus erythematosus (SLE) at an incidence that ranges from 50% to 75% of patients according to the study; however, the great

Table 1 Autoantibodies and connective tissue disease associations

Autoantibody specificity	Disease	Association (%)	Comment
dsDNA	SLE	50–75	Nephritis
Cardiolipin	SLE	20	Thrombosis, abortion
Ribosomal RNP	SLE	10	
Nuclear ribo-nucleoprotein nRNP	MCTD	>95	SLE, Raynaud's
Sm antigen [(U1-U6)RNP]	SLE	~30	Marker antibody, membraneous nephritis
SS-A (Ro) antigen	Sjögren's SLE	70–80 30–40	SS/SLE overlap, cutaneous LE, heart block
SS-B (La) antigen	Sjögren's SLE	60–70 10–15	SS/SLE overlap
Histones	SLE Rheumatoid arthritis	90 50	Drug-induced SLE
Jo-1 antigen (His-tRNA synthetase)	Myositis	10–30	Fibrosing alveolitis
Scl-70 (Topoisomerase I)	Systemic sclerosis	30–60	Marker antibody
PM/Scl	Myositis	10–30	Scleroderma features
Centromere (ACA)	Scleroderma CREST	20 70–90	Marker antibody

majority of patients with such antibodies have renal complications[5]. The obverse is that many patients with high titres of DNA antibodies do not have significant renal involvement. Similarly, antibodies against cardiolipin are found in ~20% of patients with SLE, and the association here is with thrombosis and abortion. The view is that this second group probably constitutes a separate clinical entity that can be diagnosed differentially with the assistance of an anti-cardiolipin antibody test. This is comprehensively dealt with in Chapter 14 of this book and elsewhere[6]. In other cases, the antibodies against centromere antigen(s) and Scl-70 associate with scleroderma, and the latter with the CREST disease subset. The more significant associations of autoantibodies with connective tissue diseases are summarized in Table 1.

The general application of molecular biological and biophysical methods to the analysis of autoantigens and the antibodies against them has enhanced our understanding of their role in disease processes. This chapter will deal mainly with the antibodies that react with DNA. These are a central feature of SLE and are considered to play a significant role in its pathology, although they are not unique in this. I will call them *DNA antibodies* rather than *anti-DNA antibodies* to avoid the implication that DNA is the antigen that drives their production. This is an issue that awaits clarification, although the available evidence, on balance, supports the idea.

DNA AS ANTIGEN AND THE SPECIFICITY OF DNA ANTIBODIES

For all that DNA is composed of only four basic building blocks, it is a highly plastic molecule that has many different natural forms. In resting cells it is condensed in chromatin and associated with the structural proteins (such as histones) of the cell nucleus. During transcription and replication the ordered structure of DNA is altered. This creates many different structures to which antibodies could potentially bind. Exactly which structures of DNA are antigenic is a matter of importance in defining the specificity of the antibodies themselves. When purified, DNA can take up one of several different conformations, the B form being the most commonly thought of as the basic structure of dsDNA. However, variations in pitch of the helix can be created by changes in the environmental temperature, pH and ion concentration, and although we cannot predict what the significance of these are for the binding activity of DNA antibodies *in vivo* we can say with certainty that the conditions for testing DNA antibodies *in vitro* may influence qualitatively the ways in which antibodies bind to their target antigen. The nature of DNA and other nucleic acids as antigens has been the subject of many reviews[5,7,8] and the reader is referred to these for a comprehensive account of the topic which will not be covered here in detail.

The empirical observation that antibodies against DNA react with dsDNA or with single stranded (ss) DNA or with both these physical forms has been acknowledged for many years, and a further analysis of it has been prompted largely by the intriguing association of anti-dsDNA antibodies with SLE. These are uncommon in other situations. Studies with serum antibodies are not especially illuminating with regard to the fine specificity of DNA antibodies because they are oligoclonal[9] or, in some cases, polyclonal mixtures. Thus, much of our understanding of the diversity of DNA antibody specificity comes from analysis of monoclonal antibodies (mAbs) derived from humans and mice with SLE. For convenience, I will refer to the disease in each species as SLE although it is clear that it is a greatly varied syndrome in humans. Different mouse strains are as equally diverse as individual humans in their presentation of disease. Many dozens of DNA mAbs have been analysed, and mouse and human antibodies show the same range and diversity of fine specificity. The majority can be accommodated in a classification of five Groups[10] with the characteristics shown in Table 2. Assignment to these groups depends upon the reactivity of the mAb in immunofluorescence and enzyme linked immunosorbent assay (ELISA) or radioimmunoassay (RIA). Antibodies reactive solely with dsDNA and not at all with ssDNA (Group I), and are relatively uncommon in panels of mAbs, and certainly more antibodies with specific reactivity for ssDNA but not dsDNA (Group IV) are usually isolated. The remainder react with both forms of DNA and fall into two major groups: those that react almost equally well with ssDNA and dsDNA (Group II) and those that react only

Table 2 Classification of DNA antibodies according to their fine specificity

Group	Reaction in ELISA/RIA with				Reaction in Immunofluorescence				Specificity
	dsDNA	ssDNA	Nucleotides	RNA	Phospholipids	Nucleus	Nucleolus	Cytoskeleton	
I	+++	−	−	−	++	+++	+++	−	Conformational epitopes on dsDNA groove/backbone
II	++	++/+++	−	−	++/+++	+++	+++	−	Conformational backbone epitopes
III	+	+++	++	−	+++	+++	−	−	Epitopes on ssDNA, weakly on dsDNA
IV	−	+++	+++	−	−	−	+++	−	Base dependent epitopes
V	+	++	++	++	−	−	++	++	Base dependent epitopes on DNA and RNA

Intensity of reactions are shown as semi-quantitative values.

very weakly with dsDNA (Group V) respectively. A small number that, like Group II antibodies, react equally with ssDNA and dsDNA give immunofluorescence staining patterns that spare the nucleoli in Hep-2 cells and constitute Group III antibodies.

DNA antibodies are celebrated for their cross-reactivity, this being a common feature of those isolated from lupus patients and from other individuals[11]. There has been considerable interest in the relationship of antibodies that react with phospholipids (cardiolipin especially) and with DNA. Clearly, there are antibodies that are specific for phospholipids and which do not react with nucleic acids[12,13], but from study of DNA mAbs some can be clearly identified that cross-react with cardiolipin: those examined by the author all bind significantly well to dsDNA and are found in Groups I and II of the classification. Antibodies that bind solely to ssDNA (Group IV) or to ssDNA and to RNA (Group V) do not bind cardiolipin[14]. Reactions with cytoskeletal structures are also seen in DNA antibodies and this is a feature of the polyreactive antibodies in Group V that also react to some extent with different forms of RNA.

Cross-reactive antibodies

There have been numerous other cross-reactions of DNA antibodies documented (see [7] and [15] for summaries), but it is not clear what the immunochemical basis of these is in many cases. It will be very interesting when co-crystals of DNA antibodies with their various cross-reactive ligands can be prepared and analysed by X-ray diffraction. However, the biological importance of the cross-reactions is that the DNA antibodies may have the ability *in vivo* to combine with a range of different antigens thus producing immune deposits of great antigenic diversity and complexity that could then trap antibodies of other specificity.

However, some apparent cross-reactions may be artefactual. For example, DNA antibodies that bind nuclear histone or heparan sulphate may cease to do so after they have been treated with DNase I which is an enzyme capable of digesting fragments of DNA trapped in the paratope of the antibody[16]. It is proposed that such fragments of DNA are bound naturally, especially by mAbs by virtue of the way in which the cells making them are grown, and because the DNA fragments themselves are ligands for histones or the proteoglycans, the antibodies appear to bind to the cross-reactive antigens. We might question whether DNase I can remove all trapped DNA fragments for it is thought that the presence of DNA fragments of 35–45 base pairs in the serum of SLE patients reflects the fact that antibodies protect circulating DNA from digestion by exonucleases[17]. On the other hand, it can be envisaged that immune complexes can be built up *in vivo* not only by antigen-antibody interactions but also by interactions between DNA and other cellular and extracellular antigens. One practical implication that follows and which has been stressed before[18] is that the purity of the DNA used as the target for assaying anti-DNA antibodies and the assay system itself are very important if misleading (false positive) reactions due to such bridging phenomena are to be avoided.

Epitopes on DNA

In the B form of DNA, the helix is right handed and the purine and pyrimidine bases are largely inaccessible being buried inside the helix. Thus antibodies that react with dsDNA have little if any specificity for individual base sequences: antibodies reactive with bases are found among those that react strongly with ssDNA where the unpaired bases are exposed, and indeed these particular antibodies (Group IV) do not react with dsDNA for this reason. The ability of anti-DNA antibodies to recognize base sequences is not widely documented, but there is evidence that some are sequence-specific, or at least can react specifically with particular nucleotides or nucleosides or synthetic nucleic acids implying base specificity[5,10,19]. It has also been found that the activity of some restriction endonucleases with precisely defined substrate sequence specificity can be inhibited by particular mAbs against DNA[20].

The precise antigenic sites on DNA with which DNA mAbs interact are not well defined. Obviously, the methods of epitope analysis used for protein antigens cannot be applied to nucleic acids, and so much of what is known is inferred from studies such as those mentioned above. The antibodies that interact with dsDNA, which is the major component ($\sim 85\%$) of native DNA (nDNA) as extracted from cells, interact with epitopes centred on the phosphate backbone of dsDNA. Because they can be inhibited by high salt concentrations, ionic interactions probably account for a large part of this antibody binding[21] although hydrogen bonds could also form. The importance of phosphate groups in the epitopes for these antibodies is thought to explain their cross-reactions with phospholipids and with other phosphorylated molecules including some cellular proteins[1,2]. It has been found that some DNA mAbs that show such cross-reactions can discriminate between the phosphorylated and non-phosphorylated forms of cytoplasmic and nuclear proteins[22].

Hydrogen bonding, reversible by changes in environmental pH, is probably important for many other DNA antibody interactions with DNA. For example, arginine, that is abundant in many DNA antibody V region sequences, could hydrogen bond to guanine. Other amino acids common in DNA antibody sequences that could contribute to hydrogen bonding include lysine, asparagine, glutamine, serine and threonine. These are clearly important interactions in the binding of antibodies to ssDNA where the unpaired bases present many opportunities for hydrogen bonding to antibodies. Aromatic amino acids (tyrosine and tryptophan) are found in some DNA antibodies, such as mAb V-88 which is rich in tyrosine residues[23], and these have the potential to intercalate with the stacked bases in helical DNA.

The real nature of the interaction between DNA and its antibodies will ultimately be elucidated by structural studies. In particular, the analysis by X-ray diffraction of co-crystals of mAb and DNA has commenced in several laboratories. The fact that many, if not all, DNA antibodies react with more than one ligand offers great opportunities to elucidate the structural basis of antibody cross-reaction. So far there is one reported analysis of a co-crystal from Edmundson and colleagues[24] in which it was shown that mAb # BV04-01 has a groove-like binding site for the synthetic trinucleotide $d(pT)_3$. There are numerous different contact points between antibody and antigen and all forms of bonding are employed. The flexible nature of DNA may permit it to wrap around the antibody thus involving amino acids not only in the hypervariable complementarity determining regions (CDRs) but also in the framework (FW) regions. In parallel, computer-based molecular modelling of antibody-DNA complexes may provide a way of predicting the variety of ways in which the mAbs interact with their antigens, but the real value of this approach will only be clear when more solved co-crystal structures are available.

Thus, the fine specificity of DNA antibodies is highly varied, and much greater than the classification scheme implies, and the epitopes with which the antibodies react are largely definable only by indirect means. Given that the affinity of DNA antibodies also varies considerably, we may conclude that they are highly diverse in their fine specificity. This contrasts to the situation with protein antigens where their recognition by *auto*antibodies is probably restricted to a small number of sites on each molecule. In spite of its comparative basic simplicity compared with proteins – four bases compared with 20 amino acids – the antigenic complexity of DNA may be at least as great as that of proteins because of its highly varied higher structure, its plasticity and its size. The implication is that the diversity of the repertoire of DNA antibodies is very large and arises through the use of many different primary antibody sequences. These could arise either from the use of many different germ line genes or through use of a few germ line genes that diversify through mutation. Because DNA antibodies are a major component of the response of normal B cells to polyclonal activation, for example with lipopolysaccharide, the conclusion therefore is that the potential repertoire of DNA antibodies is very large.

THE ORIGINS OF DNA ANTIBODIES

It has been alluded to earlier that DNA antibodies are not restricted to an association with SLE. In fact, they are readily detectable in sera from patients with other autoimmune diseases[7,25] and also in normal sera and can be isolated as mAbs from normal adults but especially from fetal and newborn humans and mice. The natural DNA antibodies in normal individuals, like the autoantibodies against other autoantigens that accompany them, tend to be extensively cross-reactive, of relatively low functional affinity, and to be of the IgM type. There is considerable speculation about the relationship of these antibodies to those found in association with lupus and other connective tissue diseases which tend to have higher functional affinities and to include IgG antibodies. Comparisons have been made at two levels: their cellular origins and the Ig V_H and V_L genes employed in coding them.

In fetal and young individuals there is a significant population of B cells differentiated by their expression of the CD5 molecule (synonymous with Ly-1 in the mouse) on their surface[26]. From examining mAbs reactive with

DNA derived from CD5+ and CD5− B cells respectively from human peripheral blood it is clear that the antibodies are not grossly different with regard to their specificity[27]. The suggestion that CD5+ cells can convert to CD5− cells is suggested by recent experiments[28], and this implies therefore that the usual repertoire of DNA antibodies is expressed in both types of B cell and that the cells making natural DNA antibodies, which might be supposed to have a homeostatic function[29], can convert under appropriate conditions to making antibodies that can contribute to pathology. The characteristics of pathological antibodies will be dealt with a little later, but it is germane to mention here that at least one mAb of fetal origin, assumed to originate from a CD5+ cell, has been shown to have a potential for pathology: mAb F-423 from a fetal MRL/lpr mouse has been shown to immunize MRL/n mice to induce a form of lupus disease[30].

Now that there are many sequences for DNA antibodies available for comparison, it can be tentatively concluded that the germline V_H genes used to code them are not unique in that those identified so far can also be found to code for antibodies of other specificities[31,32]. In humans, the small VH families V_H4, V_H5 and V_H6 are dedicated to coding autoantibodies and some reactive with DNA have been found in each family[33,34]. Less is known about V_L gene usage, but there is no evidence either that there is restricted V_L usage in coding DNA antibodies. It is probable that the contribution of the L chain to DNA binding is relatively small[35]. In a series of elegant studies in mice, Weigert and colleague[36] have determined the V_H gene sequences of sets of DNA antibody-secreting hybridomas from lupus mice and have shown that within one individual there is common usage of particular V_H germline genes that with time mutate to give rise to clonally related sets of cells each making DNA antibodies with slightly different functional affinity and hence fine specificity. Individual mice do not, however, use the same V_H germline genes. In these studies, and in others, variations were noted in the CDR3 sequences of the heavy chain genes implying that insertions and mutations accounted for some of the functional diversity of DNA antibodies and that the CDR3 hypervariable loop is very important in binding DNA.

So, pathological and homeostatic antibodies may come from the same cell in different states of differentiation. The question must then be asked, what are the triggers that turn a cell from making protective to making damaging antibodies? The assumption behind the question is that the antibodies *are* different in some way from each other and that disease does not arise simply from non-immunological physiological changes. In considering the high proportion of mutations that occur in DNA antibodies outside the CDRs, Diamond et al.[37] conclude that selection by antigen (either DNA or some structurally homologous molecule) is not likely to be the reason that mutated DNA antibodies are found. Rather, they invoke a defect in regulation in peripheral tolerance. In other words, self-DNA-reactive cells are not deleted or silenced and their accumulation is an essential aetiologic factor in disease.

DNA ANTIBODIES AND PATHOLOGICAL PROCESSES

The important immunopathology in SLE is generally held to centre on the deposition of immune complexes in critical sites such as the kidney, skin and blood–brain barrier. The complexes associate with basement membranes where they become lodged and induce inflammation. An excellent and comprehensive account of SLE can be found in the eponymous book by Lahita[38]. The processes of inflammation are not well understood, even in the kidney which is well studied in SLE, but the involvement of complement and the potential of the immune complexes to initiate antibody-dependent cellular cytotoxicity mechanisms involving polymorphonuclear neutrophil leucocytes and macrophages are the two major likely mechanisms. Recently, it has been realized that lymphocytes infiltrate kidney lesions in SLE and in other diseases like malaria[39]. T cells are not uncommon in infiltrates, and one can imagine that they contribute to the inflammatory process especially through the production of pro-inflammatory cytokines like IL-1, IL-6 and TNF. Clearly, more needs to be learnt about the contribution of these cells, so that their importance relative to immune complexes in initiating and perpetuating lesions can be estimated. This may be important for developing immune-based therapies, but most people would support the idea that it is the immune complexes that initiate the lesions.

Antibodies that bind DNA can be eluted from kidneys with deposited immune complexes[40,41]. However, there is every reason, as explained above, to suppose that other antigens and antibodies can participate in the formation of phlogistic complexes, but the greatest effort has been spent on the DNA antibodies. There are at least two mechanisms whereby complexes can accumulate in the kidney, and presumably also in the other target sites, and these involve either the preformation of complexes by DNA and antibodies in the circulation or the planting of antigen that then captures antibody[42,43]. Free nucleic acids survive only briefly in the circulation either because they are degraded by circulating endonucleases or because they bind with high affinity to basement membranes and endothelial cells[44,45]. For example, DNA adheres readily to fibronectin – one of the constituents of the healthy kidney mesangium – and can then in turn bind anti-DNA antibodies[43]. It is likely therefore that the sequential planting and growth of complexes in the kidney is the more important of the two mechanisms.

The characteristics of the antibodies that are found in renal deposits have been examined, and in some cases at least they tend to be relatively cationic compared with the circulating DNA antibody pool[40], implying that there is a selective localization of certain antibodies in the pathological lesions. The corollary is that not all the DNA antibodies circulating in SLE patients can be pathologically important. It might be clinically beneficial to be able to identify unequivocally the pathogenic antibodies and thus use their detection as an aid in disease assessment; flares and remissions might more easily and precisely be predicted. This so far is not possible but other analytical approaches to defining the properties of pathogenic antibodies are beginning to produce substantial amounts of information. The approaches have involved either the passive transfusion of DNA mAbs into normal mice or the creation of transgenic mice carrying the V_H and V_L genes for DNA antibodies.

Transfusion of DNA antibodies

The fact that DNA antibodies exist in normal individuals without causing symptoms of SLE is one obvious piece of evidence that not all DNA antibodies are pathogenic, but we must be aware that the amount of antibody in such situations is usually much less than that found in patients with SLE. On the other hand, amount alone is insufficient to cause nephritis. For example, mice that carry some, but not all (see below), hybridomas making DNA mAbs can have antibody at several milligrams per millilitre in their blood without evidence of immune complex nephritis[46]. Others get disease. At the least, this tells us that with antibodies that are innocuous on their own a source of antigen is necessary for inflammation to be initiated (see later) and further that DNA antibodies do not necessarily bind to kidney structures by charge interactions in the absence of (DNA) antigen to cause a lesion[11,15,18]. Several authors have reported studies in which defined mAbs have been infused under controlled conditions. Thus, we found that an IgG2bκ DNA mAb (designated IV-228) with high affinity for ssDNA caused kidney damage to young MRL/lpr mice, but that another antibody (mAb I-410) of the same isotype, with a lower affinity and reactive with both dsDNA and ssDNA, was innocuous[47]. Both antibodies could be shown to accumulate on preformed complexes but only the high affinity antibody caused changes in kidney function. In common with other authors[48–50] we found that these antibodies did not cause nephritis in normal healthy mice.

We concluded that multiple antibody–antigen interactions are involved in the formation of immune complexes in the kidney, and the same conclusion was also reached by Vlahakos et al.[51] in their more recent examination of mice implanted with hybridomas secreting DNA mAbs or directly injected with mAbs. Eight out of 24 mAbs tested in this way deposited in the kidneys of the host mice. The patterns of complex deposition (mesangial, dense, diffuse, endothelial and intramembraneous) varied with the antibody and reflected the range of patterns seen in active disease. This is an interesting method to study hybridoma antibodies that was first used to demonstrate the pathogenic properties of anti-erythrocyte autoantibodies in mice[52]. But, as the authors themselves point out[51], it is yet to be proved that the presence of the hybridoma itself does not provide critical factors that are necessary for the experimental nephritis and which are absent from the natural disease situation. In the same series of experiments it was found that five other DNA mAbs that did not participate in forming extracellular immune deposits did in fact penetrate cells and could be detected by immunofluorescence as intranuclear staining in kidney sections[53]. Intranuclear deposits were associated with morphological changes in the mesangium and functional changes expressed as proteinuria. Thus some DNA mAbs may penetrate cells *in vivo* and contribute to the physiologic changes of the lupus nephrosis.

Mice with DNA autoantibody transgenes

Although focused on tolerance studies, such mice may provide a means to study antibody pathogenicity. The approach to producing mice carrying antibody transgenes has been very valuable in studies on specific B cell development and tolerance which, by manipulation of other transgenes encoding the target antigen, can be examined in the presence or absence of the antigen[54]. However, in the case of mice with DNA antibody transgenes this luxury is not available because of the unavoidable presence of DNA as antigen[55], so the interpretation of effects seen in these mice is more difficult. In the first published study, secretion of the potentially pathogenic DNA antibody was engineered in non-autoimmune strain mice by expressing transgenes for the $V_H 3H9$ heavy chain of DNA antibody with one of several different V_L transgenes. DNA antibody production was not seen, implying that the B cells had been tolerized and that the mice were phenotypically normal[35]. Subsequently, it was reported that C57BL/6 mice with V_H and V_L transgenes for DNA mAb #A6.1 did produce small amounts of the transgenic IgG2aκ antibody and also developed a mild nephritis[56]. In this case we assume that the tolerance mechanisms were bypassed, but this approach does not yet provide a way of comparing the pathogenic properties of different anti-DNA antibodies.

The telling experiments will be those in which the antibody transgenes are established in animals with a congenital autoimmune background, like the MRL/lpr mouse. Several laboratories are working on this, but no results are yet reported. It is encouraging that it has been possible to produce mice with Ig transgenes for an anti-erythrocyte antibody, and a proportion of the transgenic animals were found to express the transgenic antibody and to develop haemolytic anaemia (also relevant to the pathology of SLE), indicating a bypass of the normal tolerance mechanisms[28]. It is relevant to the discussion above on the cellular origins of DNA autoantibodies that the cells responsible for making the pathogenic anti-erythrocyte antibody were Ly-1 + and proliferated in the peritoneal cavity where, it was assumed, they had escaped deletion through the local absence of the erythrocyte antigen.

GENETIC CONTRIBUTIONS TO DEVELOPMENT OF SLE

It is not surprising that in a disease as complex as SLE a gene or genes that universally predispose to disease have not been found. However, in common with many other autoimmune conditions, there are clear genetic influences on the development and progression of disease. In humans, the concordance rates between monozygotic twins have been reported to be between 20 and 60%[38]. It is interesting to realize, however, that it is not uncommon to find the antibodies (e.g. reactive with DNA) that characterize SLE expressed also in the unaffected spouses of patients[57]. Why, is not known.

The MHC in humans

The HLA system is clearly important but simple associations are most easily seen in defined ethnic groups: the A1,B8,DR3 haplotype gives an approximately 10 × relative risk in Caucasians[58]. The association of complement component C4 null alleles with SLE has long been recognized, and presumably operates through impaired handling of immune complexes[59]. Because MHC Class II genes can influence IgG antibody production, some effort has been put into searching for associations between them and autoantibody production in SLE. Notably the work of Arnett and colleagues[60] has shown the importance of HLA-DQ alleles, such that alleles coding DQw2.1 and DQw6 are absent from the majority of patients that make anti-Ro and anti-La antibodies. It was notable that the DQ α and β chains present in these patients had sequence variants with glutamine at position 34 in the α chain and leucine at position 26 of the β chain: both locate in the peptide binding groove of the Class II α–β heterodimer. The implication here is that these reflect the importance of an MHC Class II restricted response to an as yet unidentified peptide in the production of the autoantibodies concerned. It is easy to see how this may operate for the production of antibodies against protein antigens, but in the case of antibodies against DNA it is more difficult to envisage. Nonetheless, the HLA-DQB1 alleles *0201, *0602 and *0302 (coding for DQw2, 6 and 3 respectively) were each found to associate positively with the production of antibodies against dsDNA in SLE patients. Because there is no evidence that T cells can make MHC-restricted responses to DNA itself, one must assume that the T cells in these situations are responding to a protein component of an antigen macromolecular complex that includes the DNA to which the B cells respond. This form of linked recognition is one possible mechanism to account for effective T cell help in anti-DNA antibody production. The possibility that the B cells actually respond to cross-reactive protein antigen has not been formally excluded and could account for the MHC Class II association in view of the potential of activated B cells to present antigens.

The MHC in mice

In mice, it is also concluded that MHC genes predispose to the development of SLE. In summarizing recent work, Drake and Kotzin[61] emphasize the importance of the NZW H-2^z haplotype in (NZB × NZW)F$_1$ mice for the development of lupus disease. This is intriguing because the NZW parent of the F$_1$ hybrid is phenotypically normal, whereas it is the NZB parent that contributes to the autoimmune syndrome characterized by haemolytic anaemia and insidious lupus disease. This is an example, the *lpr* gene on the MRL background being another, of gene complementation producing an accelerated disease syndrome. The idea that it is the *I-A*^{z} or *I-E*^{z} genes that confer susceptibility to accelerated lupus in the hybrid mice is supported by studies on the H-2^{bm12} mutant gene inserted in the NZB background[62]. Such mice are like the (NZB × NZW)F$_1$ mice in that they make IgG anti-DNA antibodies and develop nephritis. The phenotypic expression of the H-2^{bm12}

mutation is in three amino acid changes in the I-Aα chain in the area involved in peptide binding. Again, we need an explanation for the help this might provide for antibody production against DNA, but it is consistent with the findings in humans where MHC Class II genes associate with lupus disease.

The *lpr* gene

There have been exciting advances recently in understanding the significance of the *lpr* gene, which in MRL strain mice will accelerate disease onset. While there is no reason to think that there is a counterpart to this gene necessarily operating in human disease, it is, as mentioned above, an example of the way in which particular genes may influence the outcome of disease in already susceptible individuals. The same *lpr* gene does not induce lupus disease in mice of other strains. MRL/lpr mice have a massive proliferation of T cells that express neither CD4 nor CD8. It has been found that the *lpr* gene is a mutant of the gene that codes the Fas antigen[63], which is a cell surface protein with predicted structural homology to the TNF receptor, the low affinity NGF receptor and the CD40 B cell marker. It is an important finding that antibodies against Fas cause programmed cell death or apoptosis of the cells with which they react. Exactly where Fas normally operates in lymphoid ontogeny is not known, but the effect of the *lpr* mutation is to permit T cells to escape from apoptosis and to accumulate in the periphery. The natural ligand for Fas has not been identified but it is possible that it is encoded by a wild type version of the *gld* gene; mice homozygous for *gld* have a generalized lymphoproliferative disorder indistinguishable from the *lpr* homozygous mice, yet *lpr* and *gld* are not allelic (reviewed in [64]).

THE IDIOTYPES OF DNA ANTIBODIES

The idiotype (Id) of an antibody is defined immunochemically by other antibodies, known as anti-idiotype antibodies, that bind to epitopes known as idiotopes in the variable regions of the heavy and/or light chains. Some idiotopes are very closely associated with the hypervariable CDRs, and others are in the FW regions. So, the Id relates in some way to the specificity of the antibody and to its protein, and may be a genetic marker of the origins of the V_H and V_L genes. Anti-Id antibodies can be produced as natural components of an antibody response and are thought to have a role in the endogenous regulation of the response; they can also be made by intentional immunization and can then be used as probes for the expression of particular antibodies bearing the Ids. In autoimmune disease in general there are thus two main areas of interest involving idiotypes: first their use as markers of pathogenic autoantibodies; second their use as therapeutic agents to control antibody-mediated pathology. The Ids of DNA antibodies have been studied intensively for these very reasons and several intriguing findings have emerged recently (for reviews see references [65] and [66], and the articles that follow them in J Autoimmunity 1990; 3(4) and Lupus 1992; 1(4) respectively).

Diversity of DNA antibody idiotype systems

Many different Id systems have been defined, in different laboratories, on DNA antibodies and over fifty have certainly been described. Most of the best studied Id systems have been reviewed by Rauch and Bell[67] and Buskila and Shoenfeld[7]. Mostly heterologous polyclonal antisera raised against mAbs or serum DNA antibodies have been used to define the Ids, although a few monoclonal anti-Id antibodies have been prepared. The great majority of the Ids have been found to be expressed on more antibodies than those used to immunize in the first place. They are thus referred to as public Ids or cross-reactive Ids (CRI). One of the most extensively studied is the 16/6 Id which has been found on many mAbs and in a high proportion of sera from SLE patients. It is interesting that Id 16/6 has been found in the sera of patients with other connective tissue diseases and infectious diseases. Because of the nature of the assay systems to detect the Ids it has not always been possible to identify the antigen specificity of Id + antibodies in sera. However, studies of various sera and antibodies have shown that the DNA antibody Ids like 16/6 can be found on antibodies of other specificities[68]. It is obvious then that DNA antibody Ids are not markers of the antibody specificity, but, as discussed below, more likely the genetic origin of the V gene segments encoding them.

Idiotypes and disease processes

Exactly how the expression of the Ids on serum immunoglobulins relates to the disease process in SLE is not well understood but there are several indications that they can be markers of disease progression. To be fair, it is also not clear exactly how the DNA antibodies themselves, especially when measured simply in the circulation, relate to the disease process.

Empirical evidence that Ids are important to disease development includes various observations that show their levels on serum antibodies fluctuate with cycles of disease activity in humans (summarized in [69]) and change with age in mice as disease develops (e.g. [70]). Antibodies eluted from deposits in lupus kidneys are not only selectively enriched for cationic immunoglobulins (above), but also may be characterized by high expression of the GN2 Id[71]. In skin and kidney immune deposits, Ids can be detected on immunoglobulins *in situ* by immunocytochemical means[72–74]. The association of DNA antibody Ids with SLE and other diseases has been demonstrated in many surveys of sera, and in a large collaboration, ten laboratories looked at 19 different Ids and found that three (3I, V-88, GN2) were especially relevant to the autoimmune features of SLE[75,76]. The study employed several anti-Id reagents raised initially against mouse DNA antibodies and these were as effective as the anti-human anti-Id reagents at identifying Ids on human serum antibodies. This emphasizes that at least some of the idiotopes of DNA antibodies are expressed across species barriers.

Genetics of DNA antibody idiotypes

In other non-autoimmune Id systems there are several examples where it appears quite obvious that there is a simple genetic basis to the expression of a particular Id that characterizes the response. However, this has been relatively difficult to identify in the more complex autoimmune SLE situation. The analysis of the gene sequences of antibodies expressing particular Ids is very complex but has indicated in the case of Id.16/6 that the CDR2 area in the H chain is highly conserved between the antibodies that express Id16/6[77]. An oligonucleotide probe for the 5' region of CDR2 has been found to hybridize with RNA from all 16/6+ hybridomas detecting the $V_H18/2$ gene that is dominant in human B cells[78]. A similar conclusion was reached by a quite different route using a pepscan method to produce synthetic peptides corresponding to the V_H and V_L sequences of mAb V-88, a mouse mAb that expresses Id.16/6. The reaction of heterologous rabbit anti-V-88 anti-Id serum with these peptides also identified a similar area of the V_H region as a site of a major idiotope, but through this approach it was concluded that the flanking FW2 sequences were also involved[23]. While these studies are not conclusive they do indicate ways in which idiotypes can be identified and analysed by relatively new molecular methods.

The pepscan approach has been used extensively in the author's laboratory to analyse also the anti-Id antibodies in sera from mice and humans with SLE. These contain antibodies that react with a variety of epitopes in the V regions of DNA antibodies[79], and some of these are the same as those recognized by the heterologous anti-Id antisera just mentioned. However, the disease sera, which are genetically autologous to the antibody sequences, tended much more to recognize epitopes in loop structures rather than those in β sheet FW areas. This emphasizes that the origin of the anti-Id antibodies influences the specificity of the idiotopes they react with. In any case, all the epitopes recognized in this way are linear sequences and not discontinuous structures; it is the latter that probably characterize the private Ids of anti-protein antibodies. An elegant crystal structure of an idiotype-anti-idiotype has been solved, and it shows quite clearly the end-to-end docking of the interacting antibodies with many amino acids contributing to the bonding between them[80]. From the sequences of reactive idiotopes identified by epitope scanning it has been possible through computer modelling of antibodies to predict their location on the V regions. In the case of V-88 we have found that the great majority of the epitopes recognized in the pepscan would be on the exposed surfaces of the parent antibody. It appears that much of the antibody V region surface is antigenically active in this way and so we conclude that it probably all contributes to the idiotype of DNA antibodies[81]. The potential for cell interactions via idiotypic connections could be very great in consequence.

The sequences identified as idiotopes are clearly not restricted to single antibodies, they are parts of the CRI. Because their distribution is so widespread they are not distributed in a strictly idiotypic way. For example, the V_H26 ($= V_H18/2$) gene that encodes Id.16/6+ antibodies exists in almost all humans so far examined, and it is known that the 16/6 idiotype is itself very widely expressed[78]. In genetic terms, this is an isotype, or possibly an allotype. Thus what have been generally thought of as idiotypes are probably not idiotypes at all – they are isotypes. This is discussed by Jefferis[82]. Clearly more needs to be done to elucidate the genetics of CRIs, and the role of somatic mutation in their expression. Private Ids are usually expressed in (highly mutated) anti-protein antibodies, and the crystal structure shows that the idiotopes are discontinuous structures. In these circumstances, they will not be coded by single gene segments in the germline DNA. CRI on the other hand are much more likely to be products of simple gene segments.

Idiotypes as molecular mimics of antigens

Some of the peptide-reactive antibodies found in anti-Id sera probably do not react with the native antibody molecules – a not uncommon finding with anti-peptide antibodies, but it does raise the question why individuals with SLE have antibodies against antibody fragments. The answer is not known, but we have noted sequence homology between the sequence of at least one V region epitope (a putative idiotope) and the sequence of the heat shock proteins Hsp60 of mammals and *E. coli* and other bacteria, and with Hsp65 of mycobacteria. We have hypothesized that this homology could underlie a functional link in that antibodies against bacterial/mammalian Hsps are also anti-idiotypic for autoantibodies against DNA[23]. One could imagine that the response to one antigen could lead to a response to the other through idiotypic linkage. Indeed this could involve T cells as well as B cells and could explain the appearance of DNA antibodies in conditions of inflammation where responses against Hsps are known to be commonplace.

Considering the great diversity of sequence that is possible in antibody V regions it is perhaps not surprising that sequences common to antibodies and other proteins might be found. Apart from the Hsp mimicry, there are other examples where V region sequences are similar to those in other proteins. Pucetti and colleagues identified a sequence of the U1RNP protein antigen in the light chain of a mAb that was anti-idiotypic to an anti-NsnRNP antibody[83], and Swanson et al. found that a sequence of C reactive protein that binds phosphorylcholine itself carries the T15 Id[84]. What is needed is experiments that address the functional link between these sequence homologies at both the B cell and the T cell level. So far, however, such experiments have not been done, but we do know that, in other experimental systems, peptides corresponding to antibody V region sequences can induce antibodies that bind to the intact parent antibody (e.g.[85,86]). Comparable activities of T cell receptor $V\beta$ peptides have been reported (e.g. [87]). It appears that V region sequences are quite strongly immunogenic – that is, they induce immune responses readily – and this can be exploited by replacing CDR sequences with foreign epitope sequences by molecular genetic means; the resulting antigenized antibodies are good immunogens to raise anti-peptide antibodies[88].

Idiotypes and induced SLE

The special immunogenicity of antibody V regions almost certainly underlies some fascinating observations that a form of SLE can be induced in mice by immunization with DNA mAbs. The ability of an antibody to induce more antibody of the same specificity when it is itself used as an immunogen has been known for some time[89], and has been one of the observations that has fuelled the idea that antibodies, and T cells too, are connected in some form of idiotype network first elegantly promoted by Jerne[90] and subsequently the subject of much speculation.

In SLE it has been found that disease and the immunologic features of it can be induced by immunizing mice of non-autoimmune strains (e.g. BALB/c) with human DNA mAbs bearing the 16/6 Id. The original observations made in two laboratories by Mozes and Shoenfeld[91] and the subsequent experiments are discussed by Buskila and Shoenfeld in Chapter 9 of this book. The explanation for this effect is that the immunizing antibody induces the production of anti-Id antibodies that in turn induce anti-anti-Id antibodies, some of which are similar enough to the first immunizing antibody to cause disease. The great importance of this model is that it demonstrates the potential to develop SLE disease in animals not noted for its idiopathic development. There are clear genetic influences on the susceptibility to induced SLE. It is not only DNA antibodies that are effective in this way because antibodies against phospholipids induce a phospholipid antibody syndrome.

There has been one study in which SLE was not induced in non-autoimmune mice by immunization with Id.16/6+ human mAbs[92]; rather the animals developed a form of adjuvant arthritis[93]. But enhanced disease has been seen in MRL/n mice immunized with mouse DNA mAbs (either IV-228 or F-423) which expressed other idiotypes[30]. In the latter experiments, it was found that serum antibodies bearing Id.V-88 were produced as a result of the immunization and, as mentioned earlier, Id.V-88 is closely related to Id.16/6, emphasizing again the central role that Id.16/6 has in SLE. The reasons why SLE disease is not equally inducible in different situations must surely be a consequence of environment, and in particular the microbial load and exposure to antigens in the diet could be particularly influential. We know from other studies that exposure through mucosal tissues to autoantigens influences the development of autoimmunity[94] and that rearing rodents in a germ-free environment will affect their susceptibility to induced arthritis[95].

Clearly the interplay between two major factors is required for the development of SLE: susceptibility genes and immune stimulation provided by environmental antigens or microbes.

Modification of disease by anti-idiotype antibodies

Therapies for controlling SLE are designed to suppress the immune system in a largely non-specific way. The possibilities for specific immunosuppression are limited: we do not know much about the important target antigens, and anyway they are probably very diverse so suppressing responses against one may be ineffective in limiting disease; we know even less about the specificity of T cells, so T cell or TCR based vaccines are not yet accessible. For these reasons there is some expectation that manipulation of DNA antibody Ids may be a route to effective disease control. There have been several reports of the immunosuppressive properties of such anti-Id antibodies[96-98], but to the extent that it has been examined, it seems that suppression is not permanent. There are cases where anti-Id antibodies stimulate rather than suppress[99], so the combined use of anti-Id antibodies and drugs like cyclosporin may be preferred[100].

Acknowledgements

The author acknowledges with thanks the support of The Arthritis and Rheumatism Council, The Wellcome Trust and The Medical Research Council for the work described here.

References

1. Chan EKL, Tan EM. Epitopic targets for autoantibodies in systemic lupus erythematosus and Sjögren's syndrome. Curr Opin Immunol. 1989; 1: 376–381.
2. Tan EM. Antinuclear antibodies: diagnostic markers for autoimmune diseases and probes for cell biology. Adv Immunol. 1989; 44: 93–151.
3. Morrow WJW, Isenberg DA. Autoimmune Rheumatic Diseases. Oxford: Blackwell Scientific Publ; 1987.
4. van Venrooij WJ, Charles P, Maini RN. The consensus workshops for the detection of autoantibodies to intracellular antigens in rheumatic diseases. J Immunol Meth. 1991; 140: 181–189.
5. Stollar BD. Anti-DNA antibodies. Clin Immunol Allergy. 1981; 1: 243–260.
6. Harris EN. Immunology of antiphospholipid antibodies. In: Lahita RG, ed. Systemic Lupus Erythematosus. New York: Churchill Livingstone; 1992: 305–325.
7. Buskila D, Shoenfeld Y. Anti-DNA antibodies. In: Lahita RG, ed. Systemic Lupus Erythematosus. New York: Churchill Livingstone; 1992: 205–26.
8. Staines NA, Denbury AN. Nucleic acids. In: Masseyeff R, Albert WA, Staines NA, eds. Methods of Immunological Analysis. 2. Reagents and Samples. VCH, Weinheim, 1993 Chapter 3.6.
9. Stott DI. Spectrotypes of anti-DNA antibodies show that anti-DNA-secreting B-cell clones of SLE patients are restricted in number, stable and long-lived. Autoimmunity. 1992; 12: 249–258.
10. Morgan A, Buchanan RRC, Lew AM, Olsen I, Staines NA. Five groups of antigenic determinants on DNA identified by monoclonal antibodies from (NZB × NZW)F₁ and MRL/*lpr/lpr* mice. Immunology. 1985; 55: 75–83.
11. Brinkman K, Termaat R, Berden JHM, Smeenk RJT. Anti-DNA antibodies and lupus nephritis: the complexity of crossreactivity. Immunol Today. 1990; 11: 232–234.
12. Harris EN, Gharavi AE, Tincani A, Chan JKH, Englert H, Mantell P, Allegro F, Ballastrieri G, Hughes GRV. Affinity purified anti-cardiolipin and anti-DNA antibodies. J Clin Lab Immunol. 1985; 17: 155–162.
13. Eilat D, Zlotnick AY, Fischel R. Evaluation of the cross-reaction between anti-DNA and anti-cardiolipin antibodies in SLE and experimental animals. Clin Exp Immunol. 1986; 65: 269–278.
14. Staines NA, Thompson HSG, Morgan A. Diversity and multispecificity of autoantibodies reactive with DNA: Some evolutionary implications. Protides Biol Fluids. 1985; 33: 241–244.

15. Eilat D. Cross-reactions of anti-DNA antibodies and the central dogma of lupus nephritis. Immunol Today. 1985; 6: 123–127.
16. Brinkman K, Termaat R-M, de Jong J, van den Brink HG, Berden JHM, Smeenk RJT. Cross-reactive binding patterns of monoclonal antibodies to DNA are often caused by DNA/anti-DNA immune complexes. Res Immunol. 1989; 140: 595–612.
17. Emlen W, Ansari R, Burdick G. DNA-anti-DNA immune complexes. Antibody protection of a discrete DNA fragment from DNase digestion *in vitro*. J Clin Invest. 1984; 74: 185–190.
18. Eilat D. Anti-DNA antibodies: problems in their study and interpretation. Clin Exp Immunol. 1986; 65: 215–222.
19. Borel H, Sasaki T, Stollar BD, Borel Y. Conjugation of DNA fragments to protein carriers by glutaraldehyde: immunogenicity of oligonucleotide-hemocyanin conjugates. J Immunol Meth. 1984; 67: 289–302.
20. Cappuro DE. Determinants on DNA identified by monoclonal DNA binding autoantibodies from lupus mice [dissertation]. London, UK: King's College London; 1993.
21. Lafer EM, Valle RPC, Möller A, Nordheim A, Schur PH, Rich A, Stollar BD. Z-DNA-specific antibodies in human systemic lupus erythematosus. J Clin Invest. 1983; 71: 314–321.
22. Bronze-da-Rocha E, Machado C, Staines NA, Sunkel CE. Systemic lupus erythematosus murine monoclonal antibodies recognize cytoplasmic and nuclear phosphorylated antigens that display cell cycle redistribution in Hep-2 cells. Immunology. 1992; 77: 582–591.
23. Staines NA, Ward FJ, Denbury AN, Mitchiner J, Hartley O, Eilat D, Isenberg DA, Bansal S. Primary sequence and location of the idiotopes of V-88, a DNA-binding monoclonal autoantibody, determined by idiotope scanning with synthetic peptides on pins. Immunology. 1993; 78: 371–378.
24. Herron JN, He XM, Ballard DW, Blier PR, Pace PE, Bothwell ALM, Voss EW, Edmundson EB. An autoantibody to single-stranded DNA: comparison of the three-dimensional structures of the unliganded Fab and a deoxynucleotide-Fab complex. Proteins: Structure Function & Genetics. 1991; 11: 159–175.
25. Wozencraft AO, Lloyd CM, Staines NA, Griffiths VJ. The role of DNA-binding antibodies in the kidney pathology associated with murine malaria infections. Infect and Immun. 1990; 58: 2156–2164.
26. Casali P, Notkins AL. CD5+ lymphocytes, polyreactive antibodies and the human B-cell repertoire. Immunol Today. 1989; 10: 364–368.
27. Suzuki N, Sakare T, Engleman E. Anti-DNA antibody production by CD5+ and CD5- B cells of patients with systemic lupus erythematosus. J Clin Invest. 1990; 85: 238–247.
28. Murakami M, Tsubata T, Okamoto M, Shimizu A, Kumagai S, Imura H, Honjo T. Antigen-induced apoptotic death of Ly-1 B cells responsible for autoimmune disease in transgenic mice. Nature. 1992; 357: 77–80.
29. Grabar P. Autoantibodies and the physiological role of immunoglobulins. Immunol Today. 1983; 12: 337–340.
30. Ravirajan CT, Staines NA. Involvement in lupus disease of idiotypes Id.F-423 and Id.IV-228 defined, respectively, upon foetal and adult MRL/*Mp/lpr/lpr* DNA-binding monoclonal autoantibodies. Immunology. 1991; 74: 342–347.
31. Diamond B, Rauch J. An idiotype systems update. Lupus. 1992; 1: 323–324.
32. Zouali M, Stollar BD. The molecular biology of anti-DNA antibodies and their idiotypes. Lupus. 1992; 1: 325–331.
33. Hillson JL, Perlmutter RM. Autoantibodies and the fetal anti-body repertoire. Int Rev Immunol. 1990; 5: 215–229.
34. Watts RA, Hillson JL, Oppliger IR, Mackenzie L, Lydyard PM, Mackworth-Young CG, Brown C, Staines NA, Isenberg DA. Sequence analysis and idiotypic relationships of BEG-2, a human fetal antibody reactive with DNA. Lupus. 1991; 1: 9–17.
35. Erikson J, Radic MZ, Camper SA, Hardy RR, Carmack C, Weigert M. Expression of anti-DNA immunoglobulin transgenes in non-autoimmune mice. Nature. 1991; 349: 331–334.
36. Shlomchik MJ, Sascelli M, Shan H, Radic MZ, Pisetsky D, Marshak-Rothstein A, Weigert M. Anti-DNA antibodies from autoimmune mice arise by clonal expansion and somatic mutation. J Exp Med. 1990; 171: 265–292.
37. Diamond B, Katz JB, Paul E, Aranow C, Lustgarten D, Scharff MD. The role of somatic

mutation in the pathogenic anti-DNA response. Annu Rev Immunol. 1992; 10: 731–757.
38. Lahita RG, ed. Systemic Lupus Erythematosus. New York: Churchill Livingstone; 1992.
39. Lloyd CM, Wozencraft AO, Williams DG. Cell mediated pathology during murine malaria associated nephritis. To be published.
40. Ebling F, Hahn BH. Restricted subpopulations of DNA antibodies in the kidneys of mice with systemic lupus erythematosus. Comparison of antibodies in serum and renal eluates. Arthritis Rheum. 1980; 23: 392–403.
41. Dang H, Harbeck RJ. The *in vivo* and *in vitro* glomerular deposition of isolated anti-double-stranded-DNA antibodies in NZB/W mice. Clin Immunol Immunopathol. 1984; 30: 265–278.
42. Izui S, Lambert PH, Miescher PA. *In vitro* demonstration of a particular affinity of glomerular membrane and collagen for DNA. A possible basis for local formation of DNA-anti-DNA immune complexes. J Exp Med. 1976; 144: 428–443.
43. Lake RA, Morgan A, Henderson B, Staines NA. A key role for fibronectin in the sequential binding of native dsDNA and monoclonal anti-DNA antibodies to components of the glomerular matrix: its possible significance in glomerulonephritis. Immunology. 1985; 54: 389–395.
44. Frampton G, Hobby P, Morgan A, Staines NA, Cameron JS. A role for DNA in anti-DNA antibodies binding to endothelial cells. J Autoimmun. 1991; 4: 463–478.
45. Chan TM, Frampton G, Staines NA, Hobby P, Perry GJ, Cameron JS. Different mechanisms by which anti-DNA MoAbs bind to human endothelial cells and glomerular mesangial cells. Clin Exp Immunol. 1992; 88: 68–74.
46. Lake RA, Staines NA. DNA-binding antibodies derived from autoimmune MRL mice fail to induce clinical changes when administered to healthy animals. Agents & Actions. 1986; 19: 306–308.
47. Lake RA, Staines NA. A monoclonal DNA-binding autoantibody causes a deterioration in renal function in MRL mice with lupus disease. Clin Exp Immunol. 1988; 73: 103–110.
48. Ben Chetrit E, Dunskey EH, Wollner S, Eilat D. *In vitro* clearance and tissue uptake of anti-DNA monoclonal antibody and its complexes with DNA. Clin Exp Immunol. 1985; 60: 159–168.
49. Cukier R, Tron F. Monoclonal anti-DNA antibodies: an approach to studying SLE nephritis. Clin Exp Immunol. 1985; 62: 143–149.
50. Jones FJ, Pisetsky DS, Kurlander RJ. The clearance of a monoclonal anti-DNA antibody following administration of DNA in normal and autoimmune mice. Clin Immunol Immunopathol. 1986; 39: 49–60.
51. Vlahakos DV, Foster MH, Adams S, Katz M, Ucci AA, Barrett KJ, Datta SK, Madaio MP. Anti-DNA antibodies form immune deposits at distinct glomerular and vascular sites. Kidney Int. 1992; 41: 1690–1700.
52. Cooke LA, Staines NA, Morgan A, Moorhouse C, Harris G. Haemolytic disease in mice induced by transplantation of hybridoma cells secreting monoclonal anti-erythrocyte autoantibodies. Immunology. 1982; 47: 569–572.
53. Vlahakos D, Foster MH, Ucci AA, Barrett KJ, Datta SK, Madaio MP. Murine monoclonal anti-DNA antibodies penetrate cells, bind to nuclei, and induce glomerular proliferation and proteinuria in vivo. J Am Soc Nephrol. 1992; 2: 1345–1354.
54. Goodnow CC. Transgenic mice and analysis of B-cell tolerance. Annu Rev Immunol. 1992; 10: 489–518.
55. Weigert M, Schwartz RS. Consideration of the transgenic and other approaches to studying DNA antibodies and their idiotypes. Lupus. 1992; 1: 333–334.
56. Tsao BP, Ohnishi K, Cheroutre H, Mitchell B, Teitell M, Mixter P, Kronenberg M, Hahn BH. Failed self-tolerance and autoimmunity in IgG anti-DNA transgenic mice. J Immunol. 1992; 149: 350–358.
57. Isenberg DA, Williams W, Le Page S, Swana G, Feldman R, Addison I, Bakimer R, Shoenfeld Y. A comparison of autoantibodies and common DNA antibody idiotypes in SLE patients and their spouses. Br J Rheumatol. 1988; 27: 431–436.
58. Worrall JG, Snaith ML, Batchelor F, Isenberg DA. SLE – a rheumatological view. Q J Med. 1990; 275: 319–330.
59. Morgan BP, Walport MJ. Complement deficiency and disease. Immunol Today. 1991; 12: 301–306.

60. Arnett FC. Genetic aspects of human lupus. Clin Immunol Immunopathol. 1992; 63: 4–6.
61. Drake CG, Kotzin BL. Genetic and immunological mechanisms in the pathogenisis of systemic lupus erythematosus. Curr Opin Immunol. 1992; 4: 733–740.
62. Chiang BL, Bearer E, Ansari A, Dorshkind K, Gershwin ME. The BM12 mutation and autoantibodies to dsDNA in NZB.H-2bm12 mice. J Immunol. 1990; 145: 1184–1194.
63. Watanabe-Fukunaga R, Brannan CI, Copeland NG, Jenkins NA, Nagata S. Lymphoproliferation disorder in mice explained by defects in Fas antigen that mediates apoptosis. Nature. 1992; 356: 314–317.
64. Cohen PL, Eisenberg RA. The *lpr* and *gld* genes in systemic autoimmunity: life and death in the *Fas* lane. Immunol Today. 1992; 13: 427–428.
65. Isenberg DA, Staines NA. Idiotypes of DNA binding antibodies: analysis of their role in health and disease. J Autoimmun. 1990; 3: 339–356.
66. Staines NA. Idiotypes of DNA-binding antibodies: recent advances. Lupus. 1992; 1: 313–316.
67. Rauch J, Bell D. The characterization of DNA antibody idiotypes – a description. J Autoimmun. 1990; 3: 357–366.
68. El-Roiey A, Sela O, Isenberg DA, Feldman R, Colaço CB, Kennedy RC, Shoenfeld Y. The sera of patients with klebsiella infections contain a common anti-DNA idiotype (16/6) Id and anti-polynucleotide activity. Clin Exp Immunol. 1987; 67: 507–515.
69. Zouali M, Diamond B. Idiotype-mediated intervention in systemic lupus erythematosus. J Autoimmun. 1990; 3: 381–388.
70. Staines NA, Ravirajan CT, Morgan A, Belcher AJ, Henry AJ, Lake RA, Smith DA, Hamblin AS, Hara M, Adu D, Morland C, Isenberg DA. Expression and relationships of seven public idiotypes of DNA-binding autoantibodies on monoclonal antibodies and serum immunoglobulins. Lupus. 1993; 2: 25–33.
71. Hahn BH, Ebling FM. Idiotype restriction in murine lupus; high frequency of three public idiotypes on serum IgG in nephritic NZB/NZW F_1 mice. J Immunol. 1987; 138: 2110–2118.
72. Isenberg DA, Collins C. Detection of cross-reactive anti-DNA antibody idiotypes on renal tissue bound immunoglobulins from lupus patients. J Clin Invest. 1985; 76: 287–294.
73. Isenberg DA, Dudeney C, Wojnaruska F, Bhogal BS, Rauch J, Naparstek Y, Duggan D, Schattner A. Detection of cross-reactive anti-DNA antibody idiotypes on tissue bound immunoglobulins from skin biopsies of lupus patients. J Immunol. 1985; 135: 261–264.
74. Watts RA, Ravirajan CT, Wilkinson LS, Williams W, Griffiths M, Butcher D, Horsfall AT, Staines NA, Isenberg DA. Detection of human and murine common idiotypes of DNA antibodies in tissues and sera of patients with autoimmune diseases. Clin Exp Immunol. 1991; 83: 267–273.
75. Isenberg DA, Williams S, Axford J, Bakimer R, Bell D, Casaseca-Grayson T, Diamond B, Ebling F, Hahn B, Harkiss G, Mackworth-Young C, Le Page S, Massicotte H, Rauch J, Ravirajan C, Schwartz R, Shoenfeld Y, Staines NA, Todd-Pokropek A, Tucker L, Watts R, Zouali M. Comparison of DNA antibody idiotypes in human sera: an international collaborative study of 19 idiotypes from 11 different laboratories. J Autoimmun. 1990; 3: 393–414.
76. Cairns E, Andrejchyshyn S, Ruach J. An inter-laboratory idiotype assay validation study. Lupus. 1992; 1: 317–322.
77. Young F, Tucker L, Rubinstein D, Guillaume T, André-Schwartz J, Barrett KJ, Schwartz RS, Logtenberg T. Molecular analysis of a germ line-encoded idiotypic marker of pathogenic human lupus autoantibodies. J Immunol. 1990; 145: 2545–2553.
78. Schwartz RS, Stewart AK, Huang CC, Stollar BD, Rubinstein D, Barrett K. A single VH gene dominates the largest human VH gene family in human B cells. Lupus. 1992; 1(Suppl 1): 4.
79. Ward FJ, Denbury AN, Bansal S, Staines NA. Epitope analysis by scanning of synthetic peptides of the specificity of antibodies against V region epitopes of DNA-binding antibodies in the sera of mice with SLE. In preparation.
80. Bentley GA, Boulot G, Riottot MM, Poljak RJ. Three-dimensional structure of an idiotype-anti-idiotype complex. Nature. 1990; 348: 254–257.
81. Hobby P, Ward FJ, Sutton BJ, Williams DG, Staines NA. Computer modelling of a three dimensional map of the V region epitopes of a DNA-binding antibody, V-88, recognized

by heterologous antisera and by antibodies in the sera of humans and mice with SLE. In preparation.

82. Jefferis R. What is an idiotype? Immunol Today. 1993; 14: 119–121.

83. Pucetti A, Koizumi T, Migliorini P, André-Schwartz J, Barrett KJ, Schwartz RS. An immunoglobulin light chain from a lupus-prone mouse induces autoantibodies in normal mice. J Exp Med. 1990; 171: 1919–1930.

84. Swanson SJ, Lin B-F, Mullenix MC, Mortensen RF. A synthetic peptide corresponding to the phosphorylcholine (PC)-binding region of human C-reactive protein possesses the TEPC-15 myeloma PC-idiotype. J Immunol. 1991; 146: 1596–1601.

85. Mazza G, Guigou V, Moinier D, Corbet S, Ollier P, Fougerau M. Molecular interactions in the 'GAT' idiotypic network. An approach using synthetic peptides. Ann Inst Pasteur/Immunol Paris. 1987; 136D: 259–269.

86. Meek K, Takei M, Dang H, Sanz I, Dauphinee MJ, Capra JD, Talal N. Anti-peptide antibodies detect a lupus-related idiotype that maps to the H chain CDR2. J Immunol. 1990; 144: 1375–1381.

87. Hashim GA, Offner H, Wang RY, Shukla K, Carvalho E, Morrison WJ, Vandenbark AA. Spontaneous development of protective anti-T cell receptor autoimmunity targeted against a natural EAE-regulatory idiotope located within the 39–59 region of the TCR Vβ8.2 chain. J Immunol. 1992; 149: 2803–2809.

88. Zanetti M. Antigenized antibodies. Nature. 1992; 355: 476–477.

89. Forni L, Coutinho A, Köhler G, Jerne NK. IgM antibodies induce the production of antibodies of the same specificity. Proc Natl Acad Sci USA. 1980; 77: 1125–1128.

90. Jerne NK. Towards a network theory of the immune system. Ann Immunol (Inst Pasteur). 1974; 125: 373–389.

91. Mendlovich S, Brocke S, Shoenfeld Y, Ben-Bassat M, Meshorer A, Bakimer P, Moyes E. Induction of a systemic lupus erythematosus-like disease in mice by a common anti-DNA idiotype. Proc Natl Acad Sci USA. 1988; 85: 2260–2264.

92. Isenberg DA, Katz DR, Le Page S, Knight B, Tucker L, Maddison P, Hutchings P, Watts R, André-Schwartz J, Schwartz RS, Cooke A. Independent analysis of the 16/6 idiotype lupus model: a role for an environmental factor. J Immunol. 1991; 147: 4172–4177.

93. Knight B, Katz DR, Isenberg DA, Ibrahim MA, Le Page S, Hutchings P, Schwartz RS, Cooke A. Induction of adjuvant arthritis in mice. Clin Exp Immunol. 1992; 90: 459–465.

94. Thompson HSG, Staines NA. Could specific oral tolerance be a therapy for autoimmune disease? Immunol Today. 1990; 11: 396–399.

95. Van Den Broek MF, Van Bruggen MCJ, Koopman JP, Hazenberg MP, Van Den Berg WB. Gut flora induces and maintains resistance against streptococcal cell wall-induced arthritis in F344 rats. Clin Exp Immunol. 1992; 88: 313–317.

96. Hahn BH, Ebling FM. Suppression of murine lupus nephritis by administration of an anti-idiotypic antibody to anti-DNA. J Immunol. 1984; 132: 187–190.

97. Mahana W, Guilbert B, Avrameas S. Suppression of anti-DNA antibody production in MRL mice by treatment with anti-idiotypic antibodies. Clin Exp Immunol. 1987; 70: 538–545.

98. Epstein A, Greenberg M, Diamond B, Grayzel AI. Suppression of anti-DNA antibody synthesis *in vitro* by a cross-reactive antiidiotypic antibody. J Clin Invest. 1987; 79: 997–1000.

99. Teitelbaum D, Rauch J, Stollar BD, Schwartz RS. *In vivo* effects of antibodies against a high frequency idiotype of anti-DNA antibodies in MRL mice. J Immunol. 1984; 132: 1282–1285.

100. Morland C, Michael J, Adu D, Kizaki T, Howie AJ, Morgan A, Staines NA. Anti-idiotype and immunosuppressant treatment of murine lupus. Clin Exp Immunol. 1991; 83: 126–132.

14
Immunology of Antiphospholipid Antibodies

S. A. KRILIS and J. E. HUNT

INTRODUCTION

Over the last few years there has been a considerable amount of interest in a group of autoantibodies known as antiphospholipid antibodies (aPL). This is due to their association with a number of clinical syndromes characterized by an increased risk of vascular thrombosis, recurrent abortion and certain neurological conditions[1,2]. Although it has been widely assumed that antiphospholipid antibodies are directed against simple anionic phospholipid molecules, it has recently been demonstrated by a number of workers that the antigens are considerably more complex. The advances made in understanding the antigenic specificity of these antibodies has given us new insights into possible mechanisms of how they could exert prothrombotic effects. In this chapter we will concentrate on these recent developments and provide direct evidence for the immunological heterogeneity of antiphospholipid antibodies, and in doing so provide the basis to re-examine the antigenic specificity of these antibodies. In order to understand the antigens to which these antibodies are directed, a review of phospholipid biochemistry is essential.

BIOCHEMISTRY OF PHOSPHOLIPIDS

Figure 1 is a schematic representation of the general structure of a phospholipid molecule. It consists of a glycerol backbone to which are attached a phosphate group on the third carbon and two esterified fatty acid chains at the first and second carbons. The phospholipid group at the third position is linked to a polar head group, the chemical nature of which determines the overall electrical charge of the phospholipid molecule.

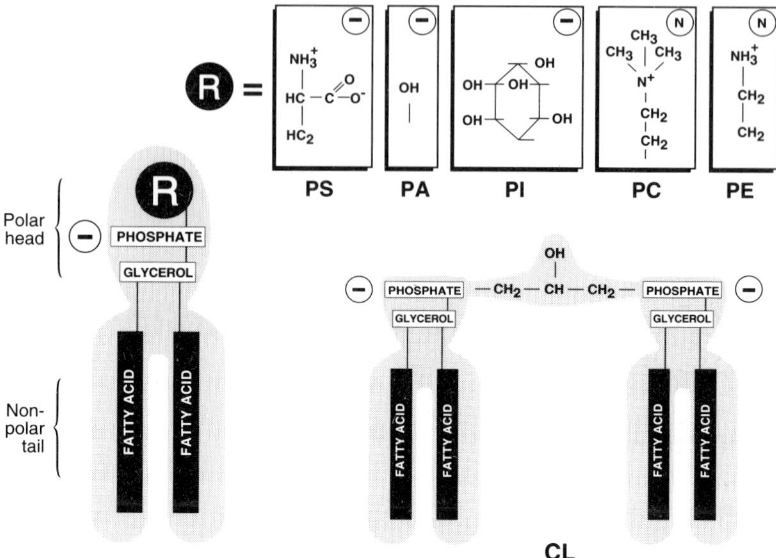

Figure 1 Schematic representation of phospholipid molecule showing basic structure consisting of a glycerol backbone to which are attached two fatty acids forming the non-polar tail and a phosphate molecule with varying head groups represented by R.
PS = phosphatidylserine, PA = phosphatidic acid, PI = phosphatidylinositol, CL = cardiolipin (− = negatively charged phospholipids), PC = phosphatidylcholine, PE = phosphatidylethanolamine (N = neutral phospholipids)

Figure 1 illustrates some of the common phospholipid molecules found in mammalian cells. The simplest structure of these is phosphatidic acid (PA) in which the alcohol is absent. Phospholipids derive their names from the type of alcohol attached to the polar head group. The negatively charged phospholipids are phosphatidylserine (PS), phosphatidic acid (PA), cardiolipin (CL) and phosphatidylinositol (PI). The neutral phospholipids are phosphatidylcholine (PC), phosphatidylethanolamine (PE) and sphingomyelin (SM). Our knowledge about the behaviour of phospholipids has been obtained from *in vitro* model membrane systems of which the simplest is where the lipid under study is dispersed in an aqueous medium. In this particular environment phospholipids, depending on the nature of their head group, length and saturation of the hydrocarbon chains, pH, temperature and divalent cation concentration, will adopt one of three phase structures. These are micellar, lamellar and hexagonal phase (Figure 2). These phase transitions are thought to be important in the induction of antibodies to phospholipids. Although it has been demonstrated that antiphospholipid antibodies can be induced experimentally following injection of bilayer forming lipids in combination with immunogenic carriers or adjuvants[3], it has been recently demonstrated that pure PE alone, in the absence of adjuvants or carriers, is immunogenic only when it is presented in the hexagonal phase[4]. It has been suggested that certain phospholipids can induce conformational changes in HLA-class II molecules that favour their

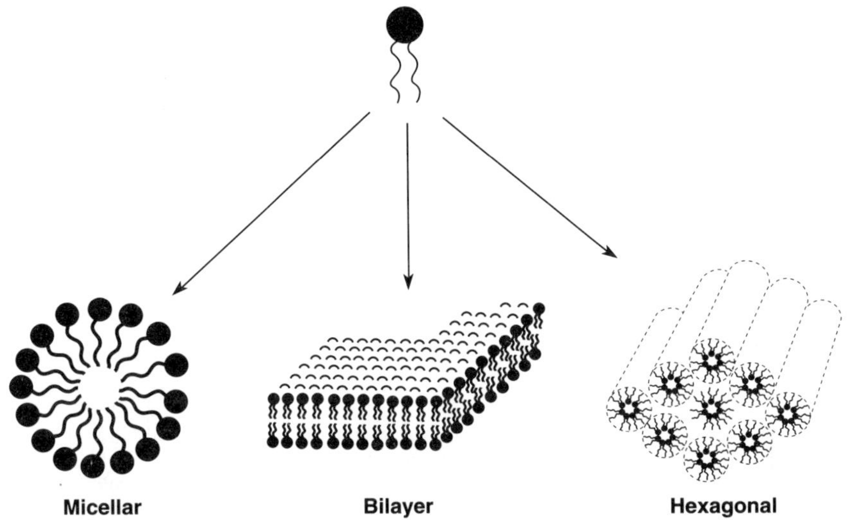

Figure 2 Schematic representation of a phospholipid molecule showing polar head group and non-polar tails and micellar, bilayer and hexagonal phase transitions

peptide binding properties[5].

Table 1 summarizes the characteristics of the major phospholipids found in human cell membranes. Cellular membranes have a common overall structure consisting of a thickness of two molecules or bilayer of fluid lipids, in which proteins are embedded traversing the whole plasma membrane or attached covalently or by charge interactions to the cell surface. Phospholipids form a major part of this bilayer and are arranged with the hydrophobic fatty acid chains directed towards the interior of the cell membrane and the hydrophilic polar head group to either side of the membrane. There is an asymmetrical distribution with respect to the phospholipids, the outer leaflet of the bilayer is rich in PC and SM, whereas the cytosolic layer is mainly composed of PE, PS and PI[6,7]. Cardiolipin is exclusively found in the inner leaflet of the mitochondrial membrane[8]. The physiological mechanisms whereby the asymmetrical distribution of membrane phospholipids is maintained is not known. The distribution of the negatively charged phospholipids to the cytosolic side of the bilayer appears to be stable, and spontaneous migration of phospholipids from the inner to the outer (flip flop) layer is a rare event[9]. However, reorientation of PS and PE can be demonstrated on platelets *in vitro* during activation, through the combined stimulus of collagen and thrombin or calcium ionophore A23187[10].

SITES OF INTERACTION OF PROCOAGULANT PHOSPHOLIPIDS WITH COAGULATION FACTORS

Although in *in vitro* model membrane systems the surface component is formed exclusively by phospholipid vesicles, the *in vivo* situation is more

Table 1 Characteristics of major phospholipids found in human cell membranes

Phospholipid	Net charge	Distribution	Preferential phase in aqueous dispersion	Function
Cardiolipin (CL)	–	Exclusive to inner mitochondria 1 membrane	L	Mitochondrial cytochromes
Phosphatidylserine (PS)	–	Cytosolic layer of plasma membrane	L	Major procoagulant phospholipid
Phosphatidylinositol (PI)	–	Cytosolic layer of plasma membrane	L	Intracellular messenger source of arachodonate
Phosphatidylcholine (PC)	N	Major component of outer plasma membrane	L	Maintain structural membrane integrity
Phosphatidylethanolamine (PE)	N	Major component of outer plasma membrane	H	
Sphingomyelin (SM)	N	Major component of outer plasma membrane	L	Maintain structural membrane integrity

complex since activated platelets, endothelial cells and most probably other cell types provide the procoagulant membrane surface. The surface of activated cells or damaged cell membranes provides procoagulant phospholipids such as PS, which is the major phospholipid with *in vitro* procoagulant activity, and other surface proteins which provide a surface for the assembly and activation of plasma coagulation proteins. Although exteriorized PS is the major procoagulant phospholipid on activated platelets, the prothrombinase activity also involves a specific binding site for factor V/V_a, and membrane bound V/V_a is the receptor for factor X_a. The intrinsic Xase complex $(IX_a/VIII_a/X/calcium)$ binds to a specific receptor at the endothelial cell membrane surface. Figure 3 is a simplified schema of the coagulation cascade, highlighting the possible sites of action of phospholipids, where they both accelerate and stimulate negative feedback reactions in the coagulation cascade (reviewed in [11]). Phospholipids bind factor X_a and V_a in the presence of calcium (prothrombinase complex) and convert prothrombin (II) to thrombin (II_a). Factor X_a and prothrombin bind the phospholipid surfaces through a calcium mediated bridging between their amino terminal gamma carboxy glutamic acid residues and the negatively charged polar head groups of the phospholipid molecules. Phospholipids are also important in the activation of factor X to X_a by the intrinsic Xase complex. Activation of factor X can occur also via the extrinsic Xase complex which consists of

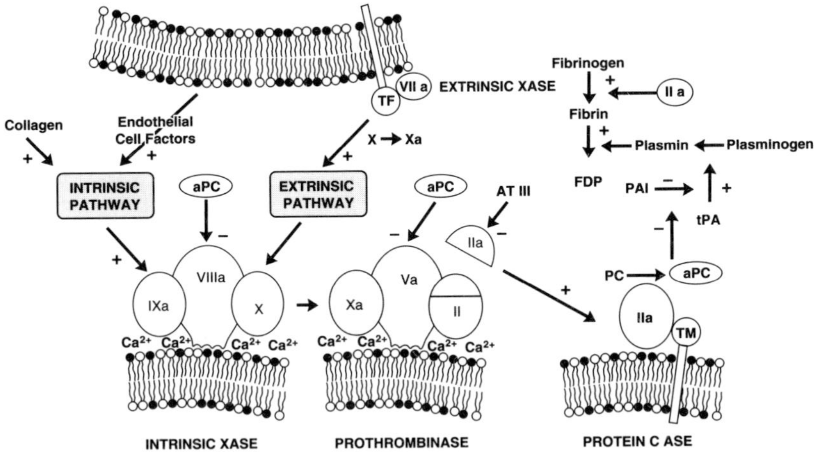

Figure 3 Schematic representation of blood coagulation cascade and sites of interaction of phospholipids with coagulation factors. Roman numerals denote blood coagulation factors. Activated form of coagulation factors is denoted by subscript a. Phospholipid head groups show either neutral or negatively charged phospholipids denoted by clear or filled in head groups, respectively.
aPC = activated protein C, PC = protein C, tPA = tissue plasminogen activator, PAI = plasminogen activator inhibitor, FDP = fibrin degradation products, ATIII = anti-thrombin III, TF = tissue factor, TM = thrombomodulin

factor VII_a, tissue factor (TF), calcium and factor X. It appears that the activation of factor X and prothrombin often occurs on the surface of the same phospholipid vesicle, which would greatly enhance the reaction, since each individual factor would not need to dissociate and reassociate from different phospholipid vesicles in order to participate in any subsequent reactions. The generation of thrombin (II_a) activates protein C in the presence of the integral membrane protein thrombomodulin (TM) (protein Case complex), which is an essential glycoprotein cofactor expressed on endothelial cells. The amplification of thrombin generation is inhibited by activated protein C (aPC). PS is also involved in the activation of protein C, which acts as a natural anticoagulant by inhibiting factor V_a and VIII_a in the presence of free protein S, a cofactor which circulates free and bound to C4b binding protein (C4bBP).

IMMUNOLOGICAL SPECIFICITY OF ANTIPHOSPHOLIPID ANTIBODIES

Assays for aPL antibodies

It has been appreciated that antiphospholipid antibodies consist of a spectrum of antibodies which can be identified using a number of assay systems. Table 2 lists the current methods used to detect these antibodies. The first of these is the ELISA which employs a negatively charged phospholipid antigen,

Table 2 Characteristics of assays for antiphospholipid antibodies

Assay type	Antibody type	Antigen
ELISA/RIA	aCL	CL
Clotting	LA	? Hexagonal PL
Agglutination/ELISA	BFP-STS	CL/PC/Cholesterol

most commonly cardiolipin (CL). Antibodies detected in this system are known as anticardiolipin antibodies (aCL). *In vitro* phospholipid dependent clotting tests are used to assay for the lupus anticoagulants (LA) which interfere by prolongation of clotting times. The exact antigen against which the LA type antibodies are directed is yet to be characterized adequately, despite an assumption that it consists of a lamellar arrangement of anionic phospholipids such as PS[12]. The serological test for syphilis (STS) which is used as a screening test for the aCL antibody occurring in syphilis (reagin) is thought to be immunologically distinct from the aCL antibodies occurring in autoimmune disease (see below). The antigen used in this system is CL, PC and cholesterol in a ratio of $1:10:30$ by weight. The current test for STS uses either an ELISA or an agglutination reaction. Antibodies reactive with the VDRL antigen can be found in patients with SLE and other related autoimmune diseases. In this circumstance it is known as the biological false positive serological test for syphilis (BFP-STS)[13]. It is most likely that the antibodies detected using the CL-ELISA are the same as those binding to the VDRL antigen. The lack of concordance between the CL-ELISA and the STS is most likely due to the fact that the VDRL antigen contains in addition to CL, PC, which would neutralize the negative charge on the CL phosphate groups thus inhibiting binding of the autoimmune aCL antibodies[1,14]. The ELISA using the VDRL antigen is much more sensitive than the agglutination reaction and is considerably more sensitive in detecting the syphilitic antibodies with aCL specificity than the CL-ELISA. Although the antigen to which the syphilitic antibodies bind is cardiolipin, it appears that the spatial presentation of cardiolipin is critical in recognition by these antibodies. Although the performance of the CL-ELISA is straightforward, some assays for aCL are quite unsatisfactory and can result in false positive results which can be due to high non-specific IgM in the serum[15]. There have been a number of attempts to standardize the CL-ELISA; however, it should be considered as a semi-quantitative measurement of circulating antibodies[16]. The initial standardization workshops recommended the use of standard units for measurement of IgG and IgM aCL antibodies. These were termed GPL, where one GPL unit equals one microgram per millilitre of affinity purified IgG aCL antibody, and MPL units, where one MPL unit equals one microgram per millilitre of affinity purified IgM aCL antibody[17]. The second anticardiolipin standardization workshop addressed the issue of inter-laboratory agreement using the semi-quantitative measurements of aCL antibodies. Six samples were distributed worldwide to sixty laboratories and the participants were broken up into groups, with additional sera exchanged between each group. Overall there was excellent agreement between laboratories in each group using the semi-quantitative measurement such that aCL antibodies levels are reported as negative, low positive, medium, or high positive corresponding to approximately GPL/MPL units of less than 5, 5 to 20, 20 to 100, or greater than 100 respectively[18]. A number of commercial CL-ELISA kits are now available. However, a comparison between six available aCL commercial kits showed considerable variation[19]. Despite an attempt to standardize the aCL assay, a recent quality assurance programme, where 20 samples were distributed to 10 different laboratories for aPL testing, revealed significant interlaboratory variation[20]. Although most published studies have only assayed for IgG and IgM aCL isotypes, it would appear that assays for aCL should include separate testing for aCL of the IgG, IgM and IgA isotypes[18,21–23]. It has been suggested that the IgG isotype correlates with predisposition to thrombosis and that the IgM isotype in the absence of either IgG or IgA is less likely to be associated with thrombosis. A number of studies have failed to find any association of clinical events such as thrombosis, fetal loss, or thrombocytopenia with any particular aCL specificity (reviewed in[1]).

aCL antibodies occurring in autoimmune disease have been found to cross-react extensively with other anionic phospholipids such as PS, PI, PG and PA but not the neutral phospholipids such as PC and PE[24]. Cardiolipin can be replaced in the ELISA by the other anionic phospholipids and it can be demonstrated that antibodies with aCL activity can bind directly to these phospholipids[14,21,24]. However, there are occasional reports of some patients who have antibodies reactive with either PE or PS alone but not CL. The polar head group of phospholipids (Figure 1) determines the overall charge which confers specificity for the aCL antibodies from autoimmune patients. In contrast the aCL antibodies occurring in syphilis are different in their specificity for cardiolipin, such that they bind optimally when CL is in the VDRL antigen and in addition recognize neutral phospholipids.

LA ANTIBODIES

The relationship between aCL antibodies and LA, which occurs in association with aCL antibodies with variable concurrence in patients with SLE or related disorders has until recently not been clearly defined. Although the LA type aPL is thought to interact with a phospholipid antigen, this is yet to be characterized adequately, despite an assumption that it consists of a lamellar arrangement of anionic phospholipids such as PS. Recently it has been demonstrated that LA antibodies fail to bind to isolated anionic phospholipids in an ELISA (see below). Other workers have presented evidence to show that LA antibodies interact with lipid structures formed in the presence of hexagonal phase PE[1]. A number of studies have shown a close relationship between the presence of anticardiolipin antibodies, LA activity and spontaneous thrombosis. Indirect evidence supports the notion that these antibodies are closely related. However, a number of studies have identified patients with LA who are aCL negative, and aCL positive patients

Table 3 Assays for identifying aPL antibodies with LA activity

Screening tests	Activator	Added phospholipid	Advantages	Disadvantages
aPTT	Surface contact	+	Convenient Simple Can be automated	Insensitive Unstandardized Less specific
KCT	Surface contact (Kaolin)	NIL	Simple Sensitive Can be used as a mixture NP:TP Not affected by presence of anticoagulants	Plasma needs to be platelet free Must be performed manually Less specific when used as mixture NP:TP
DRVVT	Activator of factor X	+	Specific Can be automated	Less sensitive

who do not show LA activity. In addition, suppression of the antibodies with immunosuppressive agents often results in discordant effects[1]. A major problem in this area is the difficulty with standardization of the variety of *in vitro* clotting tests with varying degrees of sensitivity and specificity which are used to assay for LA antibodies (Table 3). A set of criteria to define LA has been created by a working party on acquired inhibitors of coagulation of The International Committee on Thrombosis and Haemostasis[25], which some workers have found to be too stringent. Most recently a set of revised criteria for LA and guidelines for testing have been published[26]. Lupus anticoagulants are detected by the prolongation of one or more of the currently available phospholipid dependent clotting tests, activated partial thromboplastin time (aPTT), kaolin clotting time (KCT) or dilute Russel Viper Venom Time (dRVVT). Of these tests the aPTT is the most simple. However, it is less specific than the other tests, with the dRVVT being the most specific but somewhat less sensitive. It should be established that the prolongation of the phospholipid dependent clotting test is due to an inhibitor of clotting, which is normally performed by mixing normal plasma with test plasma in different ratios. The abnormality will correct if the inhibitory effect is due to a coagulation factor deficiency but will be significantly prolonged when LA is present. The confirmatory test should consist of the correction of the defect by the addition of an optimal concentration of a procoagulant phospholipid provided by either activated platelets (platelet neutralization procedure) or a pure hexagonal phase phospholipid. It should be demonstrated that the LA is an immunoglobulin although in most circumstances this is not done as a routine. The advantages and disadvantages of the currently used screening tests are outlined in Table 3. Although the aPTT is used by most laboratories as a screening test since it has a number of advantages, it suffers from nonstandardization of the added thromboplastin. The KCT has been found to be one of the most sensitive tests for detection of LA[27]. A simplified KCT screening test using a mixture of normal to test plasma of 4:1, compared to normal plasma alone, has been used and shown to be a sensitive screening test with the majority of LA plasmas[28]. Mixing studies applying the KCT using a range of plasma indicates that there is variability in the patterns, with some LA plasma having normal KCTs when tested alone but prolonged when mixed with normal plasma. This is an example of the LA cofactor effect. In this circumstance the normal plasma provides a cofactor which augments the LA mediated inhibition of *in vitro* clotting. Although originally it had been suggested that this cofactor was prothrombin, immunoglobulin or a complement-like molecule, most recently evidence has been presented that the cofactor is a phospholipid binding plasma glycoprotein (see below). When using the KCT a crucial part of the test is the preparation of the plasma, since plasma must be platelet free. Due to heterogeneity of LA, certain LAs will be missed if only one screening test is used; thus in some circumstances more than one clotting test may be required to demonstrate LA. Some workers have recommended the use of two tests, one with minimal phospholipid for sensitivity and the other with increased phospholipid for specificity[29-31].

aPL SUBSETS

Relationship of aCL and LA antibodies

There has been a general assumption in the literature that the prolonged clotting time in plasma seen with patients with LA is due to phospholipid specificity of these antibodies that presumably compete with the coagulation factors for the anionic phospholipid head groups which provide the pro-coagulant surface (reviewed in [1]). Because of this assumption aCL and LA antibodies have been thought to be closely related or identical antibodies and workers have suggested the replacement of LA tests with the more sensitive and simple phospholipid ELISA[32,33]. There is ample epidemiological and other evidence to indicate discordance between the presence of each activity. LA in the absence of aCL occur frequently and occasionally up to 40%[34]. Even when LA and aCL antibodies occur in the same patients, most reports show discordance between the levels of each[34,35]. In recent years evidence has been presented that in many cases aCL and LA are different antibody subsets. Although indirect evidence supports the notion that these antibodies are closely related, work from our laboratories and others has provided direct evidence for the separate nature of these antibodies[36,38].

A negatively charged phospholipid (CL or PS) was immobilized in a solid phase support without the need for chemical modification and provided a novel phospholipid affinity column for purification of aPL antibodies[37]. The major advantage of this technique, over the traditional affinity purification of aPL antibodies using liposomes, is that this method is simple and the purified preparation is phospholipid free. Plasma from patients with autoimmune disease that had both aCL and LA activity were subjected to purification using this phospholipid affinity column. aCL type antibodies were purified but did not possess LA activity[37]. Other workers have presented

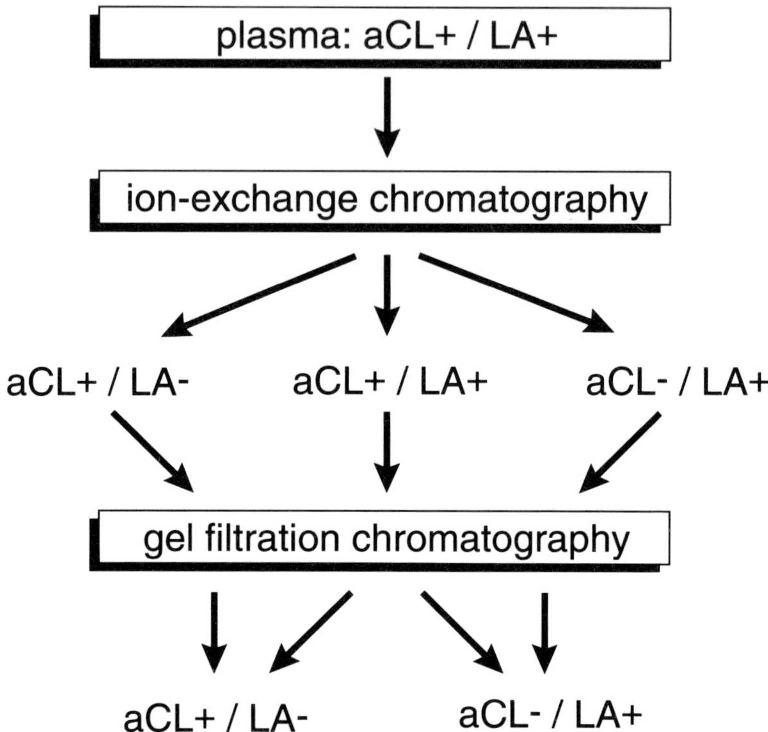

Figure 4 A flow diagram representing purification scheme used to separate aCL and LA. aCL = anticardiolipin antibody using CL-ELISA, LA = lupus anticoagulant using the KCT. + = positive − = negative

similar results using solid phase CL[38]. Subsequently we showed that plasma from patients with both activities could be separated into fractions containing aCL without LA activity and LA without aCL activity (Figure 4)[39]. Although some fractions initially contained both activities, it was possible to remove the majority of the aCL activities from these fractions without affecting the LA activity using the phospholipid affinity column. Furthermore, the fractions with aCL activity were polyspecific for all anionic phospholipids (PS, PI, CL, PA), but not neutral phospholipids (PC, SM)[39]. In addition, in this study we observed that in some patients with both activities, there was isotype discordance between aCL and LA. These experiments demonstrated heterogeneity in the aCL antibodies with at least three subtypes of IgG, aCL occurring concurrently in the same patients and resolved during ion exchange chromatography. However, other workers have shown LA activity in affinity purified aCL when these have been purified using the liposome technique[40–42]. It is possible that the preparations purified using this method contain a mixture of both LA and aCL antibody subgroups. Studies utilizing human monoclonal antibodies with LA activity have demonstrated that

Table 4 ELISA for measurement of antiphospholipid antibodies

	Standard CL-ELISA	Modified CL-ELISA
1. Antigen coated on wells	cardiolipin in ethanol	cardiolipin in ethanol
2. Blocking buffer	10% ABS/PBS	0.3% gelatine/1% milk powder
3. Sample dilution buffer	10% ABS/PBS	0.3% gelatine
4. Antigen detection	Alkaline phosphatase conjugated anti-human IgG, IgM, IgA	

some react in the CL-ELISA. Incubation of plasma with aCL and LA activity with solid phase CL resulted in concurrent reduction of both activities but with different relative reduction of LA activity versus aCL level in different patients. These results have been interpreted as indicating that LA and aCL antibodies are a heterogeneous group of antibodies with similar specificities but with different affinities or with varying affinities for different structural presentations of the lipid antigen[43]. It has also been suggested that the discordance between LA and aCL antibodies is due to a population of LA antibodies that have anti-prothrombin activity[44]. Support for this contention comes from recent work which suggests that some LA antibodies are dependent on prothrombin for their action (see below). Antiphospholipid antibodies detected by the CL-ELISA detect different antibody subgroups from those with LA activity. Thus for practical purposes, both assays should be used when assaying for the presence of aPL antibodies.

ANTIGENIC SPECIFICITY OF ANTIPHOSPHOLIPID ANTIBODIES

aCL plasma cofactor

Following purification of aCL antibodies by ion exchange chromatography or phospholipid affinity chromatography, they failed to bind to the phospholipid affinity column from which they were originally purified unless native plasma was also applied, suggesting that a cofactor present in plasma but separated from aCL during ion exchange chromatography was required for aCL to bind to negatively charged phospholipids[39]. However the purified aCL antibody could still bind in the CL-ELISA. The standard CL-ELISA uses as the diluent bovine serum, which has this cofactor activity. To purify this cofactor we developed a modified CL-ELISA (Table 4) in which all serum components were replaced with a gelatine/milk powder mixture which provided adequate blocking of non-specific binding. This cofactor was purified using sequential chromatography and the amino terminal sequence of the purified material identified it as β_2-glycoprotein I (β_2GPI)[45].

The cofactor requirement of aCL antibodies has now been independently confirmed by two other groups[46,47]. These other groups more recently have also confirmed that the aCL cofactor they reported is β_2GPI[48,49]. Binding of purified aCL antibodies to CL coated microtitre wells was found to be absolutely dependent on the presence of β_2GPI in a dose dependent manner.

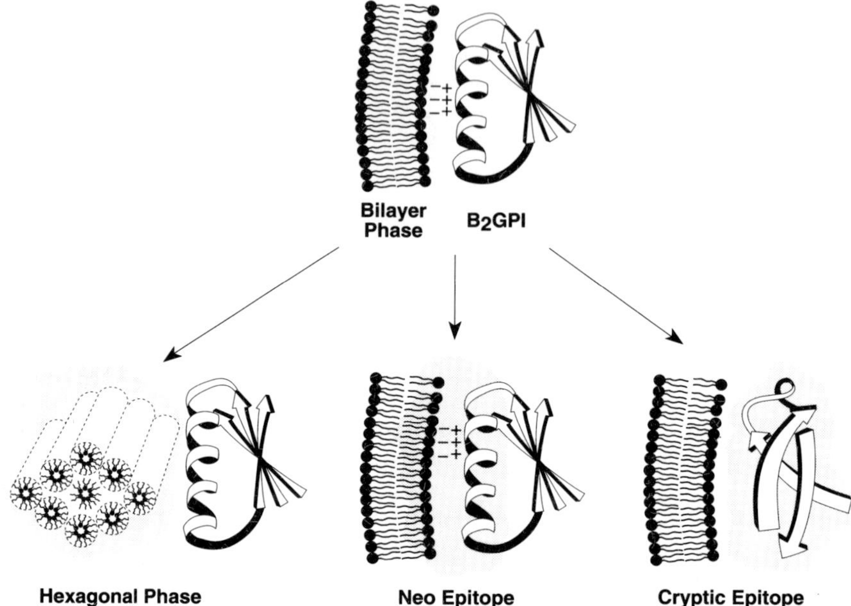

Figure 5 A schematic representation of β_2GPI interacting with negatively charged phospholipid bilayer and possible consequences of this interaction. β_2GPI is represented hypothetically as having one α helix and three β pleats. The shaded areas represent possible epitopes for aCL antibodies. Hexagonal phase phospholipid, neoepitope formed by a shared epitope of β_2GPI, and phospholipid or a cryptic epitope shown as a conformational change of β_2GPI to a hypothetical structure of 3 β pleats

β_2GPI also binds to heparin and DNA, but aCL antibodies were found not to bind to heparin, β_2GPI or β_2GPI covalently linked to Sepharose or when coated onto microtitre plates, suggesting that the β_2GPI phospholipid complex comprises the epitope to which aCL antibodies are directed.

Our results indicated that both anionic phospholipids and β_2GPI are required for binding of aCL antibodies. There are at least three hypotheses to explain the possible antigens created by the interaction of β_2GPI with negatively charged phospholipid. These are schematically represented in Figure 5.

(1) A phase change from lamellar to hexagonal occurs in the phospholipid and the aCL antibodies bind this phase.
(2) A neoepitope is formed by the interaction of phospholipid and β_2GPI or
(3) A cryptic epitope of β_2GPI is exposed which the aCL antibodies bind.

There is some experimental evidence to suggest that β_2GPI binding to negatively charged phospholipid vesicles can modify their physicochemical structure[50].

In a further study we have extended our initial observations and have examined in detail purified aCL from patients with autoimmune disease and a variety of infections including syphilis. Without exception, aCL from

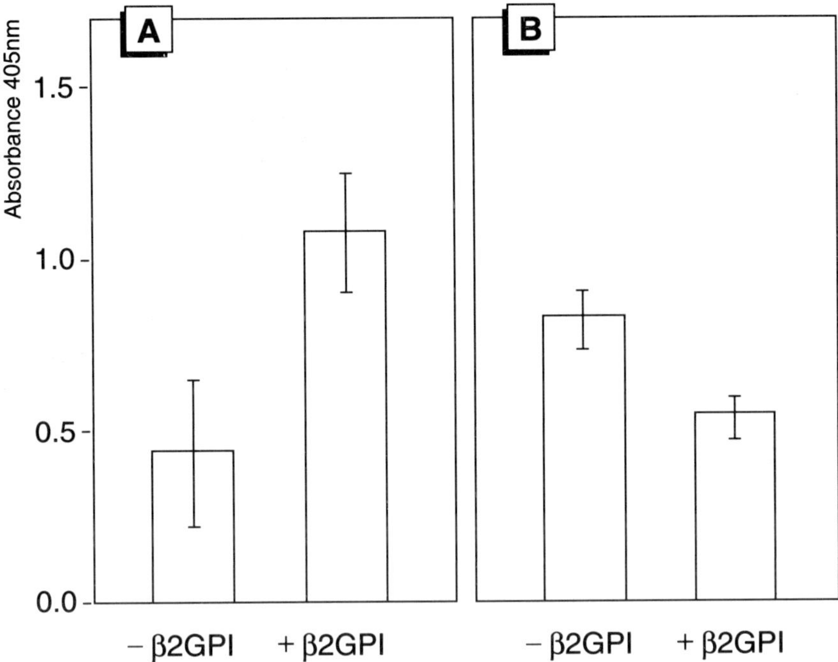

Figure 6 Results of modified CL-ELISA with and without β_2GPI.
A) IgG, aCL from patients with autoimmune disease, mean $\pm$ SD $n = 8$
B) IgG, aCL from patients with a range of infections. (Syphilis $n = 6$, malaria $n = 7$, hepatitis A $n = 1$, infectious mononucleosis $n = 1$, mean $\pm$ SD $n = 15$

patients with infections bound CL in the modified CL-ELISA without the need for added β_2GPI. In contrast, purified aCL of at least one isotype from 11 of 12 patients with autoimmune disease required the presence of β_2GPI to bind CL[51–53] (Figure 6). In one patient with autoimmune disease and aCL antibodies, binding to CL was dependent on the presence of β_2GPI only for the IgA and not for the IgG isotype. This indicates that the type of aCL antibodies occurring in infections are occasionally associated with autoimmune disease. In all samples tested from patients with infections, addition of β_2GPI resulted in a moderate reduction of aCL binding in the modified ELISA. The addition of β_2GPI inhibited binding of aCL antibodies to cardiolipin presumably because of competition for lipid binding sites. It would appear that aCL antibodies associated with infection are directed against a specific phospholipid component only and thus are not likely to display significant cross-reactivity. It is known that aCL from syphilitics recognize CL when presented as the VDRL antigen but show little or no cross-reactivity with negatively charged phospholipids. Our results provide an explanation for this phenomenon. If aCL associated with autoimmune disease recognize β_2GPI phospholipid complex as the antigen in the ELISA, then the cross-reactivity can be accounted for by the known affinity of this glycoprotein for negatively charged phospholipids. When provided in a solid

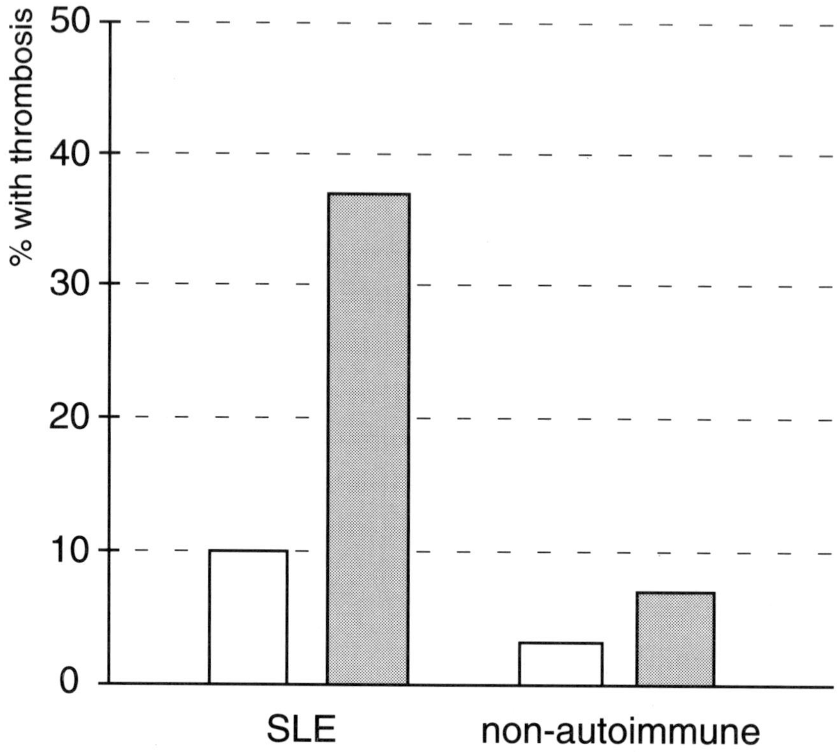

Figure 7 Incidence of thrombosis with ■ and without □ aPL antibodies. SLE = systemic lupus erythematosus, non autoimmune = patients with syphilis and certain drug therapies

phase ELISA, the β_2GPI binds to the phospholipid component and this complex in turn is bound by aCL. It would appear that aCL antibodies associated with a range of infections are directed against a specific phospholipid component only, and thus are not likely to display significant cross-reactivity. Other workers have also reported that aCL antibodies associated with syphilis can bind to CL in the absence of β_2GPI[47,54].

The fact that aCL antibodies that bind CL in the presence of β_2GPI are found only in the autoimmune group of patients may have important clinical implications. It is in this group of patients that thromboembolic complications have been reported. Most studies would indicate that patients whose aCL antibodies are associated with syphilis or other infections do not suffer from these complications. Figure 7 (summary of data from[1,2]) presents data on the risk of thrombosis in SLE and non-autoimmune associated aPL antibodies. In SLE the risk is approximately 40% in the presence compared with a risk of 15% in the absence of aPL antibodies. In marked contrast, in the non-autoimmune group (certain drug therapies and infections) there appears to be no increased risk of thrombosis in the presence of aPL antibodies. Although there is an acceptance by most workers of the importance of β_2GPI in aCL phospholipid interactions[45–47,52,54–56], there are workers who have questioned the absolute requirement of β_2GPI in the binding of aCL antibodies to anionic phospholipids[57,58]. There is still considerable controversy about the nature of the epitope to which aCL antibodies bind. A number of investigators have reported that aCL antibodies bind to β_2GPI coated plates in the absence of phospholipid[46,59,60], whereas other workers have been unable to confirm these findings[45,54–56].

β_2 – GLYCOPROTEIN I: A PROTEIN COFACTOR FOR aPL ANTIBODIES

β_2GPI is a plasma β_2 globulin first described in 1961. It is composed of 326 amino acids and has a unique sequence with abundant proline residues, multiple disulphide bonds and a high carbohydrate content of approximately 19% resulting in an apparent molecular weight of 50 kD[61]. β_2GPI is a member of the Short Consensus Repeat (SCR) or Complement Control Protein (CCP) Repeat Super Family. These proteins have in common a repeating motif of approximately 60 amino acids with a highly conserved pattern of cysteine residues. β_2GPI is composed of five of these repeats[62]. Recently Walsh et al.[63] have extensively investigated the carbohydrate residues of β_2GPI and shown that they are bi and tri antennary sugars and that all potential carbohydrate attachment sites are utilized. The concentration of β_2GPI in plasma is approximately 200 μg/ml and 40% is associated with lipoproteins of various classes[64]. Because of this, β_2GPI has also been designated apolipoprotein H[65]. β_2GPI levels are bimodally distributed and it is thought that the levels are controlled by a pair of autosomal co-dominant alleles, termed $Bg^N Bg^D$. Individuals homozygous with a common allele Bg^N have the N phenotype (normal levels greater than 140 μg/ml). Those homozygous for Bg^D have the rare D phenotype (deficient or undetectable levels) and heterozygous have type I (intermediate, less than 140 μg/ml)[66,67]. Unlike other proteins with CCP or SCR domains which are concerned with complement activation and whose genes map to chromosome one in the human, this member of the super-family maps to chromosome 17[68]. A number of workers have now determined the complete nucleotide sequence of human, bovine, rat and mouse forms of β_2GPI[62,69–71]. The sequences of interspecies (bovine, rat, mouse) β_2GPI show that they are highly homologous and are approximately 84% homologous to the amino acid sequence of human β_2GPI. Despite this homology, most aCL antibodies, however, have a preference for human β_2GPI compared to bovine[56] or mouse β_2GPI (unpublished observation). There are occasional patients whose aCL antibodies bind cardiolipin only in the presence of human and not bovine β_2GPI[56]. Although human β_2GPI inhibits CL binding by aCL antibodies from patients with infections, neither bovine nor rat β_2GPI showed this inhibition[48]. It has been suggested that the difference at position 154 in human β_2GPI might be associated with the inhibitory effect on the binding of syphilitic aCL to CL[48]. The five homologous domains of β_2GPI contain two disulphide bridges except the fifth domain which contains an additional disulphide bridge. Only six of the eleven disulphide bonds have

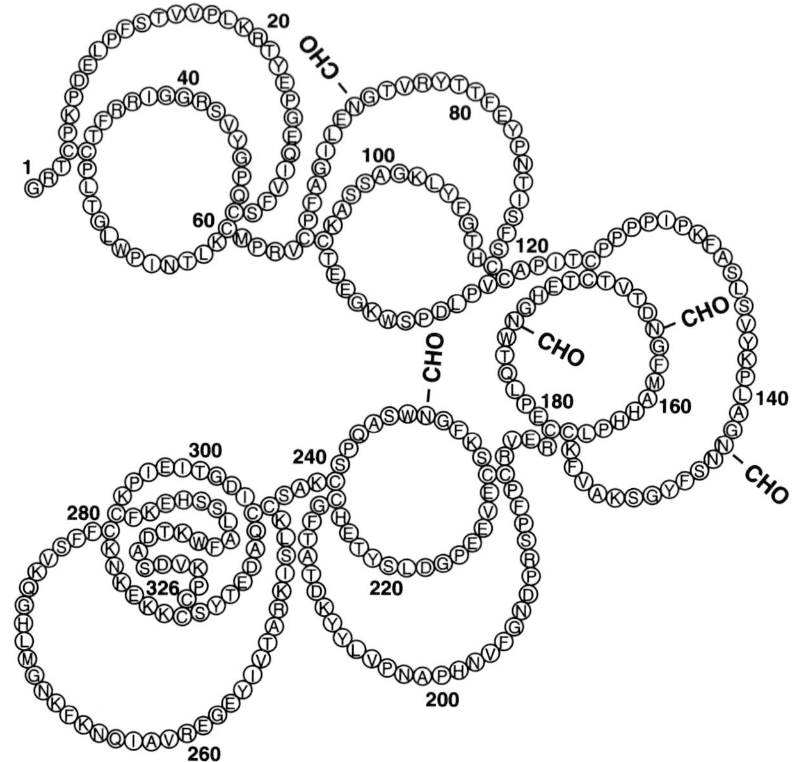

Figure 8 Proposed model of bovine β_2GPI based on the disulphide maps showing the five repeating 'sushi' domains. Letters denote different amino acids. CHO denotes N-linked glycosylation sites, 1 denotes amino terminal end, and 326 denotes carboxy terminal end. Numbers identify amino acid residues. CC denotes disulphide bonds.
Reprinted with permission from Kato H, Enjygi K-I, Biochemistry. 1991; 30: 11687–11694. Copyright 1992 American Chemical Society

been mapped for human β_2GPI and only one of these was in the fifth domain. However all disulphide bonds for bovine β_2GPI have been mapped[72] and the linkages with the proposed model depicting the five repeating domains is schematically represented in Figure 8.

The precise regions of β_2GPI involved in the interaction with negatively charged phospholipids and with other structures have not as yet been determined. The structure of β_2GPI is such that it contains a large number of basic amino acid residues in each of its domains. Out of 38 basic amino acids 15 are in domain five. A sequence of highly positively charged amino acid residues[282–287], lys-asn-lys-glu-lys-lys, is predicted to be a surface exposed turn and is a likely lipid binding site[73]. The ability of β_2GPI to bind negatively charged phospholipids is critical in its role as aCL antibody cofactor[73].

It has been suggested that ionic and hydrophobic interactions are important in the binding of lipids by β_2GPI[74]. Recently a region in the carboxy terminus of β_2GPI has been identified as a possible lipid binding site[73]. The micro heterogeneity of β_2GPI is well established and a number of isoelectric subspecies have been reported[75]. All isoelectric subspecies of β_2GPI have been reported to possess significant cofactor activity[73] despite having subspecies with a wide range of PIs. This would suggest that the carbohydrate residues are not important for aCL cofactor activity.

Although the physiological function of this glycoprotein is uncertain, it is known to be synthesized in the liver and to bind to lipoproteins and a range of negatively charged molecules such as phospholipids, heparin, DNA and mitochondrial membranes. The binding of β_2GPI to negatively charged surfaces could explain the inhibitory effect of β_2GPI in the coagulation cascade by inhibiting the phospholipid activation of a number of the coagulation factors. It has been suggested that one function of β_2GPI is to bind to and neutralize negatively charged macromolecules that might enter the bloodstream and thus diminish unwanted activation of blood coagulation[76]. This property of β_2GPI suggests that it functions as a natural anticoagulant *in vivo*.

β_2-GLYCOPROTEIN-I: A PROTEIN COFACTOR FOR LA ANTIBODIES

Recently it has been shown that β_2GPI is a cofactor not only for anticardio-lipin antibodies binding to CL but also for LA activity and that the level of LA activity is dependent on the concentration of β_2GPI in the test plasma. Using the dRVVT, Oosting et al.[77] demonstrated that LA activity in four out of six plasmas became negative when plasma was depleted of β_2GPI, and was restored once purified β_2GPI was added back to the plasma. Galli and co-workers have obtained essentially similar results[78]. However, they have also described LA that are not dependent on β_2GPI and not directed to phospholipids alone but to a complex of human prothrombin and phospholipids[79]. Using highly purified coagulation factors, these workers investigated the effect of aPL antibodies on the inhibition of β_2GPI on the procoagulant activity of PS/PC vesicles in the prothrombinase system. One type of aPL antibody, like normal IgG, had no effect in this system. In contrast, a second type of aPL antibody dramatically enhanced the inhibition of the prothrombinase reaction by β_2GPI. These authors concluded that this second type of aPL antibodies inhibited the phospholipid dependent coagulation reaction in the plasma by potentiating the inhibitory effect of β_2GPI. These studies indicate that there are at least two types of LA antibodies depending on their protein cofactor (β_2GPI or prothrombin) requirement.

These studies provide evidence for the considerable heterogeneity with respect to the immunological specificity of aPL antibodies. It is clear that there are at least two types of aCL antibodies. Type 1 are directed not to a simple phospholipid antigen but to a protein–phospholipid complex that is dependent on a protein cofactor β_2GPI and which occurs in autoimmune disease. Type 2 are directed to phospholipid antigen alone and are able to

Table 5 Characteristics and cofactor requirement of antiphospholipid antibodies

Antibody type	Antigen	Protein cofactor	Assay test	Clinical associations
aCL type 1	CL	β_2GPI	ELISA	Autoimmune disease
aCL type 2	CL	NIL	ELISA	Infections including syphilis uncommon in autoimmune disease
LA type 1	? Hexagonal PL	Prothrombin	Clotting test	Autoimmune disease
LA type 2	? Hexagonal PL	β_2GPI	Clotting test	Autoimmune disease

bind directly to CL antigen in the absence of β_2GPI. This type of aCL antibody is present in patients with various infections, including syphilis, and is occasionally present in some aCL antibody preparations from patients with autoimmune disease. Type 1 LA antibodies are directed towards lipid bound prothrombin and inhibit its conversion by prothrombinase, whereas type 2 LA antibodies recognize phospholipid bound β_2GPI and enhance the inhibition of β_2GPI in the prothrombinase assay. The characteristics and cofactor requirements of aPL antibodies are summarized in Table 5.

MECHANISM OF ACTION OF aPL ANTIBODIES

As dicussed earlier there is a high association of an increased risk of vascular thrombosis with the presence of aPL antibodies (reviewed in [1,2]). In the majority of circumstances the association of thrombosis has been studied retrospectively in different clinical groups. There are studies that question this association. However, in a review of all literature of nearly 2000 reported SLE patients, LA and aCL antibodies were found to be present in 31 and 40% respectively[1,2]. Thrombosis was present in 42% of patients with aPL antibodies as opposed to 13% in the absence of these antibodies. Fetal loss was found in 38% of patients with aPL as opposed to 16% in those that were aPL negative[1,2]. Thus it is clear that the presence of aPL antibodies, whether they be measured by LA or aCL, is associated with a significant risk of clinical syndromes characterized by thrombosis or recurrent fetal loss or thrombocytopenia. Whether the presence of these antibodies is directly pathogenic and they are involved in the thrombosis, or whether they are epiphenomena, is still yet to be established. Recent studies using a murine model for pregnancy loss have demonstrated a pathogenic role for human aPL antibodies[80-82], although no increased risk of thrombosis was demonstrated in this model.

A number of homeostatic mechanisms are involved in maintaining blood fluidity and in the formation of clotting *in vivo*. Amongst these are the vascular and endothelial surfaces, platelets and the blood coagulation cascade. aPL antibodies may act at any or all of these major components of this system (Figure 9). Alterations of the haemostatic system at these sites have

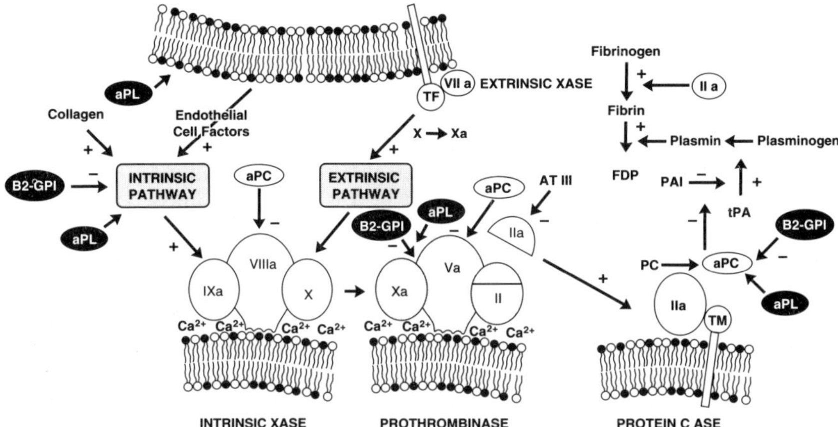

Figure 9 Same as Figure 3, but also denotes sites of action of aPL antibodies and β_2GPI, + denotes activation, − denotes inhibition

been suggested as contributing factors to the thrombotic tendency associated with antiphospholipid antibodies. These antibodies may affect endothelial cell platelet interactions, leading to increased platelet activation and changes in the endothelial cell coagulation system. Although many hypotheses have been put forward to explain a functional effect, none have been universally accepted.

EFFECT OF aPL ANTIBODIES ON ENDOTHELIAL CELLS AND PROTEIN C, PROTEIN S SYSTEM

The endothelial cell is accepted as a regulatory interphase between blood and tissues in the formation of homeostasis and thrombosis. Although anti-endothelial antibodies have been demonstrated in patients with SLE and have been reported to be correlated with antiphospholipid antibodies, it is now accepted that anti-endothelial cell antibodies are distinct from aPL antibodies[1].

A major endothelial cell product, prostacyclin, is a potent inhibitor of platelet aggregation and contributes to the endothelial cell's non-thrombogenic surface. It has been reported to be inhibited *in vitro* by plasma or purified immunoglobulin fractions from patients with LA activity and a history of either thrombosis or recurrent abortion[83–86]. The relationship between aPL antibodies and prostacyclin inhibition has been inconsistent, and these results and more detailed studies have found that inhibition of prostacyclin production does not correlate with clinical events.

The endothelial cell has two major anticoagulant pathways on its surface, one involving thrombomodulin which is an intrinsic membrane protein that forms a receptor for thrombin and alters its substrate specificity such that it becomes an anticoagulant. Thrombomodulin associated thrombin acts on protein C to activate it such that activated protein C (aPC) in association with protein S inhibits factors V_a, VIII_a. Procoagulant phospholipids significantly increase the velocity of protein C activation by thrombin and thrombomodulin complex. Patients that have either a quantitative or a qualitative reduction (greater than 60%) of protein C or protein S are at risk of recurrent thromboembolic disease[87,88]. A number of workers have reported the inhibition of soluble or endothelial bound thrombomodulin mediated protein C activation by aPL with LA activity[89–91]. Other studies have failed to find such an activity of aPL antibodies. Oosting et al.[92] were unable to demonstrate inhibition of protein C activation on endothelial cells in culture with aPL antibodies, either as IgG or as serum from 46 patients with SLE, 13 of whom had LA antibodies. In addition they could not demonstrate any effect of β_2-glycoprotein I, a protein cofactor for aPL antibodies, when this protein was added to the aPL antibodies. A number of investigators have assayed the levels of the various components of the protein C system and in general it appears that the levels of protein C and protein S are normal in patients with aPL antibodies, although spurious levels of protein S and protein C activity have been reported when certain functional assays are used[93,94]. A recent study using a thrombomodulin ELISA failed to find any autoantibodies to this protein in a large number of sera from patients with aPL antibodies[95].

Although decreased or absent fibrinolytic capacity has been demonstrated in the majority of patients with SLE, it appears to correlate with disease activity rather than with aPL antibodies.

EFFECT OF aPL ANTIBODIES ON PLATELETS

Activated platelets provide an important source of negatively charged phospholipids which provide a catalytic surface for the assembly of coagulation factors. A number of workers have demonstrated that aPL antibodies inhibit the procoagulant activity of activated platelets both in systems utilizing purified coagulation factors or plasma (see above). It is postulated that these antibodies bind directly to activated platelet plasma membranes. Khamashta and co-workers[96] have recently reported that aCL antibodies pre-incubated with freeze thawed but not intact platelets resulting in significant inhibition of cardiolipin binding activity only when serum was used as a source of antibody, and they found that the aCL activity could be eluted from these platelets. Rauch and co-workers[97] in a study on reactivities of 50 human monoclonal antibodies (all but one IgM) found a correlation between anti-platelet activity and anticardiolipin and anti-DNA activities but no correlation between LA activity and anti-platelet, and anticardiolipin activity. Furthermore, pre-treatment of platelets with phospholipases and trypsin suggested that the reactive epitopes of the platelet membrane to which these monoclonal antibodies were directed included protein and phospholipids. β_2GPI has been shown to bind to platelets[98] and the binding of some aPL antibodies to membranes of activated platelets has been shown to be β_2GPI dependent[99].

EFFECT OF aPL ANTIBODIES ON COAGULATION INHIBITORS

There are few studies that have examined the interactions of aPL antibodies with inhibitors of coagulation. Antithrombin III (ATIII) is a coagulation inhibitor whose functional integrity is dependent on vascular wall 'heparin' and heparin sulphate, both highly negatively charged molecules. It is conceivable that aPL antibodies could bind to these and inhibit the function of this molecule. Although the case of a patient with recurrent thrombosis and LA with low functional and antigenic activity of antithrombin III has been reported[100], other workers have found reduced levels of ATIII in SLE not associated with LA or with a history of thrombosis[101]. A lipoprotein associated coagulation inhibitor (LACI) which inhibits the extrinsic pathway and has been termed the extrinsic pathway inhibitor (EPI) is associated with a lipoprotein fraction of serum. It controls coagulation in a sequential way interacting with factor X_a, and then factor X_a-EPI complex can react with the tissue factor-factor VIII_a complex to block its procoagulant activity[102,103]. Since anionic phospholipids are involved in this reaction, levels of EPI have been assayed in patients with LA and found to be normal[104]. Another lipoprotein associated plasma inhibitor of coagulation is β_2GPI. Figure 9 is a simplified diagram of the coagulation cascade, illustrating the possible sites of action of this inhibitor. β_2GPI acts by inhibiting anionic macromolecular intrinsic coagulation pathway activation[76]; it acts as an anti-prothrombinase *in vitro*[105], inhibits adenosine diphosphate mediated platelet aggregation[106] and binds to aPC[107]. LA type antibodies have been shown to potentiate the inhibitory effect of β_2GPI in the prothrombinase assay[78].

Most recently monoclonal antibodies to β_2GPI, when added to normal plasma in a modified dRVVT assay, exhibited anticoagulant activity in a dose dependent manner similar to that of LA[108]. These results further support the notion that aPL antibodies act by binding to an epitope on β_2GPI. aCL antibodies from autoimmune patients are associated with thrombosis and have specificity for β_2GPI or β_2GPI phospholipid complexes. In contrast the infectious type of aCL antibodies recognize pure phospholipid antigen and are not associated with thrombotic disease. Thus it would appear that an anti-β_2GPI specificity is more likely to be prothrombotic than an anti-phospholipid specificity. Support for this contention comes from the recent clinical study that found thrombosis was associated with the presence of anti-β_2GPI antibodies (measured using a β_2GPI ELISA), and LA but not with aCL antibodies[60].

The mechanisms of thrombosis in patients with aPL antibodies still remain uncertain. However, the recent studies summarized above indicate that aPL antibodies are directed not to phospholipids alone but to protein phospholipid epitopes, which need to be taken into account when designing experiments to look at the pathogenesis of aPL antibodies *in vitro*. It may well be that some of the differences seen in different studies between LA and aCL type antibodies may relate to the availability of the protein component to which these antibodies have been shown to react. It would appear that both LA and aCL type antibodies are directed towards protein phospholipid complexes, and that aCL antibodies recognize β_2GPI after interaction with this protein with anionic phospholipids. Since β_2GPI possesses numerous inhibitory functions in multiple coagulation pathways, it is possible that aPL antibodies interfere with the function of β_2GPI *in vivo* thereby conferring a prothrombotic diathesis. In addition, since β_2GPI demonstrates homology with a number of complement receptors and some cell surface adhesion molecules[109], the possibilities of cross-reactions with these structures represents a new approach to study aPL antibody cellular interactions.

Acknowledgements

This work was funded by grants from the St George Hospital Cardiovascular Research Fund and the National Health and Medical Research Council of Australia (NH&MRC). JEH was supported by a NH&MRC scholarship. Mrs A. Coleman provided excellent secretarial assistance.

References

1. McNeil HP, Chesterman CN, Krilis SA. Immunology and clinical importance of anti-phospholipid antibodies. Adv Immunol. 199; 49: 193–280.
2. Love PE, Santoro SA. Antiphospholipid antibodies: anticardiolipin and the lupus anticoagulant in systemic lupus erythematosus (SLE) and in non-SLE disorders. Ann Intern Med. 1990; 112: 682–698.
3. Marcus DM, Schwarting GA. Immunochemical properties of glycolipids and phospholipids. Adv Immunol. 1976; 23: 203–240.
4. Rauch J, Janoff AS. Phospholipid in the hexagonal II phase is immunogenic: Evidence for immunorecognition of nonbilayer lipid phases *in vivo*. Proc Natl Acad Sci USA. 1990; 87: 4112–4114.
5. Root RW, Luescher, Unanue ER. Phospholipids enhance the binding of peptides to class II major histocompatibility molecules. Proc Natl Acad Sci USA. 1990; 87: 1735–1739.
6. Ansell GB, Spanner S. Phosphatidylserine, phosphatidylethanolamine and phosphatidylcholine. In: Kuo JF, ed. Phospholipids and Cellular Regulation. Florida: CRC Press; 1985.
7. Barenholz Y, Gatt S. Sphingomyelin: metabolism, chemical synthesis, chemical and physical properties. In: Hawthorne JN, Ansell GB, ed. Phospholipids. Amsterdam: Elsevier; 1982: 129–177.
8. Hostetler KY. Polyglycerophospholipids: phosphatidylglycerol, diphosphatidylglycerol and bis (monoacylglycero) phosphate. In: Hawthorne JN, Ansell GB, eds. Phospholipids. Amsterdam: Elsevier; 1982; 215–261.
9. Yeagle P. The Membranes of Cells. Orlando: Academic Press; 1987.
10. Zwaal RFA, Hemker HC. Blood cell membranes and haemostasis. Haemostasis. 1982; 11: 12–39.
11. Zwaal RFA, Bevers DM, Rosing J. Phospholipids and the clotting process. In: Harris EN, Exner T, Hughes GRV, Asherson RA, eds. Phospholipid-Binding Antibodies. Florida: CRC Press; 1991: 31–56.
12. Pengo V, Thiagarazan P, Shapiro SS, Heine MJ. Immunological specificity and mechanism of action of IgG lupus anticoagulants. Blood. 1987; 70: 69–76.
13. Moore JE, Mohr CF. Biologically false positive serologic tests for syphilis. JAMA. 1952; 150: 467–473.
14. Harris EN, Gharavi AE, Wasley GD, Hughes GRV. Use of an enzyme-linked immunosorbent assay and inhibition studies to distinguish between antibodies to cardiolipin from patients with syphilis or autoimmune disorders. J Infect Dis. 1988; 157: 23–31.
15. Cowchock S, Fort J, Munoz S, Norberg R, Maddrey W. False positive ELISA tests for anticardiolipin antibodies in sera from patients with repeated abortion, rheumatologic disorders and primary biliary cirrhosis: correlation with elevated polyclonal IgM and

implications for patients with repeated abortion. Clin Exp Immunol. 1988; 73: 289–294.
16. Harris EN. Antiphospholipid antibodies. Br J Haematol. 1990; 74: 1–9.
17. Harris EN, Gharavi AE, Patel SP, Hughes GRV. Evaluation of the anticardiolipin antibody test: report of an international workshop held 4 April 1986. Clin Exp Immunol. 1987; 68: 215–222.
18. Harris EN and the Kingston Anti-Phospholipid Groups (KAPS). The Second Anti-Cardiolipin Standardisation Workshop. Am J Clin Pathol. 1990; 94: 476–484.
19. Loizou S. Anticardiolipin Kits: Techniques of antiphospholipid antibody measurement. Clin Immunol Newslett. 1991; 11: 41–47.
20. Peaceman AM, Silver RK, MacGregor SN, Socol ML. Interlaboratory variation in antiphospholipid antibody testing. Am J Obstet Gynecol. 1992; 166: 1780–1787.
21. Gharavi AE, Harris EN, Asherson RA, Hughes GRV. Anticardiolipin antibodies: isotype distribution and phospholipid specificity. Ann Rheum Dis. 1987; 46: 1–6.
22. Qamar T, Levy RA, Sammaritano L, et al. Characteristics of high titre IgG antiphospholipid antibody in systemic lupus erythematosus patients with and without fetal death. Arthritis Rheum. 1990; 33: 501–504.
23. Frampton G, Winter JB, Cameron JS, Hughes RAC. Severe Guillaine-Barre syndrome: an association with IgA anti-cardiolipin antibody in a series of 92 patients. J Neuroimmunol. 1988; 19: 133–139.
24. Harris EN, Gharavi AE, Loizou S, et al. Crossreactivity of antiphospholipid antibodies. J Clin Lab Immunol. 1985; 16: 1–6.
25. Green D, Hougie C, Kazmier FJ. Report of the working party on acquired inhibitors of coagulation: studies of the 'lupus' anticoagulant. Thromb Haemostas. 1983; 49: 144–146.
26. Exner T, Triplett DA, Taberner D, Machin SJ. Guidelines for testing and revised criteria for lupus anticoagulant. SSC Subcommittee for the standardization of Lupus Anticoagulation. Thromb Haemostas. 1991; 65: 320–322.
27. Exner T, Rickard KA, Kronenberg H. A sensitive test demonstrating lupus anticoagulant and its behavioural pattern. Br J Haematol. 1978; 40: 143–151.
28. Gibson J, Starling E, Date L, Rickard KA, Kronenberg H. Simplified screening procedures for detecting lupus inhibitor. J Clin Pathol. 1988; 41: 226–231.
29. Triplett DA, Brandt JT, Maas RL. The laboratory heterogeneity of lupus anticoagulants. Arch Pathol Lab Med. 1985; 109: 946–951.
30. Triplett DA, Brandt J. Laboratory identification of the lupus anticoagulant. Br J Haematol. 1989; 73: 139–142.
31. Kelsey PR, Stevenson KJ, Poller L. The diagnosis of lupus anticoagulants by the activated partial thromboplastin time – the central role of phosphatidylserine. Thromb Haemostas. 1984; 52: 172–175.
32. Harris EN, Gharavi AE, Boey ML, et al. Anticardiolipin antibodies: detection by radioimmunoassay and association with thrombosis in systemic lupus erythematosus. Lancet. 1983; 2: 1211–1214.
33. Ware-Branch D, Rote NS, Dostal DA, Scott JR. Association of lupus anticoagulant with antibody against phosphatidylserine. Clin Exp Immunol. 1990; 80: 171–176.
34. Triplett DA, Brandt JT, Musgrave KA, Orr CA. The relationship between lupus anticoagulants and antibodies to phospholipid. JAMA. 1988; 259: 550–554.
35. Lockshin MD, Qamar T, Druzin ML, Goei S. Antibody to cardiolipin, lupus anticoagulant and fetal death. J Rheumatol. 1987; 14: 259–262.
36. McNeil HP, Chesterman CN, Krilis SA. Binding specificity of lupus anticoagulants and anticardiolipin antibodies. Thromb Res. 1988; 52: 609–619.
37. McNeil HP, Krilis SA, Chesterman CN. Purification of antiphospholipid antibodies using a new affinity method. Thromb Res. 1988; 52: 641–648.
38. Exner T, Sahman N, Trudinger B. Separation of anticardiolipin antibodies from lupus anticoagulant on a phospholipid-coated polystyrene column. Biochem Biophys Res Comm. 1988; 155: 1001–1007.
39. McNeil HP, Chesterman CN, Krilis SA. Anticardiolipin antibodies and lupus anticoagulants comprise separate antibody subgroups with different binding characteristics. Br J Haematol. 1989; 73: 506–513.
40. Harris EN, Gharavi AE, Tincani, et al. Affinity purified anti-cardiolipin and anti-DNA antibodies. J Clin Lab Immunol. 1985; 17: 155–162.

41. Violi F, Valesini G, Ferro D, et al. Anticoagulant activity of anticardiolipin antibodies. Thromb Res. 1986; 44: 543–547.
42. Pengo V, Thiagarajan P, Shapiro SS, Heine MJ. Immunological specificity and mechanism of action of IgG lupus anticoagulants. Blood. 1987; 70: 69–76.
43. McNeil HP, Chesterman CN, Krilis SA. Binding specificity of lupus anticoagulants and anticardiolipin antibodies. Thromb Res. 1988; 52: 602–619.
44. Fleck RA, Rapaport SI, Rao LVM. Anti-prothrombin antibodies and the lupus anticoagulant. Blood. 1988; 72: 512–519.
45. McNeil HP, Simpson RJ, Chesterman CN, Krilis SA. Antiphospholipid antibodies are directed against a complex antigen that includes a lipid-binding inhibitor of coagulation: β_2-Glycoprotein I (apolipoprotein H). Proc Natl Acad Sci USA. 1990; 87: 4120–4124.
46. Galli M, Comfurius P, Maassen C, et al. Anticardiolipin antibodies (ACA) directed not to cardiolipin but to a plasma protein cofactor. Lancet. 1990; 335: 1544–1547.
47. Matsuura E, Igarashi Y, Fujimoto M, et al. Anticardiolipin cofactor(s) and differential diagnosis of autoimmune disease. Lancet. 1990; 336: 177–178.
48. Matsuura E, Igarashi M, Igarashi Y, et al. Molecular definition of human β_2-glycoprotein I (β_2-GPI) by cDNA cloning and inter-species differences of β_2-GPI in alternation of anticardiolipin binding. Int Immunol. 1991; 3: 1217–1221.
49. Bevers EM, Galli M. β_2-glycoprotein-I for binding of anticardiolipin antibodies to cardiolipin. Lancet. 1990; 336: 952–953.
50. Nimpf J, Bevers EM, Bomans PHH, et al. Prothrombinase activity of human platelets is inhibited by β_2-glycoprotein I. Biochim Biophys Acta. 1986; 884: 142–149.
51. McNeil HP, Hunt JE, Krilis SA. New aspects of anticardiolipin antibodies. Clin Exp Rheumatol. 1990; 8: 525–527.
52. Hunt JE, McNeil HP, Morgan GJ, Crameri RM, Krilis SA. A phospholipid-β_2-glycoprotein I complex is an antigen for anticardiolipin antibodies occurring in autoimmune disease but not with infection. Lupus. 1992; 1: 75–81.
53. Krilis SA. Immunochemistry of antiphospholipid antibodies. Clin Immunol Newslett. 1991; 11: 34–41.
54. Matsuura E, Igarashi Y, Masao F, et al. Heterogeneity of anticardiolipin antibodies defined by the anticardiolipin cofactor. J Immunol. 1992; 148: 3885–3891.
55. Gharavi AE. Antiphospholipid cofactor. Stroke. 1992; 23 (suppl): 7–10.
56. Sammaritano LR, Lockshin MD, Gharavi AE. Antiphospholipid antibodies differ in aPL cofactor requirement. Lupus. 1992; 1: 83–90.
57. Harris EN, Peirangeli S, Barquinero J, Ordi-Ros J. Anticardiolipin antibodies and binding of anionic phospholipids and serum protein. Lancet. 1990; 336: 505–506.
58. Harris EN, Pierangeli S. What is the 'true' antigen for antiphospholipid antibodies? Lancet. 1990; 336: 1505.
59. Arvieux J, Roussel B, Jacob MC, Colomb MG. Measurement of antiphospholipid antibodies by ELISA using Beta 2 glycoprotein I as an antigen. J Immunol Meth. 1991; 143: 223–229.
60. Viard J-P, Amoura Z, Bach J-F. Association of antiβ_2 glycoprotein I antibodies with lupus-type circulating anticoagulant and thrombosis in systemic lupus erythematosus. Am J Med. 1992; 93: 181–186.
61. Lozier J, Takahashi N, Putnam FW. Complete amino acid sequence of human plasma β_2-glycoprotein I. Proc Natl Acad Sci USA. 1984; 81: 3640–3644.
62. Steinkasserer A, Estaller C, Weiss EH, Sim RB, Day AJ. Complete nucleotide and deduced amino acid sequence of human β_2-glycoprotein I. Biochem J. 1991; 277: 387–391.
63. Walsh MT, Watzlawick H, Putnam FW, Schmid K, Brossmer R. Effect of the carbohydrate moiety on the secondary structure of β_2-glycoprotein I. Implications for the biosynthesis and folding of glycoproteins. Biochemistry. 1990; 29: 6250–6257.
64. Polz E, Kostner GM. The binding of β_2-glycoprotein I to human serum lipiproteins. FEBS Lett. 1979; 102: 183–186.
65. Lee NS, Brewer HB, Osborne JC. β_2-glycoprotein I. Molecular properties of an unusual apolipoprotein, apolipoprotein H. J Biol Chem. 1983; 258: 4765–4770.
66. Propert DN. The relation of sex, smoking status, birth rank, and parental age to β_2-glycoprotein I levels and phenotypes in a sample of Australian caucasian adults. Human Genet. 1978; 43: 281–288.
67. Koppe AL, Walter H, Chopra VP, Bajatzadeh M. Investigations on the genetics and

population genetics of the β_2-glycoprotein I polymorphism. Humangenetik. 1970; 9: 164–171.

68. Haagerup A, Kristensen T, Kruse TA. Polymorphism and genetic mapping of the gene encoding human β_2-glycoprotein I to chromosome 17. Cytogenet Cell Genet. 1991; 58: 2004–2012.

69. Aoyama Y, Chan Y-L, Wool IG. The primary structure of rat β_2-glycoprotein I. Nucleic Acids Res. 1989; 17: 6401.

70. Mehdi H, Nunn M, Steel DM, et al. Nucleotide sequence and expression of the human gene apolipoprotein H (β_2-glycoprotein I). Gene. 1991; 108: 293–298.

71. Kristensen T, Schousboe I, Boel E, et al. Molecular cloning and mammalian expression of human β_2-glycoprotein I cDNA. FEBS Lett. 1991; 289: 183–186.

72. Kato H, Enjyoji K-i. Amino acid sequence and location of the disulfide bonds in bovine β_2-glycoprotein I: The presence of five sushi domains. Biochemistry. 1991; 30: 11687–11694.

73. Hunt JE, Simpson RJ, Krilis SA. Identification of a region of Beta-2-glycoprotein-I critical for lipid-binding and anticardiolipin antibody cofactor activity. Proc Natl Acad Sci USA. 1993; 90: 2141–2145.

74. Wurm H. β_2-glycoprotein-I (apolipoprotein H) interactions with phospholipid vesicles. Int J Biochem. 1984; 16: 511–515.

75. Gries A, Nimpf J, Wurm H, Kostner GM, Kenner T. Characterization of isoelectric subspecies of asialo-beta 2 glycoprotein I. Biochem J. 1989; 260: 531–534.

76. Schousboe I. β_2-glycoprotein I: a plasma inhibitor of the contact activation of the intrinsic blood coagulation pathway. Blood. 1985; 66: 1086–1091.

77. Oosting JD, Derksen RHWM, Entjes HTI, Bouma BN, de Groot PG. Lupus anticoagulant activity is frequently dependent on the presence of β_2-glycoprotein I. Thromb Haemostas. 1992; 67: 499–502.

78. Galli EM, Barbui T, Comfurius P, Zwaal RFA, Bevers EM. Anticoagulant activity of anticardiolipin antibodies is mediated by β_2-glycoprotein I. Thromb Haemostas. 1992; (in press).

79. Bevers EM, Galli M, Barbui T, Comfurius P, Zwaal RFA. Lupus anticoagulant IgG (LA) are not directed to phospholipids only, but to a complex of lipid-bound human prothrombin. Thromb Haemostas. 1991; 66: 629–632.

80. Branch DW, Dudley DJ, Mitchell MD, et al. Immunoglobulin G fractions from patients with antiphospholipid antibodies cause fetal death in BALB/c mice: a model for autoimmune fetal loss. Am J Obstet Gynecol. 1990; 163: 210–216.

81. Blank M, Cohen J, Toder V, Shoenfeld Y. Induction of anti-phospholipid syndrome in naive mice with mouse lupus monoclonal and human polyclonal anti-cardiolipin antibodies. Proc Natl Acad Sci USA. 1991; 88: 3069–3073.

82. Bakimer R, Fishman P, Blank M, Sredni B, Djaldetti M, Shoenfeld Y. Induction of primary antiphospholipid syndrome in mice by immunization with a human monoclonal anticardiolipin antibody (H3). J Clin Invest. 1992; 89: 1558–1563.

83. Carreras LO, De Freyn G, Machin SJ, et al. Arterial thrombosis, intrauterine death and 'lupus' anticoagulant: detection of immunoglobulin interfering with prostacyclin formation. Lancet. 1981; 1: 244–246.

84. Carreras LO, Vermylen JG. 'Lupus' anticoagulant and thrombosis – possible role of inhibition of prostacyclin formation. Thromb Haemostas. 1982; 48: 38–40.

85. Carreras LO, Vermylen J. 'Lupus' anticoagulant and inhibition of prostacyclin formation in patients with repeated abortion, intrauterine growth retardation and fetal death. Br J Obstet Gynaecol. 1981; 88: 890–894.

86. Watson KV, Schorer AE. Lupus anticoagulant inhibition of *in vitro* prostacyclin release is associated with a thrombosis-prone subset of patients. Am J Med. 1991; 90: 47–53.

87. Griffin JH. Clinical studies of protein C. Semin Thromb Hemostasis. 1984; 10: 109–121.

88. Comp PC, Esmon CT. Recurrent venous thromboembolism in patients with a partial deficiency of protein S. N Engl J Med. 1984; 311: 1525–1528.

89. Comp PC, DeBault LE, Esmon NL, Esmon CT. Human thrombomodulin is inhibited by IgG from two patients with non-specific anticoagulants. Blood. 1983; 62 (1 Suppl): 299A.

90. Cariou R, Tobelem G, Soria C, Caen J. Inhibition of protein C activation by endothelial cells in the presence of lupus anticoagulant. N Engl J Med. 1986; 314: 1193–1194.

91. Freyssinet J-M, Wiesel M-L, Gauchy J, et al. An IgM lupus anticoagulant that neutralizes

the enhancing effect of phospholipid on purified endothelial thrombomodulin activity – a mechanism for thrombosis. Thromb Haemostas. 1986; 55: 309–313.

92. Oosting JD, Derksen RHWM, Hackeng TM, et al. In vitro studies of antiphospholipid antibodies and its cofactor β_2-glycoprotein I, show negligible effects on endothelial cell mediated protein C activation. Thromb Haemostas. 1991; 66: 666–671.

93. Simioni P, Lazzaro A, Zanardi S, Girolami. Spurious protein C deficiency due to antiphospholipid antibodies. Am J Hematol. 1991; 36: 299–300.

94. Sthoeger ZM, Sthoeger D, Mellnick SD, Steen D, Berrebi A. Transient anticardiolipin antibodies, functional protein S deficiency and deep vein thrombosis. Am J Hematol. 1991; 36: 206–207.

95. Gibson J, Nelson M, Brown R, Salem H, Kronenberg H. Autoantibodies to thrombomodulin: development of an enzyme immunoassay and a survey of their frequency in patients with the lupus anticoagulant. Thromb Haemostas. 1992; 67: 507–509.

96. Khamashta MA, Harris EN, Gharavi AE, et al. Immune mediated mechanism for thrombosis: antiphospholipid antibody binding to platelet membranes. Ann Rheum Dis. 1988; 47: 849–854.

97. Rauch J, Meng Q-H, Tannenbaum H. Lupus anticoagulant and antiplatelet properties of human hybridoma autoantibodies. J Immunol. 1987; 139: 2598–2604.

98. Schousboe I. Binding of β_2-glycoprotein I to platelets: effect of adenylate cyclase activity. Thromb Res. 1980; 19: 225–237.

99. Chesterman CN, Chong BH, Shi W. Pathogenic potential of antiphospholipid antibodies: binding to human platelets. Thromb Haemostas. 1991; 65: 555A.

100. Cosgriff TM, Martin BA. Low functional and high antigenic anti-thrombin III level in a patient with the lupus anticoagulant and recurrent thrombosis. Arthritis Rheum. 1981; 24: 94–96.

101. Boey ML, Loizou S, Colaco CB, et al. Antithrombin III in systemic lupus erythematosus. Clin Exp Rheum. 1984; 2: 53–56.

102. Rapaport SI. Inhibition of factor VII_a/tissue factor-induced blood coagulation with particular emphasis upon a factor X_a-dependent inhibitory mechanism. Blood. 1989; 73: 359–365.

103. Hubbard AR, Jennings CA. Inhibition of the tissue factor–factor VII complex: involvement of factor X_a and lipoproteins. Thromb Res. 1987; 46: 527–537.

104. Bajaj MS, Rana SV, Wysolmerski RB, Bajaj SP. Inhibitor of the factor VIII_a-tissue factor complex is reduced in patients with disseminated intravascular coagulation but not in patients with severe hepatocellular disease. J Clin Invest. 1987; 79: 1874–1878.

105. Nimpf J, Bevers EM, Bomans PHH, et al. Prothrombinase activity of human platelets is inhibited by β_2-glycoprotein I. Biochem Biophys Acta. 1986; 884: 142–149.

106. Nimpf J, Wurm H, Kostner GM. β_2-glycoprotein I (APOH) inhibits the release reaction of human platelets during ADP-induced aggregation. Atherosclerosis. 1987; 63: 109–114.

107. Canfield WM, Kisiel W. Evidence of normal functional levels of activated protein C inhibitor in combined factor V/VII deficiency disease. J Clin Invest. 1982; 70: 1260–1272.

108. Roubey RAS, Pratt CW, Buyon JP, Winfield JB. Antibodies to β_2-glycoprotein I (β_2GPI) or to β_2GPI-phospholipid complex have lupus anticoagulant activity. Lupus. 1992; 1 (1 suppl): 149A.

109. Reid KBM, Day AJ. Structure-function relationships of the complement components. Immunology Today. 1989; 10: 177–180.

15
Autoantigens in Connective Tissue Diseases

W. J. VAN VENROOIJ

INTRODUCTION

In a number of rheumatic diseases the presence of the so-called antinuclear antibodies (ANA) is a dominant laboratory feature. These diseases include systemic lupus erythematosus (SLE), drug-induced lupus, scleroderma, mixed connective tissue disease (MCTD), polymyositis/dermatomyositis (PM/DM) and Sjögren's syndrome (SS). Patients with other rheumatic diseases like rheumatoid arthritis (RA) also produce disease-specific antibodies which are, however, of a different nature from the ANAs described here. These antigens, notably rheumatoid factor, the perinuclear factor, RA-33 and others have recently been reviewed[1] and will not be discussed here.

Autoantigens which are targets of autoantibodies in patients with rheumatic diseases are most often large cellular complexes containing protein and nucleic acid components. For example antibodies to nucleosomes, a complex of double-stranded (ds) DNA and histones are typically found in SLE patients, while antibodies to spliceosomes, the complex of small nuclear RNAs (snRNAs or U RNAs), heterogeneous nuclear RNA (hnRNA) and their associated proteins involved in the processing of RNA, are found in SLE and MCTD. An overview of the most common targets for patient autoantibodies in rheumatic diseases is given in Table 1.

These antibodies have two striking and most helpful characteristics. First, a large number of them are disease-specific. Therefore the presence of a certain 'marker' autoantibody in a patient's serum may help the clinician considerably in reaching a diagnosis. In cases where a clinical diagnosis has already been reached, the presence of an autoantibody activity is not only a confirmation of the diagnosis but may also point to a disease subset with a particular prognosis (Table 1). Secondly, some autoantibody specificities appear to be present very early in disease, long before a clinical diagnosis

Table 1 Cellular complexes targeted by autoantibodies

	Antigenic components	*Disease correlation*	*Reference*
Nucleosomes	dsDNA	SLE	70–77
	histones	SLE, drug-induced SLE	8, 14, 19, 90
Other DNA-binding proteins	Topoisomerase I	Scleroderma	7, 8, 127
	Centromere proteins	CREST	8, 127
	Ku (p70/p80)	SLE, scleroderma, myositis	13, 14, 91, 92
	PCNA (cyclin)	SLE	8
Spliceosomes	U1RNA	MCTD, SLE	84, 85, 89
	U1RNP	MCTD, SLE	7, 8, 35
	Sm	SLE	7, 8, 35
	U1,U2RNP	SLE	35, 105
	hnRNP	SLE, RA	113–116
Nucleolus	U3RNP	Scleroderma	127, 131–133
	Th (To)	Scleroderma	140, 141, 146
	Pm/Scl	PM/Scleroderma overlap	148
	NOR-90	Scleroderma	152
	RNA polymerase I	Scleroderma	127, 147
	Nucleolin	SLE	150
Cytoplasmic complexes	Ro/SS-A	SS, SLE	7, 8, 160
	La/SS-B	SS, SLE	7, 8, 160
	Jo-1 (His-tRNA synthetase)	PM	190, 192
	ribRNP	SLE	183, 187

Abbreviations: SLE: Systemic lupus erythematosus
CREST: Syndrome of calcinosis, Raynaud's, oesophageal disorder, sclerodactyly, telangiectasias
(scleroderma with limited skin involvement)
MCTD: Mixed connective tissue disease
RA: Rheumatoid arthritis
PM: Polymyositis

has been reached[2–5]. In such cases an antibody profile can be helpful in differentiating the future development of a certain type of disease (reviewed in [6]).

In this review I will discuss the various nuclear antigens most commonly targeted by patient autoantibodies. I will describe methods for the detection of these antibodies and the correlation they appear to have with the disease. As part of the source material for this chapter I relied also upon several reviews, particularly the chapter by Craft and Hardin in the 4th Edition of the Textbook of Rheumatology[7], the review on ANAs by Tan[8] and the special issue of the journal Molecular Biology Reports discussing the B-cell epitopes on autoantigens in connective tissue disease[9–15].

METHODS FOR DETECTION OF ANTINUCLEAR ANTIBODIES

The LE observed by Hargraves and colleagues in 1948 was the first recognition of an antinuclear antibody (ANA). The LE cell test, shown to depend on the presence of antibodies to deoxyribonucleoprotein[16], is after more than 40 years still in use but the assay is now considered to be tedious, insensitive and not very specific. Several other specific tests for individual ANAs have been developed since then and their use will be discussed below. Technical details of the methods, as well as specific and reliable protocols, will be published elsewhere[17].

Indirect immunofluorescence (IF)

Most laboratories rely on IF as the initial screening test for ANAs[17]. This method is highly sensitive and detects all ANA specificities whose target antigens reside in sufficient quantities within substrate cells. Originally tissue sections, but more recently cultured cells fixed on a microscope slide are used as a source of nuclear antigen. After incubation with diluted (1:30 or 1:40) patient serum and washing with buffer, the bound ANA can be detected with a fluorescently labelled second antibody. When a serum does contain ANA, various patterns can be distinguished. Most often a positive IF pattern is homogeneous, speckled or nucleolar but patterns showing nuclear dots[18] or nuclear rims[19] can be observed as well. However, specific antibody activities are definable only in a few cases, for example when anti-centromere antibodies are present[19,20]. Another problem in the interpretation of IF data is the fact that staining patterns may vary as sera are diluted. For example, sera containing anti-histone or anti-RNP antibodies may produce the homogeneous pattern at lower dilutions and a speckled pattern at higher dilutions. In addition, a negative IF pattern does not necessarily mean that antibodies are not present. It is known that some rather frequently occurring antibody specificities such as anti-56K[21] and low titred anti-cytoplasmic antibody activities such as anti-Ro, anti-ribRNP and anti-Jo-1 are relatively difficult to detect in the IF assay[20]. Other factors such as quality of reagents and microscope used may also add to an inconsistency between results from various laboratories in this assay.

Immunodiffusion (ID) and counter-immunoelectrophoresis (CIE)

Autoantibodies against many nuclear antigens can be detected by immuno-precipitation in double diffusion (ID) or by counter-immunoelectrophoresis (CIE)[17,19]. Mostly a commercially available rabbit thymus extract (ENA, extractable nuclear antigen) is used and for some antibodies, in particular those against nRNP, Sm, La, Jo-1 and Scl-70, these are reliable and relatively easy methods widely used in clinical laboratories[20]. Some new antibody specificities such as PCNA[22], Ku[23] and PM-Scl or PM-1[24] can also be detected with this method. In contrast, antibodies which bind less abundant or less stable ribonucleoproteins, such as the nucleolar Th and U3 RNPs, are not routinely detectable in these assays[7]. A disadvantage of the method is that only soluble antigen complexes can form precipitation lines and that several important autoantibodies, notably those against DNA, histones and centromere antigens, cannot be detected. In some cases one needs an extract from another tissue, as in the case of anti-Ro where a human spleen extract should be used[25].

Nuclear autoantigens are mostly complexes of a nucleic acid, DNA or RNA, associated with several antigenic proteins. In some cases it might be important to distinguish which antigenic proteins are targeted by the patient antibodies[26–29]. In those cases ID or CIE techniques fail, and more sophisticated methods, such as immunoblotting or immunoprecipitation, should be used.

Immunoblotting (IB)

The main advantage of the immunoblotting technique[17,30] is that almost all specificities, even when mixed, can be detected in a sensitive and relatively easy way. Since the antigenic protein targets of ANAs are visualized directly after electrophoretic separation, information is obtained about which polypeptide carries the specific epitope that is being recognized. For certain antibodies, such as anti-Ro60, which often target conformational epitopes that are disrupted by gel electrophoresis[31], immunoblots are less effective[20]. Besides that, the technique is more laborious than ID or CIE, and the interpretation of the blot profiles is more difficult. Experience is essential since ascribing an antibody specificity to a band of known molecular weight requires practice. For example, histone bands can easily be misjudged as a centromeric antigen and there are a variety of 50 kDa bands which are not the La antigen. Another problem is the occurrence of protein degradation in the cell extract which may lead to antigenic degradation products and hence to more complicated immunoblot profiles[20]. Finally, there is the possibility that antigens comigrate in the electrophoresis system used, as has been shown to occur for example with the Ro52 and La antigens[26–28].

Immunoprecipitation (IP)

Radioimmunoprecipitation is one of the most sensitive methods for the detection of autoantibodies[17]. One of the earliest assays based on this method is the Farr assay for detection of antibodies to native DNA[17,32,33]. In more recent years, radioimmunoprecipitation assays have been used for detection of antibodies directed to ribonucleoprotein (RNP) particles. Using these methods[17,34] it was possible to distinguish anti-U1RNP and anti-U1/U2RNP activities in anti-nRNP sera, and to define anti-Sm as an activity directed to a protein complex (Sm) bound to the single-stranded region of the abundant U RNAs (U1, U2, U4/U6 and U5) (reviewed in [35]).

The main advantages of the method are its sensitivity and specificity, and the fact that it detects antigens in *native* complexes. Disadvantages are that the method may require the use of radioactivity and that it is more laborious than immunoblotting, counter-immunoelectrophoresis or ELISA methods.

Enzyme-linked immunosorbent assay (ELISA)

The technique most adequate for clinical laboratories is an ELISA using highly purified autoantigen preparations. Several of such ELISAs have

Table 2 Autoantigens that have been cloned

	Cloned antigenic polypeptides	Reference
DNA-binding antigens		
Ku	Ku-p70	64
	-p80	65
PCNA	PCNA (cyclin)	69
Scl-70	Topoisomerase 1	51, 52
Centromere proteins	CENP-B	53, 128
	CENP-C	222
RNA-binding antigens		
U1RNP	70 K	46, 47
	A	48
	C	49
U2RNP	A'	55
	B"	56
Sm	B'/B	41, 43–45, 58, 199
	D1	40
	E	42
hnRNP	A1	66, 67
	A2	67, 68
Nucleolar antigens		
U3RNP	fibrillarin	61
PM-Scl	PM-Scl-75	59
	PM-Scl-100	220
Nucleolin	Nucleolin	60
NOR-90	hUBF	221
Cytoplasmic antigens		
La(SS-B)	La protein	39, 57, 156
Ro(SS-A)	Ro60	36, 57, 63
	Ro52	37, 38
ribRNP	P0, P1, P2	62
Jo-1	his-tRNA synthetase	50

already been described but the main problem still is the reproducible and adequate purification of the antigens[17,20]. In general it can be said that the ELISA technique probably detects an additional 5–10% of ANA-positivity compared with the other techniques described. The future trend appears to be the use of recombinant antigens. Most of the 'marker' autoantigens have been cloned by now (see Table 2) and the expression of the recombinant antigens in bacteria is generally very good, facilitating their purification. Furthermore, most of the bacterially expressed antigens are recognized very well by the autoantibodies. A possible disadvantage of an ELISA procedure is the fact that when more proteins are present in the antigenic complex, as in the case of the U1RNP antigen, for example, the ELISA should be performed with all antigens, either separately or in a mixture.

COMPLEXITY OF AUTOANTIGENS

In this review I will divide the autoantigens to be discussed into the following groups:

1. *Nucleic acids*
   Autoantibodies directed to the naked nucleic acid components of cellular complexes are frequently found in the connective tissue diseases. They are not only important diagnostic markers for diseases like SLE (anti-dsDNA), MCTD (anti-U1RNA) or PM (anti-tRNA) but changes in the level of the antibodies appear to have a useful correlation with the severity of disease as well.
2. *DNA-associated proteins*
   DNA-associated proteins are an important and large group of autoantigens which can be divided into two subgroups. Firstly, autoantigens like histones, Ku and PCNA which are typical targets of antibodies in SLE patients. Secondly, the scleroderma-specific autoantigens, including topoisomerase I, the centromere proteins and nucleolar antigens such as RNA polymerase I, nucleolin and NOR-90.
   It should be noted, however, that there are also a few reports on autoantibodies directed to other chromatin-associated autoantigens such as HMG 14 and 17, lamins or poly(ADP-ribose)polymerase that will not be dealt with (see [8]).
3. *RNA-associated proteins*
   The RNA-associated autoantigens can be divided into at least three groups depending on their cellular localization. The first group includes the small nuclear ribonucleoproteins (snRNPs) present in the nucleoplasm. These antigens are mostly referred to as the URNPs (excluding U3RNP) and the corresponding antibodies are known as anti-U1RNP (or anti-nRNP), anti-U1,U2RNP and anti-Sm. The hnRNP complex as an autoantigen also belongs in this group.
   The second group is the nucleolar RNPs which include U3RNP and the Th complex. They will be discussed in the paragraph on scleroderma-specific antigens.
   The third group that will be discussed includes the RNPs with a predominantly cytoplasmic localization, such as the Ro (SS-A) and La (SS-B) RNPs, the ribosomal RNPs and the tRNA-synthetases.
4. *Heat-shock proteins*
   There will be a short paragraph on the heat shock proteins as autoantigen.

Nucleic acids

DNA

The presence of anti-native DNA is one of the most helpful markers for diagnosing SLE (reviewed in [70,71]). Antibodies to single-stranded DNA occur in a wide variety of disorders, including drug-induced lupus, chronic active hepatitis, infectious mononucleosis and RA[72-74], and have poor diagnostic specificity. There are many reviews on various aspects of anti-DNA antibodies. The four methods most relevant for the measurement of anti-dsDNA antibodies (the ELISA, the indirect immunofluorescence test on *Crithidia luciliae*, the PEG assay and the Farr assay) have been discussed recently by Smeenk and Hylkema[33]. The possible role of these antibodies in the pathophysiology of connective tissue diseases has been extensively reviewed as well[7,8,19,75-77].

RNA

Traditionally, the anti-RNA antibody response has mostly been measured using heterogeneous populations of single-stranded (ss) and double-stranded (ds) RNAs, or various synthetic polynucleotides as substrates. The antibodies detected in this way generally reacted with a broad spectrum of different RNAs and were almost exclusively present in SLE patients' sera. In this way, antibodies to synthetic dsRNA (poly A–poly U, poly I–poly C, poly G–poly C), synthetic ssRNA (poly A, poly U, poly(ADP-ribose) and native RNAs (transfer RNA (tRNA), ribosomal (rib)RNA and viral RNA) have been described (reviewed in [15]). Most of these early studies already indicated that there was hardly any cross-reaction between anti-RNA and anti-DNA antibodies. In contrast to these broadly reactive anti-RNA autoantibodies, specific anti-RNA antibodies directed to a distinct RNA have been found as well. Typical examples are anti-tRNA antibodies in myositis patients' sera[78-80], autoantibodies against the GTPase activity centre of 28S ribRNA in SLE patients[81,82] and anti-U1RNA antibodies in patients with SLE overlap syndromes containing anti-(U)RNP autoantibodies[78,83-85]. These specificities have been discussed in more detail in a recent review[15].

It is noteworthy that the titres of anti-dsDNA and anti-U1RNA antibodies tend to fall after successful treatment and often become undetectable during periods of sustained remission[86-89].

DNA-associated proteins

Histones

The five major histones are small DNA-binding proteins rich in basic amino acids that are highly conserved in evolution. Eukaryotic histones have a well defined function in packing DNA in nucleosomes. Nucleosomes consist of an octameric core complex containing two molecules each of the histones H2A, H2B, H3 and H4, which is tightly associated with 146 bp of DNA wound in two superhelical turns around it. Nucleosomes are connected by variable lengths of linker DNA to which the histone H1 is bound. The highly basic C-terminal region of H1 is likely to play a role in chromatin condensation. Autoantibodies directed to histones occur in a number of diseases including SLE, drug-induced lupus, juvenile rheumatoid arthritis and RA (reviewed in [7,8,14,19]). The frequency of autoantibodies to individual histones varies according to the type of autoimmune disease. In general, anti-H1 antibodies are the most frequent in SLE, followed by anti-H2B, anti-H2A, anti-H3 and anti-H4 antibodies, respectively[90]. A recent review on the antigenic determinants localized on histone polypeptides has been written by Chou and co-workers[14].

Ku (p70/p80) antigen

Anti-Ku antibodies, named after the prototype patient, were first described in Japanese patients with scleroderma-polymyositis overlap syndromes[91]. Subsequently, these antibodies were also found in patients with SLE, scleroderma and MCTD[92]. The antibodies can be detected by their fine speckled staining of the nucleus in IF, but also by CIE, ID and immuno-blotting[7].

The Ku antigen is a 10S particle consisting of two noncovalently linked proteins of 70 and 80 kDa that bind DNA (reviewed in [14]). The antigen appears to be identical with nuclear factor IV (NF IV), a protein which is thought to play a role in DNA replication, repair or recombination[93]. The cDNA and amino acid sequences of human p70 (609 amino acids)[64] and p80 (732 amino acids)[65] have been determined. Epitope mapping studies indicate that most of the major autoepitopes are conformational[13,14]. Certain anti-Ku autoimmune sera inhibit the binding of Ku antigen to DNA *in vitro*, suggesting that the autoantibodies bind at or near the active site[14].

Proliferating cell nuclear antigen (PCNA)

PCNA (or cyclin[94]) is the target antigen for autoantibodies in the sera of about 3% of patients with SLE[8,22,95]. It can be detected by the characteristic speckled IF pattern in dividing cells because the bulk of its expression occurs during late G and early S phase of the cell cycle just before DNA synthesis[96]. However, PCNA does not disappear in noncycling cells. Rather, it appears to associate with different compartments of the cell nucleus during different phases of the cell cycle, making the antigen more or less readily extractable during methanol fixation[14].

The antibody can also be detected by CIE or ID and shows a 36 kDa band on immunoblots although the deduced amino acid sequence gives a molecular weight of 29 kDa[69]. Because the antigen is primarily present in dividing cells, it will be prominent in the cytoplasmic fraction after biochemical fractionation. PCNA has been identified as an auxiliary protein of DNA polymerase δ[97,98], a multisubunit particle which is required for DNA replication.

Anti-PCNA antibodies inhibit the function of the protein, and epitope mapping studies have revealed that the major autoepitopes are conformational[99] (reviewed in [14]).

RNA-associated proteins

RNP and Sm

All eukaryotic cells contain a number of distinct small RNAs which can be broadly divided into two classes: the capped small nuclear RNAs (snRNAs or U RNAs) and the non-capped small cytoplasmic RNAs (scRNAs). At present at least 14 U RNAs have been identified in mammalian cells, which account for about 1% of the total cellular RNA. The U RNAs are nuclear, metabolically stable RNAs and contain unique cap structures at their 5'-ends in addition to several internal modifications. They are all organized into ribonucleoprotein particles (U snRNPs). Whereas U1, U2, U3 and U5 snRNPs contain just one kind of snRNA, U4 and U6 usually reside together in the same snRNP particle in a base-paired state. The U1-U6 snRNPs, with the exception of U3 snRNP, have an important function in messenger RNA processing (reviewed by Lührmann and co-workers[100]).

So far, 26 polypeptides have been identified as constituents of the major nucleoplasmic snRNPs U1, U2, U5, and U4/U6 from HeLa cells[100]. Nine of these proteins are present in each of the individual snRNPs and hence are designated as Sm or 'core' proteins (see Figure 1). These include the B/B' doublet, the D1/D2/D3 triplet and the E,F and G polypeptides. One or more of these proteins have a strong affinity for a single-stranded sequence present in most U RNAs, refered to as Sm-binding site. Anti-Sm antibody from SLE patients are directed to the D proteins (either to all three or to a subset of them[101]) and to the B'/B doublet[102], but in some sera, antibody against the E, F and G proteins can be detected as well[103].

Fractionation of the individual snRNPs further revealed that in addition to the core polypeptides, most of the snRNPs contain characteristic proteins. Thus U1 snRNPs contain at least three unique polypeptides with apparent molecular weights 70 kDa (U1-70 K), 32 kDa (U1A) and 22 kDa (U1C), which are found in this particle only[35,100]. Characteristic of U2 snRNP particles is the presence of two unique proteins of 31 kDa and 28.5 kDa, termed U2A' and U2B", respectively[35,100,104,105]. Specific protein components have been described for U5 snRNP as well[100], but none of these proteins has so far been identified as a major target for autoantibodies. Recently, two research groups reported the existence of patient antibodies directed to polypeptides specifically contained in the U4/U6 RNP complex[106,107].

Autoantibodies against snRNPs occur predominantly in sera from patients with SLE or mixed connective tissue disease (MCTD). Whereas antibodies to the Sm complex are exclusively found in patients with SLE and therefore are disease-specific (reviewed by Van Venrooij and Sillekens[35]), antibodies to U1RNP are considered as a 'marker' antibody for MCTD[8,19], although they can be present in sera from SLE patients as well[29]. As discussed above, most anti-Sm sera contain antibodies reacting with the core proteins B'/B

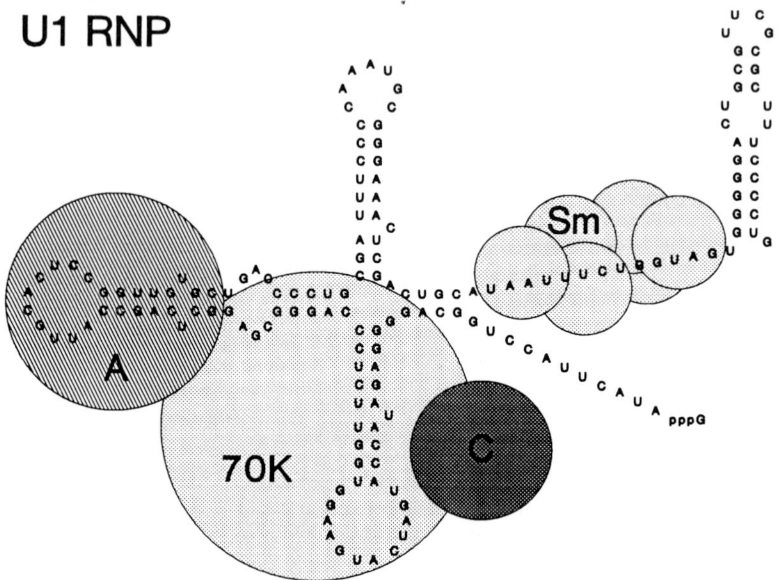

Figure 1 Schematic representation of the U1RNP and U2RNP complexes.
A. U1RNP is a complex of one U1 snRNA molecule (165 nt) containing 4 stemloops and a single-stranded region, mostly referred to as the Sm-binding site[200], and a number of proteins. The specific proteins are the U1-70K protein[46,47], associated with stemloop I[201], the U1A protein[48], associated with stemloop II[202], and the U1C protein[49] associated with the U1RNP complex via protein-protein interactions[203]. The Sm proteins, B'/B, D1, D2, D3, E, F, and G[100], are associated with the Sm-binding site.
B. U2RNP is a complex of one U2 snRNA molecule (188–189 nt) containing 4 stemloops and an Sm-binding region, and several proteins. The specific proteins are the U2A"[55] and the U2B"[56] polypeptides which are associated with the fourth stemloop[201]. The Sm proteins (see above) are associated with the Sm-binding site[100]

and D1, D2 and D3. Since these proteins are common to all major snRNPs, except U3, anti-Sm antibodies precipitate U1, U2, U4, U5 and U6 snRNPs. Anti-U1RNP sera, which selectively precipitate U1 snRNPs, predominantly recognize the U1 snRNP-specific polypeptides U1A and U1-70K, and with lower frequency also U1C. About 60% of the anti-U1RNP sera also show a weak but evident reaction with the proteins B'/B on immunoblots. This is probably due to the presence of anti-U1A or anti-U1C antibodies cross-reacting with B'/B[108].

Anti-U1RNP sera of MCTD patients mostly react with three closely spaced polypeptides of 70 kDa on immunoblots[109]. In SLE the frequency of anti-70K antibodies is much lower. In fact, it has been suggested that the *absence* of anti-70K antibodies in anti-U1RNP sera points to a diagnosis of SLE[29].

Apart from the anti-Sm and anti-U1RNP antibody systems, one more autoantibody specificity reacting with snRNP proteins has been described. These so-called anti-U1/U2RNP sera contain mostly antibodies against the U2 snRNP-specific B" protein and in some cases also antibodies against

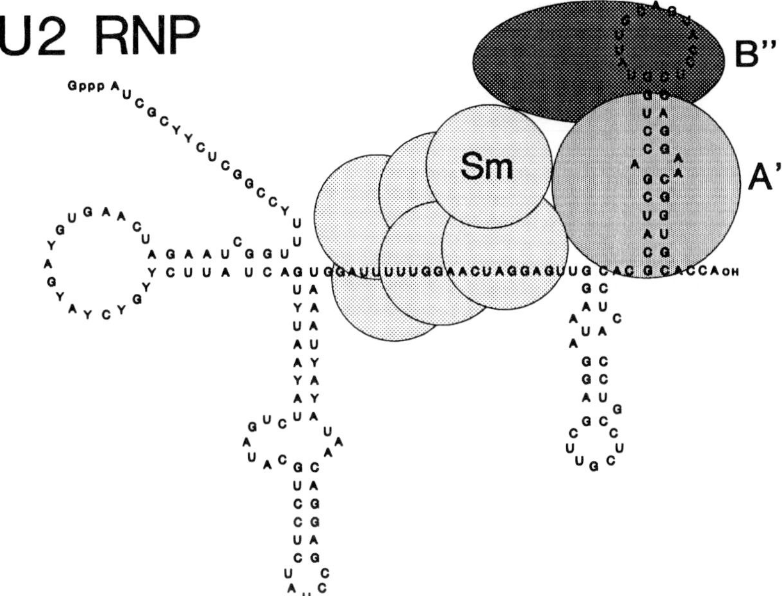

Figure 1b

the U2A' protein[104,105]. Immunoblotting studies revealed that the anti-U1/U2RNP reactivity is due to anti-U2B" antibodies that cross-react with the U1A protein[104]. Such antibodies are present in about 10% of all anti-RNP sera. Recent reviews appeared discussing the B-cell epitopes on the snRNP proteins targeted by anti-Sm antibodies[11], and anti-U1 RNP antibodies[10].

Heterogeneous nuclear RNP proteins (hnRNP)

In eukaryotic cells, RNA polymerase II transcripts are associated with a specific set of proteins forming heterogeneous nuclear ribonucleoprotein (hnRNP) complexes. The processing of a subset of heterogeneous nuclear RNAs into mature mRNAs occurs within these RNPs[110]. The hnRNP complexes contain at least 20 major polypeptides, the most abundant ones being the A1, A2, B1, B2, C1 and C2 proteins[111]. Their best known function is the packaging of pre-mRNA, although recently an RNA-transport function of the hnRNP-A1 protein has been proposed[112]. Although hnRNP complexes, just like snRNPs, are essential components of spliceosomes[100], they have only rarely been described as targets for human autoantibodies. The hnRNP-A1 protein[66,67] has been identified as an autoantigen in a variety of autoimmune diseases[113–115] and recently it was shown that the hnRNP-A2 protein[67,68] is identical to the RA-specific autoantigen RA-33[116]. Future research will teach us whether other hnRNP proteins, all being components

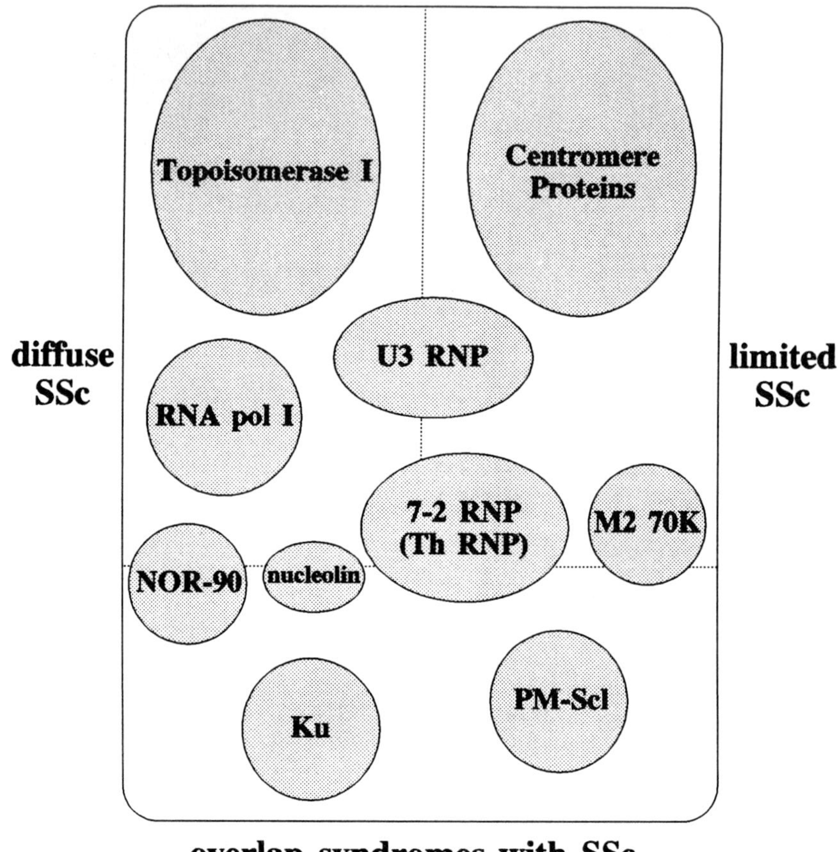

Figure 2 Relation between the antigenic specificities and the main scleroderma subgroups. (Taken from [13] with permission). SSc: systemic sclerosis

of the same dynamic spliceosome structure, are also targeted by human autoantibodies.

The scleroderma-specific antigens

There are several antigens which are specifically targeted by autoantibodies in scleroderma patients. The most common autoantigens are the enzyme DNA-topoisomerase I, the centromere complex and several nucleolar complexes (see Figure 2).

Topoisomerase I

Topoisomerase I is a protein of 110 kDa (in human cells) which has now been cloned by several groups[51,52]. The enzyme is involved in the modulation of the topological state of DNA duplices, being responsible for the relaxation of supercoiled DNA by nicking and resealing one strand of the DNA duplex[117]. This process is an important step in unwinding the DNA strands during DNA replication and transcription. Antibodies against topoisomerase I (in earlier literature the antigen has been referred to as Scl-70[118] and Scl-86[119]) are found in more than 50% of the sera of patients with diffuse cutaneous systemic sclerosis and are specific and important diagnostic markers for this disease. The antibody activity can be detected by CIE or ID in about 30% of the diffuse scleroderma patients[120,121], a proportion that can be increased to about 35–40% when immunoblots or ELISAs are used for detection[52,121,122]. It should be noted, however, that in smaller series of European scleroderma patients with diffuse disease up to 70% will have anti-topo I antibodies[52,122–124]. The presence of this antibody in patients with Raynaud's phenomenon that eventually develop scleroderma suggest that this marker antibody may have prognostic significance[2–4]. A detailed overview of the B-cell epitopes on topoisomerase I targeted by these antibodies has been given by Verheijen[13].

Centromere proteins

The centromere complex (reviewed in [125]) contains at least three antigenic proteins, the 17–19 kDa protein CENP-A, the 80 kDa protein CENP-B and the 140 kDa CENP-C[126]. Antibodies directed to CENP-A and CENP-B are most common and can be found in about 50–70% of patients with limited sclerosis (CREST phenomenon) (reviewed in [8,127]). In diffuse scleroderma they are much more rare. These antibodies thus are important diagnostic markers for scleroderma with limited skin involvement and appear to have prognostic significance as well[2–5]. Data concerning the antigenic relationship between the three proteins are limited, although cross-reactivities between the three proteins have been shown to occur[13]. The CENP-B protein has been cloned[53], and Verheijen et al. demonstrated that the C-terminal 60 amino acids of CENP-B constitute an important autoantigenic domain[13,128].

Nucleolar antigens

Antibodies against nucleolar components include the U3 snRNP associated fibrillarin antigen[129], the Th RNP complex[130], RNA polymerase I[127] and the PM/Scl antigen[59].

Fibrillarin, a 34 kDa protein[61,129], reacts well in Western blots with about 5–10% of scleroderma sera[131–133]. The antigen is associated with the nucleolar U3RNP particle[134], a complex shown to be involved in the processing of pre-ribosomal RNA[135,136]. Interestingly, the production of anti-fibrillarin antibodies can be induced when mercury chloride is given orally to mice from susceptible strains[137,138]. Since these induced murine autoantibodies as well as scleroderma-specific human anti-U3 RNP antibodies reacted with nucleoli from a wide variety of species in immunofluorescence, it can be concluded that both types of antibodies recognize evolutionarily highly conserved epitopes on fibrillarin. However, this does not necessarily mean that they recognize the same epitopes. The Hg-mediated induction of autoantibodies is an important observation and may allow studies of the genetic and immunopathological mechanisms leading to autoantibody production in scleroderma.

The Th RNP or To complex[139,140] consists of a small RNA (7–2S RNA, 267 nt long) and at least six associated polypeptides[130]. The major antigenic protein has a molecular weight of about 40 kDa[141]. The Th RNP is identical to the human mitochondrial RNA processing (MRP) ribonucleo-protein[142,143] and thus responsible for the sequence-specific cleavage of mitochondrial RNA that generates an RNA primer that is used during mitochondrial DNA replication[144]. The Th particle also shares an antigenic polypeptide with a nuclear ribonucleoprotein particle called RNase P[141–143]. The RNase P complex is an endoribonuclease that processes precursor tRNA transcripts to generate their mature 5′termini[145]. So, anti-Th sera precipitate H1 RNA, the RNA component of eukaryotic RNase P, and the MRP/7-2 RNA from crude cell extracts[139,141,142]. Anti-Th antibodies are found in about 8% of the scleroderma patients[141,146].

The RNA polymerase I complex transcribes the ribosomal RNA genes to produce the ribosomal RNAs. These antibodies are present in about 3% of scleroderma patients, reportedly in patients with diffuse scleroderma characterized by high prevalence of internal organ involvement including renal crisis[132]. The antibody cannot be detected by routine assays such as CIE or ID but is readily detected via immunoprecipitation procedures. The enzyme complex is composed out of at least 13 polypeptides with molecular weights ranging from 210 kDa to 12.5 kDa, with the 210 kDa polypeptide being the antigenic target[127,147].

Autoantibodies to the PM/Scl antigen are produced predominantly by patients with features of scleroderma and polymyositis[132]. The composition of this nucleolar antigen is very complex. It contains at least 11–16 polypeptides ranging in apparent molecular mass from 20–110 kDa[148,149]. In immunoblotting studies, reactivity with a 110 kDa antigen was reported in all PM/Scl sera examined[149] while only some recognized an antigen of about 70 kDa[132]. This latter protein has recently been cloned and was shown to be a 39 kDa polypeptide which migrates in sodium dodecylsulphate-polyacrylamide gels at about 70 kDa[59]. Very recently the 110 kDa component of the PM/Scl complex has been cloned as well[220].

Certain scleroderma sera have been shown to contain antibody to other nucleolar component such as nucleolin, a highly conserved protein of 110 kDa molecular weight with multiple functions in the nucleolus of rapidly dividing cells[60,150]. It is thought to be shuttling between nucleolus and cytoplasm during ribosome biogenesis[151]. Antibodies to a 90 kDa component of the nucleolar-organizing region of the chromosomal satellites (NOR-90) have been described as well[152]. The antigenic component has been cloned and was shown to be identical to the human upstream binding protein, hUBF[221].

The cytoplasmic antigens

Cellular localization

It is questionable whether it is correct to define an antigen such as La as a cytoplasmic antigen. The protein clearly has an important nuclear function and there is no doubt that part of the cellular La molecules, at least 30%[153], are localized in the nucleus. The same holds for the Ro proteins of which also about 30% is localized in the nucleus[153] giving rise to the nuclear immunofluorescent patterns of anti-Ro and anti-La antibodies. However, the Y-RNAs to which the Ro and La proteins are bound to form the antigenic Ro RNP complex are predominantly cytoplasmic. Recent data from our laboratory indicate that the Ro and La proteins bind to the newly synthesized Y RNA in the nucleus, and the matured Ro RNP complex is then transported to the cytoplasm. Assuming that the Ro RNP complex is the antigenic target of the antibodies[8] and knowing that more than 95% of the Y-RNAs are in the cytoplasm[153], we think it justified to classify Ro and La as predominantly cytoplasmic antigens.

The La(SS-B) antigen complex

La RNPs are composed of an RNA polymerase III transcript complexed with a 47 kDa antigenic phosphoprotein, hereafter referred to as La. The transcripts include (precursors of) 7S RNA, 5S RNA, tRNA, U6RNA and the Y(Ro)RNAs as well as a number of virus encoded RNAs (reviewed by Pruijn et al.[154]). The common sequence motif present in these RNAs, a short sequence of uridylate residues at the 3' terminus, appears to be the site of interaction with the La antigen[155,57]. Since this 3' sequence motif is mostly lost upon maturation of the transcripts (but not by the Y RNAs), the La protein in most cases binds to precursor-RNAs only transiently.

The La protein (Figure 3) contains a domain of approximately 80 amino acids termed the RNP-80 or RNA-recognition motif, shown to be essential for RNA binding[57]. Other structural features of La include an α-helical central domain and two presumed ATP-binding sites. There are also three so-called PEST-regions (PEST: sequences rich in the amino acids P, E, S and T), known to be susceptible to protease digestion. These PEST regions may explain the susceptibility of the La protein to proteolytic degradation, often leading to characteristic degradation products of 43 and 28 kDa[156].

One of the functions of the La protein has been elucidated. Gottlieb and Steitz[157,158] demonstrated that La is required for efficient and correct termination of RNA polymerase III transcription. The finding that La might function as an ATP-dependent helicase able to melt RNA-DNA hybrids[159], thereby resembling the prokaryotic transcription-termination factor rho, has not yet been confirmed.

Anti-La antibodies are not completely disease-specific since they can be found in SLE (10–40%), SS (40–80%), and RA (0–20%) patients (reviewed in [7,8,19,160]). The variance in the percentages can be explained in part by the use of different methods for the detection of these antibodies[161].

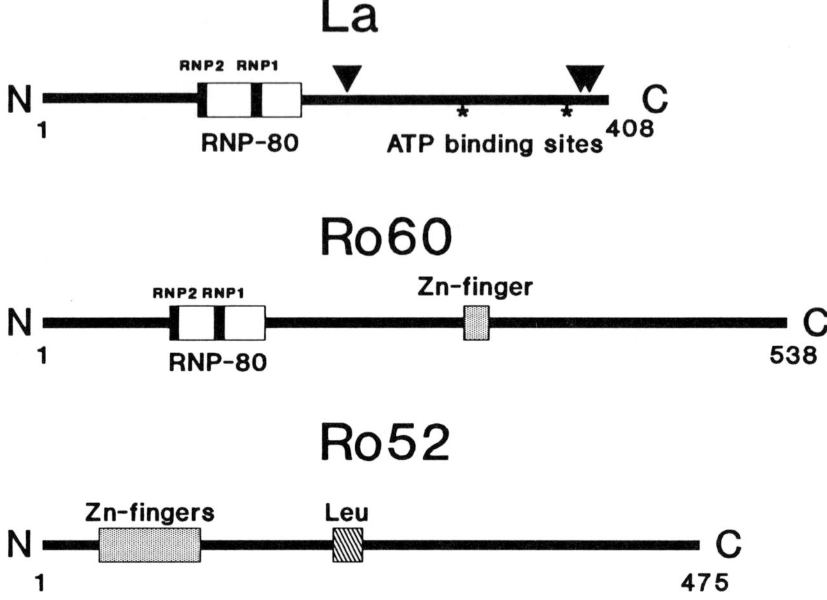

Figure 3 Structural features of La, Ro60 and Ro52 polypeptides.
RNP-80: RNP-80 motif, RNA-recognition motif or RNA-binding region, a sequence present in a large number of RNA-binding proteins[201–204].
Leu: leucine zipper[174–176].
RNP1 and RNP2: most highly conserved sequences within the RNP-80 motif[201,204]. Arrowheads indicate the so-called PEST regions that are susceptible to protease digestion (see text). Numbers refer to the amino acids of the respective proteins. N is the amino-terminus, C the carboxy-terminus.
(Taken from [160] with permission)

The Ro(SS-A) antigen complex

Ro RNPs[162] are composed of several proteins complexed with a subset of the La associated RNAs, the RNA polymerase III transcribed Ro or Y RNAs. In human cells four different Ro RNAs, all about 100 nucleotides in length, have been identified as well as two autoimmune reactive Ro proteins, Ro60 and Ro52 (reviewed in [154,160]). However, in contrast to La RNPs, Ro RNPs show heterogeneity at several levels. First, the total number of cellular Ro RNAs differs among species, varying from two in mouse and duck cells to four in human and bovine cells. Second, differences in Ro RNP complexity between cells within a species have been observed for human lymphocytes, erythrocytes and thrombocytes[163,165]. Ro protein from red blood cells and platelets exists in association with only two small RNAs as opposed to four in other human cell types (reviewed in [154,164]). In red blood cells immunoreactive Ro proteins of 60 kDa and 54 kDa have been detected while in lymphocytes, platelets and other human cells 60 kDa (Ro60, immunologically distinct from the red blood cell 60 kDa protein) and 52 kDa (Ro52) proteins were found[165,166].

Third, within a cell, different Ro RNPs can be distinguished. During fractionation of a cytoplasmic HeLa cell extract the Ro RNPs segregate into distinct subpopulations with characteristic physicochemical properties[167]. Recent results suggest that Y RNP particles consist of their constituent RNA plus three 'core' polypeptides, La, Ro60 and Ro52, plus an unknown number of specific proteins. First of all, the Ro RNAs contain the La-binding region in the mature RNA and, therefore, the La protein is considered to bind these RNAs in a stable manner[57,153,168,169]. Immunoprecipitations with monospecific anti-Ro52 and anti-Ro60 antibodies indicate that all Y RNAs are associated with both proteins[153,170]. The specific, and as yet hypothetical proteins are probably no major antigens and may be only transiently associated with their cognate RNAs.

Several cDNAs encoding Ro60 have been isolated and characterized (Table 2). It is peculiar that some differences exist in all sequences obtained so far, suggesting that the transcript of the Ro60 gene can be spliced in several alternative ways leading to a further heterogeneity of the Ro RNPs. The common part of the deduced Ro60 proteins contains an RNP-80 motif and a putative zinc finger (Figure 3). Although the RNP-80 domain is thought to dominate the RNA-Ro60 interaction (see legend Figure 3), it has become clear that the conformation of Ro60 is extremely important for the binding to the Y RNAs[57] as well as for its antigenicity[171].

Ro52 was not detected by immunoblotting until recently, because it comigrates in the traditional SDS-polyacrylamide gels with the more abundant La protein. However, altering the cross-linking level of the polyacrylamide gels enables the separation of the Ro52 and La polypeptides and their subsequent detection by immunoblotting[26-28]. Recently, two cDNA clones coding for Ro52 were isolated and characterized (Table 2). The deduced amino acid sequence revealed the presence of a number of putative zinc-finger motifs in the amino-terminal part and a leucine zipper motif in the central part of the Ro52 protein[37,38] (see Figure 3). These motifs were originally described in DNA-binding proteins, but are now known to participate in protein–protein interactions and dimer formation as well[172-176]. The Ro52 protein does not contain an RNP-80 motif and indeed, no direct association of Ro52 with Ro RNAs has been found.

In 1990, the cDNA sequence of another putative Ro protein was published by McCauliffe and co-workers[177,178]. This protein is most likely the human homologue of the calcium binding protein calreticulin. Recent data from two other groups, however, strongly indicate that calreticulin is not a Ro/SS-A antigen[179,180], although anti-calreticulin antibodies can be found in some sera of patients with SLE[179].

Anti-Ro antibodies often occur alone in SLE and SS; however, the converse finding of isolated anti-La antibodies is unusual[181,182]. In this respect, the anti-Ro and anti-La antibody systems mimic that of anti-U1RNP and anti-Sm, where the latter antibody specificity rarely occurs alone. Lupus patients with anti-Ro alone have a greater frequency of renal disease, whereas patients with anti-Ro and anti-La have a greater frequency of sicca complex (reviewed in [7,8]). Most of the studies mentioned above could not discriminate between anti-Ro60 and anti-Ro52 antibodies. Ben-Chetrit et al.[26] and Slobbe et al.[27]

...(a/k)**KEESEESD(D/E)DMGFGLDF**-COOH

Figure 4 Homologous carboxy-terminal amino acid sequence of ribosomal proteins P0, P1 and P2. Amino acids in bold constitute the defined epitope[62,185].

reported recently the presence of both anti-Ro60 and anti-Ro52 antibody in SLE and SS patients' sera. The presence of anti-Ro60 alone, however, appeared to be indicative of SLE, whereas the presence of anti-Ro52 alone was found in SS sera only. It is possible, however, that such findings are dependent on the method employed for the detection of the antibodies (see [171]).

Ribosomal RNP

P-proteins (phosphorylated acidic ribosomal proteins) are generally present in multiple copies on the ribosome and have isoelectric points in the range of pH 3 to 5, in contrast to most ribosomal proteins which are single copy and basic. In eukaryotes two slightly different proteins, analogous to the *E. coli* proteins L7/L12, have been named P1 and P2 and these proteins interact with eukaryotic elongation factors EF1 and EF2 and are required for aminoacyl-tRNA binding and EF2-dependent GTPase activity as well as polypeptide synthesis (reviewed in [62]). These proteins share an identical 22-amino-acid sequence at their C-termini that contains an epitope that is recognized by autoantibodies in about 10% of SLE patients[62,183–185]. Antibodies reactive with this C-terminal epitope of mammalian P1 and P2 also recognize a neutral phosphoprotein (P0) with a molecular weight of about 37 kDa that is found in the large subunit of ribosomes and most probably is the analogue of *E. coli* protein L10[62]. On immunoblots, loaded with a preparation of ribosomal proteins, the anti-ribRNP antibody therefore recognizes three bands which migrate at molecular weights of about 37 kDa (P0, predicted M_r: 34 kDa[62]), and a doublet of P1 and P2 that migrates in the 15 kDa to 18 kDa range (predicted M_r of both proteins about 12 kDa[62]). Using a synthetic peptide based on the identical C-terminal sequence of the three proteins (Figure 4) a sensitive ELISA technique can also be used for the detection of these antibodies[185].

Recently another ribosomal protein, the small subunit protein S10 (molecular weight about 20 kDa) was identified as a target of antibodies in about 10% of SLE patients[186,187].

In addition to antibody reacting with the P proteins, sera may contain often (up to 75% of the cases) antibody against 28S ribosomal RNA as well. The antigenic region has been identified as the GTPase activity centre, localized between nucleotides 1922 and 2020[81,82], (reviewed in [15]).

The tRNA synthetases

There is a striking association of anti-tRNA synthetase antibodies with polymyositis (reviewed in [188]). The aminoacyl-tRNA synthetases are a group of cytoplasmic enzymes that catalyse the binding of tRNA to their respective amino acids, with a unique enzyme for each amino acid. The most common anti-tRNA synthetase autoantibody in PM is anti-Jo-1[189]. The Jo-1 antigen is identical to the enzyme His-tRNA synthetase (mol. wt. 54 kDa) which is responsible for the linkage of the amino acid histidine to its tRNA. Since the synthetase is associated with a tRNA during this process, the Jo-1 antigen is a ribonucleoprotein. Antibody to Jo-1 is found in 25–30% of patients with adult PM[190–192].

Other antigenic tRNA synthetases in PM are those of alanine, often referred to as the PL-12 system (mol. wt. 110 kDa)[80,188,193], threonine or PL-7 (mol. wt. 80 kDa)[194–196], isoleucine (mol. wt. 139 kDa) and glycine (mol. wt. 77 kDa)[188]. These latter activities, however, occur in only 1–4% of the myositis patients.

In the PL-12 system, separate antibody populations were found that reacted with alanyl-tRNA synthetase as well as with naked $tRNA^{ala}$[79,80]. The antibodies recognize at least six distinguishable human $tRNA^{ala}$ species grouped into two sequence families. The antigenic determinant could be identified as a 7–9 nucleotide sequence comprising the anticodon loop plus one or two additional bases at its 3′ side[79,15]. Preliminary studies indicate that about 20% of the sera with antibody to Jo-1 or histidyl-tRNA synthetase and glycine-tRNA synthetase also contain antibodies which specifically recognize the cognate tRNA[9]. Finally, a tRNA autoantibody specificity directed to initiator methionine tRNA has been found in two sera from myositis patients[78]. These studies indicate that the antibody response is directed to all components of the synthetase-tRNA complex. Other reports suggest that the production of anti-Jo-1 antibodies appears to be driven by this antigenic complex[197,198], as indeed also has been suggested for other anti-ribonucleoprotein antibodies including anti-Sm/RNP, anti-ribRNP and anti-Ro/La (reviewed in [9]).

The heat shock proteins

Heat shock proteins (HSPs) are produced when a cell is confronted with a sudden increase in temperature (reviewed in [205,206]). When it was found that many insults other than heat can also induce HSP synthesis, the term 'stress proteins' was introduced. HSP synthesis is known to be induced by environmental stress conditions (heat, heavy metals, oxidants and organic reagents) and by pathophysiological stress conditions (e.g. microbial infections) but can also occur under normal conditions (hormonal stimulation, cell differentiation, cell cycle). It is clear that HSPs serve important physiological functions and that many of them are present and active in normal cells[207,208]. The designation 'molecular chaperone' was coined to account for their more general role as house-keeping proteins in the cell[207,208].

The initial studies on cloned heat shock genes and purified proteins showed that the HSPs are incredibly highly conserved among widely divergent organisms. For example, the major heat shock protein, hsp70, has about 50% of its sequence conserved between *E. coli* and human, and some domains are 96% similar[205]. Several of the major HSPs are members of gene (protein) families that include proteins normally present. Some of these families are the hsp70, the hsp90 and the hsp60 family. One of the functions of the hsp70 proteins is that they are needed for import of proteins into other eukaryotic cell organelles including the endoplasmic reticulum, the mitochondrion and the lysosome. The hsp70 proteins are thought to unfold partially folded polypeptides so that they can be translocated through membrane pores. Hsp70 proteins are also able to disassemble protein complexes. The hsp60 proteins participate in the folding and assembly of polypeptides. Based on this property, they have been referred to as chaperonins[208]. The hsp90 protein function as chaperones in that they can form complexes with a number of cellular proteins, notably kinases, and can activate or inactivate their functions (reviewed in [205,206]).

A number of other proteins have been reported to be HSPs, based on their enhanced rate of synthesis after stress. Some of these stress proteins, mostly of low molecular mass (15–30 kDa) have been identified as proteins with normal functions in the cell, e.g. glycolytic enzymes. Ubiquitin, the highly conserved polypeptide that marks a protein for degradation, is also considered to be one of these smaller HSPs[209].

Increasing evidence from studies with experimental animals and patients indicates that HSPs may have a role in autoimmunity (reviewed in [210–212]). Antibodies to hsp65 have been described in rheumatoid arthritis[213,214] and those to ubiquitin, hsp70 and hsp90 in SLE[215–217]. It has also been shown that monoclonal antibodies generated against human hsp60 show reactivity with synovial membranes of patients with juvenile chronic arthritis[218]. These studies have been reviewed extensively by Kaufmann[212,219] and by Winfield[210,211].

Acknowledgements

I am grateful to my colleagues Ger Pruijn, Ron Verheijen, René Hoet and Joe Craft for critically reading the manuscript. The research of the author has been generously supported by grants from Het Nationaal Reumafonds of the Netherlands.

References

1. Smolen J, Maini RN, Kalden J, eds. In: Rheumatoid Arthritis – Recent Research Advances. Springer Verlag: Heidelberg; 1992.
2. Weiner E, Hildebrandt S, Senecal J-L, Daniels L, Noell S, Joyal F, Roussin A, Earnshaw WC, Rothfield N. Prognostic significance of anticentromere antibodies and anti-topoisomerase I antibodies in Raynaud's disease: A prospective study. Arthritis Rheum. 1991; 34: 68–77.
3. Kallenberg CGM, Wouda AA, Hoet MH, Van Venrooij WJ. Development of connective tissue disease in patients presenting with Raynaud's phenomenon: a six year follow up with emphasis on the predictive value of antinuclear antibodies as detected by immunoblotting.

Ann Rheum Dis. 1988; 47: 634–641.

4. Wollersheim H, Thien Th, Hoet MH, Van Venrooij WJ. The diagnostic value of several immunological tests for antinuclear antibody in predicting the development of connective tissue disease in patients presenting with Raynaud's phenomenon. Eur J Clin Invest. 1989; 19: 535–541.

5. Sarkozi J, Bookman AAM, Lee P, Keystone EC, Fritzler MJ. Significance of anticentromere antibody in idiopathic Raynaud's syndrome. Am J Med. 1987; 83: 893–898.

6. Van Venrooij WJ, Van De Putte LBJ. The clinical significance of anti-nuclear antibodies in connective tissue diseases. Seminars in Clin Immunol. 1991; 3: 27–32.

7. Craft JE, Hardin JA. Antinuclear and Anticytoplasmic Antibodies. In: Textbook of Rheumatology, 4th edition. Kelley WN, Harris ED, Ruddy S, Sledge C, eds. Philadelphia: WB Saunders, 1992: in press.

8. Tan E. Antinuclear antibodies: Diagnostic markers for autoimmune diseases and probes for cell biology. Adv Immunol. 1989; 44: 93–151.

9. Plotz PH. The role of autoantigens in the induction and maintenance of autoimmunity. Mol Biol Rep. 1992; 16: 127–133.

10. Guldner HH. Mapping of epitopes recognized by anti-(U1)RNP autoantibodies. Mol Biol Rep. 1992; 16: 155–165.

11. Rokeach LA, Hoch SO. B-cell epitopes of Sm autoantigens. Mol Biol Rep. 1992; 16: 165–175.

12. Whittingham S. B-cell epitopes of La and Ro autoantigens. Mol Biol Rep. 1992; 16: 175–183.

13. Verheijen R. B-cell epitopes of scleroderma-specific autoantigens. Mol Biol Rep. 1992; 16: 183–191.

14. Chou C-H, Satoh M, Wang J, Reeves WH. B-cell epitopes of autoantigenic DNA-binding proteins. Mol Biol Rep. 1992; 16: 191–199.

15. Hoet RM, Van Venrooij WJ. B-cell epitopes of RNA autoantigens. Mol Biol Rep. 1992; 16: 199–207.

16. Holman HR, Kunkel HG. Affinity between the lupus erythematosus serum factor and cell nuclei and nucleoprotein. Science. 1957; 126: 162–163.

17. Van Venrooij WJ, Maini RN, eds. Manual of Biological Markers of Disease. Section A: Methods of Autoantibody Detection. Dordrecht: Kluwer Academic Publishers; 1993

18. Andrade LEC, Chan EKL, Raska I, Peebles CL, Roos G, Tan EM. Human autoantibody to a novel protein of the nuclear coiled body: Immunological characterization and cDNA cloning of p80-coilin. J Exp Med. 1991; 173: 1407–1419.

19. Tan EM. Autoantibodies to nuclear antigens (ANA): Their immunobiology and medicine. Adv Immunol. 1982; 33: 167–240.

20. Van Venrooij WJ, Charles P, Maini RN. The consensus workshops for the detection of autoantibodies to intracellular antigens in rheumatic diseases. J Immunol Methods. 1991; 140: 181–189.

21. Van Venrooij WJ, Wodzig KW, Habets WJ, De Rooij DJ, Van De Putte LBA. Anti-56K: a novel, frequently occurring autoantibody specificity in connective tissue disease. Clin Exp Rheumatol. 1989; 7: 277–282.

22. Miyachi K, Fritzler MJ, Tan EM. Autoantibody to a nuclear antigen in proliferating cells. J Immunol. 1978; 121: 2228–2234.

23. Mimori T, Akizuki M, Yamagata H, Inada S, Yoshida S, Homma M. Characterization of a high molecular weight acidic nuclear protein recognized by autoantibodies in sera from patients with polymyositis-scleroderma overlap. J Clin Invest. 1981; 68: 611–620.

24. Reichlin M, Maddison PJ, Targoff IN, Bunch T, Arnett FC, Sharp G, Treadwell E, Tan EM. Antibodies to a nuclear/nucleolar antigen in patients with polymyositis-overlap syndrome. J Clin Immunol. 1984; 4: 40–44.

25. Provost TT, Levin LS, Watson RM, Mayo M, Ratrie H. Detection of anti-Ro(SS-A) by gel double diffusion and a 'sandwich' ELISA in systemic and subacute cutaneous lupus erythematosus and Sjögren's syndrome. J Autoimmun. 1991; 4: 87–96.

26. Ben-Chetrit E, Fox RI, Tan EM. Dissociation of immune responses to the SS-A (Ro) 52-kD and 60-kD polypeptides in systemic lupus erythematosus and Sjögren's syndrome. Arthritis Rheum. 1990; 33: 349–355.

27. Slobbe RL, Pruijn GJM, Damen WGM, Van Der Kemp JWCM, Van Venrooij WJ.

Detection and occurrence of the 60- and 52-kD Ro(SS-A) antigens and of autoantibodies against these proteins. Clin Exp Immunol. 1991; 86: 99–105.

28. Buyon JP, Slade SG, Chan EKL, Tan EM, Winchester R. Effective separation of the 52 kDa SS-A/Ro polypeptide from the 48 kDa SS-B/La polypeptide by altering conditions of polyacrylamide gel electrophoresis. J Immunol Methods. 1990; 129: 207–210.

29. Reichlin M, Van Venrooij WJ. Autoantibodies to the URNP particles: relationship to clinical diagnosis and nephritis. Clin Exp Immunol. 1991; 83: 286–290.

30. Stott DI. Immunoblotting and dot blotting. J Immunol Methods 1989; 119: 153–187.

31. Boire G, Lopez-Longo F-J, Lapointe S, Ménard H-A. Sera from patients with autoimmune disease recognize conformational determinants on the 60-kD Ro/SS-A protein. Arthritis Rheum. 1991; 34: 722–730.

32. Wold RT, Young FE, Tan EM, Farr RS. Deoxyribonucleic acid antibody: A method to detect its primary interaction with deoxyribonucleic acid. Science. 1968; 161: 806–807.

33. Smeenk R, Hylkema M. Detection of antibodies to DNA: a technical assessment. Mol Biol Rep. 1992; 17: 71–79.

34. Craft J, Hardin JA. Immunoprecipitation assays for the detection of soluble nuclear and cytoplasmic nucleoproteins. In: Manual of Clinical Laboratory Immunology, 4th Edition. N Rose, H. Friedman, J. Fahey, eds. American Society of Microbiology, Washington, DC. 1992; 747–754.

35. Van Venrooij WJ, Sillekens PTG. Small nuclear RNA associated proteins: autoantigens in connective tissue diseases. Clin Exp Rheumatol. 1989; 7: 635–645.

36. Ben-Chetrit E, Gandy BJ, Tan EM, Sullivan KF. Isolation and characterization of a cDNA clone encoding the 60-kD component of the human SS-A/Ro ribonucleoprotein autoantigen. J Clin Invest. 1989; 83: 1284–1292.

37. Chan EK, Hamel JC, Buyon JP, Tan EM. Molecular definition and sequence motifs of the 52-kD component of human SS-A/Ro autoantigen. J Clin Invest. 1991; 87: 6876.

38. Itoh K, Itoh Y, Frank MB. Protein heterogeneity in the human Ro/SSA ribonucleoproteins. The 52- and 60 kD Ro/SSA autoantigens are encoded by separate genes. J Clin Invest. 1991; 87: 177–186.

39. Chambers JC, Kenan D, Martin BJ, Keene JD. Genomic structure and amino acid sequence domains of the human La autoantigen. J Biol Chem. 1988; 263: 18043–18051.

40. Rokeach L, Haselby J, Hoch S. Molecular cloning of a cDNA encoding the human Sm-D autoantigen. Proc Natl Acad Sci USA. 1988; 85: 4832–4836.

41. Rokeach LA, Jannatipour M, Haselby JA, Hoch SO. Primary structure of a human small nuclear ribonucleoprotein polypeptide as deduced by cDNA analysis. J Biol Chem. 1989; 264: 5024–5030.

42. Stanford DR, Kehl M, Perry CA, Holicky E, Harvey SE, Rohleder AM, Rehder K, Lührmann R, Wieben ED. The complete primary structure of the human snRNP E protein. Nucleic Acids Res. 1988; 16: 10593–10605.

43. Ohosone Y, Mimori T, Griffith A, Akizuki M, Homma M, Craft J, Hardin JA. Molecular cloning of cDNA encoding Sm autoantigen: derivation of a cDNA for a B polypeptide of the U series of small nuclear ribonucleoprotein particles. Proc Natl Acad Sci USA. 1989; 86: 4249–4253.

44. Ohosone Y, Mimorit T, Griffith A, Akizuki M, Homma M, Craft J, Hardin JA. Molecular cloning of cDNA encoding Sm autoantigen: derivation of a cDNA for a B polypeptide of the U series of small nuclear ribonucleoprotein particles (correction). Proc Natl Acad Sci USA. 1989; 86: 8982.

45. Van Dam A, Winkel I, Zijlstra-Baalbergen J, Smeenk R, Cuypers HT. Cloned human snRNP proteins B and B' differ only in their carboxy-terminal part. EMBO J. 1989; 8: 3853–3860.

46. Theissen H, Etzerodt M, Reuter R, Schneider C, Lottspeich F, Argos P, Lührmann R, Philipson L. Cloning of the human cDNA for the U1 RNA-associated 70K protein. EMBO J. 1986; 5: 3209–3217.

47. Spritz RA, Strunk K, Surowy CS, Hoch SO, Barton DE, Francke U. The human U1-70K protein: cDNA cloning, chromosomal localization, expression, alternative splicing and RNA-binding. Nucleic Acids Res. 1987; 15: 10373–10391.

48. Sillekens PTG, Habets WJ, Beijer RP, Van Venrooij WJ. cDNA cloning of the human U1 snRNP associated A protein: extensive homology between U1 and U2 snRNP-specific

proteins. EMBO J. 1987; 6: 3841–3848.
49. Sillekens PTG, Beijer RP, Habets WJ, Van Venrooij WJ. Human U1 snRNP-specific C protein: complete cDNA and protein sequence and identification of a multigene family in mammals. Nucleic Acids Res. 1988; 16: 8307–8321.
50. Ramsden D, Chen J, Miller F, Misener V, Bernstein R, Siminovitch K, Tsui FWL. Epitope mapping of the cloned human autoantigen, histidyl-tRNA synthetase: analysis of the myositis-associated anti-Jo-1 autoimmune response. J Immunol. 1989; 143: 2267–2272.
51. D'Arpa P, Machlin P, Ratrie H, Rothfield NF, Cleveland DW, Earnshaw WC. cDNA cloning of the human DNA topoisomerase I: Catalytic activity of a 67.7-kDa carboxyl-terminal fragment. Proc Natl Acad Sci USA. 1988; 85: 2543–2547.
52. Verheijen R, Van Den Hoogen F, Beijer R, Richter A, Penner E, Habets WJ, Van Venrooij WJ. A recombinant topoisomerase I used for autoantibody detection in sera from patients with systemic sclerosis. Clin Exp Immunol. 1990; 80: 38–43.
53. Earnshaw WC, Sullivan KF, Machlin PS, Cooke CA, Kaiser DA, Pollard TD, Rothfield NF, Cleveland DW. Molecular cloning of cDNA for CENP-B, the major human centromere autoantigen. J Cell Biol. 1987; 104: 817–829.
54. McNeilage LJ, Whittingham S, McHugh N, Barnett AJ. A highly conserved 72,000 dalton centromeric antigen reactive with autoantibodies from patients with progressive systemic sclerosis. J Immunol. 1986; 137: 2541–2547.
55. Sillekens PTG, Beijer RP, Habets WJ, Van Venrooij WJ. Molecular cloning of the cDNA for the human U2 snRNA-specific A' protein. Nucleic Acids Res. 1989; 17: 1893–1906.
56. Habets WJ, Sillekens PTG, Hoet MH, et al. Analysis of a cDNA clone expressing a human autoimmune antigen: full-length sequence of the U2 small nuclear RNA-associated B'' antigen. Proc Natl Acad Sci USA. 1987; 84: 2421–2425.
57. Pruijn GJM, Slobbe RL, Van Venrooij WJ. Analysis of protein-RNA interactions within Ro ribonucleoprotein complexes. Nucleic Acids Res. 1991; 19: 5173–5180.
58. Sharpe NG, Williams DG, Howarth DN, Coles B, Latchman DS. Isolation of cDNA clones encoding the human Sm B'/B autoimmune antigen and specifically reacting with human anti-Sm autoimmune sera. FEBS Lett. 1989; 250: 585–590.
59. Alderuccio F, Chan EKL, Tan EM. Molecular characterization of an autoantigen of PM-Scl in the polymyositis/scleroderma overlap syndrome: a unique and complete human cDNA encoding an apparent 75-kD acidic protein of the nucleolar complex. J Exp Med. 1991; 173: 941–952.
60. Lapeyre B, Bourbon H, Amalric F. Nucleolin, the major nucleolar protein growing eukaryotic cells: An unusual protein structure revealed by the nucleotide sequence. Proc Natl Acad Sci USA. 1987; 84: 1472–1476.
61. Aris JP, Blobel G. cDNA cloning and sequencing of human fibrillarin, a conserved nucleolar protein recognized by autoimmune antisera. Proc Natl Acad Sci USA. 1991; 88: 931–935.
62. Rich BE, Steitz JA. Human acidic ribosomal phosphoproteins P0, P1 and P2: Analysis of cDNA clones, in vitro synthesis and assembly. Mol Cell Biol. 1987; 7: 4065–4074.
63. Deutscher SL, Harley JB, Keene JD. Molecular analysis of the 60-kDa human Ro ribonucleoprotein. Proc Natl Acad Sci USA. 1988; 85: 9479–9483.
64. Reeves WH, Sthoeger ZM. Molecular cloning of cDNA encoding the p70 Ku Lupus autoantigen. J Biol Chem. 1989; 264: 5047–5052.
65. Yaneva M, Wen J, Ayala A, Cook R. cDNA-derived amino acid sequence of the 86 kDa subunit of the Ku antigen. J Biol Chem. 1989; 264: 13407–13411.
66. Cobianchi F, SenGupta DN, Zmudzka BZ, Wilson SH. Structure of rodent helix-stabilizing protein revealed by cDNA cloning. J Biol Chem. 1986; 261: 3536–3543.
67. Kumar A, Williams KR, Szer W. Purification and domain structure of core hnRNP proteins A1 and A2 and their relationship to single-stranded DNA-binding proteins. J Biol Chem. 1986; 261: 11266–11273.
68. Burd CG, Swanson MS, Görlach M, Dreyfuss G. Primary structures of the heterogeneous nuclear ribonucleoprotein A2, B1 and C2 proteins: A diversity of RNA binding proteins is generated by small peptide inserts. Proc Natl Acad Sci USA. 1989; 86: 9788–9792.
69. Almendral JM, Huebsch D, Blundell PA, Macdonald-Bravo H, Bravo R. Cloning and sequence of the human nuclear protein cyclin. Proc Natl Acad Sci USA. 1987; 84: 1575–1579.
70. Stollar BD. Immunochemistry of DNA. Int Rev Immunol. 1989; 5: 1–22.

71. Stollar BD. Antibodies to DNA. CRC Crit Rev Biochem. 1986; 20: 1–36.
72. Koffler D, Carr R, Agnello V, Feizi T, Kunkel HG. Antibodies to polynucleotides: Distribution in human serum. Science. 1969; 166: 1648–1649.
73. Ballou SP, Kushner I. Anti-native DNA detection by the Crithidia luciliae method: An improved guide to the diagnosis and clinical management of systemic lupus erythematosus. Arthritis Rheum. 1979; 22: 321–327.
74. Koffler D, Carr RI, Agnello V, Thoburn R, Kunkel HG. Antibodies to polynucleotides in human sera: Antigenic specificity and relationship to disease. J Exp Med. 1971; 134: 294–312.
75. Carson DA. The specificity of anti-DNA antibodies in systemic lupus erythematosus. J Immunol. 1991; 146: 1–2.
76. Smeenk R, Brinkman K, Van Den Brink H, Termaat RM, Berden J, Nossent H, Swaak T. Antibodies to DNA in patients with systemic lupus erythematosus. Their role in the diagnosis, the follow-up and the pathogenesis of the disease. Clin Rheum. 1990; suppl. 1: 100–110.
77. Brinkman K, Termaat R, Berden JHM, Smeenk RJT. Anti-DNA antibodies and lupus nephritis: the complexity of crossreactivity. Immunol Today. 1990; 11: 232–233.
78. Wilusz J, Keene JD. Autoantibodies specific for U1 RNA and initiator methionine tRNA. J Biol Chem. 1986; 261: 5467–5472.
79. Bunn CC, Mathews MB. Autoreactive epitope defined as the anticodon region of alanine transfer of RNA. Science. 1987; 238: 1116–1119.
80. Bunn CC, Bernstein RM, Mathews MB. Autoantibodies against alanyl tRNA synthetase and tRNA^{ala} coexist and are associated with myositis. J Exp Med. 1986; 163: 1281–1291.
81. Chu J-L, Brot N, Weissbach H, Elkon K. Lupus antiribosomal P antisera contain antibodies to a small fragment of 28S rRNA located in the proposed ribosomal GTPase center. J Exp Med. 1991; 174: 507–514.
82. Uchiumi T, Traut RR, Elkon K, Kominami R. A human autoantibody specific for a unique conserved region of 28S ribosomal RNA inhibits the interaction of elongation factors 1α and 2 with ribosomes. J Biol Chem. 1991; 266: 2054–2062.
83. Deutscher SL, Keene JD. A sequence-specific conformational epitope on U1RNA is recognized by a unique autoantibody. Proc Natl Acad Sci USA. 1988; 85: 3299–3304.
84. Van Venrooij WJ, Hoet R, Castrop J, Hageman B, Mattaj IW, Van De Putte LB. Anti-(U1) small nuclear RNA antibodies in anti-small nuclear ribonucleoprotein sera from patients with connective tissue diseases. J Clin Invest. 1990; 86: 2154–2160.
85. Hoet RM, De Weerd P, Klein Gunnewiek J, Koornneef I, Van Venrooij WJ. Epitope regions on U1 small nuclear RNA recognized by anti-U1RNA-specific autoantibodies. J Clin Invest. 1992; 90: 1753–1762.
86. Swaak AJG, Aarden LA, Van Epps LWS. Anti-dsDNA and complement profiles as prognostic guides in systemic lupus erythematosus. Arthritis Rheum. 1979; 22: 226–235.
87. Swaak AJG, Groenwold J, Bronsveld W. Predictive value of complement profiles and anti-dsDNA in systemic lupus erythematosus. Ann Rheum Dis. 1986; 45: 359–366.
88. Ter Borg EJ, Horst G, Hummel EJ, Limburg PG, Kallenberg CGM. Predictive value of rises in anti-dsDNA antibody levels for disease exacerbation in systemic lupus erythematosus: a long term prospective study. Arthritis Rheum. 1990; 33: 634–643.
89. Hoet RM, Koornneef I, De Rooij DJ, Van De Putte LBA, Van Venrooij WJ. Changes in anti-U1RNA antibody levels correlate with disease activity in patients with SLE overlap syndrome. Arthritis Rheum. 1992; 35: 1202–1210
90. Gohill J, Cary PD, Couppez M, Fritzler MJ. Antibodies from patients with drug-induced and idiopathic lupus erythematosus react with epitopes restricted to the amino and carboxyl termini of histone. J Immunol. 1985; 135: 3116–3121.
91. Mimori T, Akizuki M, Yamagata H, Inada S, Yoshida S, Homma M. Characterization of a high molecular weight acidic nuclear protein recognized by autoantibodies in sera from patients with polymyositis-scleroderma overlap. J Clin Invest. 1981; 68: 611–620.
92. Reeves WH. Use of monoclonal antibodies for the characterization of novel DNA-binding protein recognized by human autoimmune sera. J Exp Med. 1985; 161: 18–39.
93. Stuiver MH, Coenjaerts FEJ, Van Der Vliet PC. The autoantigen Ku is indistinguishable from NF IV, a protein forming multimeric protein-DNA complexes. J Exp Med. 1990; 172: 1049–1054.

94. Mathews MB, Bernstein RM, Franze BR Jr, Garrels JI, Identity of the proliferating cell nuclear antigen and cyclin. Nature. 1984; 309: 374–376.
95. Ogata K, Ogata Y, Nakamura RM, Tan EM. Purification and N-terminal amino acid sequence of proliferating cell nuclear antigen (PCNA/cyclin) and development of ELISA for anti-PCNA antibodies. J Immunol. 1985; 135: 2623–2627.
96. Kurki P, Vanderlaan M, Dolbeare F, Gray J, Tan EM. Expression of Proliferating Cell Nuclear Antigen (PCNA/Cyclin) during the cell cycle. Exptl Cell Res. 1986; 166: 209–219.
97. Bravo R, Frank R, Blundell PA, Macdonald-Bravo H. Cyclin/PCNA is the auxiliary protein of DNA polymerase-d. Nature. 1987; 326: 515–517.
98. Prelich G, Tan C-K, Kostura M, Mathews MB, So AG, Downey KM, Stillman B. Functional identity of proliferating cell nuclear antigen and a DNA polymerase-d auxiliary protein. Nature. 1987; 326: 517–520.
99. Huff JP, Roos G, Peebles CL, Houghten R, Sullivan KF, Tan EM. Insights into native epitopes of proliferating cell nuclear antigen using recombinant DNA protein products. J Exp Med. 1990; 172: 419–429.
100. Lührmann R, Kastner B, Bach M. Structure of spliceosomal snRNPs and their role in pre-mRNA splicing. Biochim Biophys Acta. 1990; 1087: 265–292.
101. Lehmeier T, Foulaki K, Lührmann R. Evidence for three distinct D proteins, which react differentially with anti-Sm antibodies, in the cores of the major snRNPs U1, U2, U4/U6 and U5. Nucleic Acids Res. 1990; 18: 6475–6484.
102. Habets WJ, Berden JHM, Hoch SO, Van Venrooij WJ. Further characterization and subcellular localization of Sm and U1 ribonucleoprotein antigens. Eur J Immunol. 1985; 15: 992–997.
103. Reuter R, Roth S, Habets W, Van Venrooij WJ, Lührmann R. Autoantibody production against the U small nuclear ribonucleoprotein particle proteins E, F and G in patients with connective tissue diseases. Eur J Immunol. 1990; 20: 437–440.
104. Habets WJ, Hoet M, Bringmann P, Lührmann R, Van Venrooij WJ. Autoantibodies to ribonucleoprotein particles containing U2 small nuclear RNA. EMBO J. 1985; 4: 1545–1550.
105. Craft J, Mimori T, Olsen TL, Hardin JA. The U2 small nuclear ribonucleoprotein particle as an autoantigen. Analysis with sera from patients with overlap syndrome. J Clin Invest. 1988; 8: 1716–1724.
106. Okano Y, Medsger TA Jr. Newly identified U4/U6 snRNP-binding proteins by serum antibodies from a patient with systemic sclerosis. J Immunol. 1991; 146: 535–542.
107. Fujii T, Mimori T, Hama N, Suwa A, Akizuki M, Tojo T. Characterization of autoantibodies that recognize U4/U6 small ribonucleoprotein particles in serum from a patient with primary Sjögren's syndrome. J Biol Chem. 1992; 267: 16412–16416
108. Habets WJ, Sillekens PTG, Hoet MH, McAllister G, Lerner MR, Van Venrooij WJ. Small nuclear RNA-associated proteins are immunologically related as revealed by mapping of autoimmune reactive B-cell epitopes. Proc Natl Acad Sci USA. 1989; 86: 4674–4678.
109. Van Venrooij WJ. Autoantibodies against small nuclear ribonucleoprotein components. J Rheum. 1987, suppl. 13, 14: 78–82.
110. Dreyfuss G, Swanson MS, Pinol-Roma S. Heterogeneous nuclear ribonucleoprotein particles and the pathway of mRNA formation. Trends Biochem Sci. 1988; 13: 86–91.
111. Pinol-Roma S, Choi YD, Matunis MJ, Dreyfuss G. Immunopurification of heterogeneous nuclear ribonucleoprotein particles reveals an assortment of RNA-binding proteins. Genes Dev. 1988; 2: 215–227.
112. Pinol-Roma S, Dreyfuss G. Shuttling of pre-mRNA binding proteins between nucleus and cytoplasm. Nature. 1992; 355: 730–732.
113. Gelpi C, Rodriquez-Sanchez JL, Hardin JA. Purification of hnRNP from HeLa cells with a monoclonal antibody and its application in ELISA: detection of autoantibodies. Clin Exp Immunol. 1988; 71: 281–288.
114. Astaldi-Ricotti CGB, Bastagno M, Cerini A, Negri C, Caporali R, Cobianchi F, Longhi M, Montecucco C. Antibodies to hnRNP core protein A1 in connective tissue diseases. J Cell Biochem. 1989; 40: 1–5.
115. Montecucco C, Caporali R, Negri C, DeGennaro F, Cerino A, Bestango M, Cobianchi F, Astaldi-Ricotti G. Antibodies from patients with rheumatoid arthritis and systemic lupus erythematosus recognize different epitopes of a single heterogeneous nuclear RNP core

protein. Arthritis Rheum. 1990; 33: 180–186.

116. Steiner G, Hartmuth K, Skriner K, Maurer-fogy I, Sinski A, Thalmann E, Hassfeld W, Barta A, Smolen J. Purification and partial sequencing of the nuclear autoantigen RA-33 shows that it is indistinguishable from the A2 protein of the heterogeneous nuclear ribonucleoprotein complex. J Clin Invest. 1992; 90: 1061–1066

117. Osheroff N. Biochemical basis for the interactions of type I and type II topoisomerases with DNA. Pharmacol Ther. 1989; 41: 223–241.

118. Douvas A, Achten M, Tan EM. Identification of a nuclear protein (Scl-70) as a unique target of human antinuclear antibodies in scleroderma. J Biol Chem. 1979; 254: 10514–10522.

119. Van Venrooij WJ, Stapel SO, Houben H, Habets WJ, Kallenberg CGM, Penner E, Van De Putte LB. Scl-86, a marker for diffuse scleroderma. J Clin Invest. 1985; 75: 1053–1060.

120. Steen VD, Powell DL, Medsger TA Jr. Clinical correlations and prognosis based on serum autoantibodies in patients with systemic sclerosis. Arthritis Rheum. 1988; 31: 196–203.

121. Weiner ES, Earnshaw WC, Senecal JL, Bordwell B, Johnson P, Rothfield NF. Clinical associations of anticentromere antibodies and antibodies to topoisomerase I. Arthritis Rheum. 1988; 31: 378–385.

122. Kumar V, Kowalewski C, Koelle M, Qutaishat S, Chorzelski T, Beutner EH, Jarzabek-Chorzelska M, Kolacinska Z, Jablonska S. Scl-70 antigen stability and its effect on antibody detection in scleroderma. J Rheum. 1988; 15: 1499–1502.

123. Jarzabek-Chorzelska M, Blaszczyk M, Jablonska S, Chorzelski T, Kumar V, Beutner EH. Scl-70 antibody, a specific marker of systemic sclerosis. Brit J Derm. 1986; 115: 393–401.

124. Meesters TM, Hoet MH, Van Den Hoogen FHJ, Habets WJ, Van Venrooij WJ. Analysis of an immunodominant epitope of Topoisomerase I in patients with systemic sclerosis. Mol Biol Rep. 1992; 16: 117–123.

125. Pluta AF, Cooke CA, Earnshaw WC. Structure of the human centromere at metaphase. TIBS. 1990; 15: 181–185.

126. Earnshaw WC, Bordwell BJ, Marino C, Rothfield N. Three human chromosomal autoantigens are recognized by sera from patients with anti-centromere antibodies. J Clin Invest. 1986; 77: 426–430.

127. Reimer G. Autoantibodies against nuclear, nucleolar and mitochondrial antigens in systemic sclerosis (scleroderma). In: Rheumatic disease clinics of North America, Scleroderma. LeRoy EC, Guest Editor. Philadelphia: Saunders; 1990; 16: 169–182.

128. Verheijen R, De Jong BAW, Oberijé EHH, Van Venrooij WJ. Molecular cloning of a major CENP-B epitope and its use for the detection of anticentromere autoantibodies. Mol Biol Rep. 1992; 16: 49–59.

129. Lischwe MA, Ochs RL, Reddy R, Cook RG, Yeoman LC, Tan EM, Reichlin M, Busch H. Purification and partial characterization of a nucleolar scleroderma antigen ($M_r = 34,000$; pI, 8.5) rich in N^G N^G dimethylarginine. J Biol Chem. 1985; 260: 14304–14310.

130. Craft J, Gold H. New RNPs in higher eukaryotes. Mol Biol Rep. 1990; 14: 97–101.

131. Kipnis RJ, Craft J, Hardin J. The analysis of antinuclear and antinucleolar autoantibodies of scleroderma by radioimmunoprecipitation assays. Arthritis Rheum. 1990; 33: 1431–1437.

132. Reimer G, Steen VD, Penning CA, Medsger TA Jr, Tan EM. Correlates between autoantibodies to nucleolar antigens and clinical features in patients with systemic sclerosis (scleroderma). Arthritis Rheum. 1988; 31: 525–532.

133. Okano Y, Steen VD, Medsger TA Jr. Autoantibody to U3 nucleolar ribonucleoprotein (fibrillarin) in patients with systemic sclerosis. Arthritis Rheum. 1992; 35: 95–100.

134. Baserga SJ, Yang XDW, Steitz JA. An intact Box-C sequence in the U3 snRNA is required for binding of fibrillarin, the protein common to the major family of nucleolar snRNPs. EMBO J. 1991; 10: 2645–2651.

135. Parker KA, Steitz JA. Structural analyses of the human U3 ribonucleoprotein particle reveal a conserved sequence available for base pairing with pre-rRNA. Mol Cell Biol. 1987; 7: 2899–2913.

136. Kass S, Tyc K, Steitz JA, Sollner-Webb B. The U3 small nucleolar ribonucleoprotein functions in the first step of preribosomal RNA processing. Cell. 1990; 60: 897–908.

137. Reuter R, Tessars G, Vohr H, Gleichmann E, Lührmann R. Mercuric chloride induces

autoantibodies against U3 small nuclear ribonucleoprotein in susceptible mice. Proc Natl Acad Sci USA. 1989; 86: 237–241.

138. Hultman P, Eneström S, Pollard KM, Tan EM. Anti-fibrillarin autoantibodies in mercury-treated mice. Clin Exp Immunol. 1989; 78: 470–477.

139. Hashimoto C, Steitz JA. Sequential association of nucleolar 7-2 RNA with two different autoantigens. J Biol Chem. 1983; 258: 1379–1382.

140. Reddy R, Tan EM, Henning D, Nohga K, Busch H. Detection of a nucleolar 7-2 ribonucleoprotein and a cytoplasmic 8-2 ribonucleoprotein with autoantibodies from patients with scleroderma. J Biol Chem. 1983; 258: 1383–1387.

141. Gold HA, Craft J, Hardin JA, Bartkiewicz M, Altman S. Antibodies in human sera that precipitate ribonuclease P. Proc Natl Acad Sci USA. 1988; 85: 5483–5487.

142. Gold HA, Topper J, Clayton D, Craft J. The human RNA processing enzyme RNase MRP is identical to the Th ribonucleoprotein autoantigen and related to RNase P. Science. 1989; 245: 1377–1380.

143. Yuan Y, Tan E, Reddy R. The 40-kilodalton To autoantigen associates with nucleotides 21 to 64 of human mitochondrial RNA processing/7-2 RNA *in vitro*. Mol Cell Biol. 1991; 11: 5266–5274.

144. Chang DD, Clayton DA. Mouse RNase MRP RNA is encoded by a nuclear gene and contains a decamer sequence complementary to a conserved region of mitochondrial RNA substrate. Cell. 1989; 56: 131–139.

145. Altman S, Gold HA, Bartkiewicz M. Ribonuclease P as a snRNP. In: Structure and function of small ribonucleoproteins. Birnstiel M, ed. Berlin: Springer-Verlag; 1988; 183–195.

146. Okano Y, Medsger T. Autoantibody to Th ribonucleoprotein (nucleolar 7-2 RNA protein particle) in patients with systemic sclerosis. Arthritis Rheum. 1990; 33: 1822–1828.

147. Reimer G, Rose KM, Scheer U, Tan EM. Autoantibody to RNA polymerase I in scleroderma sera. J Clin Invest. 1987; 79: 65–72.

148. Reimer G, Scheer U, Peters JM, Tan EM. Immunolocalization and partial characterization of a nucleolar autoantigen (PM-Scl) associated with polymyositis/scleroderma overlap syndromes. J Immunol. 1986; 137: 3802–3808.

149. Gelpi C, Alguero A, Angeles Martinez M, Vidal S, Juarez C, Rodriguez-Sanchez JL. Identification of protein components reactive with anti-PM/Scl autoantibodies. Clin Exp Immunol. 1990; 81: 59–64.

150. Minota S, Jarjour WN, Suzuki N, Nojima Y, Roubey RAS, Mimura T, Yamada A, Hosoya T, Takaku F, Winfield JB. Autoantibodies to nucleolin in systemic lupus erythematosus and other diseases. J Immunol. 1991; 146: 2249–2252.

151. Borer RA, Lehner CF, Eppenberger HM, Nigg EA. Major nucleolar proteins shuttle between nucleus and cytoplasm. Cell. 1989; 56: 379–390.

152. Rodriguez JL, Gelpi C, Juarez C, Hardin JA. Anti-NOR-90: a new autoantibody in scleroderma that recognizes a 90-kDa component of the nucleolus-organizing region of chromatin. J Immunol. 1987; 139: 2579–2584.

153. Peek R, Pruijn GJM, Van Der Kemp AM, Van Venrooij WJ. Subcellular distribution of Ro RNPs and their constituents. J. Cell Sci. 1993; in press.

154. Pruijn GJM, Slobbe RL, Van Venrooij WJ. Structure and function of La and Ro RNPs. Mol Biol Rep. 1990; 14: 43–48.

155. Stephano JE. Purified lupus antigen La recognizes an oligouridylate stretch common to the 3′ termini of RNA polymerase III transcripts. Cell. 1984; 36: 145–154.

156. Chan EKL, Sullivan KF, Tan EM. Ribonucleoprotein SS-B/La belongs to a protein family with consensus sequences for RNA-binding. Nucleic Acids Res. 1989; 17: 2233–2244.

157. Gottlieb E, Steitz JA. The RNA binding protein La influences both the accuracy and the efficiency of RNA polymerase III transcription *in vivo*. EMBO J. 1989; 8: 841–850.

158. Gottlieb E, Steitz JA. Function of the mammalian La protein: evidence for its action in transcription termination by RNA polymerase III. EMBO J. 1989; 8: 851–861.

159. Bachmann M, Pfeifer K, Schröder HC, Müller WEG. Characterization of the autoantigen La as a nucleic acid-dependent ATPase/dATPase with melting properties. Cell. 1990; 60: 85–89.

160. Slobbe RL, Pruijn GJM, Van Venrooij WJ. Ro(SS-A) and La(SS-B) ribonucleoprotein complexes: structure, function and antigenicity. Ann Med Intern. 1991; 142: 592–600.

161. Slobbe RL, Van Esch B, Kveder T, Van Venrooij WJ. The use of adenovirus-infected cells for the detection of low titer autoantibodies. J Immunol Methods. 1991; 138: 237–244.
162. Hendrick JP, Wolin SL, Rinke J, Lerner MR, Steitz JA. Ro small cytoplasmic ribonucleoproteins are a subclass of La ribonucleoproteins: further characterization of the Ro and La small ribonucleoproteins from uninfected mammalian cells. Mol Cell Biol. 1981; 1: 1138–1150.
163. Rader MD, O'Brien C, Liu YS, Harley JB, Reichlin M. Heterogeneity of the Ro/SSA antigen. Different molecular forms in lymphocytes and red blood cells. J Clin Invest. 1989; 83: 1293–1298.
164. Pruijn GJM, Wingens P, Peters S, Thijssen J, Van Venrooij WJ. RoRNP associated Y-RNAs are highly conserved among mammals. Biochim Biophys Acta 1993; in press.
165. Itoh Y, Reichlin M. Ro/SS-A antigen in human platelets. Arthritis Rheum. 1991; 34: 888–893.
166. Ben-Chetrit E, Chan EKL, Sullivan KF, Tan EM. A 52-kDa protein is a novel component of the SS-A/Ro antigenic particle. J Exp Med. 1988; 167: 1560–1571.
167. Boire G, Craft J. Biochemical and immunological heterogeneity of the Ro ribonucleoprotein particles: analysis with sera specific for the Ro^{hY5} particle. J Clin Invest. 1989; 84: 270–278.
168. Boire G, Craft J. Human Ro ribonucleoprotein particles: Characterization of native structure and stable association with the La polypeptide. J Clin Invest. 1990; 85: 1182–1189.
169. Wolin SL, Steitz JA. Genes for two small cytoplasmic Ro RNAs are adjacent and appear to be single copy in the human genome. Cell. 1983; 32: 735–744.
170. Slobbe RL, Pluk W, Van Venrooij WJ, Pruijn GJM. Ro ribonucleoprotein assembly *in vitro*: Identification of RNA-protein and protein-protein interactions. J Mol Biol. 1992; 227: 361–366
171. Bozic B, Pruijn GJM, Rozman B, Van Venrooij WJ. Sera from patients with autoimmune diseases recognize different epitope regions on the 52 kDa Ro/SS-A protein. Clin Exp Immunol. 1993; in press.
172. Klug A, Rhodes D. 'Zinc fingers': a novel protein motif for nucleic acid recognition. TIBS. 1987; 12: 464–469.
173. Berg JM. Zinc fingers and other metal-binding domains. J Biol Chem. 1990; 265: 6513–6516.
174. Landschultz WH, Johnson PF, McKnight SL. The leucine zipper: a hypothetical structure common to a new class of DNA-binding proteins. Science. 1988; 240: 1759–1764.
175. Sassone-Corsi P, Ransone LJ, Lamph WW, Verma IM. Direct interaction between fof and jun nuclear oncoproteins: role of the 'leucine zipper' domain. Nature. 1988; 336: 692–695.
176. Kouzarides T, Ziff E. The role of the leucine zipper in the fos-jun interaction. Nature. 1988; 336: 646–651.
177. McCauliffe DP, Lux FA, Lieu TS, Sanz I, Hanke J, Newkirk MM, Bachinski LL, Itoh Y, Siciliano MJ, Reichlin M. Molecular cloning, expression, and chromosome 19 localization of a human Ro/SS-A autoantigen. J Clin Invest. 1990; 85: 1379–1391.
178. McCauliffe DP, Zappi E, Lieu T-S, Michalak M, Sontheimer RD, Capra JD. A human Ro/SS-A autoantigen is the homologue of calreticulin and is highly homologous with onchocercal RAL-1 antigen and an Aplysis 'memory molecule'. J Clin Invest. 1990; 86: 332–335.
179. Rokeach L, Haselby JA, Meilof JF, Smeenk RJT, Unnasch TR, Greene BM, Hoch SO. Characterization of the autoantigen calreticulin. J Immunol. 1991; 147: 3031–3039.
180. Pruijn GJM, Bozic B, Schoute F, Rokeach LA, Van Venrooij WJ. Refined definition of the 56 K and other autoantigens in the 50–60 kDa region. Mol Biol Rep. 1992; 16: 267–276.
181. Wasicek CA, Reichlin M. Clinical and serological differences between systemic lupus erythematosus patients with antibodies to Ro versus patients with antibodies to Ro and La. J Clin Invest. 1982; 69:835–843.
182. Wasicek CA, Reichlin M. Clinical and serological differences between systemic lupus erythematosus patients with antibodies to Ro versus patients with antibodies to Ro and La. J Clin Invest. 1982; 69: 835–843.

183. Bonfa E, Elkon K. Clinical and serologic associations of the anti-ribosomal P protein response. Arthritis Rheum. 1986; 29: 981–985.
184. Franceour A-M, Peebles CL, Heckman KJ, Lee JC, Tan EM. Identification of ribosomal protein autoantigens. J Immunol. 1985; 135: 2378–2384.
185. Elkon K, Skelly S, Parnassa A, Möller W, Danho W, Weissback H, Brot N. Identification and chemical synthesis of a ribosomal protein antigenic determinant in systemic lupus erythematosus. Proc Natl Acad Sci USA. 1986; 83: 7419–7423.
186. Bonfa E, Parnasa AP, Rhoades DD, Roufa DJ, Wool IG, Elkon KB. Anti-ribosomal S10 antibodies in humans and MRL/lpr mice with systemic lupus erythematosus. Arthritis Rheum. 1989; 32: 1252–1261.
187. Sato T, Uchiumi T, Ozawa T, Kikuchi M, Nakano M, Kominami R, Arakawa M. Autoantibodies against ribosomal proteins found with high frequency in patients with systemic lupus erythematosus with active disease. J Rheum. 1991; 18: 1681–1684.
188. Targoff IN. Autoantibodies to aminoacyl-transfer RNA synthetases for isoleucine and glycine. J Immunol. 1990; 144: 1737–1743.
189. Nishikai M, Reichlin M. Heterogeneity of precipitating antibodies in polymyositis and dermatomyositis. Characterization of the Jo-1 antibody system. Arthritis Rheum. 1980; 23: 881–888.
190. Reichlin M, Arnett FC. Multiplicity of antibodies in myositis sera. Arthritis Rheum. 1984; 27: 1150–1156.
191. Targoff IN, Reichlin M. Measurement of antibody to Jo-1 by ELISA and comparison to enzyme inhibitory activity. J Immunol. 1987; 138: 2874–2882.
192. Arnett FC, Hirsch TJ, Bias WB, Nishikai M, Reichlin M. The Jo-1 antibody system in myositis: relationships to clinical features and HLA. J Rheum. 1981; 8: 295–939.
193. Targoff IN, Arnett FC. Clinical manifestations in patients with antibody to PL-12 antigen (alanyl-tRNA synthetase). Am J Med. 1990; 88: 241–251.
194. Mathews MB, Reichlin M, Hughes GRV, Bernstein RM. Anti-threonyl-tRNA synthetase, a second myositis related autoantibody. J Exp Med. 1984; 160: 420–434.
195. Okada N, Mukai R, Harada F, Kabashima T, Nakao Y, Yamane K, Ohshima Y, Sakamoto K, Kashiwagi H, Hamaguchi H. Isolation of a novel antibody which precipitates ribonucleoprotein complex containing threonine tRNA from a patient with polymyositis. Eur J Biochem. 1984; 139: 425–429.
196. Targoff IN, Arnett FC, Reichlin M. Antibody to threonyl-transfer RNA synthetase in myositis sera. Arthritis Rheum. 1988; 31: 515–524.
197. Miller FW, Waite KA, Biswas T, Plotz P. The role of an autoantigen, histidyl-tRNA synthetase, in the induction and maintenance of autoimmunity. Proc Acad Natl Sci USA. 1990; 87: 9933–9937.
198. Miller FW, Twitty SA, Biswas T, Plotz P. Origin and regulation of a disease-specific autoantibody response. J Clin Invest. 1990; 85: 468–475.
199. Chu J-L, Elkon KB. The small nuclear ribonucleoproteins SmB and B' are products of a single gene. Gene. 1991; 97: 311–312.
200. Reddy R, Busch H. Small nuclear RNAs: RNA sequences, structure and modifications. In: Structure and Function of Major and Minor Small Nuclear Ribonucleoprotein Particles. Birnstiel ML. ed. Heidelberg: Springer Verlag; 1988: 1–38.
201. Query CC, Bentley RC, Keene JD. A common RNA recognition motif identified within a defined U1 RNA binding domain of the 70K U1 snRNP protein. Cell. 1989; 57: 89–101.
202. Scherly D, Boelens W, Dathan NA, Van Venrooij WJ, Mattaj IW. Major determinants of the specificity of interaction between small nuclear ribonucleoproteins U1A and U2B″ and their cognate RNAs. Nature. 1990; 345: 502–506.
203. Nelissen RLH, Henrichs V, Habets WJ, Simons F, Lührmann R, Van Venrooij WJ. Zinc finger-like structure in U1-specific protein C is essential for specific binding to U1 snRNP. Nucleic Acids Res. 1991; 19: 449–454.
204. Bandziulis RJ, Swanson MS, Dreyfuss G. RNA-binding proteins as developmental regulators. Genes Develop. 1989; 3: 431–437.
205. Schlesinger MJ. Heat shock proteins. J Biol Chem. 1990; 265: 12111–12114.
206. Ellis RJ, Van Der Vies SM. Molecular chaperones. Ann Rev Biochem. 1991; 60: 321–347.
207. Pelham H. Heat shock proteins; coming in from the cold. Nature. 1987; 332: 776–777.
208. Hemmingsen SM, Woolford C, Van Der Vies SM, Tilly K, Dennis DT, Georgopoulos

CP, Hendrix RW, Ellis RJ. Homologous plant and bacterial proteins chaperone oligomeric protein assembly. Nature. 1988; 333: 330–334.

209. Schlesinger M, Hershko A. The ubiquitin system. Current Communications in Molecular Biology. Cold Spring Harbor Laboratory Press; 1988.

210. Winfield JB. Stress proteins, arthritis and autoimmunity. Arthritis Rheum. 1989; 32: 1497–1504.

211. Winfield J, Jarjour W. Do stress proteins play a role in arthritis and autoimmunity? Immunol Rev. 1991; 121: 193–220.

212. Kaufmann SHE. Heat shock proteins in health and disease. Int J Clin Lab Res. 1992; 22: 221–226.

213. Bahr GM, Rook GAW, Al-Saffar J. Clin Exp Immunol. 1988; 74: 211–215.

214. Tsoulfa G, Rook GA, Van Embden JD, Young DB, Mehlert A, Isenberg DA, Hay FC, Lydyard PM. Raised serum IgG and IgA antibodies to mycobacterial antigens in rheumatoid arthritis. Ann Rheum Dis. 1988; 48: 118–123.

215. Muller S, Briand JP, Van Regenmortel MH. Presence of antibodies to ubiquitin during the autoimmune response associated with systemic lupus erythematosus. Proc Natl Acad Sci USA. 1988; 8176–8180.

216. Minota S, Cameron B, Welch WJ, Winfield JB. Autoantibodies to the constitutive 73 kDa member of the hsp70 family of heat shock proteins in systemic lupus erythematosus. J Exp Med. 1988; 168: 1475–1480.

217. Minota S, Koyasu S, Yahara I, Winfield JB. Autoantibodies to the heat shock protein hsp90 in systemic lupus erythematosus. J Clin Invest. 1988; 81: 106–109.

218. Boog CJP, De Graeff-Meeder ER, Lucassen MA, Van Der Zee R, Voorhorst-Ogink MM, Van Kooten PJS, Geuze HJ, Van Eden W. Two monoclonal antibodies generated against human hsp60 show reactivity with synovial membranes of patients with juvenile chronic arthritis. J Exp Med. 1992; 175: 1805–1810.

219. Kaufmann SHE. Heat shock proteins and the immune response. Immunol Today. 1990; 11: 129–136.

220. Bluthner M, Bautz FA. Cloning and characterization of the cDNA coding for a polymyositis-scleroderma overlap syndrome-related nucleolar 100-kD protein. J Exp Med. 1992; 176: 973–980.

221. Jantzen HM, Admon A, Bell SP, Tjian R. Nucleolar transcription factor hUBF contains a DNA-binding motif with homology to HMG proteins. Nature. 1990; 344: 830–836.

222. Saitoh H, Tomkiel J, Cooke CA, Rothfield NF, Earnshaw WC. CENP-C, an autoantigen in scleroderma is a component of the human inner kinetochore plate. Cell. 1992; 70: 115–124.

16
Sjögren's Syndrome: From Polyclonal B Cell Activation to Monoclonal B Cell Proliferation

A. G. TZIOUFAS, N. TALAL and H. M. MOUTSOPOULOS

INTRODUCTION

Sjögren's syndrome (SS) is a chronic autoimmune disease of unknown aetiology, characterized by lymphocyte infiltration of exocrine glands resulting in xerostomia (XS) and keratoconjunctivitis sicca (KCS). SS is particularly interesting among the autoimmune diseases for two reasons. First, it has a broad clinical spectrum extending from autoimmune exocrinopathy to extraglandular (systemic) disease affecting the lungs, kidneys, blood vessels and muscles; it may be found alone (primary SS, pSS) or in association with other autoimmune diseases (secondary SS). Finally, it is a disorder in which a benign autoimmune process can terminate in a lymphoid malignancy[1].

In fact, the relationship between SS and lymphoma has been known since 1964[2]. Kassan et al.[3] subsequently showed that patients with SS have a 44 times greater relative risk of developing lymphoma than age-, sex- and race-matched control populations. SS, a chronic, slowly progressive autoimmune disease, is characterized by immune system hyperreactivity, as illustrated by hypergammaglobulinaemia, multiple organ and non-organ specific autoantibodies and focal lymphocytic infiltrations of the exocrine glands[1]. Hence, SS is at the crossroads of autoimmune diseases and lymphoid malignancy. Although monoclonal gammopathy and lymphoma have been described in other autoimmune diseases[4], SS remains a powerful model for potential insights into the pathogenetic mechanisms leading from immune dysregulation (as observed in autoimmune diseases) to monoclonal B cell expansion.

In this chapter, the immunological abnormalities and the monoclonality which are observed in SS are described and the pathogenetic mechanisms are discussed.

Table 1 Autoantibodies in Sjögren's syndrome

Organ specific	Percent	Non-organ specific	Percent
Anti-thyroid antibodies	50	Rheumatoid factor	80
Antibodies to gastric mucosa	5–15	Antinuclear antibodies	80
		Antibodies to Ro/SSA	60
		Antibodies to La/SSB	50
		Anti-mitochondrial antibodies	10

IMMUNOLOGICAL ABNORMALITIES OF SJÖGREN'S SYNDROME

Sera of patients with SS are usually hypergammaglobulinaemic, containing numerous autoantibodies directed against organ and non-organ specific autoantigens (Table 1). The most common autoantibodies to cellular antigens recognize the ribonucleoproteins Ro/SSA and La/SSB which are composed of proteins (60 kD and 52 kD for Ro/SSA and 47 kD for La/SSB) in conjunction with cytoplasmic (hy) RNAs[5]. These autoantibodies are not specific for SS and may be found in other autoimmune diseases, especially systemic lupus erythematosus (SLE)[6]. Although sera of patients with SS contain high amounts of autoantibodies, peripheral blood B lymphocytes of SS patients are not overtly activated. In fact, peripheral B lymphocytes from patients with SS, unlike those from patients with SLE, do not spontaneously secrete increased amounts of immunoglobulins[7]. Thus, while the activated B cells in patients with SLE are widely distributed, in patients with SS these cells are probably localized to the infiltrated tissues, such as the affected salivary glands. In this regard, it has been previously demonstrated that the B cells infiltrating the minor salivary glands of SS patients synthesize large amounts of immunoglobulins with rheumatoid factor activity[8]. Thus, it appears that the exocrine glandular tissues of SS patients are a major site of B lymphocyte activation.

Histopathological studies of exocrine glands from patients with primary SS revealed that infiltration of the glands is gradual and that the infiltrates contain very few monocytes[9-11]. Most of the infiltrating cells are T-cells (Figure 1A), while B cells are found in approximately 20% of the total cell number[12]. Natural killer cells are very rarely observed. The majority of T-cells belong to the CD4+ helper-inducer phenotype, while the remainder express the CD8 phenotype[12,13]. Most of these T cells are activated, since they express DR antigens on their surface. These T cells secrete large quantities of interleukin-2 (IL-2)[14] and γ-interferon[13]. The activated CD4+ T cell population in the infiltrate consists of about two-thirds memory cells (4B4+) and one-third naive or suppressor-inducer cells (2H4+)[15] (Figure 1B). The former are thought to be the actual helper-inducer cells for the growth and differentiation of B lymphocytes into antibody secreting cells. As mentioned previously, the B lymphocytes in the exocrine gland infiltrates of patients with primary SS secrete large amounts of immunoglobulins, rheumatoid factors, and various antibodies, such as anti-Ro and anti-La[16]. These factors indicate an *in situ* immune response with a significant autoantigen specific component. The lack of monocytes, the classical antigen presenting cells, in the lesion makes this proposition problematic. On the other hand, the epithelial cells in the infiltrated exocrine glands show hyperexpression of HLA-A, B and C antigens, as well as *de novo* inappropriate expression of HLA-DR antigens on their surface. Since γ-interferon has been shown to induce expression of both histocompatibility antigen classes on the surface of epithelial and other cells, one is faced with the chicken-and-egg problem; that is, whether the DR expression and possible antigen presentation by epithelial cells predates or is a consequence of the lymphocytic infiltration. In addition, acinar epithelial cells express the protooncogene c-*myc*[17] (Figure 1C) while translocation and membrane localization of the nuclear antigen La/SSB has been observed in conjunctival epithelial cells of SS patients[18]. Furthermore, the infiltrating lymphocytes express lymphocytic function associated antigen-1 (LFA-1) on their surface. This antigen, which is found on activated lymphocytes, binds to the intracellular adhesion molecule (ICAM-1) found on the surface of epithelial and endothelial cells. This adhesion molecule, which is also found on T lymphocytes, is the ligand for LFA-3. The latter belongs to a group of proteins known as integrins, which play a significant role in cell-to-cell contact[19,20]. The molecules LFA-3 and ICAM-1 have been found on epithelial cells of the infiltrated exocrine glands in primary SS adjacent to the sites of intense infiltration[21]. These changes of epithelial cells in SS suggest an *in situ* immune response with the epithelial cell playing the role of an antigen presenting cell. As a consequence, T-cells are attracted, become activated and secrete various cytokines, which activate B lymphocytes to secrete antibodies (Table 2).

MONOCLONAL EXPANSION OF B LYMPHOCYTES

Knowing that SS patients can develop B cell lymphomas prompted a study of the serum and urine of SS patients. It was shown that patients with extraglandular manifestations very often present monoclonal immunoglobulins and/or light chains in their serum and urine[22,23]. In the case of lymphoma development, the level of urinary free light chains may correlate with disease activity[24]. Furthermore, one-third of patients with primary SS have cryoglobulins in their serum. These are mixed cryoglobulins containing an IgMκ monoclonal rheumatoid factor (RF). Interestingly, the presence of the cryoglobulins was associated with a higher prevalence of extraglandular disease and autoantibodies to Ro/SSA and RF, as compared to patients without cryoglobulins[25]. These findings suggest that patients with SS express monoclonal immunoglobulins in the circulation along with polyclonal B cell activation very early in the disease course. Monoclonality is observed more often in SS patients with systemic extraglandular disease. The latter is of particular interest, since SS patients with extraglandular manifestations are at higher risk of developing malignancy[3]. In fact, a long-term follow up of SS patients with type II cryoglobulinaemia showed that these patients are more likely to develop lymphoma (unpublished data).

The observation that the activated B lymphocyte is located mainly in the

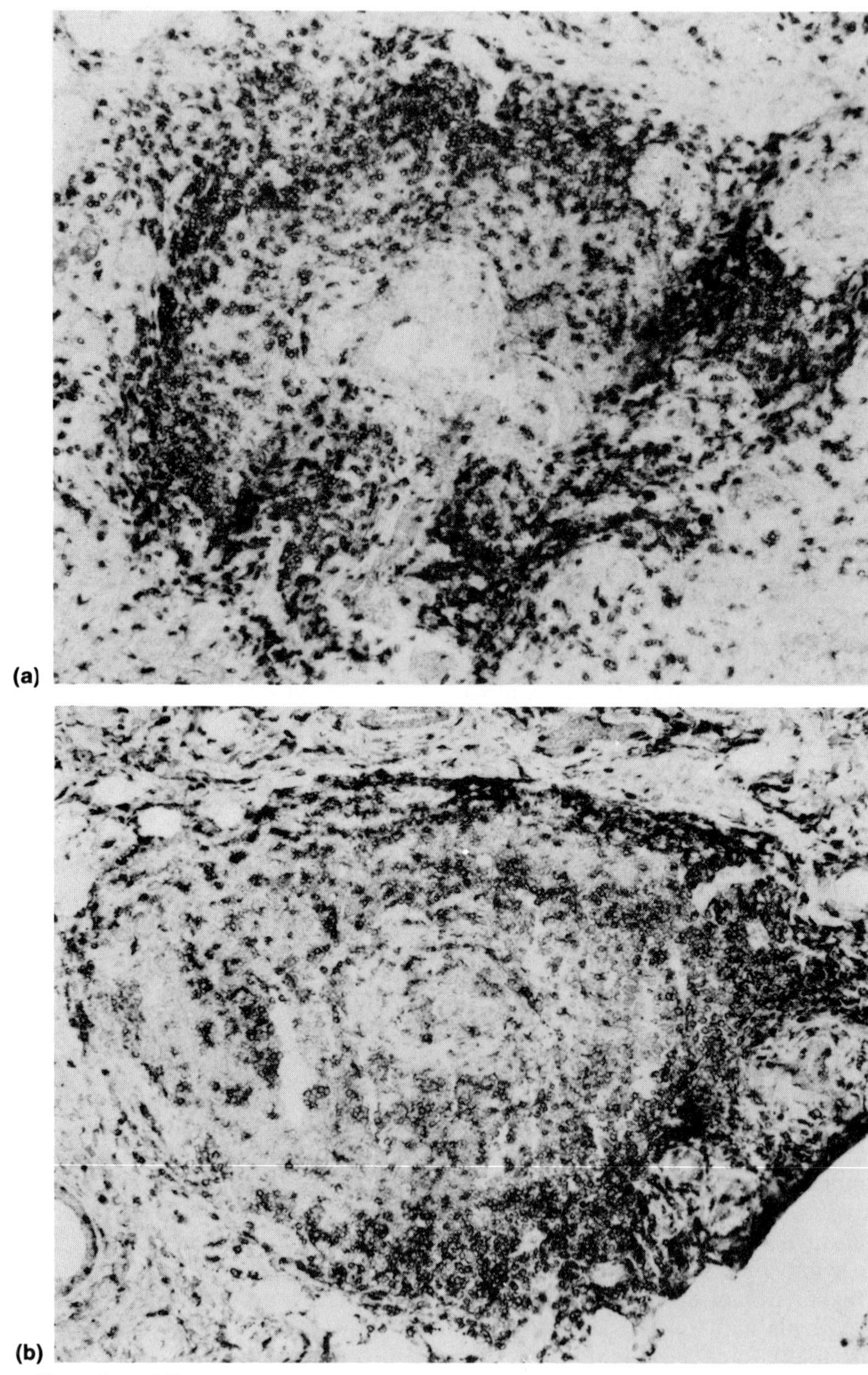

Figure 1a and 1b

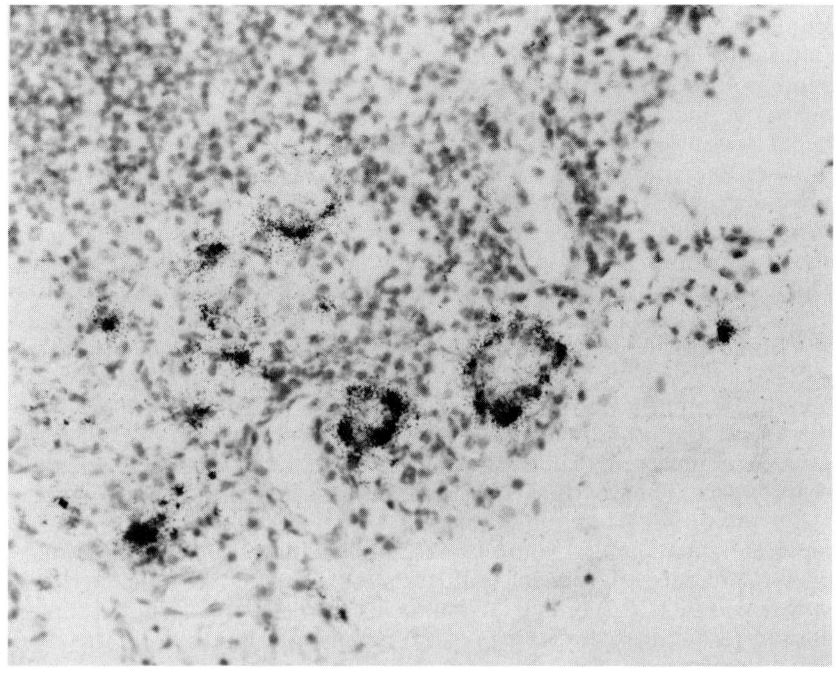

(c)

Figure 1 Labial minor salivary gland biopsy from a patient with primary Sjögren's syndrome.
A. Immunostained with anti-CD3 monoclonal antibody (Leu4) recognizing all T-cells.
B. Immunostained with anti-CD45RO (UCHL-1) recognizing memory T-cells.
C. *In situ* hybridization with an oligonucleotide probe from the 3rd exon of the c-*myc* gene. Pictures A and B are serial sections of the same sample. The majority of cells infiltrating the tissue are memory T cells. The c-*myc* expression is restricted to the epithelial acinar cells (Courtesy of Dr F. N. Skopouli)

Table 2 Immunological abnormalities in Sjögren's syndrome

Peripheral blood	*Infiltrated exocrine glands*
Autoantibodies	Infiltration by T and B lymphocytes
Immune complexes	T-cells are activated
Normal B- and T-cell count	HLA-DR expression
B-cells not activated	IL-2 expression
	γ-interferon production
	LFA-1, ICAM expression
	B-cells are activated
	production of immunoglobulins
	Epithelial cell
	Inappropriate HLA-DR expression
	c-*myc* protooncogene expression
	La(SSB) and heat shock protein membrane expression

salivary glands, in association with other factors which may promote neoplasia in the salivary gland lesion (e.g. the absence of NK cells), prompted studies for the detection of monoclonal B cell subsets in the minor salivary gland infiltrates of SS patients responsible for the production of monoclonal immunoglobulins. In 1982, Schmid et al. suggested that the benign lymphoepithelial lesion of SS salivary glands with areas of confluent lymphoid proliferation contains plasma cells with cytoplasmic monoclonal IgMκ immunoglobulins and represent an *in situ* malignant lymphoma (in fact, these were all immunocytomas)[26]. The above immunological study is consistent with the findings of Fishleder et al. in 1987[27] who, using restriction fragment length polymorphism (RFLP), found clonal immunoglobulin rearrangements in all the salivary gland specimens that contained lymphoepithelial lesions. Furthermore, Freimark and co-workers in 1989 showed that 5 of 9 SS patients with circulating monoclonal immunoglobulins had oligoclonal immunoglobulin gene rearrangements in their salivary gland lymphocytes (the κ gene in four patients and λ gene in one). Two additional SS patients revealed oligoclonal rearrangements of the β chain of the T-cell antigen receptor gene. Three of these SS patients developed non-Hodgkin's lymphoma 2 to 8 years after the initial biopsy[28].

We evaluated paraffin embedded sections of minor salivary gland biopsies for the presence of monoclonal B cell subsets[29]. Using the peroxidase-antiperoxidase (PAP) bridge technique for the detection of intracytoplasmic immunoglobulins in the salivary gland lymphocyte infiltrates, it was demonstrated that seven of 12 SS patients with circulating IgMκ monoclonal cryoglobulins also had in their minor salivary glands a ratio of κ light chain positive plasma cells to λ light chain positive plasma cells greater than 3. The above immunohistological picture is consistent with a monoclonal plasma cell subpopulation. Two of these patients had immunocytomas in the minor salivary glands (Figure 2). In contrast, none of the SS patients without cryoglobulins or with polyclonal cryoglobulins (type III) had a ratio of κ:λ positive plasma cells greater than 3, suggesting a polyclonal plasma cell pattern in the minor salivary glands (Table 3). The above data lead to the speculation that the salivary glands in SS patients may serve as the initial site of B cell neoplastic transformation. However, B cells from other organs, such as the peripheral blood and bone marrow, must be carefully evaluated for the presence of transformed B cells.

In order to delineate the origin and the mechanisms of monoclonal rheumatoid factor production, several studies concentrated on the idiotypes of rheumatoid factors. Monoclonal RFs have been shown to share cross-reactive idiotypes extensively. Monoclonal RF from Waldenstrom's patients have been categorized into three groups, the groups Wa and Po to which 60% and 20% of monoclonal RFS belong respectively, and the minor subgroup Bla which is characterized by multispecificity[30,31]. The light chains of the monoclonal RF which reacted with the anti-Wa antibodies were further shown to belong to the VKIIIb subgroup[32]. Subsequently, Carson and Fong showed that 50% of monoclonal RFs reacted with the 17.109 monoclonal antibody. The 17.109 idiotypes were shown to react with 25% of κ bearing CD5+ B cells of chronic lymphocytic leukaemia and to be

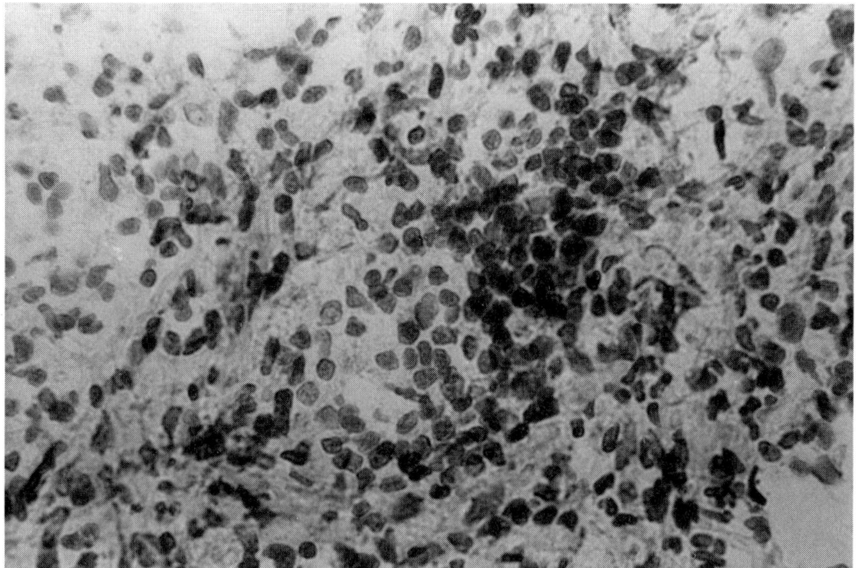

Figure 2 A minor salivary gland biopsy stained with goat anti-human κ light chains, using the avidin-biotin-peroxidase method, showed heavy infiltration by B lymphocytes containing exclusively κ light chains

associated with the expression of the Humkv 325 germ line gene[33,34].

Cross-reactive idiotypes are also shared by SS and rheumatoid arthritis[35,36], while others such as 17.109 are found only in RFs from SS patients[37]. Fox et al. reported that 12 of 15 monoclonal RFs from patients with SS reacted with the 17.109 antiidiotype. B cells containing immunoglobulins reactive with the 17.109 monoclonal antibody were detected in the salivary gland biopsies in 11 of 12 SS patients at high frequencies. Interestingly, in one patient with pre-existing SS who developed non-Hodgkin's lymphoma, the malignant cell producing the RF paraprotein reacted with anti-17.109 monoclonal antibody[37]. Further analysis of the 17.109 bearing idiotype B cells in the salivary gland of SS patients revealed a multiclonal origin in which somatic mutations accumulated in a non-random fashion, strongly suggesting an antigenic and T-cell driven process in the expansion of these cells[38].

Recently, we developed a polyclonal antiidiotype raised against a monoclonal IgMκ RF from the cryoglobulin of a patient with SS. Utilizing the F(ab)$_2$ fragment of this polyclonal antiidiotype, we investigated with a highly specific ELISA the serum of 32 patients with SS, 33 patients with rheumatoid arthritis, 30 patients with SLE, 6 patients with Waldenstrom's macroglobulinaemia and 20 normal individuals. The cross-reactive idiotype detected by the rabbit polyclonal antiidiotypic antibody was found in 20 patients with SS (62.5%) and in nine patients with rheumatoid arthritis (27%). Two patients with Waldenstrom's macroglobulinaemia were also found positive for the idiotype. The idiotype levels were significantly higher in SS patients

Table 3 Incidence and type of monoclonicity in sera and minor salivary gland biopsies of SS patients

Patients	Age (years) $(x \pm SD)$	Disease duration (years) $(x \pm SD)$	Cryoglobulinaemia (total protein; mg/dl) $(x \pm SD)$	Minor salivary gland biopsy (κ:λ infiltrating B cells ratio >3) (Percent)
SS with IgMκ mixed monoclonal cryoglobulins (Type II) ($n = 11$)	55 ± 12	11 ± 6	160 ± 130	55
SS without cryoglobulinaemia ($n = 7$)	58 ± 16	6 ± 4	—	0
Secondary SS (associated with rheumatoid arthritis) with polyclonal cryoglobulins (Type III) ($n = 4$)	60 ± 32	14 ± 8	100 ± 65	0

Table 4 Clinical spectrum of Sjögren's syndrome

Organ specific	Systemic	Lymphoma
Exocrine glands	Musculoskeletal	Exocrine glands
lacrymal	Lungs	Lymphoid tissue
salivary	Kidneys	Extra-lymphoidal
	Vessels	
	Lymph nodes (pseudolymphoma)	
	SEROLOGICAL	
	B-cell hyperreactivity	
Polyclonal	Polyclonal	Monoclonal
	Oligoclonal	
	Monoclonal	
Benign		Malignant

with monoclonal expansion of the B-cells in the minor salivary gland infiltrates and in patients with monoclonal type II cryoglobulinaemia[39]. Family studies of 17.109 and polyclonal rabbit antiidiotype showed that the idiotypes are not inherited, but they may be present on immunoglobulins of first degree family members of SS probands who also present autoimmune serological abnormalities, such as antinuclear antibodies or rheumatoid factor[40]. The findings imply that immunoglobulins bearing the cross-reactive idiotypes in SS are probably acquired during the disease process as a result of environmental factors, and that their presence is associated with autoimmune serological abnormalities.

CLINICAL PICTURE

Lymphoproliferation in SS follows a multistep process (Table 4). The local exocrine gland lesions produce sicca manifestations, such as xerostomia, keratoconjunctivitis sicca, xerorhinia, dyspareunia and dry skin. As the disease evolves, an aggressive polyclonal B cell activation often accompanied with lymphocytic infiltration of other organs is observed. In many instances, monoclonal immunoglobulins can be seen in sera of these patients. At this stage, patients present with extraglandular manifestations (Table 5) which are attributed to two main pathophysiological mechanisms. First, an extension of lymphocytic infiltration to several parenchymal organs results in their functional impairment and, second, in immune complex mediated injury. Extraglandular features usually observed are skin vasculitis, lung involvement, kidney involvement, hepatic involvement, Raynaud's phenomenon, and non-erosive arthritis. It should be noted, however, that Raynaud's phenomenon is an extraglandular feature which may be present even before the sicca manifestations[41].

Some of the patients develop a clinical picture suggestive of malignancy, which, however, cannot be classified as malignant, even using modern molecular pathology techniques, such as immunophenotyping and immuno-

Table 5 Incidence of extraglandular manifestations in primary Sjögren's syndrome

Clinical manifestations	Percent
Arthralgias/arthritis	50–60
Raynaud's phenomenon	30–40
Lymphadenopathy	10–15
Vasculitis	5–12
Lung involvement	15–25
Kidney involvement	10–20
Liver involvement	5–10
Splenomegaly	5–10
Peripheral neuropathy	5–10
Myositis	1–5
Lymphoma	5–8

genotyping[42]. The term 'pseudolymphoma' has been applied to such cases[43]. The course of these patients is variable. Some of them respond to corticosteroid and immunosuppressive drug therapy, while some later develop a frank malignant lymphoma. The autoimmune disorder may precede the development of lymphoma by up to 20 years[44]. Certain extraglandular manifestations, such as splenomegaly and lymphadenopathy, as well as parotid swelling are more often observed in patients predisposed to lymphoma. Lymphomas may affect salivary glands or major parenchymal organs, such as the lungs, the kidneys or the gastrointestinal tract (Figure 3). Lymphomas may differ by location and grading. In our patient population, among eight lymphomas of SS patients, six were low grade immunocytomas and two intermediate grade non-Hodgkin's lymphomas[44]. Five of the immunocytomas affected the minor salivary or lacrimal glands. Two of patients with immunocytomas showed spontaneous regression, while two others (one with immunocytoma and one with an intermediate grade) developed a high grade lymphoma after 3 and 5 years respectively. Therefore, the clinical picture of SS lymphoma appears to be diverse, suggesting that the therapeutic approach should be guided according to the stage and the grade of the disease.

PATHOGENETIC ASPECTS

Experimental models

Monoclonal expansion of B lymphocytes has been observed in ageing animals (C57BL/KaL WRij mice)[45]. Long-term antigenic stimulation by multiple antigens (pneumococcal polysaccharide, ovalbumin) also resulted in the development of monoclonal gammopathy in high frequencies[46].

The monoclonal B cell proliferation of SS has been studied in Scid mice. The CB17 Scid/Scid mice are born with severe combined immunodeficiency and lack mature T and B lymphocytes. Injection of peripheral blood mononuclear cells from anti-La/SSB positive SS patients into these mice

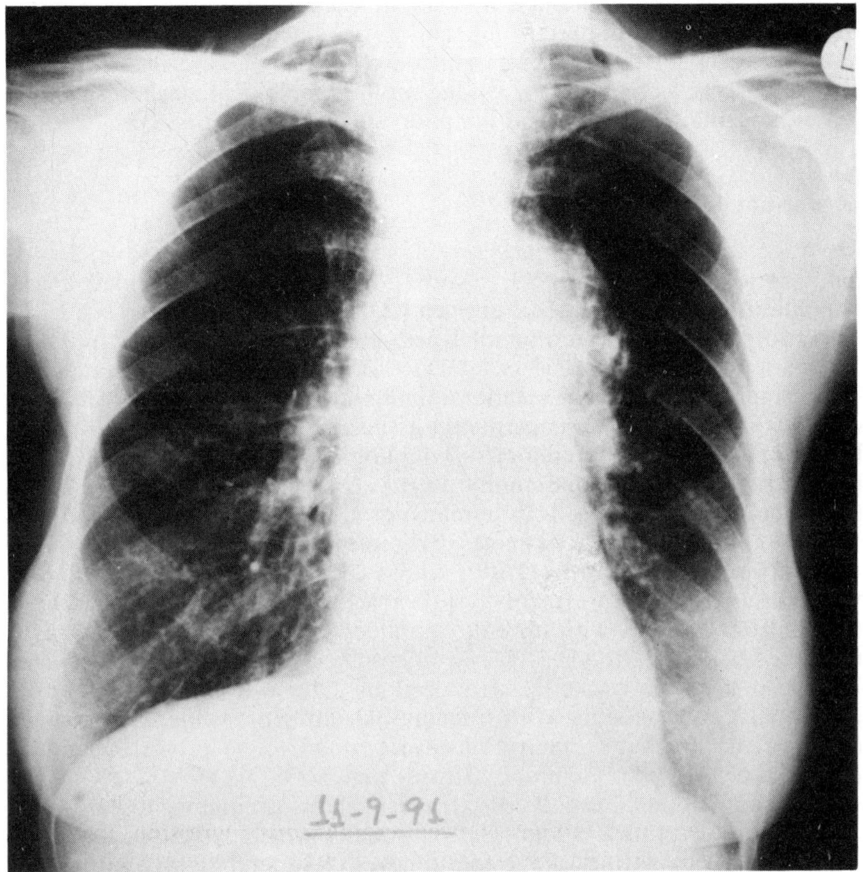

Figure 3 Chest roentgenogram of a patient with Sjögren's syndrome and lymphoma shows a lymph node block in the left hilar and right paratracheal regions

resulted in the development of lymphoid infiltrates in several tissues consistent with disseminated lymphoid neoplasia[47]. DNA from these infiltrates tested by polymerase chain reaction contained both A and B Epstein-Barr virus (EBV) strains, suggesting that the cells were of human origin. In another study, salivary gland biopsies were implanted under the kidney capsule of Scid mice[48]. These biopsies maintained their histological features, including lymphoid infiltrates and HLA-DR expression in epithelial cells, for at least 4 weeks. The proportion of human CD4+ T-cells gradually decreased, while the number of CD19+ B cells increased. Human immunoglobulins were detected after 3 weeks in these Scid/SS chimeric mice and their levels increased until the animals died with lymphoid tumours at 6–12 weeks. These tumours, of human B cell origin, histologically resembled non-Hodgkin lymphoma, expressed oligoclonal immunoglobulin gene arrangements, transcribed high levels of cytokines IL-6 and IL-10 (which are not found in normal B cells) and contained EBV DNA encoded antigens. These results suggest that in an immunoincompetent environment, B cells of SS patients have the tendency to proliferate and develop malignancy. Therefore, Scid mice may serve as a model for studies on immunological mechanisms for B cell monoclonal expansion and lymphoma development in SS.

Lymphocyte studies

In order to address the question of which cell is responsible for the monoclonal expansion in SS, research has focused on a small B cell population bearing the surface antigen CD5. The CD5 molecule is a 67 kD glycoprotein which is found on all T-cells and in a small percentage (3%) of B cells in normal individuals[49,50]. CD5+ B cells have been associated with both lymphoid malignancies and autoimmunity. While these cells were first described and since then consistently associated with chronic lymphocytic leukaemia and small lymphocytic lymphoma[51,52], they may also play a pathogenetic role in autoimmunity. Ly-1+ B cells in NZB mice (the mouse equivalent to CD5+ B cells in humans) produce anti-erythrocyte and anti-ssDNA antibodies[53]. In humans EBV infected CD5+ B cells produce RF and anti-ssDNA antibodies[54], whilst CD5+ B cells stimulated with *Staphylococcus aureus* are mainly responsible for IgM RF production. CD5+ B cells from patients with chronic lymphocytic leukemia produce *in vitro* multispecific autoantibodies[55,56]. Multispecific low affinity autoantibodies have also been shown to be produced by CD5+ B cells from normal individuals and patients with rheumatoid arthritis while, interestingly, monospecific and high affinity RFs were found to be produced only by CD5+ B cells from rheumatoid arthritis patients[57].

Peripheral blood CD5+ B cells are elevated in autoimmune diseases, such as rheumatoid arthritis[58] and SS[59,60], diseases which are characterized by high levels of circulating RFs. Interestingly, in SS there are high numbers of CD5+ B cells in salivary gland infiltrates, a site considered a candidate for the initiation of lymphoproliferative and B cell malignancies in SS. SS patients with monoclonal gammopathy also have increased levels of circulating CD5+ B cells, showing a possible association of these cells with the monoclonal process in SS[59]. The above observations, as well as the findings that B lymphomas in mice are Ly-1+[61,62] and that the malignant clone in chronic lymphocytic leukaemia and different lymphomas in humans is of CD5+ B cell origin[51,52], suggest that a small CD5+ B cell subpopulation may be expanded under selective pressure through an antigenic or T cell driven process and is responsible for the monoclonal expansion observed in SS.

Cytokine studies

Several cytokines play an important role in B cell differentiation. In fact, resting B cells enter into DNA synthesis using IL-4[63], proliferate with IL-5[64] and differentiate into plasma cells via IL-6[65]. Recent experimental evidence suggests that patients with multiple myeloma have circulating mononuclear cells which can be considered as malignant cell precursors since their growth and terminal differentiation to malignant plasma cells are governed by the synergistic action of IL-3 and IL-6[66]. Transgenic mice carrying the human IL-6 gene in association with an immunoglobulin enhancer developed polyclonal plasma cells[67]. Therefore, it appears that the constitutive expression of IL-6 induces a polyclonal plasma cell proliferation and that a second event, such as a viral infection or an altered oncogene expression or even the synergistic action of another cytokine, may transform the cells into a monoclonal population. Assessment of serum IL-6 levels in SS patients did not reveal important differences between patients who developed lymphoma and those who did not[68]. A role for other cytokines in SS, such as IL-3, IL-4 and IL-5, has not yet been determined. Since the affected salivary glands of SS patients are considered the major site of B cell proliferation, the measurement of cytokines in salivary gland biopsies using molecular biology techniques, such as mRNA expression or *in situ* hybridization, should provide useful new information.

Molecular cytogenetic studies

Several cytogenetic and molecular alterations can be seen in patients with monoclonal gammopathies. These include chromosomal abnormalities such as hyperdiploidy[69] and translocations[70]. The B cell monoclonal process may be associated with altered protooncogene expression. In lymphomas, chromosomal transformations involving the juxtaposition of growth related protooncogenes c-*myc* and bcl-1 to the immunoglobulin heavy chain gene locus 14q32 result in the transcriptional deregulation of these genes and the subsequent neoplastic transformation of B lymphocytes[71]. Furthermore, retroviral vector used to introduce H- or N-*ras* oncogenes into human B lymphoblasts, which were previously immortalized by EBV, led to malignant transformation of these cells as indicated by clonogenicity and tumorogenicity in immunodeficient mice[72].

Although patients with SS may have increased c-*myc* protooncogene expression in both peripheral lymphocytes and salivary glands, there is no evidence that this is associated with the development of lymphoid malignancy since: a) there was no correlation between c-*myc* expression and monoclonal gammopathy[17] and b) analysis of SS lymphomas with Southern blot revealed no translocations of c-*myc*[73]. In contrast, Fox et al., using both Southern blot and the polymerase chain reaction, demonstrated that 50% of SS lymphomas present with translocation of the protooncogene bcl-2t (14;18)[73]. This translocation was not detected in SS patients without lymphoma and those with pseudolymphoma. The authors postulate that lymphoma arising in SS develops as a multistep process where prolonged B cell stimulation leads to karyotypic error associated with neoplastic transformation.

Viral studies

EBV is a ubiquitous human herpes virus which remains latent in the stomatopharyngeal cavity in immunologically intact humans[74]. EBV is the aetiologic agent for Burkitt's lymphoma[75], a B cell neoplasm. This virus may play a role in SS, since antibodies to the EBV capsid antigen are more frequently found in SS patients[76] and EBV is a potent polyclonal activator of B cells which can induce autoantibodies *in vitro*[77]. One of them, the anti-La/SSB antibody found in sera of SS patients, precipitates a cytoplasmic protein complexed with EBV encoded small RNAs termed EBER 1 and EBER 2[78]. Recently, EBV DNA has been detected in the salivary gland biopsies of 50% of SS patients by *in situ* hybridization and polymerase chain reaction[79]. Although the role of EBV in activating B lymphocytes is well known and the presence of EBV in SS patients well established, at present one cannot postulate that infection of salivary glands cells by this virus initiates the autoimmune process in SS.

Recent experimental data suggest that retroviruses may be responsible for the initiation of the autoimmune damage in SS. Transgenic mice bearing the *tax* gene from human T cell leukaemia/lymphoma virus type I (HTLV-I) produced a histopathological picture in the salivary and lachrimal glands resembling that of primary SS: initially, epithelial cells proliferate, followed by gradual infiltration of lymphocytes and plasma cells and, finally, gradual destruction of the acinus[80]. The extent of histopathological change in various glands of these transgenic mice correlated directly with the concentration of the tax protein expressed in the nuclei of the epithelial cells. The tax protein is a trans-acting gene activator that in transfected T lymphocytes increases the expression of the genes for IL-2, IL-2 receptor, IL-3 (which is responsible for B cell growth) and granulocyte/monocyte colony stimulating factor. In addition, it is clear from this study that the HTLV-I virus has a tropism for the ductal epithelium of the salivary and lachrimal glands. Another report has shown that EBV and adult T cell leukaemia derived factor were present in the salivary glands in 10 out of 11 patients with SS[81]. HTLV-I was not detected in these samples. In another study, minor salivary gland biopsies of patients with pSS and SS associated with other connective tissue diseases were examined with three monoclonal antibodies to core (gag) proteins of HTLV-1 and two monoclonal antibodies to HIV-1. Sections from 31% of patients with pSS contained an epithelial cytoplasmic protein reactive with a monoclonal antibody to the p19 group specific antigen of HTLV-1. The antigen was detected also in a lower percentage in patients with secondary SS. All other monoclonal antibodies gave negative reactions. All patients had no serum antibodies to HTLV-1, indicating that the antigen was not part of HTLV-1; this antigen had endogenous retroviral properties since it was absent from healthy tissues but inducible by stimulation with phytohemagglutinin or IFN-γ[82]. Experiments with affinity purified rabbit antibodies to p25 protein of HTLV-related endogeneous sequences (HRES-1) showed that this antigen is distinct from the HRES-1, although the open reading frame of HRES-1 has sequence similarities both to p19 gag of HIV-1[83]. In another study, however, 30% of SS patients had serum antibodies that reacted with the capsid antigen p24 of HIV. One to four percent of healthy individuals matched for age had such autoantibodies in their sera[84].

Recently, it was suggested that a putative viral agent infecting the salivary glands of patients with primary SS could be identified by culturing extracts for lip biopsy specimens of patients with RH9 lymphoblastoid cells. This particle is different from the HIV particle by several physicochemical and ultrastructural criteria[85]. These findings have some implications concerning the pathogenesis of primary SS. Retroviral infection could cause significant changes in the behaviour of the epithelial cells of exocrine glands, such as *de novo* expression of HLA-DR antigens[86], expression of autoantigen on their surface, and heightened expression of lymphocytic adhesion molecules on the proximal endothelium. This may mean that retroviral infection of exocrine epithelial cells in subjects with a susceptible genetic and environmental background may predispose the glands to infiltration by immunocytes and the development of a localized autoimmune response with all the pathological consequences that ensue.

The infection of the epithelial cell by a virus, however, does not address the monoclonal expansion of B lymphocytes. This phenomenon can be explained by one of three mechanisms. First, a consistent neoantigen expression as a result of viral infection may lead to a chronic antigenic stimulation and subsequent expansion of particular B cell clones. Second, the viral infection may augment the synthesis of certain B cell growth factors (e.g. IL-3 by the tax gene of HTLV-I) while the cytokines produced locally promote virus activation. Indeed, IL-6 acting synergistically with TNF can activate HIV-I in chronically infected promonocytic cells[87], hence perpetuating the viral infection. Finally, a secondary infection of salivary glands following gland injury by another 'innocent bystander', such as EBV, cannot be excluded.

Acknowledgements

The authors are grateful to Dr E.O. Johnson for helpful suggestions, and to Mr G.E. Papanikolaou for secretarial assistance.

References

1. Moutsopoulos HM, Chused TM, Mann DL et al. Sjögren's syndrome (sicca syndrome): Current issues. Ann Intern Med. 1980; 92: 212–226.
2. Talal N, Bunim JJ. Development of malignant lymphoma in the course of Sjögren's syndrome. Am J Med. 1964; 36: 529–540.
3. Kassan SS, Thomas T, Moutsopoulos HM et al. Increased risk of lymphoma in sicca syndrome. Ann Intern Med. 1978; 89: 888–892.
4. Kyle RA, Lust JA. The monoclonal gammopathies (paraproteins). Adv Clin Chem. 1990; 28: 145–218.
5. Harley JB. Autoantibodies in Sjögren's syndrome. In: Sjögren's Syndrome: Clinical and Immunological Aspects N Talal, HM Moutsopoulos, SS Kassan), eds. Berlin: Springer Verlag; 1987: 218–234.
6. Moutsopoulos HM, Zerva LV. Anti-Ro(SSA)/La(SSB) antibodies and Sjögren's syndrome. Clin Rheumatol. 1990; 1 (Suppl) 123–131.
7. Fauci AS, Moutsopoulos HM. Polyclonally triggered B-cells in the peripheral blood of normal individuals and in patients with SLE and primary Sjögren's syndrome. Arthritis Rheum. 1981; 24: 577–584.
8. Anderson LG, Cummings NA, Asofsky R et al. Salivary gland immunoglobulin and rheumatoid factor synthesis in Sjögren's syndrome. Natural history and response to

treatment. Am J Med. 1972; 53: 456–463.

9. Daniels TE. Labial salivary gland biopsy in Sjögren's syndrome: assessment as a diagnostic criterion in 362 suspected cases. Arthritis Rheum. 1984; 27: 147–156.

10. Lindahl G, Hedfors E, Klareskog L, Forsum U. Epithelial HLA-DR expression and T-lymphocyte subsets in salivary glands in Sjögren's syndrome. Clin Exp Immunol. 1985; 61: 475–482.

11. Moutsopoulos HM, Hooks JJ, Chan C, Dalavanga YA, Skopouli FN, Detrick B. HLA-DR expression in labial salivary gland tissues in Sjögren's syndrome. Ann Rheum Dis. 1986; 54: 677–683.

12. Fox R, Carstens S, Fong S, Robinson CA, Howell P, Vaughan JH. Use of monoclonal antibodies to analyse peripheral blood and salivary gland lymphocyte subsets in Sjögren's syndrome. Arthritis Rheum. 1982; 25: 419–422.

13. Dalavanga YA, Drosos AA, Moutsopoulos HM. Labial salivary gland immunopathology in Sjögren's syndrome. Scand J Rheumatol. 1986; 61 (Suppl): 67–70.

14. Fox RI, Theophilopoulos AN, Altman AA. Production of interleukin-2 (Il-2) by salivary gland lymphocytes in Sjögren's syndrome. Detection of reactive cells by using antibodies directed to synthetic peptides of IL-2. J Immunol. 1985; 135: 3109–3115.

15. Skopouli FN, Fox PC, Galanopoulou V, Atkinson JC, Jaffe BC, Moutsopoulos HM. T-cell subpopulations in the labial minor salivary gland histopathologic lesion in Sjögren's syndrome. J Rheumatol. 1991; 18: 210–214.

16. Talal N, Asofsky R, Lightbody P. Immunoglobulin synthesis by salivary gland lymphoid cells in Sjögren's syndrome. J Clin Invest. 1970; 49: 49–54.

17. Skopouli FN, Kousvelari EE, Mertz P, Jaffe ES, Fox PC, Moutsopoulos HM. c-myc mRNA expression in minor salivary glands of patients with primary Sjögren's syndrome. J Rheumatol. 1992; 19: 693–699.

18. Giannopoulos D, Moutsopoulos HM, Roncin S, Youinou P, Pennec YL, et al. Conjunctival epithelial cells of patients with primary Sjögren's syndrome express inappropriately major histocompatibility molecules, La/SSB and heat shock proteins. J Clin Immunol. 1992; 12: 259–265.

19. Albelda SM, Buck CA. Integrins and other adhesion molecules. FASEB J. 1990; 4: 2868–2880.

20. Springer TA. Adhesion receptors of the immune system. Nature. 1990; 346: 425–434.

21. St Clair EW, Angellilo JC, Singer KH. Expression of cell adhesion molecules in the salivary gland microenvionment of Sjögren's syndrome. Arthritis Rheum. 1992; 35: 62–66.

22. Moutsopoulos HM, Steinberg AD, Fauci AS, Lane HC, Papadopoulos NM. High incidence of free monoclonal light chain in the sera of patients with Sjögren's syndrome. J Immunol. 1983; 130: 2263–2265.

23. Moutsopoulos HM, Costello R, Drosos AA, Mavridis AK, Papadopoulos NM. Demonstration and identification of monoclonal proteins in the urine of patients with Sjögren's syndrome. Ann Rheum Dis. 1985; 44: 109–112.

24. Walters MT, Stevenson FK, Hervert A, Cawley MID, Smith JL. Urinary monoclonal free light chains in primary Sjögren's syndrome: an aid to the diagnosis of malignant lymphoma. Ann Rheum Dis. 1986; 45: 210–219.

25. Tzioufas AG, Manoussakis MN, Costello R, Silis M, Papadopoulos NM, Moutsopoulos M. Cryoglobulinemia in autoimmune rheumatic diseases; evidence of circulating monoclonal cryoglobulins in patients with primary Sjögren's syndrome. Arthritis Rheum. 1986; 29: 1098–1104.

26. Schmidt V, Helbron D, Lennert K. Development of malignant lymphoma in myoepithelial sialadenitis (Sjögren's syndrome). Pathol Anat. 1982; 395: 11–43.

27. Fishleder A, Tubbs R, Hesse B, Levine H. Uniform detection immunoglobulin gene rearrangements in benign lymphoepithelial lesions. N Engl J Med. 1987; 316: 1118–1121.

28. Freimark B, Fantozzi R, Bone R, Bording G, Fox R. Detection of clonally expanded salivary gland lymphocytes in Sjögren's syndrome. Arthritis Rheum. 1989; 32: 859–869.

29. Moutsopoulos HM, Tzioufas AG, Bai M, Papadimitriou C. Primary Sjögren's syndrome: serum monoclonality is associated with a monoclonal B cell subset infiltrating the minor salivary glands. Ann Rheum Dis. 1990; 49: 929–931.

30. Kunkel HG, Agnello V, Joslin FG, Winchester RJ, Capra JD. Cross-idiotypic specificity among monoclonal IgM proteins with anti-gamma globulin activity. J Exp Med. 1973;

331–342.
31. Agnello V, Arbetter A, Ibanez A, et al. Evidence for a subset of rheumatoid factors that cross react with DNA-histone and have a distinct cross-idiotype. J Exp Med. 1980; 151: 1514–1527.
32. Kunkel HG, Winchester RJ, Joslin FG, Capra JD. Similarities in the light chains of anti-γ globulins showing cross-reactive specificities. J Exp Med. 1974; 149: 128–136.
33. Carson DA, Fong S. A common idiotype on human rheumatoid factors identified by a hybridoma antibody. Molec Immunol. 1983; 20: 1081–1087.
34. Kipps TJ, Fong S, Tomhave E, Chen PP, Goldfien RD, Carson DA. High frequency expression of a conserved kappa light-chain variable region gene in chronic lymphocytic leukemia. Proc Natl Acad Sci USA. 1987; 2916–2920.
35. Mageed RA, Dearlove M, Goodall DM, Jefferis R. Immunogenic and antigenic epitopes of immunoglobulins, XVII-monoclonal antibodies reactive with common and restricted idiotypes to the heavy chain of human rheumatoid factors. Rheumatol Int. 1986; 6: 179–183.
36. Gharavi AE, Patel EM, Hughes GRV, Elkon KG. Common IgA and IgM rheumatoid factor idiotypes in autoimmune diseases. Ann Rheum Dis. 1985; 44: 155–158.
37. Fox RI, Chen P, Carson DA, Fong S. Expression of a cross-reactive idiotype on rheumatoid factor in patients with Sjögren's syndrome. J Immunol. 1986; 136: 477–483.
38. Kipps TJ, Tomhave E, Chen PP, Fox RI. Molecular characterization of a major autoantibody associated cross-reactive idiotype in Sjögren's syndrome and rheumatoid factor associated cross-reactive idiotype. J Immunol. 1989; 142: 4261–4268.
39. Katsikis PD, Youinou PY, Galanopoulou V, Tzioufas AG, Moutsopoulos HM. Monoclonal process in primary Sjögren's syndrome and rheumatoid factor associated cross reactive idiotype. Clin Exp Immunol. 1990; 82: 509–514.
40. Tzioufas AG, Boumba DS, Skopouli FN, Carson DA, Moutsopoulos HM. Inheritance of monoclonal rheumatoid factor cross-reactive idiotypes in primary Sjögren's syndrome. Comparative studies of a rabbit polyclonal antiidiotype and 17109 monoclonal antiidiotype. Eur J Clin Invest; 22: 475–481
41. Skopouli FN, Talal A, Galanopoulou V, Tsampoulas CG, Drosos AA, Moutsopoulos HM. Raynaud's phenomenon in primary Sjögren's syndrome. J Rheumatol. 1990; 17: 618–620.
42. Cleary ML, Galili N, Levy N, Talal N, Sklar J. Detection of lymphoma in Sjögren's syndrome by analysis of immunoglobulin gene rearrangements. In: Tadal N, Montsopoulos HM, Kassan SS, eds. Sjögren's Syndrome: Clinical and Immunological Aspects. Berlin: Springer Verlag; 1987: 137–143.
43. Talal N, Sokoloff L, Barth WF. Extrasalivary lymphoid abnormalities in Sjögren's syndrome (reticulin-cell-sarcoma, 'pseudolymphoma', macroglobulinemia). Am J Med. 1967; 43: 50–65.
44. Pavlidis NA, Drosos AA, Papadimitriou C, Talal N, Moutsopoulos HM. Lymphoma in Sjögren's syndrome. Med Ped Oncol. 1992; 20: 279–283.
45. Radl J, Hollander CF, Van den Berg P, de Glopper E. Idiopathic paraproteinemia I. Studies in an animal model – The aging C57BL/kaLWRij mouse. Clin Exp Immunol. 1978; 33: 395–402.
46. Van den Akker TW, Brondijk R, Radl J. Influence of long term antigenic stimulation started in young C57BL mice on the development of age-related monoclonal gammopathies. Int Arch Allergy Appl Immunol. 1988; 87: 165–170.
47. Whittingham S, Nasseli G, Hicks JD, O'Brien C, Sculley TB. Studies on Sjögren's syndrome in Scid mice. Clin Exp Rheumatol. 1991; 9: 332 (Abstract).
48. Kang H, Pisa P, Moore K, Abrams J, Fox RI. Sjögren's syndrome pseudolymphoma induced in Scid/hu mice chimeras. Clin Exp Rheumatol. 1991; 9: 334 (Abstract).
49. Reinherz EL, Kung PC, Golstein C, Schlossman SF. A monoclonal antibody with selective reactivity with functionally mature human thymocytes and all peripheral human T-cells. J Immunol. 1979; 128: 1312–1317.
50. Hardy RR, Hayakawa K, Shimizu M, Yamasaki K, Kishimoto T. Rheumatoid factor secretion from human Leu-1 + B-cells. Science. 1987; 236: 81–83.
51. Wang CY, Good RA, Ammirati P, Dymbort G, Evans RI. Identification of a 69,71 complex expressed on human-T cells sharing determinants with B-type chronic lymphatic leukemic cells. J Exp Med. 1980; 151: 1538–1544.

52. Martin PJ, Hanson JA, Siadak AW, Nowinski RC. Monoclonal antibodies recognizing normal human T-lymphocytes and malignant human B-lymphocytes. A comparative study. J Immunol. 1981; 127: 1920–1923.

53. Hayakawa K, Hardy RR, Honda M, Herzenberg LA, Steiberg AD, Herzenberg LA. Ly-1B cells: functionally distinct lymphocytes that secrete IgM autoantibodies. Proc Natl Acad Sci USA. 1984; 81: 2494–2498.

54. Casali P, Burastero SE, Nakamura M, Inghirami G, Notkins AL. Human lymphocytes making rheumatoid factor and antibody to ssDNA belong to leu-1 + B-cell subset. Science. 1987; 236: 77–81.

55. Broker BM, Klajman A, Youinou P, et al. Chronic lymphocytic leukemia (CLL) cells secrete multispecific autoantibodies. J Autoimmunity. 1988; 1: 469–481.

56. Sthoeger ZM, Wakai M, Tse DB, et al. Production of autoantibodies by CD5-expressing leukemia. J Exp Med. 1989; 169: 255–268.

57. Burastero SE, Casali P, Wilder RL, Notkins AL. Monoreactive high affinity and polyreactive low affinity rheumatoid factor are produced by CD5 + B-cells from patients with rheumatoid arthritis. J Exp Med. 1988; 168: 1979–1992.

58. Plater-Zyberk C, Maini RN, Lam K, Kennedy RD, Janossy G. A rheumatoid arthritis B-cell subset expresses a phenotype similar to that in chronic lymphocytic leukemia. Arthritis Rheum. 1985; 28: 971–976.

59. Youinou P, Mackenzie L, Le Masson G, et al. CD5-expressing B-lymphocytes in blood and salivary glands of patients with primary Sjögren's syndrome. J Autoimmunity. 1988; 1: 185–194.

60. Dauphinee M, Tovar Z, Talal N. B-cells expressing CD5 are increased in Sjögren's syndrome. Arthritis Rheum. 1988; 31: 642–647.

61. Lanier LL, Warner NL, Ledbetter JA, Herzenberg LA. Expression of lyt-1 antigen on certain murine B-cell lymphomas. J Exp Med. 1981; 153: 998–1003.

62. Davidson WF, Frederickson TN, Rudikoff EK, Coffman RL, Hartley JW, Morse HC. A unique series of lymphomas related to the Ly-1 + lineage of B-lymphocytes differentiation. J Immunol. 1984; 133: 744–753.

63. Rabin EM, Mond JJ, Ohara J, Paul WE. B cell stimulatory factor 1 (BSF1) prepares resting B cells to enter phase in response to IgM and lipopolysaccharide. J Exp Med. 1986; 164: 517–531.

64. Kishimoto T. Factors affecting B cell growth and differentiation. Ann Rev Immunol. 1985; 3: 133–157

65. Hirano T, Yasukawa K, Harada H, et al. Complementary DNA for a novel human interleukin (BSF-2) that induces B-lymphocytes to produce immunoglobulins. Nature (London). 1986; 324: 73–76.

66. Bergui L, Schena M, Gaidano G, Riva M, Caligaris-Cappio F. Interleukin-3 and Interleukin-6 synergistically promote the proliferation and differentiation of malignant plasma cells precursors in multiple myeloma. J Exp Med. 1989; 170: 613–618.

67. Kishimoto T. The biology of interleukin-6. Blood. 1989; 74: 1–10.

68. Germanidis GS, Manoussakis MN, Tzioufas AG, Drosos AA, Moutsopoulos HM. Interleukin-6 in serum of patients with primary Sjögren's syndrome and other rheumatic diseases. Clin Exp Rheumatol. 1991; 9: 334 (Abstract).

69. Latreille J, Barlogie B, Johnston D, Drewinko B, Alexanian R. Ploidy and proliferative characteristics in monoclonal gammopathies. Blood. 1982; 59: 43–51.

70. Gould J, Alexanian R, Goodacre A, Pathak S, Hecht B, Barligie B. Plasma cell karyotype in multiple myeloma. Blood. 1988; 71: 453–456.

71. Showe LC, Croce CM. Oncogene probes in the detection of human cancer. Clin Physiol Biochem. 1987; 5: 227–237.

72. Seremetis S, Inghirami G, Ferrero D, et al. Transformation and plasmacytoid differentiation of EBV infected human B-lymphoblasts by ras oncogenes. Science. 1989; 243: 660–663.

73. Fox RI, Robinson C, Pisa P, Pisa E. Detection of BCL-2t(14,18) translocations in Sjögren's syndrome lymphoma. Clin Exp Rheumatol. 1991; 9: 333 (Abstract).

74. Chang RS, Lewis JL, Abilgaard CF. Prevalence of oropharyngeal excreters of leukocyte-transforming agents among a human population. N Engl J Med. 1973; 289: 1325–1329.

75. Epstein MA, Achong BG. The Epstein-Barr Virus. Berlin: Springer Verlag; 1979.

76. Venables PSW, Ross MGR, Charles PJ, Melsom RD, Griffiths PD, Maini RN. A

seroepidemiplogical study of cytomegalovirus and Epstein Barr virus in rheumatoid arthritis and sicca syndrome. Ann Rheum Dis. 1985; 44: 742–746.

77. Slaughter A, Carson DA, Jensen FC, Holbrook TL, Vaughan JH. *In vitro* effects of Epstein-Barr virus on peripheral blood mononuclear cells from patients with rheumatoid arthritis and normal subjects. J Exp Med. 1978; 148: 1429–1434.

78. Lerner MR, Andrews NC, Miller G, Steitz JA. Two small RNAs encoded by Epstein-Barr virus and complexed with protein are precipitated by antibodies from patients with systemic lupus erythematosus. Proc Natl Acad Sci USA. 1981; 78: 805–809.

79. Mariette X, Gozlan J, Clerk D, Bisson M, Morinet M. Detection of Epstein-Barr virus DNA by *in situ* hybridization and polymerase chain reaction in salivary gland biopsy specimens from patients with Sjögren's syndrome. Am J Med. 1991; 90: 286–294.

80. Green JB, Hinricks SH, Vogel J, Jay G. Exocrinopathy resembling Sjögren's syndrome in HTLV-I tax transgenic mice. Nature. 1989; 341: 72–74.

81. Saito I, Nishimura S, Kudo I, et al. Adult T-cell leukemia-derived factor (ADF) in Sjögren's syndrome (Abstract). Clin Exp Rheumatol. 1991; 9: 336.

82. Shattles WR, Brookes SM, Venables PJW, Clark DA, Maini RN. Expression of antigen reactive with a monoclonal antibody to HTLV-I p19 in salivary glands in Sjögren's syndrome. Clin Exp Immunol. 1992; 89: 46–51.

83. Perl A, Rosenblat JD, Chen ISY, et al. Detection and cloning of new HTLV-related endogenous sequences in man. Nucl Acids Res. 1989; 17: 6841–6854.

84. Talal N, Dauphinee MJ, Dang H, Alexander SS, Hart DJ, Garry RF. Detection of serum antibodies to retroviral proteins in patients with primary Sjögren's syndrome (autoimmune exocrinopathy). Arthritis Rheum. 1990; 33: 774–781.

85. Garry RF, Fermin CD, Hart DJ, Alexander SS, Donebower LA, Luo-Zhang H. Detection of a human intracisternal A-type retroviral particle antigenically related to HIV. Science. 1990; 250: 1127–1129.

86. Majello B, LaMantia G, Simeone A, Boncinelli E, Lania L. Activation of major histocompatibility complex Class I mRNA containing an Alu-like repeat in polyoma virus transformed rat cells. Nature. 1985; 314: 457–459.

87. Rosenberg ZF, Fauci AS. Immunopathologic mechanisms of human immunodeficiency virus (HIV) infection. In: The Human Retroviruses. Gallo RC, Jay J, eds. London: Academic Press; 1991: 141–161.

17
Immunotherapy

G. H. KINGSLEY and G. S. PANAYI

INTRODUCTION

As described in earlier chapters in this book, our understanding of the pathogenesis of connective tissue diseases has increased rapidly over the last ten years. Although the causative antigens remain, for the most part, unknown many of the immune mechanisms and genetic associations involved have been identified. In this chapter, we will examine how this newly acquired knowledge can be applied to the treatment of patients. The main emphasis will be on rheumatoid arthritis (RA) because of the extensive human studies in this disease although the ideas put forward are applicable to any T cell-mediated disease. Most attention will be devoted to biological agents such as monoclonal antibodies or peptides, which have been developed as a result of rational understanding of the disease, rather than new drugs, which have not yet been used in human connective tissue diseases and which have been identified as a result of the time-honoured techniques of screening animal or *in vitro* systems. For the latter, the reader is referred to recent reviews[1-3]. An exception will be made for cyclosporin because of the extensive human experience with this agent in RA. The article also confines itself strictly to immunological targets. Other approaches such as interfering with angiogenesis[4] or inhibiting enzymes in the synovium[5] are also valid perhaps in combination with the immunologically based therapies described here.

RA[6] is a chronic inflammatory disease primarily affecting the joints although there may be involvement of other systems such as the lungs, skin and nervous system. The disease affects many joints resulting in severe disability for the patient; it may even be fatal. The drugs currently used in treatment were developed on an empirical basis and most have been used unchanged in clinical practice for between thirty and fifty years. Even methotrexate and sulphasalazine, introduced over the last ten years, are old drugs borrowed from other diseases. All of them are toxic, their effect on symptoms is unpredictable and, more seriously, it is doubtful whether they can substantially alter the outcome of the disease. For all these reasons, new therapies are sorely needed.

THE PATHOGENESIS OF RA

Although we still do not have a complete understanding of the pathogenesis of RA, we are now in a position to build a hypothesis so that appropriate targets for immunotherapy can be identified[6-8]. RA is initiated by an unknown antigen; the disease may be perpetuated by the same or a different antigen. It is also unclear whether the initiating and perpetuating antigens are exogenous or autoantigens. After processing by antigen presenting cells (APC), the putative antigen is presented by MHC (major histocompatibility complex) class II molecules, probably HLA-DR4 and DR1 which are strongly associated with RA[9], to arthritogenic CD4+ T cells. The important question of whether these latter are polyclonal or use a restricted T cell receptor (TCR) repertoire remains unanswered[10]. Activation of the arthritogenic CD4+ T cells induces the production of cytokines including interleukin-1 (IL-2) which leads to clonal T cell expansion and interferon-gamma (IFN-γ) which activates monocytes. In this way a cascade of inflammatory interactions is triggered resulting in joint inflammation and destruction and, in some patients, systemic disease. The effector mechanisms include T cells, macrophages, synoviocytes and B cells and involve a variety of mediators including cytokines, notably interleukin-1 (IL-1) and tumour necrosis factor alpha (TNFα), growth factors, proteolytic enzymes and antibodies. Another important aspect of the arthritic process is cell migration since the inflammatory cells not normally resident in the joint must traffic into it. Migration is enhanced during inflammation since cytokines stimulate synovial endothelial cells to upregulate adhesion molecules such as E-selectin and ICAM-1[11-13]; these molecules thus also represent rational therapeutic targets as do their ligands on T cells. Finally, all immune processes are regulated by natural immunoregulatory mechanisms although they are, as yet, little understood. If methods of enhancing them could be identified, they would clearly represent a safe and specific mode of therapy.

It is beyond the scope of this chapter to discuss in detail the data supporting the hypothesis and, in particular, the central role of the T cell[8]. Much of it is reviewed in earlier chapters; the five key points are briefly outlined below. First, in animal models of RA such as adjuvant arthritis the disease can be transferred to naive animals by T cell lines specific for the inducing antigen. Second, in reactive arthritis, the T cells in the joint are specific for the triggering antigen[14,15]. Third, immunohistological studies of the RA synovium have shown a predominance of activated CD4+ T cells clustered around macrophages[16] which is strong, albeit indirect, evidence for a close interaction between these cell types. Fourth, since the major function of class II MHC molecules is to present antigen to CD4+ T cells, the strong association of RA in most populations with HLA-DR4 and HLA-DR1[9] argues persuasively for a role for T cells in the disease. Perhaps the most convincing evidence comes from the early studies of immunotherapy where inhibition of T cell function by, for example, cyclosporin or anti-T cell antibodies can lead to improvement in the disease; this forms the subject of the remainder of the chapter.

TARGETS FOR IMMUNOTHERAPY

It is clear that therapeutic targets exist at all levels of the pathogenetic pyramid. In general, the nearer the target is to the apex of the pyramid, the more likely it is to be able to switch off most aspects of the disease and the less likely it is to be generally immunosuppressive. For example, if it were possible to devise a therapy targeted at the arthritogenic antigen, this would be highly specific for RA; furthermore, since the antigen triggers the entire inflammatory cascade, its inhibition would abort the disease. Conversely, non-steroidal anti-inflammatory drugs (NSAID) have as their main target a group of mediators, the prostaglandins (PG), at the end of the inflammatory cascade. NSAID therapy affects joint inflammation whilst having no effect on joint damage; even the effect on inflammation may only be partial because of the existence of other inflammatory pathways. Furthermore, PGs are involved in other physiological pathways, for example in the kidney, so their inhibition inevitably has adverse effects.

One aspect not considered so far is the timescale over which the disease evolves. It is possible that all the processes described occur continuously during the course of RA. In this case any therapeutic target would be appropriate at any stage of disease. Another scenario is that the disease matures from an initiating stage where cognate antigen-MHC-TCR interactions are important to a later stage in which specific T cells no longer play a role, the disease being perpetuated by monocyte–macrophage and synoviocyte interactions[17]. In that case, in late disease, only targets low down in the pyramid would be relevant.

A final important point to bear in mind is the distinction between active and passive forms of immunotherapy. In passive immunotherapy, for example MHC-binding peptides used to block the MHC groove, continuous administration is required or the effect wears off. By contrast the idea of active immunotherapy, for example vaccination with T cell receptor peptides, is to generate an ongoing immune response by the patient against a part of the disease process. In this latter situation, a single course of treatment would suffice, which is clearly a major advantage.

EARLY IMMUNOTHERAPY

Early attempts at immunotherapy provided the first definitive evidence for the cell-mediated pathogenesis of synovitis in RA. Whilst disease remission could be induced by techniques directed at mononuclear cells, such as thoracic duct drainage (TDD), lymphocytapheresis or total lymphoid irradiation (TLI), removal of antibodies by plasmapheresis had no effect on synovitis. Later studies with the first practical T cell suppressive agent, cyclosporin, have lent further weight to the concept of a T cell-mediated disease.

Thoracic duct drainage

The advantage of TDD is that the duct contains mainly recirculating lymphocytes permitting manipulation of the lymphocyte pool without affecting other white blood cells. In one study of TDD[18], the thoracic duct was cannulated in nine patients and lymphocytes were drained from it for between 3 and 15 weeks, the patient's cell-free lymph being reinfused daily to prevent protein depletion. Clinical improvement began about seven days after treatment was initiated though it became more obvious with time. The remission lasted between 2 and 12 weeks after stopping TDD but lymphocyte counts did not return to pretreatment levels for 15 weeks. In some patients, lymphocytes drained from the thoracic duct were reinfused intravenously and this precipitated an immediate relapse. A small proportion of the reinfused lymphocytes could be shown to re-enter the synovium although many more entered the spleen and liver. Those which re-entered the joints persisted there longer than those in the reticulo-endothelial tissue, suggesting that they may have been selectively retained within the joint; however, this specific homing subset constituted a very small fraction of the thoracic duct lymphocytes. Since the effect of TDD is only temporary yet it has high costs and a serious risk of complications, it is not a realistic proposition for therapy. The importance of the TDD studies was the unequivocal support they gave to the concept of a central role for lymphocytes in the pathogenesis of RA.

Lymphocytapheresis

Lymphocytapheresis[19,20] represented an attempt to improve the practical aspects of lymphocyte drainage therapy since it can be performed as an outpatient through a central venous catheter. The blood removed is centrifuged to separate the buffy coat which contains both lymphocytes and monocytes; thus the therapy, unlike TDD, is not lymphocyte specific. The procedure does result in clinical remission which persists for at least 3 months[20] although the results may be best in the subset of RA patients who have pre-existing poor cell-mediated immune responses[21]. The procedure is associated with circulating lymphopenia but recent studies[22] suggest that downregulation of monocyte activation may be an additional mechanism.

Total lymphoid irradiation

An alternative anti-lymphoid therapy, derived from the treatment of Hodgkin's disease, is TLI, in which 'mantle' lymphoid tissue (cervical, axillary, mediastinal and hilar lymph nodes and thymus) and then the 'inverted-Y' field (para-aortic, iliac and inguinal lymph nodes) are irradiated in separate courses of fractionated treatments to a total dose of 750–2000 rads to each field. Though predominantly affecting T cells, TLI cannot be said to be T cell specific. Studies have demonstrated remission for 6 to 10 months but long-term follow up shows that all the patients have relapsed clinically by 40 months and progression of joint damage is not inhibited[23]. The depletion of circulating lymphocytes outlasts clinical improvement, being still detectable at 40 months. The exact mechanism of clinical improvement is unknown; studies[24] have shown a marked decrease in circulating CD4 + T cells and an impairment of *in vitro* T cell function as assessed by proliferation to mitogens, mixed lymphocyte responses and the ability to provide help for immunoglobulin secretion. In contrast, the synovial inflammatory infiltrate, including the numbers of T cells, was little changed by TLI although spontaneous IL-1 production by synovial biopsies was much decreased. Unfortunately, side-effects were severe. While infection was a major problem, especially in those receiving higher doses, the most serious concern was the development of malignant disease which occurred particularly in patients who later needed therapy with cytotoxic immunosuppressive drugs.

Cyclosporin

Cyclosporin (CyA) represented the first practical and relatively specific anti-T cell therapy. It suppresses an early step in T cell activation inhibiting cytokine gene transcription and hence production of cytokines, notably interleukin-2 (IL-2). Its mode of action at a molecular level has been the subject of much recent research and some of the details are still contentious[25,26]. The most widely accepted model is that CyA binds to an endogenous receptor called cyclophilin; the resulting cyclophilin-CyA complex binds to another intracytoplasmic protein, calcineurin, which is calcium and calmodulin dependent. This complex modulates calcineurin phosphatase activity thus inhibiting dephosphorylation of NF-ATc, the cytoplasmic subunit of the transcription factor NF-AT. Normally NF-ATc translocates to the nucleus where it joins with the nuclear NF-AT subunit, NF-ATn, to form functional NF-AT. NF-AT, whose effect is restricted to T cells, is one of the transcription factors which cooperate to activate transcription of the IL-2 gene. Interference with NF-ATc dephosphorylation inhibits the action of NF-AT and in turn IL-2 gene transcription and IL-2 production. Although the major therapeutic action of CyA appears to be via its action on T cells, it may also have direct effects on other tissues such as bone and cartilage[27] which may be relevant in RA.

CyA was first used in renal transplantation and rapidly became standard therapy. After this success, initial studies at doses of 5–6 mg/kg confirmed its effectiveness in RA[28] but treatment was hampered by toxicity. RA patients seem peculiarly vulnerable to the renal side effects of CyA; hypertension and renal impairment are common, and permanent renal damage has been reported[29]. Several explanations for the particular susceptibility to nephrotoxicity in RA patients have been advanced. These include concurrent therapy with nephrotoxic drugs, especially NSAIDs, and a high frequency of undetected underlying renal disease. Although subsequent studies have reduced nephrotoxicity by modifying the dose regimes used, efficacy has been compromised[28]. Furthermore concern about the induction of malignancy with CyA remains, although the risk has proved difficult to quantify[30]. For all these reasons, CyA has not been generally adopted as therapy for RA; guidelines have been proposed restricting its use to refractory disease and delineating patients in whom it should not be considered[31]. One way in which CyA may prove useful in RA is in combination with other immunomodulatory therapies but there is little experience of this.

ANTI-T CELL MONOCLONAL ANTIBODY THERAPY

Although murine monoclonal antibodies (MAb), such as OKT3, directed against the pan-T cell marker CD3, had been used in the treatment of renal transplant rejection, their use in a chronic disease like RA posed very different problems. Renal transplant recipients were severely immunocompromised, first, by their preceding renal failure and, second, by intense anti-rejection therapy including steroids and cytotoxic drugs. In contrast, RA patients have little general immunosuppression and so are much more likely to develop an immune response against a murine MAb. In addition, whilst MAb were used in transplantation to treat rejection which is a single event, the disease process in RA is chronic and any solution has to demonstrate long-term tolerability or long-term effectiveness. For ethical reasons, most studies in RA to date have been carried out in patients with long-standing disease unresponsive to other therapies. This is unavoidable but the disease process in such patients may be especially resistant to therapy and any change will be difficult to detect in the context of their overall status. On the positive side, it is important to remember that, even if MAb themselves do not turn out to be practical therapies, their use will considerably enhance our knowledge of pathogenesis and help identify appropriate therapeutic targets for new drugs.

Murine monoclonal antibodies

Murine MAb are produced by the fusion of a non-secreting immortal mouse myeloma cell line with spleen cells from a mouse previously immunized with the relevant antigen. The fused hybridoma cells are screened to select those producing antibodies with an Fab portion specific for the chosen antigen and an Fc isotype suitable for the desired function. Many therapeutic trials of murine MAb have now been reported in RA; because of the central role proposed for T cells in the pathogenesis of RA, most have involved MAb against T cell surface markers but MAb against adhesion molecules and cytokines have also been used.

From the earliest studies, it became clear that administration of murine protein to non-immunosuppressed patients virtually always induced an anti-mouse immune response. Such responses were expected to be less prominent in the case of anti-CD4 MAb therapy because this antibody has been shown to tolerize mice against neoantigens[32]; this effect did not prove to be significant in practice, perhaps by virtue of the doses used, since, in mice, there is a threshold dose of MAb below which tolerance is not induced. Whilst the human anti-mouse antibody response was primarily directed against the Fc portion of the murine MAb, anti-Fab responses also occurred. After a single course of MAb, there was clinical evidence of an anti-mouse immune response in only a minority of patients, although antibodies could be detected in most. However, because the benefits of MAb therapy were often only transient, patients required further treatment courses and this presented more of a problem. Although some patients were re-treated with murine MAb for two or even three courses of therapy apparently safely, anti-mouse antibody levels tended to rise and it was clear that long-term use of murine MAb would risk allergic side-effects or even anaphylaxis. In addition, anti-Fab responses could block binding of the MAb to its target and thus interfere with its therapeutic effect. Attempts were therefore made to redesign MAb to render them less immunogenic (reviewed in [33]).

Redesigning antibodies

Because of the prevalence of anti-Fc antibodies, the first attempt to get round this problem was to substitute a human Fc portion for the murine sequence, a so-called chimeric MAb. An additional benefit of such alterations is that the most appropriate Fc isotype can be selected; for example, IgG1 can be chosen if complement mediated cytotoxicity is desired. MAb which have been altered in this way include CD7 and CD4. Next, further molecular substitutions were then made to produce humanized MAb, where parts of the Fab portion were also altered to make them human in sequence. In this way, virtually the entire MAb, with the exception of the regions which combine with the antigen, has a human sequence. Unfortunately, alterations of this type are often associated with a loss of affinity of the MAb and, despite these manipulations, treatment with chimeric and even humanized MAb still induces an immune response although mostly against the Fab rather than the Fc portion of the MAb.

More recently still, other variations on standard antibodies have been produced, for example proteins comprising only the heavy chain variable region or target-specific antibody fragments generated by molecular recombination techniques[33]. None have yet been used in humans for therapy but they may well prove to be very important possibilities in the future. Perhaps even more important to consider is the idea that, if MAb therapy can identify a particular molecule as a useful therapeutic target, blocking drugs could be developed which avoid many of the toxicities of proteins. For example, in the field of anti-adhesion molecule therapy, small molecules which can block the carbohydrate binding sites on selectin molecules have recently been identified.

One of the major problems involved in the generation of 'designer' antibodies is the lack of a suitable *in vitro* model which enables prediction of, for example, which antibody isotype is most effective in therapy. This is compounded by our lack of knowledge of the mode of action of even those antibodies which are effective. Early ideas that these antibodies worked solely by depleting the relevant T cell subset are clearly much too simplistic, as discussed elsewhere in this chapter. One question which is often raised is whether the clinical effects seen with these antibodies are simply due to a non-specific immunoglobulin effect, especially in view of the promising results reported in some connective tissue diseases for polyclonal immunoglobulin therapy. This is unlikely, first, because some antibodies have proved ineffective and, second, because no convincing benefit for immunoglobulin in RA has been demonstrated.

Appropriate targets on T cells

Three different types of T cell antigen have been targeted in devising therapy for RA: T cell activation markers such as CD25 (IL-2 receptor) and CD7, pan-T cell markers such as CD3, CD5 and CDw52 and T cell subset markers such as CD4. The possibility of targeting the arthritogenic T cells themselves with anti-TCR monoclonal antibodies is obviously the most selective possibility of all and will be discussed in the section on therapy against the trimolecular complex below.

Monoclonal antibodies against CD7

One of the first studies[34] used RFT2, a murine MAb against CD7 previously shown to be effective in transplantation. CD7 is a 40 kD protein which is upregulated on the surface of activated T cells, and MAb against CD7 are immunosuppressive *in vitro*[35]. In this pilot clinical study, six patients with refractory RA were treated in hospital with daily intravenous (iv) injections of 10 mg RFT2 for 14 days. Only two patients showed any clinical improvement and these relapsed as soon as treatment was withdrawn. Importantly for the future of this type of therapy, side effects were minimal, with two patients developing chills and mild fever. Despite the lack of clinical effect, the peripheral blood and synovial membrane of these patients were depleted of CD7+ cells. It was thought that these disappointing results might be due to inability to achieve sustained high levels of the antibody. Therefore a further study with a chimeric anti-CD7 MAb which had a far longer half-life was undertaken, the antibody being given twice weekly instead of daily. Sadly, the clinical results were no better[36]. Interestingly, later *in vitro* studies[37] suggested that the primary role of CD7 was in the CD45RA + T cell subset whereas the majority of synovial T cells are CD45RO + CD45RA-; this may explain the lack of efficacy of anti-CD7 therapy in RA.

Targeting the IL2 receptor

MAb against the IL2 receptor were predicted to be an effective treatment for autoimmune diseases on theoretical grounds since the IL2 receptor is found on activated T cells and thus on T cells involved in the ongoing immune response *in vivo*. Studies of anti-IL2 receptor MAb therapy in animal models of arthritis, such as collagen arthritis[38], confirmed their efficacy and led to a pilot study in humans. Campath 6, a rat IgG_{2b} MAb against the p55 chain of the interleukin 2 receptor (CD25), was used in three patients, two of whom improved although they later relapsed[39]. No immunological data were reported in this study. Whilst further studies with a humanized or chimerized anti-IL2 receptor MAb would be one way to extend this work, alternative ways of targeting IL2 receptor positive cells could be considered. For example IL2 itself could be used to home to the receptor since it has a higher affinity for its target than a MAb.

The molecule, $DAB_{486}IL2$[40], is a fusion toxin in which the native receptor binding domain of diphtheria toxin is replaced by sequences from human IL2 whilst the membrane-translocating and enzymatic (toxic) portions of the diphtheria toxin molecule remain intact. The molecule binds specifically to the high affinity IL2 receptor and kills cells bearing it utilizing the potent cytotoxicity of the diphtheria toxin. $DAB_{486}IL2$ was originally devised for use in therapy of leukaemias and lymphomas but has now been used in various autoimmune diseases including RA and diabetes mellitus (DM). An initial open uncontrolled study in 19 patients with RA showed that some 40% of patients improved at the two higher doses used and that repeat dosing was associated with further improvement. Adverse effects, none severe, included fever, nausea and minor reversible transaminase elevations replicating the experience in cancer therapy where $DAB_{486}IL2$ has been used since 1989. Similar results have recently been obtained in a larger placebo-controlled study where the response has been shown to last from 4 to 30 weeks. An improved version of the IL2 fusion toxin, $DAB_{389}IL2$, has been developed by deleting 97 amino acids, which results in a five times greater binding to the high affinity IL2 receptor and, in murine collagen arthritis, a ten times greater potency with a wider ratio between therapeutic and toxic effects than its predecessor. A study using $DAB_{389}IL2$ in RA is in progress.

$DAB_{486}IL2$ has also been used, followed by maintenance low-dose cyclosporin, in diabetic patients symptomatic for less than sixteen weeks. In about half the patients, the insulin dose could be reduced to minimal levels for at least three months; a few patients remained in remission at 18 months. The use of $DAB_{486}IL2$ as an induction agent, followed by maintenance therapy with another drug, would also be an appropriate approach in RA.

Therapy with a CD5-ricin conjugate

The CD5 molecule was initially of interest in autoimmunity because it identified a subset of B cells thought to be associated with autoantibody production. However, it later became clear that the effect of anti-CD5 therapy was due to the ubiquitous distribution of the CD5 molecule on T cells. The agent used for therapy was CD5-Plus™ which is an immunoconjugate of a murine IgG_1 anti-CD5 MAb with two chains of ricin-A, added to enhance cytotoxicity. Since no studies of anti-CD5 alone have been performed in RA, the contribution of ricin to the effect of CD5-Plus[TM] remains a matter for speculation. Unusually for a biological therapy, the drug has been studied[41] in both late disease (mean 10.7 years after onset) and early disease (mean 1.8 years after onset). Patients in the late group had failed a mean of 4.3 DMARDs and were thus roughly comparable to those used in other biological studies whereas those in the early group had failed a mean of only 1.7 DMARDs. The maximal improvement in both groups was seen at four weeks and at this stage patients in the early arthritis group were approximately twice as likely to respond. However, this difference had largely disappeared by three months when only a quarter of patients still showed a response; by one year only 10% could be considered as responders.

The mechanism by which CD5-Plus[TM] is effective is far from clear. As expected, it induces a fall in circulating T cells which is less severe or persistent than that with some other anti-T cell MAbs. However, recent work by Verwilghen et al.[42] may also be relevant. As in previous studies, these workers found that anti-CD5 antibody was a costimulator for IL2-stimulated peripheral blood T cells. Conversely, synovial T cells stimulated by IL2 were inhibited by additional stimulation with anti-CD5 antibody.

CD5-Plus[TM] has also been used in four patients with lupus nephritis unresponsive to prednisolone and cyclophosphamide[43]. All patients showed a transient fall in CD5+ T cells but only one showed a sustained clinical response whilst two had a response lasting about six months and one did not respond at all. Only the patient who showed the sustained response had a persistent decrease in CD5+ T cells.

CDw52 as a therapeutic target

Campath-1H is a humanized IgG_1 MAb specific for CDw52, an antigen of unknown function found on all lymphocytes and some monocytes. Campath-1H has been used in vasculitis[44] and in an open study in RA[45,46]. In the RA study, eight patients with active disease who had failed at least two DMARDs were treated with intravenous MAb for ten days (total dose 60 mg). Seven out of eight showed a clinical response, maximal at four weeks, which was said to last for three to eight months. The degree of remission was not so impressive at later time points; for example, as a percentage of pretreatment value, the median joint score was 53% at four weeks and 44% at eight weeks but had risen to 75% by three months. Four patients were treated with 40 mg Campath-1H daily for five days, although one could only tolerate a single 40 mg dose. In all, a further remission occurred. No change in erythrocyte sedimentation rate (ESR) or C-reactive protein (CRP) was observed in any patient.

Campath-1H induced a marked and persistent decrease in the total lymphocyte count; in three of the initial five patients treated, the total lymphocyte count remained at or below 400–500 cells/μl at 9 to 12 months. NK cells were unaffected by Campath-1H, B cell numbers had recovered by two months and CD8 cells by six months but CD4 counts remained low although no serious infections were seen. Antiglobulin responses were not detected after a single course of treatment but three of the four re-treated patients developed a response, in two a pure anti-Id response, which was able to block Campath-1H binding. The most serious side-effect seen was a severe first dose reaction lasting 2–3 hours and consisting of fever up to 40°C, rigors and hypotension lasting 2–3 hours; this appeared similar to the cytokine release syndrome seen with OKT3 therapy.

Following this initial pilot study, Campath-1H, now licensed by Wellcome, is undergoing multicentre studies using two regimes, a single intravenous infusion protocol[47] and a ten day subcutaneous protocol[48]. The single intravenous infusion study demonstrated only transient clinical benefit although CD4+ T cell counts were still reduced after three months. More than 75% of the patients developed the first dose reaction described above and 50% became hypotensive. In the subcutaneous study, the acute first dose effect still occurred but was associated with hypotension in only a very small number of patients; there was a local reaction at the site of injection. Approximately half the patients treated subcutaneously improved by more than 50% although this level of remission lasted only a few weeks. Unfortunately different outcome scores were used in these studies and that by Isaacs et al.[45]; where comparison is possible, the benefit appears similar in degree and duration. Anti-idiotypic responses to Campath-1H have occurred in about half the patients whether treated subcutaneously or intravenously. Most worryingly of all, two fatal opportunistic infections have been reported; although these occurred in sick patients on additional immunosuppressive therapy a connection between this and the antibody therapy must be considered particularly in view of the sustained decrease in lymphocyte counts (J Johnston, personal communication).

Campath-1H has also been used in patients with vasculitis unresponsive to steroids and cytotoxic drugs[44]. Interestingly, Campath-1H alone was not able to induce a sustained remission but, in combination with anti-CD4 antibody a prolonged effect was seen. It is not clear what the mechanism of the additive effect is, since the two MAb both appear to have CD4+ T cells as their primary target. It will be interesting to see if this combination is effective in other diseases.

Therapy with murine anti-CD4 monoclonal antibodies

The greatest experience of MAb therapy in RA has been gained with anti-CD4 MAb, initially murine and more recently chimeric. The CD4 molecule is an obvious therapeutic target in view of the central role proposed for CD4+ T cells in the pathogenesis of RA and the effectiveness of anti-CD4 MAb in animal models of arthritis[49]. However, investigators were reluctant to embark on studies of anti-CD4 MAb because of possible parallels between MAb-induced CD4 cell depletion and AIDS. There was even the theoretical possibility of generating an idiotypic network centred on CD4 in which case the depletion could have been permanent and irreversible. Fortunately, these fears proved unfounded. The initial pilot study of two murine IgG_{2a} anti-CD4 MAbs, M-T151 (five patients) and VIT4 (three patients) demonstrated benefit in all patients although, in some, the improvements were short-lived[50-52]. The CD4 antigen was not modulated from the T cell surface but circulating CD4+ T cells were depleted and there was some reduction in *in vitro* T cell function.

Further open studies using M-T151[53] or another murine IgG$_1$ anti-CD4 MAb, MAX 16H5[54], demonstrated clinical benefit, albeit sometimes short-lived, in about 70% of refractory RA patients. Surprisingly, some patients who did not benefit from their first MAX 16H5 treatment responded to re-treatment. The ESR and CRP did not fall after M-T151, even in patients who improved clinically; there was some reduction in about half the MAX 16H5 patients. Other murine anti-CD4 MAb have been used in pilot studies. Treatment with B-F5, an IgG$_1$ MAb[55,56], led to improvement in the majority of patients. However, the IgG$_{2a}$ MAb, BL4[57], and the IgG$_{2a}$ MAb, OKT4A[58], were much less promising. It has so far proved impossible to predict whether a particular anti-CD4 MAb will be clinically effective by looking at either its isotype or the domain of CD4 it recognizes although it is clear that the pharmacokinetics of various anti-CD4 MAb differ considerably[59]. The lack of an *in vitro* model or surrogate marker for predicting efficacy is a serious handicap in developing more effective antibodies. It is equally difficult to predict which patients will respond, particularly since a patient's response may differ on different occasions[54] though, again, patients vary in their metabolism of these MAb[59]. It should be emphasized that none of these studies were placebo-controlled and therefore their clinical results have to be interpreted with caution. Controlled studies have recently been performed with chimeric anti-CD4 MAb and will be discussed below.

How does murine anti-CD4 MAb therapy work? Initially the effect was thought to be due simply to a reduction of CD4+ T cells, other lymphocyte subsets being largely unaffected. Consistent with this idea, treatment with MAX 16H5 induced a persistent depression of CD4+ T cells (40% of pre-treatment levels after two months) and modulated CD4 off the T cell surface. In contrast, however, with M-T151 therapy there was no CD4 modulation and CD4+ T cells returned to normal after 24 hours. Since the clinical effects of M-T151 lasted for more than 24 hours, a decrease in CD4+ T cells cannot be the sole explanation. The *in vitro* response to T cell mitogens was diminished by treatment but the effect on recall antigen responses varied, partly because these are decreased or absent in many RA patients. Other potential mechanisms of action will be discussed further in the section on chimeric anti-CD4 MAb therapy.

In view of animal experiments showing that a neoantigen given at the same time as anti-CD4 was tolerogenic rather than immunogenic[32], it was hoped that patients given an adequate dose of anti-CD4 MAb would not produce an anti-mouse response. However, anti-mouse antibodies could be detected in more than half the patients in most studies. After a single course, they are often at a lower level than with other MAbs, allowing for re-treatment. However, antibody levels usually rose after repeat courses of therapy suggesting that the number of courses which could be safely given was limited. No other serious adverse effect was observed although some patients developed mild fever, nausea and, rarely, allergic manifestations. In one patient[60], M-T151 treatment was associated with the development of transient acute renal failure secondary to interstitial nephritis although no causative effect could be proved.

Therapy with chimeric anti-CD4 monoclonal antibody

Following the successful studies with murine anti-CD4 MAb, a chimerized MAB against CD4 was used in therapy in the hope of reducing immunogenicity. The MAB selected was cM-T412 which was chimerized by Centocor Inc from a murine MAb M-T412 conjugated to a human IgG_1 Fc region. M-T412 itself was not used clinically so no direct comparison between murine and chimeric studies can be made. cM-T412, which has a half-life some 5–6 times longer than murine MAb, has been used in studies in Holland[61], in the USA[62] and in the UK[63,64] using a variety of doses and regimens. Comparison of the various results may allow some generalizations about the way in which MAb therapy, and especially anti-CD4 MAb, may be most effectively used. Most patients treated with MAb to date have been taking only NSAIDs and perhaps low-dose steroids but, in some of these studies, the possibility of using concurrent DMARDs, notably methotrexate, has also been explored.

Initial studies in Leiden replicated the regimes found effective in murine studies, that is to say seven days therapy with 10, 50 or 100 mg daily as an intravenous infusion[61]. The effects of the 50 mg and 100 mg regimes were very similar, with significant improvement of some 30% in all clinical parameters for several weeks; the 10 mg regime was substantially less effective. The lymphopenia was much more persistent than the clinical effect; there was an immediate fall in CD4 + T cells to 25% of baseline and, at 12 months, they were still only 60% of normal. The acute phase response was unchanged. Following on these studies, which were conducted in patients with refractory disease, the group has embarked on a study of early RA.

Initial studies at Guy's Hospital[63] were undertaken using an intermittent pulsed regime which was felt to be more practical for long-term therapy in general clinical use. Unfortunately, neither the patients who received a single 50 mg intravenous infusion of MAb nor those who received four such doses once a week for four weeks demonstrated any clinical improvement. In the single-infusion patients, there was only a transient decrease in CD4 + T cells but the patients receiving four doses demonstrated a lymphopenia which persisted for up to two months[63]. Currently we are investigating[64] the effects of an induction course of five daily infusions of 50 mg of cM-T412 followed either by an identical re-treatment course after five weeks or by weekly maintenance infusions of 50 mg. Preliminary results suggest that some patients do improve significantly. This usually occurs after a few days of the induction regime; the degree of improvement appears to correlate with the extent of cM-T412 coating of the CD4 cells in the joint.

The studies in Alabama[62] focused, for the most part, on single-dose regimens at doses ranging from 10 to 200 mg cM-T412. A small number of patients were treated with thrice weekly or daily infusions of 100 mg of MAb.

These patients differed from those in the European chimeric and murine studies in that, in addition to the NSAIDs and low-dose steroids permitted in those studies, the Alabama patients were all on a stable low dose of methotrexate. All the patients were followed up for six months and virtually all for as long as eighteen months[65]. Multiple-infusion regimes resulted in more profound CD4+ T cell depression than the single-dose schedules. With the former, CD4+ T cells fell to 50% of normal initially and were still at that level at eighteen months; with the latter, the initial fall was to 25% of normal and by eighteen months CD4+ T cells had risen to only 30% of normal. The fall affected both the CD45RA+ and CD45RO+ T cells but, at least in those patients who began to repopulate their CD4 population fairly rapidly, the CD45RO+ cells recovered more quickly. Though the initial fall was similar to that seen by the Dutch investigators with their multiple-dose regime, the CD4+ T cells in the Alabama patients remained much lower; the reason is unknown but may well relate to concurrent methotrexate. Following the promising results seen above in the pilot studies from all three groups, a randomized controlled trial of cM-T412 is in progress.

The side-effects of cM-T412 were similar to those seen with the murine anti-CD4 MAbs discussed above. Approximately 60% of patients had a mild 'flu-like' syndrome which in a few has been associated with mild vasomotor instability. Out of the 150 patients so far treated, only four have had severe hypotension. There has been one death[65] in a patient who received a single 100 mg dose in addition to treatment with steroids and methotrexate. Eighteen months after receiving cM-T412, at a time when his CD4+ T cells had returned to 70% of normal levels, this patient contracted a fatal pneumocystis pneumonia. Varying percentages of patients have developed human anti-chimeric antibodies but these, generally at low titre, have not prevented retreatment.

These chimeric studies have thrown further light on the mechanism of action of anti-CD4 MAb in humans. CM-T412 tended to induce a more profound and prolonged CD4 lymphopenia than the murine anti-CD4 MAb though it does not modulate the CD4 antigen off the surface of the T cell. Typically, the CD4 cells are depressed below $200/\mu l$ and may remain low for months; CD45RA cells remain particularly suppressed. CD8 cells may be transiently depleted for less than 72 hours. The study of intermittent infusions of cM-T412 by Choy et al.[63] found a depletion of circulating CD4+ T cells equivalent to that induced in other studies with the same MAb[61,62] yet unlike them found no therapeutic benefit. This strongly suggests that decreasing peripheral blood CD4+ T cells alone is not sufficient to lead to benefit. Since it is not known how many CD4+ T cells are required to induce arthritis, it is possible that a complete removal of CD4 T cells (which has not been achieved by any study) would be sufficient to induce remission; however, it would very likely be toxic in terms of subsequent opportunistic infections. It may be that the crucial issue is the degree of depletion of CD4 cells in the joint. For example, intermittent infusions may fail to achieve persistent high levels of MAb in the joint so that synovial CD4 cells are not depleted. Alternatively other extra-vascular sites such as bone marrow or lymphoid tissue may be the most relevant. Little is known, as yet, about these tissues although studies using a radiolabelled anti-CD4 MAb[59] have shown that it enters the joint rapidly.

However, if CD4 T cell depletion is not the mechanism by which anti-CD4 MAb is effective, there are a number of other ways in which ligation of CD4 on T cells by anti-CD4 MAb could affect T cells. By binding first to the CD4 molecule, the MAb could act (i) by interfering with binding of the MHC-antigen complex to the TCR, (ii) by preventing the physical association of CD4 to the CD3/TCR complex required for T cell activation[59], (iii) by inducing an anergic state preventing further triggering via the TCR[59] or (iv) by inducing apoptosis[64,66]. Whilst most of these mechanisms would apply equally to all T cells and are not disease specific, the possibility of apoptosis is of particular interest because it might introduce an element of specificity as to which CD4+ cells are inhibited. In the original work by Newell et al.[66], pre-incubation of murine CD4+ T cells with MAb against CD4 followed by activation via the TCR can induce apoptosis (programmed cell death). This has also been demonstrated *in vitro* using human lymphocytes and cM-T412[64]. Since apoptosis only occurs when the cM-T412 coated T cell meets its cognate antigen, one can conceive of a scenario where cells were coated in the blood and those migrating to the joint underwent apoptosis in synovium when they met their antigen. Thus there would be selective apoptosis of arthritogenic T cells.

In addition to T cells, cells of the monocyte–macrophage lineage also bear the CD4 antigen. It has been argued, drawing on new information about the pathogenesis of AIDS, that they could be a major therapeutic target. Relatively little is known about the effect of anti-CD4 MAb on these cells. Most studies have shown that there is only a transient depletion of monocytes as identified by the CD14 antigen[61,63,64]. In contrast, it has been shown that at least one MAb, MAX 16H5, induced marked decreases in monocyte activation markers such as neopterin, TNFα and IL1[67]. This may be peculiar to this MAb since it has a more profound effect than other anti-CD4 MAb on the acute phase response which is largely monokine-dependent. In support of this, one study[62,65] with cM-T412, a MAb which has little effect on the acute phase response, was not able to demonstrate any change in IL1 or TNF. There was a transient marked elevation in IL6 levels in these patients, particularly notable in those who had fever, which returned to normal within 24 hours.

These studies, demonstrating, in the main, transient improvements, produce little support for the concept propounded by Waldmann et al.[68] that therapy with anti-CD4 would result in a permanent 'reprogramming' of the immune system. Nonetheless, a very small minority of patients do get a very prolonged remission. One such, a girl of 25 who had had juvenile-onset seropositive RA since the age of 11 unresponsive to any second-line agent singly or in combination, has been in a virtually complete clinical remission for over three years following a single course of M-T151[64]. The difference between such patients and the vast majority who experience only a short-lived effect is very important but a complete enigma.

MONOCLONAL ANTIBODIES AGAINST ADHESION MOLECULES

The experience with MAb against non-T cell targets is much less extensive. Adhesion molecules represent an attractive therapeutic target but the only clinical study to date in RA is a preliminary dose-escalating study using five daily doses of BIRR1, a murine IgG_{2a} MAb to ICAM-1/CD54 previously used in renal allograft rejection[69]. ICAM-1 was chosen as a target because the ligand pair LFA-1/ICAM-1 is involved both in generating stable adhesion and in transendothelial migration; in animal studies, an anti-ICAM-1 antibody led to much less infection than an antibody against the LFA-1 β chain. The appropriate MAb dose was determined from pilot studies including *in vitro* functional studies with patients' serum[69,70]. Of the thirteen refractory RA patients treated, eight showed a good response lasting in most for one to two months; side-effects were transient and moderate, allowing treatment to continue. The antibody bound to circulating ICAM-1 in the peripheral blood so that this needed to be saturated before therapy could be effective. Patients developed a peripheral lymphocytosis (whether they developed a clinical response or not) and their peripheral blood T cells bound better to cultured endothelial cells than those of untreated patients; both observations are consistent with an inhibitory effect of anti-ICAM MAb on the migration of T cells out of the circulation. However, this may not be the only, or even the main, mode of action of the MAb since patients' T cells also respond poorly to mitogen after therapy, and ICAM-1 is, of course, involved in many immune processes. Patients did develop an anti-mouse antibody response; since blocking of adhesion processes is likely to induce only transient remission, the antibody would need to be chimerized or humanized if long-term therapy is to be considered.

Another group of adhesion molecules which are being considered as therapeutic targets are the selectins. These mediate the initial rolling phase of adhesion which is required before the stable integrin-mediated bond can be established[11,12]. Selectins bind to their ligands using their terminal carbohydrate domains. There are three members of the family, L-selectin which is found on leukocytes and P- and E-selectins which are found on endothelial cells. P-selectin, which is activated by thrombin, free radicals and histamine, is mainly involved in hyperacute states like reperfusion injury whilst E-selectin, which is induced by cytokines and endotoxin, is involved in acute and chronic inflammation. Anti-P-selectin has been shown to inhibit reperfusion injury and cobra-venom-induced lung injury whilst anti-E-selectin inhibits late bronchoconstriction in asthma. One very encouraging development is that an analogue of the terminal carbohydrate moiety of selectins has been synthesized which is able to block the rolling stage of adhesion. Such a small non-protein molecule represents a considerable advance since it is likely to be free of many of the undesirable features of MAb. RA is one of the disease targets for this molecule particularly in view of the high levels of E-selectin in synovial tissue[71].

The Holy Grail of adhesion scientists is to discover organ-specific adhesion mechanisms allowing the inhibition of migration into the joint, for example, whilst having no effect on migration required for other immune responses.

Although it is now clear that lymphoid organs do have tissue-specific adhesion molecules, no organ-specific molecule has been identified with certainty for peripheral tissues, with the possible exception of the cutaneous lymphocyte antigen (CLA) which may be a specific homing receptor for a subset of skin-homing lymphocytes[72].

MONOCLONAL ANTIBODIES AGAINST CYTOKINES AND OTHER ANTI-CYTOKINE THERAPIES

Cytokines are another target for monoclonal antibody therapy in RA although there must be reservations with regard to both the redundancy of the cytokine network (the ability of one cytokine to perform the role of another) and their importance in many different immune processes. It is also unclear whether anti-cytokine therapy could alter the long-term outlook of the disease. Further difficulties include the existence of physiological inhibitors of cytokine action including natural anti-cytokine antibodies and specific antagonists such as IL1ra and TNF binding proteins. The effect of therapeutic blockade may be difficult to measure because binding to inhibitors may prolong serum cytokine half-life resulting in apparently raised levels of the cytokine (although it will be in an inactive bound form). Specific natural inhibitors also need to be considered in obtaining a true picture of the role of any cytokine *in vivo* since their presence will, at least partially, antagonize the effect of the active cytokine.

One target cytokine is TNFα because of *in vitro* studies in which it appears to act as the 'boss' cytokine in RA, being responsible for the release of all others, and because of its efficacy in collagen-induced arthritis[73]. In further support of this theory, a recently developed TNFα-transgenic mouse develops arthritis which can be inhibited by anti-TNF Ab[74]. The acid test for the 'boss' cytokine theory is, however, therapeutic; if TNFα is truly the primary generator of inflammation in RA, then treatment directed against it should switch off all the markers of inflammation in these patients. In a recent pilot clinical trial of ten patients with refractory RA treated with cA2, a chimeric IgG$_2$ anti-TNFα MAb, has shown promising results[75]. Patients were given a total of 20 mg/kg as two or four intravenous infusions over two weeks. Nine of the ten patients improved with a marked reduction in disease activity to approximately 25% of pre-treatment levels. Unlike the studies with anti-T cell reagents, there was a concomitant significant decrease in the acute phase response often to within the normal range. Although these patients were selected on a similar basis to those in the other biological studies, they may have been somewhat less active as their mean ESR prior to therapy was only 34 mm/h. Maximum response was seen at four weeks and the longest remission lasted for four months. In terms of the effect of cA2, there could simply be a general decrease in circulating TNFα or a specific neutralization of TNFα in the joint. It is also unclear which action of TNFα it is most important to antagonize. Whilst there are many possibilities, the very rapid onset of action may suggest that an important target is the TNFα-induced upregulation of adhesion proteins since inhibition of this process will rapidly decrease migration of leucocytes into inflammatory sites. No results on anti-human antibody responses are yet available; this is particularly important with anti-cytokine MAb because long lasting remission cannot be anticipated. For this reason, in the long term, other anti-TNFα agents such as soluble TNF receptors, discussed below, will probably be preferable.

There are several other ways of targeting cytokines which may be equally effective yet avoid some of the risks of therapy with MAb. Drugs which suppress IL1 have been developed but, as yet, none have reached the market, being withdrawn for toxicity. For IL1, a specific antagonist against the IL1 receptor has been discovered. This molecule, IL1ra, which has no agonist action, has been given by daily subcutaneous injection in preliminary clinical studies in RA; it induces a marked reduction in clinical symptoms by seven days[76]. An idea which is more generally applicable is to make soluble cytokine receptors. A monomeric form of the soluble IL1 receptor has been used in studies of allergic disease and is now being studied in RA. Soluble TNF receptor is also being studied, this time as a complex of two soluble TNF molecules complexed to an Ig molecule; this form has increased affinity compared to the monomer.

THERAPY AGAINST THE TRIMOLECULAR COMPLEX

The therapies discussed above, whilst more rational than those in common use today, are far from specific for RA. In order to produce a truly specific therapy for the disease, it is necessary to focus on the components of the trimolecular complex, that is the antigenic peptide, the disease-associated MHC and the TCR of the arthritogenic T cell. Whilst theoretically attractive and certainly feasible in animal models, too little is known in RA (except perhaps about the MHC) to allow clinical trials using these molecules as targets. Consequently, whilst the foregoing discussion reviewed practical therapy in humans, this section consists mainly of theoretical discussion and some results from animal studies. Because of the lack of concrete data in humans, not to mention the unfortunate tendency of such innovative therapies to fail in the development stage, the review is brief.

One essential distinction is whether the technique is passive or active. An example of a passive technique is the use of MHC-binding peptides to block the MHC; the effect will wear off when the peptide is removed. In an active technique, the therapy induces a permanent change in the patient's immune system; techniques exemplifying this include T cell and TCR peptide vaccination, anti-MHC immunization and tolerance induction.

THE ANTIGEN AS A TARGET

Despite intensive study, there is no convincing information about the causative antigen in RA, not even whether it is a single or multiple associated antigen or whether it is an autoantigen. The situation in many other connective tissue diseases is the same. Thus the effective and non-toxic approach of antigen-specific tolerance cannot easily be adopted. Nevertheless, one technique, T cell receptor antagonism[77], which could be used to induce tolerance if the antigen were identified, will be discussed in the TCR section below.

However, one tolerance technique has already been used in human autoimmune diseases, oral tolerance. Oral tolerance relies on the special properties of the gut immune system by which an antigen given orally may not induce an immune response but rather anergy; this is obviously required to prevent food proteins inducing an immune response. In animal models[78], feeding the causative antigen can suppress autoimmune disease; for example, oral collagen suppresses collagen arthritis and myelin basic protein (MBP) inhibits experimental autoimmune encephalomyelitis (EAE). Active suppression with CD8+ T cells appears to be involved and transforming growth factor β may mediate the effect. Antigen given nasally by aerosol is also tolerogenic although the underlying mechanism may differ; mechanisms postulated include a role for a switch in the T cell response from Th1 to Th2 T cells with the concomitant change in cytokines and antibodies which that implies.

One very important fact which came out of the animal studies was that it was not only the aetiological antigen which could induce oral tolerance. For example, collagen is able to suppress not only collagen arthritis but also adjuvant arthritis and pristane arthritis. Similarly, MBP-induced EAE can be inhibited not only by MBP itself but also by other nervous system proteins. Most interestingly of all, the spontaneous diabetes which occurs in the non-obese diabetic (NOD) mouse can be suppressed by feeding oral insulin, which is, of course, not metabolically active. Thus it appears that tolerance is not causative antigen-specific but rather target organ-specific. This offers hope in conditions like RA where the aetiological agent remains unknown. The only double-blind study of oral tolerance reported in humans to date is a one year trial of daily bovine myelin 300 mg in patients with acute relapsing multiple sclerosis[79]. There was no clear beneficial benefit; the most significant result was a reduction in the frequency of MBP-specific T cells. However, a larger group of patients needs to be studied. A double-blind study using collagen type II as a tolerogen in RA is near completion.

However, it must be recalled that, if the initiating antigen were a foreign antigen, simpler possibilities such as antigen-specific chemotherapy or vaccination might be more appropriate paths to follow. In this regard, studies of antibiotic therapy in RA are of greater interest particularly in view of the recent data suggesting that tetracyclines may shorten and reduce the severity of arthritis in patients with chronic chlamydial reactive arthritis[80]. The issue of long-term antibiotic therapy in the treatment of rheumatoid arthritis is a contentious one, with investigators claiming success with several agents including rifampicin and tetracyclines[81]. Although these studies can be interpreted as supporting a bacterial aetiology for RA, many antibiotics, including those mentioned above, have profound immunoregulatory effects which are perhaps more likely to be responsible for the effect.

The MHC as target

It has been known for many years that RA is strongly associated in many, although not all populations, with particular class II MHC antigens notably

HLA-DR1 and DR4. It has also become clear more recently that HLA-DR4 in particular is associated with more severe disease, more erosions and a poorer functional outcome. This area is reviewed in more detail elsewhere in this book. Thus the MHC molecule is an obvious therapeutic target. Two approaches to targeting the MHC molecule exist, allele-specific MAb and MHC-binding peptides.

The technically simpler approach to targeting the MHC would be to use MAb yet there has been surprisingly little work in this area. In part, this may be because early studies using anti-MHC MAb in monkeys were associated with severe side-effects but later studies in other breeds did not confirm these poor results. Ferrone and his colleagues[82] immunized patients intramuscularly with an anti-HLA DR4 antibody hoping to generate an anti-anti-HLA DR4 response which would recognize HLA DR4. Thus the patient would generate his own ongoing anti-HLA DR4 response. Only a small number of patients were studied and, whilst there were no major side-effects, no clinical responses were seen and there was little evidence of an anti-idiotypic network. Further studies of the therapeutic potential of anti-HLA DR MAb appear long overdue.

The approach of using MHC-binding peptides initially appeared very promising. Animals could be protected against autoimmune diseases such as EAE by treating them, prior to inducing the disease, with a peptide which bound to the disease-associated MHC[83] although the effect in established disease was less certain. Subsequent studies confirmed that there was indeed *in vivo* MHC blockade preventing T cell activation[84] and also investigated the treatment in situations more similar to that required to treat established human disease[85]. At first, the mechanism was considered simply to be blockade of the disease-related MHC which inhibited access for the disease-inducing peptide. When it became clear that binding peptides which were analogues of the antigen were more effective than non-homologous blockers, it was realized that the situation was more complex. Subsequent studies have confirmed that therapy with blockers which are antigen-analogues involves other mechanisms including TCR antagonism (see below).

Two major problems have become obvious over time. Increasing experience of using peptides for therapy has confirmed their very short half-life. This is a particular problem for passive therapies where a sustained plasma level of peptide is required; however, it may be possible to make peptide mimetics which are less easily metabolized by substituting non-critical sites with non-natural structures. A more fundamental objection to this mode of therapy is that it depends on the association between HLA and disease being due to an ongoing role in antigen presentation as described at the beginning of the chapter. However, if the MHC association were due, for example, to a particular MHC biasing the thymic repertoire or to a non-MHC linked gene then the MHC would not be an appropriate therapeutic target.

The T cell as target

In many ways this cannot be separated from the use of the MHC as a target. The most obvious example of this is the use of MHC-binding peptides as

TCR antagonists (reviewed in [77]). TCR antagonism was first identified when it was observed that an MHC-binding peptide inhibited a T cell clone 1000 times more effectively when it was an analogue of the antigenic peptide than when it was a non-homologous blocker capable only of MHC blockade although the affinity of both peptides for the MHC was the same. What is the mechanism of TCR antagonism? The interaction of the antigenic peptide with the TCR is a high-affinity interaction in which first binding and then signalling occurs (agonist effect). In contrast, the interaction of the analogue blocking peptide with the TCR is a low-affinity interaction where the TCR is engaged but some intracellular signalling pathways, notably that involving protein kinase C, are not induced (antagonist effect). The use of TCR antagonism as therapy is still at the *in vitro* experimental stage. The most important hurdle to overcome is to identify the antigen; in this regard recent technical advances allowing the elution and sequencing of peptides bound to specific MHC molecules *in vivo* may represent a great advance.

An alternative approach to targeting the T cell is to stimulate the patient to develop an immune response against the disease-inducing T cells. This has been done in two ways, by vaccination with whole T cells (T cell vaccination; TCV) and by vaccination with peptides derived from the TCR. Both approaches have now been used in humans. The first to be developed was TCV (reviewed in [86] and [87]) in which pathogenic T cells, in an attenuated form, are injected into an animal to induce a specific immune response against them. This approach has been shown to be effective in protecting and treating animal models of T cell mediated autoimmune disease including induced conditions like EAE and adjuvant arthritis and spontaneous ones like diabetes in NOD mice. The vaccines were initially made from T cell lines or clones but, in an attempt to imitate the situation in human disease where causative-antigen specific T cell lines are not available, lymph node cells from primed animals were also shown to be effective. Most interestingly, it became apparent that TCV does not create an immunoregulatory network *de novo* but amplifies a naturally existing one which is either pre-formed or forms as the disease develops. The mechanism of TCV involves the generation of a CD4 and CD8 T cell response directed primarily at the TCR (anti-idiotypic) but also against activation markers (anti-ergotypic) on the vaccinating T cells. TCV has recently been tested in humans with MS and RA[88]. These studies differed from those in animals in that they used T cells from the lesions (synovium or spinal fluid) because it was thought that the pathogenic T cells would be at the highest concentration at these sites. These studies demonstrated that the technique was feasible and side-effect free but convincing clinical effects occurred infrequently. Worse, because the antigen was unknown, it was impossible to assess the effects of therapy on disease-specific immune processes so the dose and regime selected may not have been appropriate.

TCV, however successful, will always suffer from the difficulty that it needs to be customized to each individual patient. Since the main immune response in TCV is directed against the TCR, it was reasonable to assume that vaccination with peptides from the TCR itself would be equally effective and, if there was a common oligoclonal TCR usage among patients with a particular disease, the therapy could be standardized (reviewed in [87] and [89]). Vaccination with a TCR peptide from the TCR used by the encephalitogenic T cells has been shown to be effective in EAE, both in preventing and in treating the condition. The TCR peptide was shown to induce regulatory T cells and antibodies which downregulated the function of the encephalitogenic T cells but did not delete them. The current hypothesis is that these regulatory cells recognize naturally processed TCR epitopes expressed in association with the MHC on the surface of the encephalitogenic T cells. Following studies in animals, TCR peptide vaccination has been studied in MS, in which MBP is a candidate autoantigen. The same restricted TCR usage of $V\beta5.2$ and $V\beta6$ has been observed both in MS brain tissue and in MBP-specific T cell clones from the blood of MS patients. A pilot study has used TCR peptides from either $V\beta5.2$ or $V\beta6$ to treat patients with chronic progressive MS[89]. It has demonstrated that these peptides are not toxic and can induce increased frequency of $V\beta5.2$ and $V\beta6$ specific T cells. Tantalizingly, the therapy also decreases the frequency of MBP-specific T cells but numbers are too small to assess efficacy. This approach is very promising, being selective and non-toxic but, until either a candidate autoantigen or a restricted TCR usage has been convincingly shown, it cannot be used in RA.

THE FUTURE

Over the last few years, it has been very exciting to watch the application of our new knowledge of immunopathogenesis to therapy. Now the honeymoon is over and real practical difficulties have to be overcome. These may be pharmacological, for example the poor bioavailability of peptides or the residual immunogenicity of even chimerized and humanized MAb. They may relate to toxicity since effective immunosuppression, unless absolutely specific for some unique aspect of disease pathogenesis, will inevitably result in opportunistic infection. Only now are sufficient numbers of patients being studied to evaluate such problems. Some difficulties have been financial; the small biotechnology companies do not have the reserves of the large pharmaceutical concerns which are required for an industry with such a long lead time and such a high failure rate. This has resulted in potentially effective agents being withdrawn and, more seriously, may mean that if a single agent against a particular target is unsuccessful, the target will be abandoned. The inappropriateness of this is clear when one considers the different properties of the various anti-CD4 MAb. It will also be difficult, for commercial reasons, to conduct comparative studies of two biological agents and even more problematic to do combination studies. Patient selection is also a problem; for ethical reasons most studies of new agents are done in refractory patients yet in these patients, the immunologically active stage of their disease may be past and certainly their disease has proved unresponsive to conventional therapy. Most seriously of all, when an agent proves ineffective, how do we know whether this is simply that the particular biological agent does not inhibit the target effectively or whether this means that our assumptions about the disease are wrong. Ultimately, the use of biologicals will allow us to learn still more about the disease process and to identify even more closely the most appropriate therapeutic targets. The jury is still out on whether, in the final analysis, these targets will be most effectively targeted biologically or by standard pharmaceutical preparations.

References

1. Veys EM, Mielants H, Verbruggen G, de Keyser F. Intervention with immunomodulatory agents: new pharmacological developments. In: Emery P, ed. Baillière's Clinical Rheumatology Volume 6: management of early inflammatory arthritis. London: Baillière Tindall; 1992: 455–484.
2. Thomson AW. The spectrum of action of new immunosuppressive drugs. Clin Exp Immunol. 1992; 89: 170–173.
3. Kingsley GH, Lanchbury J, Panayi GS, eds. Proceedings of the Second International Symposium on the Immunotherapy of the Rheumatic Diseases; 1993 April 1–4; Brighton, England. Clin Exp Rheumatol. 1993; 11 (Suppl 8).
4. Moses M. A cartilage-derived inhibitor of neovascularization and metalloproteinases. Clin Exp Rheumatol. 1993; 11 (Suppl 8): 67–69.
5. Gordon JL, Drummond AH, Galloway WA. Metalloproteinase inhibitors as therapeutics. Clin Exp Rheumatol. 1993; 11 (Suppl 8): 91–94.
6. Panayi GS. The immunopathogenesis of rheumatoid arthritis. Rheumatology Review. 1992; 1: 63–74.
7. Panayi GS, Kingsley GH, Lanchbury JS. Immunotherapy of Immune-mediated Diseases. Q J Med. 1992; 84: 489–495.
8. Panayi GS, Lanchbury JS, Kingsley GH. The importance of the T cell in initiating and maintaining the chronic synovitis of rheumatoid arthritis. Arthritis Rheum. 1993; 35: 729–735.
9. Lanchbury JS. Genetic aspects of rheumatoid arthritis. Clin Exp Rheumatol. 1993; 11 (Suppl 8): 9–11.
10. Marguerie C, Lunardi C, So A. PCR based analysis of TCR repertoire in human autoimmune diseases. Immunol Today. 1992; 13: 336–338.
11. Keelan E, Haskard DO. CAMs and anti-CAMs, the clinical potential of cell adhesion molecules. J R Coll Phys Lond. 1992; 26: 17–24.
12. Pitzalis C. Adhesion and migration of inflammatory cells. Clin Exp Rheumatol. 1993; 11 (Suppl 8): 71–76.
13. Elices MJ, Tamraz S, Tollefson V, Vollger LW. The integrin VLA-4 mediates leukocyte recruitment to skin inflammatory sites in vivo. Clin Exp Rheumatol. 1993; 11 (Suppl 8): 77–80.
14. Sieper J, Kingsley G, Palacios-Boix A, Pitzalis C, Treharne J, Keat A, Panayi GS. Synovial T lymphocyte-specific immune response to Chlamydia trachomatis in Reiter's disease. Arthritis Rheum. 1991; 34: 588–598.
15. Sieper J, Braun J, Wu P, Kingsley G. T cells are responsible for the enhanced synovial cellular immune response to triggering antigen in reactive arthritis. Clin Exp Immunol. 1993; 91: 96–102.
16. Janossy G, Panayi G, Duke O, Bofill M, Poulter LW, Goldstein G. Rheumatoid arthritis: a disease of T-lymphocyte macrophage immunoregulation. Lancet. 1981; 2: 839–842.
17. Firestein GS, Zvaifler NJ. How important are T cells in chronic synovitis? Arthritis Rheum. 1990; 33: 768–773.
18. Paulus HE, Machleder HI, Levine S, Yu DTY, MacDonald NS. Lymphocyte involvement in rheumatoid arthritis. Studies during thoracic duct drainage. Arthritis Rheum. 1977; 20: 1249–1262.
19. Karsh J, Klippel JH, Plotz PH, Wright DG, Flye MW. Lymphapheresis in rheumatoid arthritis: a randomised trial. Arthritis Rheum. 1981; 24: 867–873.
20. Emery P, Smith GN, Panayi GS. Lymphocytapheresis – a feasible treatment for rheumatoid arthritis. Br J Rheumatol. 1986; 25: 40–43.
21. Wahl SM, Wilder RL, Katona IM et al. Leukapheresis in rheumatoid arthritis. Arthritis

Rheum. 1983; 26: 1076–1084.
22. Burmester GR, Hahn G, Stuhlmuller B, Kalden JR, Pfizenmaier K. Modulation of monocyte activation in patients with rheumatoid arthritis (RA) by leukapheresis therapy. Arthritis Rheum. 1993; 35: S199.
23. Soden M, Hassan J, Scott DL, Hanly JG, Moriarty M, Whelan A, Feighery C, Bresnihan B. Lymphoid irradiation in intractable rheumatoid arthritis. Arthritis Rheum. 1989; 32: 523–530.
24. Gaston JSH, Strober S, Solovera JJ, Gandour D, Lane N, Schurman D, Hoppe RT, Chin RC, Eugui EM, Vaughan JH, Allison AC. Dissection of the mechanisms of immune injury in rheumatoid arthritis, using total lymphoid irradiation. Arthritis Rheum. 1988; 31: 21–30.
25. Schreiber SL, Crabtree GR. The mechanism of action of cyclosporin A and FK506. Immunology Today. 1992; 13: 136–142.
26. Erlanger BF. Do we know the site of action of cyclosporin? Immunology Today. 1992; 13: 487–490.
27. Russell RGG, Graveley R, Skjodt H. The effects of cyclosporin on bone and cartilage. Br J Rheumatol. 1993; 32 (Suppl 1): 42–46.
28. Tugwell P. Cyclosporine in rheumatoid arthritis: documented efficacy and safety. Seminars in Arthritis and Rheumatism. 1992; 21: 30–38.
29. Ludwin D, Alexopolou I. Cyclosporin A nephropathy in patients with rheumatoid arthritis. Br J Rheumatol. 1993; 32 (suppl 1): 60–65.
30. Arellano F, Krupp P. Malignancies in rheumatoid arthritis patients treated with cyclosporin A. Br J Rheumatol. 1993; 32 (suppl 1): 72–75.
31. Cohen DJ, Appel GB. Cyclosporine: nephrotoxic effects and guidelines for safe use in patients with rheumatoid arthritis. Seminars in Arthritis and Rheumatism. 1992; 21: 43–48.
32. Waldmann H. Manipulation of T-cell responses with monoclonal antibodies. Annu Rev Immunol. 1989; 7: 407–444.
33. Mayforth RD, Quintans J. Designer and catalytic antibodies. N Engl J Med. 1990; 323: 173–178.
34. Kirkham BW, Pitzalis C, Kingsley GH, Chikanza IC, Sabharwal C, Barbatis C, Grahame R, Gibson T, Amlot PL, Panayi GS. Monoclonal antibody treatment in rheumatoid arthritis: the clinical and immunological effects of a CD7 monoclonal antibody. Br J Rheumatol. 1991; 30: 459–463.
35. Costantinides I, Kingsley G, Pitzalis C, Panayi GS. Inhibition of proliferation by a monoclonal antibody (RFT2) against CD7. Clin Exp Immunol. 1991; 85: 164–167.
36. Kirkham BW, Thien F, Pelton BK, Pitzalis C, Amlot P, Denman AM, Panayi GS. Chimeric CD7 monoclonal antibody therapy in rheumatoid arthritis. J Rheumatol. 1992; 19: 1348–1352.
37. Lazarovits AI, White MJ, Karsh J. CD7- Tcells in rheumatoid arthritis. Arthritis Rheum. 1992; 35: 615–624.
38. Banerjee S, Wei B-Y, Hillman K, Luthra HS, David CS. Immunosuppression of collagen-induced arthritis in mice with an anti IL2 receptor antibody. J Immunol. 1988; 141: 1150–1154.
39. Kyle V, Coughlan RJ, Tighe H, Waldmann H, Hazleman BL. Beneficial effect of monoclonal antibody to interleukin-2 receptor on activated T cells in rheumatoid arthritis. Ann Rheum Dis. 1989; 48: 428–429.
40. Woodworth TG. Early clinical studies of IL-2 fusion toxin in patients with severe rheumatoid arthritis and recent onset diabetes mellitus. Clin Exp Rheumatol. 1993; 11 (Suppl 8): 177–180.
41. Strand V, Lee ML and the CD5 Plus RA Investigators Group. Differential patterns of response in patients with rheumatoid arthritis following administration of an anti-CD5 immunoconjugate. Clin Exp Rheumatol. 1993; 11 (Suppl 8): 161–164.
42. Verwilghen J, Kingsley GH, Ceuppens JL, Panayi GS. Inhibition of synovial fluid T cell proliferation by anti-CD5 monoclonal antibodies: a potential mechanism for their immunotherapeutic action in vivo. Arthritis Rheum. 1992; 35: 1445–1452.
43. Wacholtz MC, Lipsky PE. Treatment of lupus nephritis with CD5 PLUS, an immunoconjugate of an anti-CD5 monoclonal antibody and ricin A chain. Arthritis Rheum. 1992; 35: 837–838.

44. Mathieson PW, Cobbold SP, Hale G, Clark MR, Oliveira DBG, Lockwood CM, Waldmann H. Monoclonal antibody therapy in systemic vasculitis. N Engl J Med. 1990; 323: 250–254.
45. Isaacs JD, Watts RA, Hazleman BL, Hale G, Keogan MT, Cobbold SP, Waldmann H. Humanised monoclonal antibody therapy for rheumatoid arthritis. Lancet. 1992; 340: 748–752.
46. Watts RA, Isaacs JD, Hale G, Hazleman BL, Waldmann H. Campath-1H in inflammatory arthritis. Clin Exp Rheumatol. 1993; 11 (Suppl 8): 165–167.
47. Weinblatt ME, Johnston JM, Hazleman BL, Manna VK and the CAMPATH-1H RA Investigators. Treatment of rheumatoid arthritis (RA) with single-dose infusion of Campath-1H. Arthritis Rheum. 1992; 35 (Suppl): S105.
48. Johnston JM, Hays AE, Heitman CK, St Clair EW, Jacobs MR, Yocum DE, Thakor MS, Achkar AA, Matteson EL. Treatment of rheumatoid arthritis (RA) patients by subcutaneous infusion of Campath-1H. Arthritis Rheum. 1992; 35 (Suppl): S105.
49. Ranges GE, Sriram S, Cooper SM. Prevention of type II collagen-induced arthritis by in vivo treatment with anti-L3T4. J Exp Med. 1985; 162: 378–391.
50. Herzog C, Walker C, Pichler W, Aeschlimann A, Wassmer P, Stockinger H, Knapp W, Rieber P, Muller W. Monoclonal anti-CD4 therapy in arthritis. Lancet. 1987; 2: 1461–1462.
51. Herzog C, Walker C, Muller W, Rieber P, Reiter C, Riethmuller G, Wassmer P, Stockinger H, Madic O, Pichler WJ. Anti-CD4 antibody treatment of patients with rheumatoid arthritis: I Effect on clinical course and circulating T cells. J Autoimmunity. 1989; 2: 627–642.
52. Walker C, Herzog C, Rieber P, Riethmuller G, Muller W, Pichler WJ. Anti-CD4 antibody treatment of patients with rheumatoid arthritis: II Effect of in vivo treatment on in vitro proliferative response of CD4 cells. J Autoimmunity. 1989; 2: 643–649.
53. Reiter C, Kakavand B, Rieber EP, Schattenkirchner M, Riethmuller G, Kruger K. Treatment of rheumatoid arthritis with monoclonal CD4 antibody M-T151. Arthritis Rheum. 1991; 34: 525–536.
54. Horneff G, Burmester GR, Emmrich F, Kalden JR. Treatment of rheumatoid arthritis with an anti-CD4 monoclonal antibody. Arthritis Rheum. 1991; 34: 129–140.
55. Wendling D, Wijdenes J, Racadot E, Morel-Fourier B. Therapeutic use of monoclonal anti-CD4 antibody in rheumatoid arthritis. J Rheumatol. 1991; 18: 325–327.
56. Didri C, Portales P, Andary M, Brochier J, Combe B, Clot J, Sany J. Treatment of rheumatoid arthritis with monoclonal anti-CD4 antibodies. Clinical results. Arthritis Rheum. 1991; 34 (Suppl). S92.
57. Goldberg D, Morel P, Chatenoud DL, Boitard C, Menkes CJ, Bertoye PH, Revillard JP, Bach JF. Immunological effects of high dose administration of anti-CD4 antibody in rheumatoid arthritis patients. J Autoimmunity. 1991; 4: 617–630.
58. Chatenoud L, Goldberg D, Viard J-P, Dain M-P. A pilot study using an anti-CD4 monoclonal antibody (OKT4A) in rheumatoid arthritis. Arthritis Rheum. 1992; 35 (Suppl): S106.
59. Burmester GR, Emmrich F. Anti-CD4 therapy in rheumatoid arthritis. Clin Exp Rheumatol. 1993; 11 (Suppl 8): 139–145.
60. Choy EHS, Kingsley GH, Panayi GS. Treatment with anti-CD4 monoclonal antibody and interstitial nephritis. Arthritis Rheum (in press).
61. van der Lubbe PA, Reiter C, Riethmuller G, Breedveld FC. Anti-CD4 therapy in rheumatoid arthritis. Arthritis Rheum (in press).
62. Moreland LW, Bucy RP, Tilden A, Pratt PW, LoBuglio AF, Khazaeli M, Everson MP, Daddona P, Ghrayeb J, Kilgariff, Sanders ME, Koopman WJ. Use of a chimeric monoclonal anti-CD4 antibody in patients with refractory rheumatoid arthritis. Arthritis Rheum. 1993; 36: 307–318.
63. Choy EHS, Chikanza IC, Kingsley GH, Corrigall V, Panayi GS. Treatment of rheumatoid arthritis with single dose or weekly pulses of chimeric anti-CD4 monoclonal antibody. Scand J Immunol. 1992; 36: 291–298.
64. Choy EHS, Kingsley GH. Anti-CD4 therapy in rheumatoid arthritis. Clin Exp Rheumatol. 1993; 11 (Suppl 8): 147–149.
65. Moreland LW, Pratt PW, Sanders ME, Koopman WJ. Experience with a chimeric monoclonal anti-CD4 antibody in the treatment of refractory rheumatoid arthritis. Clin Exp Rheumatol. 1993; 11 (Suppl 8): 153–159.

66. Newell MK, Haughn LJ, Maroun CR, Julius MH. Death of mature T cells by separate ligation of CD4 and the T cell receptor for antigen. Nature. 1990; 347: 286–289.
67. Horneff G, Sack U, Kalden JR, Emmrich F, Burmester GR. Reduction of monocyte-macrophage markers upon anti-CD4 treatment. Decreased levels of IL-1, IL-6, neopterin and soluble CD14 in patients with rheumatoid arthritis. Clin Exp Immunol. 1993; 91: 207–213.
68. Cobbold SP, Martin G, Waldmann H. The induction of skin graft tolerance in major histocompatibility complex mismatched or primed recipients: primed T cells can be tolerised in the periphery with anti-CD4 and anti-CD8 antibodies. Eur J Immunol. 1990; 20: 2747–2755.
69. Kavanaugh AF, Nichols LA, Lipsky PE. Treatment of refractory rheumatoid arthritis with an anti-CD54 (intercellular adhesion molecule-1, ICAM-1) monoclonal antibody. Arthritis Rheum. 1992; 35: S43.
70. Kavanaugh AF, Norris S, Rothlein R, Nichols LA, Lipsky PE. Pharmacokinetic analysis of rheumatoid arthritis patients treated with an anti-CD54 (intercellular adhesion molecule-1, ICAM-1) monoclonal antibody. Arthritis Rheum. 1992; 35: S106.
71. Corkill MM, Kirkham BW, Haskard DO, Barbatis C, Gibson T, Panayi GS. Gold treatment of rheumatoid arthritis decreases synovial expression of the endothelial leukocyte adhesion receptor ELAM-1. J Rheumatol. 1991; 18: 1453–1460.
72. Picker LJ, Michie SA, Rott LS, Butcher EC. A unique phenotype of skin associated lymphocytes in humans. Am J Pathol. 1990; 136: 1053–1067.
73. Williams RO, Feldmann M, Maini RN. Anti-tumour necrosis factor ameliorates joint disease in murine collagen induced arthritis. Proc Natl Acad Sci USA. 1992; 9784–9788.
74. Keffer J, Probert L, Cazlaris H, Georgopoulos S, Kazlaris E, Kioussis D et al. Transgenic mice expressing tumour necrosis factor: a predictive genetic model of arthritis. EMBO J. 1991; 10: 4025–4031.
75. Elliot MJ, Maini RN, Feldmann M, Charles P. Treatment of rheumatoid arthritis with chimaeric monoclonal antibodies to TNF-α. Safety, clinical efficacy and control of the acute phase response. Clin Rheumatol. 1993; 12: 34.
76. Lebsack ME, Paul CC, Bloedow DC, Burch FX, Sack MA, Chase W, Catalano MA. Subcutaneous IL-1 receptor antagonist in patients with rheumatoid arthritis. Arthritis Rheum. 1992; 34 (Suppl): 545.
77. Grey HM, Alexander L, Snoke K, Sette A, Ruppert J. Antigen analogues as antagonists of the T cell receptor. Clin Exp Rheumatol. 1993; 11 (Suppl 8): 47–50.
78. Miller A, Lider O, Weiner H. Antigen-driven bystander suppression after oral administration of antigens. J Exp Med. 1991; 174: 791–798.
79. Weiner HL, Mackin GA, Matsui M, Orav EJ, Khoury SJ, Dawson DM, Hafler DA. Double blind trial of oral tolerisation with myelin antigens in early relapsing-remitting multiple sclerosis. Science. 1993; 259: 1321–1324.
80. Lauhio A, Leirisalo-Repo M, Lahdevirta J, Saikku P, Repo H. Double-blind placebo-controlled study of three-month treatment with lymecycline in reactive arthritis with special reference to chlamydial arthritis. Arthritis Rheum. 1991; 34: 6–14.
81. Kloppenburg M, Breedveld FC, Miltenburg AMM, Dijkmans BAC. Antibiotics as disease modifiers in arthritis. Clin Exp Rheumatol. 1993; 11 (Suppl 8): 113–115.
82. Fiocco U, Cozzi L, Cozzi E, Fagiolo U, Ferrone S. Murine monoclonal antibodies to HLA antigens in the treatment of rheumatoid arthritis: a phase 1 clinical trial. Eur J Clin Invest. 1991; 21: 64.
83. Lamont AG, Sette A, Fujinami R, Colon SM, Miles C, Grey HM. Inhibition of experimental autoimmune encephalomyelitis induction in SJL/J mice by using a peptide with high affinity for I-A^s. J Immunol. 1990; 145: 1687.
84. Guery JC, Sette A, Leighton J, Dragomir A, Adorini L. Selective immunosuppression by adminstration of major histocompatibility complex (MHC) class II binding peptides. I. Evidence for in vivo MHC blockade preventing T cell activation. J Exp Med. 1992; 175: 1345.
85. Adorini L, Nagy ZA. Peptide competition for antigen presentation. Immunol Today. 1990; 11: 21.
86. Mor F, Cohen IR. Experimental aspects of T cell vaccination. Clin Exp Rheumatol. 1993; 11 (Suppl 8): 55–57.

87. Kingsley GH, Panayi GS. Intervention with immunomodulatory agents: T cell vaccination. In: Emery P, ed. Baillière's Clinical Rheumatology Volume 6: management of early inflammatory arthritis. London: Baillière Tindall; 1992: 435–454.
88. Kingsley GH, Verwilghen J. T cell vaccination in humans. Clin Exp Rheumatol. 1993; 11 (Suppl 8): 63–64.
89. Vandenbark AA, Bourdette DN, Whitham R, Chou YK, Hashim GA, Offner H. T cell receptor peptide therapy in EAE and MS. Clin Exp Rheumatol. 1993; 11 (Suppl 8): 51–53.

18
Immune Reactions Against Heat Shock Proteins and Arthritis

P. RES, J. THOLE, F. BREEDVELD and R. DE VRIES

INTRODUCTION

During the last decade our insight into the aetiology and pathogenesis of supposedly autoimmune diseases like rheumatoid arthritis made considerable progress: they seem to be helper T lymphocyte (T cell) mediated; possible triggering and/or target antigens have been identified and aberrant expression of human leucocyte antigens (products of the HLA system, the human major histocompatibility complex) may be involved in the presentation of these antigens to helper T cells. The helper T cell, which is a class II-restricted CD4 positive T cell, plays a central role in orchestrating the immune response. The way it does so is by producing cytokines or lymphokines, which regulate, at least, all the other activated (by antigen) players of the immune system. Thus the most specific and efficient immunotherapy for an autoimmune disease is to shut off the button that specifically turns on the autoreactive helper T cell. That button is the HLA molecule presenting an autoantigen to the T cell receptor of an autoreactive helper T cell. How this button for autoreactive helper T cells (Th) may indeed be turned off very efficiently, has been shown in experimental animal models and has been further discussed in the previous chapter by Kingsley and Panayi on Immunotherapy. One such animal model that has stimulated a lot of research in this direction has been adjuvant arthritis (AA), which is induced in susceptible animals (Lewis rats) by the injection of *Mycobacterium tuberculosis* in oil. In this model, helper T cells from affected Lewis rats have been isolated that are capable of transferring the disease to naive animals. These T cells recognize epitopes on a mycobacterial heat shock protein of 65 kDa (hsp65). In this chapter we will review the studies performed in the last 6 or 7 years, that have addressed the possible role of heat shock proteins, and in particular hsp65, in the pathogenesis of, respectively, reactive and rheumatoid arthritis.

HEAT SHOCK PROTEINS

hsp belong to some of the most conserved and abundant proteins throughout nature. On the basis of their approximate molecular mass, hsp can be divided into a number of families, and members of the hsp65, hsp70 and hsp90 families are probably present in all prokaryotes and eukaryotes[1,2]. At the amino acid level, extreme conservation between members of the same family in distantly related organisms exists. For example, hsp65 of *Mycobacterium tuberculosis* is approximately 50% identical to human homologue in mitochondria and displays 20% conservative replacements[3].

Under physiological conditions hsp65, hsp70 and hsp90 function as so-called molecular chaperons that, by transient binding to proteins, guide their assembly into oligomeric structures, their folding and unfolding during transport into various compartments, or their degradation by proteolytic enzymes[4]. Other hsp are in fact proteases that degrade misfolded or 'foreign' proteins. The ATPase activity of many hsp probably assists in these functions. Different hsp families interact with a variety of different proteins. For example, hsp70 members bind to immunoglobulin heavy chains, clathrin baskets and tumour antigen p53, whereas hsp90 binds to steroid hormone receptors, to DNA replication complexes, to actin and to tubulin.

Under a variety of stress stimuli such as heat – hence the term hsp – but also nutrient deprivation, oxygen radicals, viral, bacterial and parasitic infections, cells respond by increasing the production of specific hsp. For example, in the bacterium *Escherichia coli*, hsp65 accounts for approximately 1% of the total cell protein when grown at 37°C, but accumulates up to 15% soon after the cells are shifted to 46°C[5]. In eukaryotic cells, hsp do not generally accumulate to such extreme levels, and some members are probably not inducible. In both prokaryotes and eukaryotes, each hsp family probably consists of multiple members. In mycobacteria very recently a second member of the hsp65 family was identified[6]. The relative expression of both members under physiological and under stress conditions is currently not known. Within the hsp70 family of *Drosophila*, seven copies of inducible hsp genes were identified[2]. In addition, seven non-inducible related genes (heat-shock cognates) were found. These are constitutively expressed in the cell under normal conditions. Upon heat shock, the intracellular localization of hsp in eukaryotes often changes, and some of them may even become expressed at the cell surface[7,8]. hsp65 of the mycobacteria has been shown to be present in the cell wall fraction and in culture medium under conditions of stress[9,10]. hsp probably protect the cell during adverse conditions by maintaining a functional conformation of essential proteins, and by assisting in the removal of denatured proteins.

IMMUNE REACTIVITY TO HEAT SHOCK PROTEINS: FRIEND OR FOE?

A number of studies have indicated that hsp are major targets for the host immune response against pathogenic micro-organisms. In particular, hsp65, hsp70 and hsp90 are frequently recognized[11,12]. For example, hsp65 is a dominant antigen for serum antibodies in individuals infected with bacteria such as *Coxiella, Legionella, Treponema* and *Borrelia*[13-16]. In man and mice exposed to mycobacteria, a high proportion of T cells and antibodies were found to respond to mycobacterial hsp65[17-21]. In sera of patients with malaria and trypanosomiasis, antibodies were identified which recognized hsp70 and hsp90[22-24].

However, hsp-reactive T cells and antibodies can also be demonstrated in healthy controls. This has been most extensively studied using the human and mycobacterial hsp65 molecules and derived peptides. About 20% of all human T cell lines generated with purified protein derivative (PPD) or BCG displayed cytotoxicity against targets pulsed with mycobacterial hsp65, indicating the immunodominance of this hsp in the normal repertoire[25]. Proliferative and cytotoxic T cell clones responding to the mycobacteria hsp65 have been isolated from normal controls (Ottenhoff, personal communication)[26]. One of the proliferative clones also recognized the human homologue, indicating the presence of autoreactive T cells in normal individuals[26]. Other evidence that supported the recognition of self hsp65 came from Munk et al.[27], who studied the specificity of *M. tuberculosis*-induced T cell lines from normal individuals. Eight out of nine of these lines expressed DR-restricted cytotoxicity, not only against monocytes pulsed with trypsinized mycobacterial hsp65, but also against monocytes pulsed with synthetic peptides identical to shared parts of human hsp65. Evidence for recognition of self hsp65 was also obtained from studies demonstrating lysis of antigen-unloaded macrophages by mycobacterial hsp65-induced human T cell lines[25,28]. In this case self hsp65 on the surface of the macrophages is probably recognized. Namely, hsp65 cell surface expression, that could be markedly induced by interferon (IFN)-γ treatment, was found on murine bone marrow macrophages by staining with ML30, an antibody reactive to mycobacterial and human hsp65[29]. The effector cells within the lines responsible for the cytolysis were predominantly CD4$^+$ and major histocompatibility complex (MHC) cells II restricted[25,28,30]. Also, in mice, mycobacterial hsp65-reactive T cells were found that recognized autologous hsp65; spleen T cell lines induced with tryptic fragments of the mycobacterial hsp65, lysed bone marrow macrophages stressed by IFN-γ treatment or by infection with murine cytomegalovirus[31]. In addition such cytotoxic T lymphocytes (CTL) lysed Schwann cells after a stress treatment[32]. In mice, the 65-kDa-reactive CTL were CD8+ and MHC class I restricted[31,32]. hsp may be immunodominant in both healthy and infected individuals, because these are proteins abundantly present not only in pathogenic but also non-pathogenic micro-organisms, especially under the adverse conditions imposed upon them by the host environment. In addition, the presence of stressed or transformed autologous cells and a variety of micro-organisms in the host environment ensures the almost continuous restimulation of immunological memory for hsp. Finally, some hsp may be intrinsically antigenic, because they are easily processed and presented to the immune system. The fact that some of the hsp65, hsp70 and hsp90 are naturally 'sticky' may be of some significance in this respect. The function of the immune response to hsp is probably twofold. Firstly, it may be used to eliminate pathogenic microorganisms. The rapidity of this immune response provides a first line of defence before immunity to pathogen-specific antigens is mounted. Secondly, the response to self epitopes on hsp may function in eliminating stressed or transformed autologous cells because of a sufficient concentration of self hsp epitopes on their surface, whereas normal cells do not generate this density of self epitopes at their outer membranes. If either the stress response or immunity to hsp is not properly regulated at certain sites in the host, immunopathology and/or autoimmunity may arise.

Before discussing the role of hsp65 in human arthritis, we will briefly discuss the role of this molecule in an animal model.

Adjuvant arthritis

Adjuvant arthritis (AA) is a type of arthritis that can be induced in a genetically susceptible strain of female Lewis rats by immunization with complete Freund's adjuvant, i.e. a sonicate of *M. tuberculosis* in an emulsion of oil. The clinical symptoms in affected animals resemble the ones found in RA patients and, therefore, investigation of AA has directed a lot of attention towards mycobacteria as possible inducing agents of RA.

An AA-inducing T cell clone, A2b, has been isolated from a rat with AA induced by *M. tuberculosis*. A2b responds to hsp65 of *M. tuberculosis* and to proteoglycans, but not to mammalian hsp65[33-35]. Immunization with hsp65 induces resistance to subsequent attempts to induce AA either by immunization with *M. tuberculosis* or transfer of A2b cells[33,36]. The epitope on hsp65 recognized by A2b has been identified, and a peptide analogue binding to the presenting MHC-molecule was shown to prevent AA after immunization before disease induction[37]. In addition, a T cell clone M1 recognizing a different T cell epitope on hsp65 was identified that could be used as a vaccine: upon immunization with these cells the recipient rat becomes resistant to AA, probably resulting from activation of T cells responding to the idiotype of the M1 cells. The balance in a network formed by idiotype-specific helper and suppressor T cells was found to determine whether resistance or susceptibility to AA is developed after a certain treatment. Whatever the mechanism may be, it is clear that responses to the *M. tuberculosis* hsp65 play a crucial role in AA.

Reactive arthritis

ReA is a joint disease that starts after an infection of the gastrointestinal or the genitourinary tract with bacteria such as *Salmonella, Yersinia, Campylobacter* or *Chlamydia*[38]. HLA B27 confers an increased risk to develop ReA.

Synovial fluid mononuclear cells (SFMNC) of ReA patients display a clear reactivity against the triggering organisms[39-41]. Antigens of the bacteria which induce the ReA can be demonstrated in the affected joint, although attempts to culture organisms from the joint thus far have been unsuccessful[42,43]. Nevertheless, the above suggest a direct stimulation of joint T cells by bacterial antigens as a cause of joint inflammation in ReA, although in this case it would be difficult to explain the specific localization of the disease in the joints and the association of ReA with HLA B27. A direct stimulation of T cells by components of the triggering organism itself in the joint is also supported by the work of Stagg et al.[44]. In this study, *Chlamydia*- and PPD-reactive T cell lines were generated from SFMNC of a patient with a *Chlamydia*-induced ReA, whose SFMNC responded better to both antigen preparations than the peripheral blood mononuclear cells (PBMNC). The *Chlamydia*-reactive line did not cross-react with PPD and vice versa, indicating that the responses to the *Chlamydia*-reactive line are caused by different joint T cell populations. Synovial fluid dendritic cells (SFDC) from the same patient were found to induce proliferation of the *Chlamydia*-reactive T cell line but not of the PPD-reactive T cell line. Probably the SFDC carried *Chlamydia* antigens, although the possibility cannot be excluded that *Chlamydia*-reactive T cells recognized self antigens presented by the SFDC. The latter possibility is supported by Hermann et al.[45], who studied *Yersinia*-induced ReA. A T cell clone was identified that reacted to *Yersinia* hsp65, but also to mycobacterial and human hsp65. In addition, unstimulated SFMNC and heat shocked PBMNC were recognized by this clone. These data clearly indicate that T cells induced to bacterial hsp65 in ReA may also respond to autologous (human) hsp65.

From the studies of Gaston et al.[46-48] it is also evident that the bacterial hsp65 can be a protein recognized by synovial T cells. DR3-restricted T cell clones responsive to amino acids (aa) 1–15 of the mycobacterial hsp65 could be isolated from SFMNC cells of a patient with the clinical picture of ReA. However, this patient had no known history of a preceding infection of the gastrointestinal or the genitourinary tract and it was suggested that mycobacteria might have caused the arthritis. Using mycobacterial hsp65, the cloning procedure specifically selected for T cells responsive to this particular mycobacterial hsp.

SFMNC of a *Salmonella*-infected ReA patient were found to proliferate optimally to those *Salmonella* immunoblot fractions which contain hsp65[46]. From another patient with a *Salmonella*-associated arthritis, SFMNC were cloned in an antigen-specific manner with either *Salmonella* antigens or mycobacterial hsp65. The cloning procedure with *Salmonella* yielded *Salmonella*-specific and mycobacterial hsp65 cross-reactive clones. All clones obtained using the mycobacterial hsp65 were cross-reactive, responding to both the mycobacterial hsp65 and *Salmonella*. Further analysis of the antigen specificity of four cross-reactive clones revealed that they may not recognize the mycobacterial hsp65 but *E. coli* contaminants present in the recombinant preparation. In fact, one of these clones responded to the *E. coli* hsp65, and this cross-reactive clone may also recognize the hsp65 of *Salmonella*[48,49]. It would be interesting to know whether the other *Salmonella*-specific and *E. coli* cross-reactive clones also respond to hsp.

The proliferative responses of SFMNC from 13 patients with ReA against the triggering bacteria correlated significantly with the recombinant mycobacterial hsp65, whereas the responses to this latter preparation did not correlate with PPD, which is known to contain hsp65[48]. This finding indicates that the SFMNC responses to the recombinant mycobacterial hsp65 preparation were perhaps directed to *E. coli* contaminants, which would better explain the correlation between the SFMNC responses to the triggering bacteria and the recombinant hsp65 preparation, since *E. coli* is closely related to some of the bacteria implicated in ReA. Furthermore, SFMNC usually respond to *E. coli* in addition to the triggering bacteria. Hence, at least part of the SFMNC responses to antigens present in the bacteria associated with ReA and to *E. coli* antigens are exerted by the same T cells, as was the case in the above-mentioned patient. In addition to epitopes on hsp65, the epitopes involved may well be part of other conserved bacterial molecules.

Rheumatoid arthritis

Within the synovium, T cells are found in close contact with the extensions of dendritic-like cells[50]. The joint T cells are mainly CD4+, CDw29+ and HLA-DR+, and dendritic cells (DC) are known to be excellent APC[51-53]. Thus it is conceivable that T cells are activated in the joint after recognition of peptides presented by DC. Obviously, it is of major importance to detect which antigens/epitopes are responsible for the induction of joint T cell activation. In the next paragraphs we will discuss the experimental findings which are in favour of, or in contradiction with, a role of mycobacterial antigens, in particular hsp65, in the pathogenesis of RA.

Assuming that the number of T cells in the joint responding to antigens present in the joint is increased as a result of local proliferation, then elevated *in vitro* reactivity of SFMNC compared to PBMNC against certain antigens could well be a reflection of a specific expansion of the T cells recognizing those antigens or cross-reactive ones in the joint. The finding that SFMNC of patients with RA or other forms of chronic arthritis displayed an enhanced *in vitro* response to an acetone-precipitate of *M. tuberculosis* was therefore interpreted as an important indication that *M. tuberculosis* reactive T cells, in analogy to the AA model, could also be involved in the pathogenesis of RA[54-56].

In a follow-up study we demonstrated that the increased antigen reactivity of SFMNC is not specifically directed to *M. tuberculosis* antigens, but was also measured with about the same magnitude and frequency of positive responses (SI > 3) against *E. coli* antigens[57]. Moreover, the increased antigen reactivity seems to be a general feature of cells from sites of chronic inflammation, because pleural exudate mononuclear cells (PEMNC) from non-RA patients with a pulmonary disorder other than tuberculosis also displayed the same elevated responses to *M. tuberculosis* and *E. coli* when compared to PBMNC from the same individuals. *M. tuberculosis* and *E. coli* are not unique in their capacity to provoke strong SFMNC responses; also *M. bovis* BCG, collagen type II, and *Salmonella* have this ability[46,58,59]. Thus far tetanus toxoid has been the only exception; SFMNC of RA patients often display a decreased response to this antigen[55,58,59]. It is not conceivable that the elevated responses of SFMNC to all of the above antigen preparations are the outcome of enhanced numbers within the SF of T cells which specifically recognize these antigens. Also the possibility of a single set of T cells responding to epitopes contained within all preparations seems unlikely, since none of our *M. tuberculosis* reactive T cell lines and clones generated from SFMNC of different RA patients cross-react with *E. coli*[60]. Thus at least these two bacterial antigen preparations are recognized by different synovial T cells. The observed difference between the *in vitro* reactivity to antigens by SFMNC and PBMNC, often interpreted as an indication that these antigens might be involved in the aetiology of RA, demands other explanations.

One explanation could be related to the finding that more than 90% of joint T cells are CDw29 + compared to 50% of the peripheral blood T cells. CDw29 + are memory T cells, which respond better to soluble antigen than the CDw29 − cells. CD29 + cells may selectively home in the joint, because of a stronger ability to adhere to endothelial cells of the venules than CDw29 − cells[51]. Another possibility is that CDw29 − cells in the joint convert into CDw29 + cells after an aspecific stimulation by IL released at the site of inflammation, such as IL-2 or IL-4, which can cause this effect[61].

Another explanation concerns an increased frequency of SFDC. DC are excellent APC and have been shown to have higher capacity to present PPD, herpes simplex virus antigen and *Chlamydia trachomatis* to purified T cells than monocytes, on a cell-to-cell basis[52,53]. Peripheral blood T cells of ReA and RA patients cultured in the presence of SFDC display responses to antigens, which are not observed testing unseparated PBMNC[27]. The above data demonstrate that a specific role for *M. tuberculosis* antigens in the pathogenesis of RA cannot be deduced from the strong SFMNC responses to this antigen preparation.

Other investigators have focused on the role of γ/δ T cells reactive to mycobacteria in RA. BCG-stimulated SFMNC lines contained significantly higher numbers of γ/δ T cells than BCG-stimulated PBMNC lines, and γ/δ T cell clones recognizing mycobacterial antigens have been generated from SFMNC[59,62]. In the RA synovium and the synovial fluid the V δ 1$^+$ subset of γ/δ T cells predominates[63,64]. In contrast, in the peripheral blood of both patients and healthy individuals most γ/δ T cells are Vδ2 + and Vγ9 +. This could mean that specifically the Vδ1 positive T cells in the joints are locally activated by antigens, possibly mycobacterial antigens. However, thus far all human mycobacteria reactive γ/δ T cell clones, including the clones derived from the inflamed joint, were shown to be Vγ9/Vδ2^{+}[65,66]. Furthermore, the Vδ1 subset is also dominant in the thymus and in the inflamed gut of patients with coeliac disease. In addition, among patients with RA, higher numbers of γ/δ T cells in the SF compared to the peripheral blood were only present in a few patients[64]. The preponderance of Vδ1 T cells in the joint, thymus and gut may therefore not reflect an *in vivo* activation, but perhaps only a homing of this subset into these tissue compartments. This would fit the finding that six Vδ1 cDNA clones derived from SFMNC of an RA patient all have different V−J junction sequences, indicating a polyclonal population of Vδ1 cells in the joint[67]. Activation of γ/δ T cells in the joint or in BCG-induced lines might also be caused by IL which result from an antigen driven proliferative response of $\alpha\beta$ T cells. Namely, IL-2 stimulated T cell lines from RA patients display an increased frequency of γ/δ T cells compared to unstimulated T cell lines[59]. Thus, the role of mycobacteria in relation to specific activation of γ/δ T cells in the joint remains unclear.

Significantly increased IgG and IgA antibody levels to the recombinant mycobacterial hsp65 were detected in sera of RA patients as compared with the titres in sera of healthy individuals and patients with SLE, tuberculosis, ankylosing spondylitis or Crohn's disease. The response seemed to be specific for this hsp65, since IgG and IgA antibody levels to hsp65 of *E. coli* were not significantly different between these sera and sera from RA patients. Binding of IgG and IgA to mycobacterial *E. coli* and human hsp70 was about equal in RA, SLE and tuberculosis seria, but increased with regard to the remaining sera[68].

A possible role for the mycobacterial hsp65 as a target for T cells in RA was indicated by the finding that SFMNC from many RA patients recognized the recombinant *M. bovis* BCG hsp65 (identical to the *M. tuberculosis* hsp65) and *M. leprae* hsp65. Furthermore, as mentioned before, Holoshitz et al.[62] isolated *M. tuberculosis* specific T cell clones from SF cells. Some of these clones carried the γ/δ receptor and one γ/δ T cell clone reacted to the mycobacterial hsp65. The antigen recognition of the clones is not restricted by certain MHC class II gene products but may require presentation by a nonpolymorphic determinant of class II molecules.

That the mycobacterial hsp65 is presumably not a dominant mycobacterial protein recognized by SFMNC was demonstrated in a recent study[69]. No increase in frequency of anti-hsp65 reactive T cells was found in SFMNC compared to PBMNC from RA patients. Another study showed that *E. coli* contaminants within the recombinant mycobacterial hsp65 preparations are at least partly responsible for the induction of the previously demonstrated responses of SFMNC against these preparations. We considered this possibility when, in the process of trying to generate T cell lines and clones against the hsp65, unexpected responses were observed to *E. coli* contaminants, present within this preparation. Gaston et al.[49] encountered the same problems with *E. coli* components present in the *M. leprae* hsp65 preparation, when this preparation was used in the cloning of SF T cells of ReA patients. We wondered whether the previously demonstrated responses of SFMNC to the recombinant BCG hsp65 were actually, at least partly, caused by *E. coli* determinants within this preparation. Therefore, in the study in which the responses of SFMNC and PEMNC were compared, we included a more purified recombinant hsp65 BCG preparation (more than 96% purified versus 80% in the preparation previously used) apart from *M. tuberculosis*, *E. coli* and the previously used recombinant BCH hsp65 preparation. The purified hsp65 induced a positive response in only 1 out of 26 SFMNC samples, but in 5 out of 22 PEMNC samples. SFMNC and PEMNC responded more frequently to the unpurified hsp65 and responses to this preparation coincided with responses to *E. coli*[57]. Thus we have found that the hsp65 antigen is not an immunodominant antigen recognized on bulk level by SFMNC of RA patients. These results have now been confirmed by

Life et al.[48] testing a high number of RA patients. In contrast, two other recent studies still claim a high frequency of SFMNC responses to the mycobacterial hsp65[58,59]. Whether components of the *E. coli* lysate in the recombinant hsp65 were involved in these responses is unclear, moreover, because these studies did not include *E. coli* as a control.

Our finding that none of 30 *M. tuberculosis* reactive clones isolated from the synovial fluid of four RA patients recognized the hsp65 was in agreement with the low incidence of hsp65 responses observed by us in samples of SFMNC[60]. However, as mentioned before, responses to whole *M. tuberculosis* were often present in SFMNC. An absence of T cell clones responsive to the hsp65 was also observed by Quayle et al.[70] in a panel of 26 SF T cell clones generated against BCG. In contrast, with the use of hsp65 as a selecting agent in the cloning procedure they succeeded in isolating hsp65 reactive T cell clones. One of these clones was tested in more detail and was found to recognize an epitope contained within aa 241–255 on the mycobacterial hsp65 in the context of DQ. This clone also lysed autologous monocytes pulsed with hsp65[70] (and Quayle, personal communication). Gaston et al.[71] generated hsp65 reactive SF T cell clones from a patient homozygous for DR4. These clones were restricted via DP. However, these clones do not respond to aa 241–255 but to an epitope localized on the C-terminal part of the molecule. Thus, both epitopes recognized by the above-described human hsp65-reactive SF T cell clones are located on another part of the molecule than the aa 180–188 epitope recognized by the disease-inducing T cell clone in AA[35]. The *in vivo* relevance of these hsp65 reactive SF T cell clones is unclear, especially since mycobacterial hsp65 reactive T cells are also present in healthy individuals. However, the DP/DQ restriction of the above clones is interesting, since none of the thus far detected 26 T cell epitopes on the mycobacterial hsp65 is recognized in the context of HLA-DR4; the HLA antigen conferring the highest risk to develop RA. In the possible absence of DR4 restricted hsp65 T cell responses, DP/DQ restricted hsp65 specific-T cells may be of more significance *in vivo*.

We have investigated the possibility that mycobacterial antigens other than the hsp65 are involved in RA. If certain *M. tuberculosis* reactive T cells would cross-react in the joint with autoantigens, a dominant recognition by synovial T cells of only a few *M. tuberculosis* proteins should be expected, since in all probability only a few *M. tuberculosis* proteins will share homologous aa-stretches with autoantigens which are also T cell epitopes. In this case we particularly addressed the possibility of cross-reaction by the *M. tuberculosis* reactive T cells with joint specific auto-antigens rather than self hsp which will probably share a high number of T cell epitopes with *M. tuberculosis* hsp. A dominant recognition of only a limited number of *M. tuberculosis* proteins could also occur if only certain *M. tuberculosis* proteins end up in the joint and directly stimulate *M. tuberculosis* reactive T cells. The data we have obtained did not support a selective expansion of only particular *M. tuberculosis* reactive T cells in the joint. In a set of 15 T cell clones generated from *M. tuberculosis* induced SF T cell lines of four RA patients at least 12 different antigenic specificities were distinguished. This was determined by testing the proliferative response of the clones to SDS-

PAGE separated *M. tuberculosis* immunoblot fractions, each representing a specific molecular mass range[60].

These immunoblot fractions are excellent tools for assigning an unknown *M. tuberculosis* protein recognized by a T cell clone to a certain molecular mass range, as we have demonstrated for several proteins. Two *M. tuberculosis* reactive clones were eventually shown to recognize the 85 complex of secreted 30–31 kDa proteins, which was tested as a putative antigen after these clones were found to recognize an *M. tuberculosis* immunoblot fraction calculated to contain proteins in the molecular mass range of 30–33 kDa. In the same way, an *M. leprae* reactive T cell clone was shown to respond to hsp 70 of *M. leprae* (Ottenhoff, personal communication). In another study, using immunoblot separated *M. tuberculosis* fractions as antigens, a 47 kDa fraction was demonstrated to contain a major antigen recognized by PBMNC of DR4+ RA patients and controls[72]. However, only one of our 13 DR4+ *M. tuberculosis* reactive clones responded to an immunoblot fraction in this molecular mass range[60].

Based on the sequence identity in aa of the third hypervariable region of the β chain between DR1, Dw4, Dw14 and Dw15, all associated with an increased risk for developing RA, the so-called shared epitope hypothesis was put forward some years ago by Silver and Goyert[73]. This hypothesis implies that this particular part of the β chain, which distinguishes the above mentioned HLA antigens from other HLA molecules, plays a critical role in the restriction of those T cell peptide-HLA complex interactions which are directly involved in the pathogenesis of RA[73,74].

To investigate this hypothesis we used our *M. tuberculosis* reactive SF T cell clones which were isolated from three DR1,DR4 heterozygous patients and from one DR4 homozygous patient. Two DR1,DR4 positive patients were positive for the Dw14 subtype of DR4 and the other was positive for the Dw4 subtype. The DR4,DR4 positive patient was typed as Dw4,Dw14 heterozygous. The clones obtained were either DR1 or DR4 restricted and 11 out of 13 DR4 restricted clones were specifically restricted via Dw4 or Dw14. The other two DR4 restricted clones responded equally well to *M. tuberculosis* whether Dw4+ or Dw14+ APC were used[60]. The restriction of our clones, being either DR1 or DR4 (Dw4 or 14), and their variety in antigen recognition do not support a most likely implication of the hypothesis, which is that the crucial effector T cells responding to autoantigens will be restricted via both DR1 and DR4 and/or recognize the same peptides. Thus far, only one T cell determinant on a mycobacterial antigen has been shown to be recognized in the context of both DR1 and DR4. This epitope, present on aa 1–15 of the 19 kDa antigen of *M. tuberculosis*, was immunodominant since PBMNC of four out of four DR1 positive and four out of four DR4 positive individuals responded to the corresponding synthetic peptide[75]. We found that only one Dw14 restricted T cell clone responded to an immunoblot fraction with *M. tuberculosis* proteins in this molecular mass range. This clone almost certainly does not recognize this epitope, since it does not respond to *M. tuberculosis* presented by DR1.

ANTI-hsp T CELL REACTIVITY AND ARTHRITIS: THREE HYPOTHESES

Three models, which are not mutually exclusive, can be proposed with regard to the antigen recognition of effector T cells in the affected joint(s) of arthritis patients.

1. The effector T cells in the joint may respond to endogenous antigen(s) only. The site specificity of arthritis makes joint components likely to be the relevant targets for such T cells. Possible targets are collagen and proteoglycans. T cell clones and lines responding to collagen and/or proteoglycans have been derived from joint tissue and fluid of RA patients. However, T cells specific for these molecules are also present in healthy individuals[76-78].

   Other possible targets are self specific epitopes on autologous hsp produced and/or presented by cells from affected tissues. Although the hsp are ubiquitous proteins in the body, their expression might be increased in cells at the site of inflammation due to stress stimuli caused by the ongoing inflammatory process. Significant expression of self hsp65 was demonstrated in the cartilage–pannus junction in rheumatoid joints and in rheumatoid nodules, but not in normal joints or in normal or inflamed kidney or liver[79]. Certain cytokines, such as IFN-γ, secreted by activated T cells can upregulate expression of hsp. Thus, hsp expression and recognition may also be secondary to activation of T cells by other antigens; such hsp may well be bystander antigens for a T cell response that perpetuates the inflammation. This concept excludes the involvement of exogenous (mycobacterial) antigens.

2. The effector T cells responding to self molecules in the joint may cross-react with exogenous antigens such as products from infectious micro-organisms. An infection somewhere in the body might have pretriggered the disease inducing T cells. This is what presumably happens in AA. One of the T cell clones (A2b) responding to the mycobacterial 65 kDa also responds to proteoglycans *in vitro*[33]. Such T cells are activated somewhere in the body after immunization with *M. tuberculosis* and may selectively or aspecifically enter the joint and induce arthritis after recognition of proteoglycans. Because of their extreme sequence homology with endogenous hsp, it is tempting to speculate the exogenous hsp are candidates to induce T cell cross-reactivity in arthritis. In this respect, it is unlikely that the mycobacterial 180–186 epitope of hsp65 identified in AA evokes such cross-reactivity, since this epitope differs considerably from the corresponding sequence on the rat hsp65.

   In man, the occurrence of T cells reacting with both the mycobacterial and human hsp65 was demonstrated in normal individuals. Of course, detection of cross-reactivity of T cells between endogenous and exogenous antigens *in vitro* does not necessarily imply that the T cells concerned have encountered antigens of both preparations *in vivo*. Analysis of the recognition of bulk SFMNC and *M. tuberculosis* reactive T cell clones derived from the joint showed that the mycobacterial hsp65 is not an immunodominant antigen, arguing against a role for this molecule in inducing cross-reactive T cells in RA[57,60]. So far no evidence has been found that other mycobacterial antigens are predominantly recognized by joint T cells.

3. Effector T cells in the joint may be stimulated by exogenous antigens only. This model implies the presence of exogenous antigens in the joint. Antigens of bacteria inducing ReA have been demonstrated in the affected joints[42,43]. Furthermore, freshly isolated SFDC were shown to carry antigens of the triggering bacteria. These SFDC stimulated joint T cells specific for these bacteria without adding exogenous antigens[44]. This implied that such T cells are stimulated by exogenous antigens in the joint. Although T cells specific for the bacteria implicated in ReA have been cloned, the individual antigens recognized have not yet been defined. One T cell clone recognized hsp65, but a specific role for this hsp in ReA remains to be elucidated[49].

CONCLUDING REMARKS

T cells and antibodies against self and non-self heat shock proteins are present in both arthritis patients and healthy controls. T cells responding to hsp65 can cause arthritis as was demonstrated in an animal model: adjuvant arthritis (AA) in Lewis rats. In human reactive arthritis there is evidence for a direct stimulation of joint T cells by antigens of the organisms causing the infection which precedes the joint inflammation. The individual antigens of the triggering bacteria still have to be defined, but hsp65 may be of importance since this is one of the molecules recognized by synovial T cells in reactive arthritis patients. Although in rheumatoid arthritis, T cells recognizing hsp65 and other mycobacterial antigens are present in the joint, a specific involvement of one or a limited set of (myco)bacterial antigens in the pathogenesis of this disease is unlikely.

Acknowledgement

Parts of this chapter are based on a review by Res et al published in Springer Semin Immunopathol. 1991; 13: 81–98.

References

1. Lindquist S. The heat shock response. Ann Rev Biochem. 1986; 55: 1151–1191.
2. Lindquist S. The heat shock proteins. Ann Rev Genet. 1988; 22: 631–637.
3. Jindal S, Dudani AK, Singh B, Harley CB, Gupta RS. Primary structure of a human mitochondrial protein homologous to the bacterial and plant chaperonines and to the 65-kilodalton mycobacterial antigen. Mol Cell Biol. 1989; 9: 2279–2283.
4. Ellis J. Proteins as molecular chaperones. Nature. 1987; 328: 378–379.
5. Neidhardt FC, Philips TA, Van Bogelen RA, Smith MW, Georgalis Y, Subramanian AR. Identity of the B56.5 protein, the A protein, and the gro E gene product of *Escherichia coli*. J Bacteriol. 1981; 145: 513–520.

6. Rinke de Wit TF, Bekelie S, Osland A, Miko TL, Hermans PWM, Van Soolingen D, Drijfhout JW, Schöningh R, Janson A, Thole JER. Mycobacteria contain two *groEL* genes: the second *Mycobacterium leprae groEL* gene is arranged in an operon with *groES*. Mol Microbiol. 1992; 6: 1995–2007.

7. Jarjour W, Tsai V, Woods V, Welch W, Pierce W, Shaw M, Mehta H, Dillmann W, Zwaifler N, Winfield J. Cell surface expression of heat shock proteins. Arthritis Rheum. 1989; 32: S44.

8. Lakey EK, Margoliash E, Pierce SK. Identification of a peptide binding protein that plays a role in antigen presentation. Proc Natl Acad Sci USA. 1987; 84: 1659–1663.

9. De Bruyn J, Bosmans R, Nyabenda J, Turneer M, Weckx M, van Vooren J-P, Falmagne P, Wiker HG, Harboe M. Purification, partial characterization and identification of a skin reactive protein antigen of *Mycobacterium bovis*, BCG. Infect Immun. 1987; 55: 245–252.

10. Gillis TP, Miller RA, Young DB, Kanolkar SR, Buchanan TM. Immunochemical characterization of a protein associated with *Mycobacterium leprae* cell wall. Infect Immun. 1985; 49: 371–377.

11. Young DB, Lathigra R, Hendrix R, Sweetser D, Young RA. Stress proteins are immune targets in leprosy and tuberculosis. Proc Natl Acad Sci USA. 1988; 85: 4267–4270.

12. Young RA. Stress proteins and immunology. Ann Rev Immunol. 1990; 8: 401–420.

13. Hansen K, Bangsdorf JM, Fjordvang H, Pedersen NS, Hinderssen P. Immunochemical characterisation of, and isolation of the gene for a Borrelia burgdorferi immunodominant 60 kDa antigen common to a wide range of bacteria. Infect Immun. 1988; 56: 2047–2053.

14. Hindersson P, Knudson JD, Axelsen NH. Cloning and expression of *Treponema pallidum* common antigen (Tp-4) in *E. coli* K-12. J Gen Microbiol. 1987; 133: 587–596.

15. Plikaytis BB, Carlone GM, Pau CP, Wilkinson HW. Purified 60 kD *Legionella* protein antigen with *Legionella*-specific and non-specific epitopes. J Clin Microbiol. 1987; 25: 2080–2084.

16. Vodkin MH, Williams JC. A heat shock protein operon in *Coxiella burnetti* produces a major antigen homologous to a protein in both mycobacteria and *Escherichia coli*. J Bacteriol. 1988; 170: 1227–1234.

17. Engers HD. Results of a World Health Organization-sponsored workshop to characterize antigens recognized by mycobacterium-specific monoclonal antibodies. Infect Immun. 1986; 51: 718–720.

18. Emmrich B, Thole J, van Embden J, Kaufmann SHE. A recombinant 64 kilodalton protein of *Mycobacterium bovis* Bacillus Galmette-Guérin specifically stimulates human T4 clones reactive to mycobacterial antigens. J Exp Med. 1986; 163: 1024–1029.

19. Kaufmann SHE, Vath U, Thole JER, Van Embden JDA, Emmrich F. Enumeration of T cells reactive with Mycobacterium tuberculosis organisms and specific for the recombinant 64-kDa protein. Eur J Immunol. 1987; 17: 351–357.

20. Oftung F, Mustafa AS, Husson R, Young RA, Godal T. Human T cell clones recognize two abundant *Mycobacterium tuberculosis* protein antigens expressed in *Escherichia coli*. J Immunol. 1987; 138: 927–931.

21. Thole JER, Dauwerse HG, Das PK, Groothuis DG, Schouls LM, van Embden JDA. Characterization, sequence determination and immunogenicity of a 64-kilodalton protein of *Mycobacterium bovis* BCG expressed in *Escherichia coli* K-12. Infect Immun. 1987; 55: 1466–1475.

22. Ardeshir F, Flint JE, Richman J, Reese RT. A 75 kD merozoite surface protein of *Plasmodium falciparum* which is related to the 70 kD heat-shock proteins. EMBO J. 1987; 6: 493–499.

23. Bianco AE, Favaloro JM, Burkof TR, Culnevor JG, Crewther PE, Brown GV, Anders RF, Coppel RL, Kemp DJ. A repetitive antigen of *Plasmodium falciparum* that is homologous to heat shock protein 70 of *Drosophila melanogaster*. Proc Natl Acad Sci USA. 1986; 83: 8713–8717.

24. Engman DM, Kirchoff LV, Henkle K, Donelsen JE. A novel hsp 70 cognate in trypanosomes. J Cell Biochem. 12D 1988; Supplement: 290.

25. Ottenhoff THM, Kaleab B, Van Embden JDA, Thole JER, Kiessling R. The recombinant 65-kD heat shock protein of mycobacterium bovis bacillus calmette guerin/M. tuberculosis is a target molecule for CD4+ cytotoxic T lymphocytes that lyse human monocytes. J Exp Med. 1988; 168: 1947–1952.

26. Lamb JR, Bal V, Rothbard JB, Mehlert A, Mendez-Samperio P, Young DB. The

mycobacterial Groel stress protein: a common target of T-cell recognition in infection and autoimmunity. J Autoimmunol. 1989; 2 (suppl): 93–100.

27. Munk ME, Schoel B, Modrow S, Karr RW, Young RA, Kaufmann SHE. T lymphocytes from healthy individuals with specificity to self-epitopes shared by the mycobacterial and human 65-kilodalton heat shock protein. J Immunol. 1989; 143: 2844–2849.

28. Kaleab B, Ottenhoff T, Converse P, Halapi E, Tadesse G, Rottenberg M, Kiessling R. Mycobacterial antigen-induced cytotoxic T cells as well as nonspecific killer cells derived from healthy individuals and leprosy patients. Eur J Immunol. 1990; 20: 2651–2659.

29. Wand-Wurttenberger A, Schoel B, Ivanyi J, Kaufmann SHE. Surface expression by mononuclear phagocytes of an epitope shared with mycobacterial heat shock protein 60. Eur J Immunol. 1991; 21: 1089.

30. Kaleab B, Kiessling R, Van Embden JDA, Thole JER, Kumararatne DS, Pisa P, Wondimu A, Ottenhoff THM. Induction of antigen-specific CD4+ HLA-DR-restricted cytotoxic T lymphocytes as well as nonspecific nonrestricted killer cells by the recombinant mycobacterial 65-kDa heat-shock protein. Eur J Immunol. 1990; 20: 369–377.

31. Koga T, Wand-Wurttenberger A, De Bruyn J, Munk ME, Schoel B, Kaufmann SHE. T cells against a bacterial heat shock protein recognize stressed macrophages. Science. 1989; 245: 1112–1115.

32. Steinhof U, Schoel B, Kaufmann SHE. Lysis of interferon-α activated Schwann cell by cross-reactive CD8+δ T cells with specificity for the mycobacterial 65 kD heat shock protein. Int Immunol. 1990; 3: 279–284.

33. Cohen IR. Autoimmunity to chaperonins in the pathogenesis of arthritis and diabetes. Ann Rev Immunol. 1991 (in press).

34. Holoshitz J, Matitau A, Cohen IR. Arthritis induced in rats by cloned T lymphocytes responsive to mycobacteria but not to collagen type II. J Clin Invest. 1984; 73: 211–215.

35. Van Eden W, Thole JER, van der Zee R, Noordzij A, van Embden JDA, Hensen EJ, Cohen IR. Cloning of the mycobacterial epitope recognized by T lymphocytes in adjuvant arthritis. Nature. 1985; 331: 171–173.

36. Lider O, Karin N, Shinitzky M, Cohen IR. Therapeutic vaccination against adjuvant arthritis using autoimmune T lymphocytes treated with hydrostatic pressure. Proc Natl Acad Sci USA. 1987; 84: 4577–4580.

37. Wauben MHM, Boog CJP, Van der Zee R, Joosten I, Schlief A, Van Eden W. Disease inhibition by major histocompatibility complex binding peptide analogues of disease-associated epitopes: More than blocking alone. J Exp Med. 1992; 667–677.

38. Aho K, Leirisalo-Repo M, Repo H. Reactive arthritis. Clin Rheum Dis. 1985; 11: 25–40.

39. Gaston JSH, Life PF, Granfors K, Merilahto-Palo R, Bailey L, Consalvey S, Toivanen A, Bacon PA. Synovial lymphocyte recognition of organisms which trigger reactive arthritis. Clin Exp Immunol. 1989; 76: 348–353.

40. Hermann E, Fleischer B, Mayet WJ, Poralla T, Meyer zum Buschenfelde KH. Response of synovial fluid T cell clones to *Yersinia enterocolitica* antigens in patients with reactive arthritis. Clin Exp Immunol. 1989; 73: 365–370.

41. Stagg AJ, Harding B, Hughes RA, Keat A, Knight SC. Peripheral blood and synovial fluid T cells differ in their responses to alloantigens and recall antigens presented by dendritic cells. Clin Exp Immunol. 1991; 84: 72.

42. Granfors K, Jalkanen S, Lahesmaa-Rantala R, Isomaki O, Pekkola-Heino K, Merilahti-Palo R, Saario R, Isomaki H, Toivanen A. Yersinia antigens in the synovial fluid from patients with reactive arthritis. N Engl J Med. 1989; 320: 216–221.

43. Granfors K, Jalkanen S, Lindberg AA, Maki-Ikola O, von Essen R, Lahesmaa-Rantala R, Saario R, Isomaki H, Arnold W, Toivanen A. Salmonella lipopolysaccharide in synovial cells from patients with reactive arthritis. Lancet. 1990; 1: 685–688.

44. Stagg AJ, Harding B, Hughes R, Keat A, Knight SC. Antigen presenting cells indicate the causative antigen in reactive arthritis. Arthritis Rheum. 1990; 33: S106.

45. Hermann E, Lohse AW, Van der Zee R, Van Eden W, Mayet WJ, Probst P, Poralla T, Meyer zum Büschenfelde K-H, Fleischer B. Synovial fluid-derived *Yersinia*-reactive T cells responding to human 65-kDa heat shock protein and heat-stressed antigen-presenting cells. Eur J Immunol. 1991; 21: 2139–2143.

46. Gaston JSH, Life PF, Bailey LC, Bacon PA. In vitro responses to a 65-kilodalton mycobacterial protein by synovial T cells from inflammatory arthritis patients. J Immunol.

1989; 143: 2494–2500.
47. Gaston JSH, Life PF, Jenner PJ, Colston MJ, Bacon PA. Recognition of a mycobacteria-specific epitope in the 65 kilodalton heat-shock protein by synovial fluid derived T cell clones. J Exp Med. 1990; 171: 831–834.
48. Life PF, Viner NJ, Bacon PA, Gaston JSH. Synovial fluid antigen-presenting cells unmask peripheral blood T cell responses to bacterial antigens in inflammatory arthritis. Clin Exp Immunol. 1990; 79: 189–194.
49. Gaston JSH (1991) Heat shock proteins and autoimmunity. Seminars in Immunology (in press).
50. Duke O, Panayi GS, Janossy G, Poulter LW. An immunohistochemical analysis of lymphocyte subpopulations and their microenvironment in the synovial membranes of patients with rheumatoid arthritis using monoclonal antibodies. Clin Exp Immunol. 1982; 49: 22–30.
51. Pitzalis C, Kingsley G, Haskard D, Panayi G. The preferential accumulation of helper-inducer T lymphocytes in inflammatory lesions: evidence for regulation by selective endothelial and homotypic adhesion. Eur J Immunol. 1988; 18: 1397–1404.
52. Waalen K, Førre O, Teigland J, Natvig JB. Human rheumatoid synovial and normal blood dendritic cells as antigen-presenting cells: comparison with autologous monocytes. Clin Exp Immunol. 1987; 70: 1–9.
53. Zembala M, Uracz W, Ruggiero I, Mytar B, Pryjma J. Isolation and functional characteristics of FcR + and FcR − human monocyte subsets. J Immunol. 1984; 133: 1293–1299.
54. Holoshitz J, Klajman A, Drucker I, Lapidot Z, Yaretzky A, Frenkel A, van Eden W, Cohen IR. T lymphocytes of rheumatoid arthritis patients show augmented reactivity to a fraction of mycobacteria cross-reactive with cartilage. Lancet. 1986; 2: 305–309.
55. Pope RM, Pahlavani MA, LaCour E, Sambol S, Desai BV. Antigenic specificity of rheumatoid synovial fluid lymphocytes. Arthritis Rheum. 1989; 32: 1371–1379.
56. Res PCM, Schaar CG, Breedveld FC, van Eden W, van Embden JDA, Cohen IR, de Vries RRP. Synovial fluid T cell reactivity against the 65 kD heat shock protein of mycobacteria in early chronic arthritis. Lancet. 1988; 2: 478–480.
57. Res PCM, Telgt D, van Laar JM, Oudkerk Pool M, Breedveld FC, de Vries RRP. High antigen reactivity in mononuclear cells from sites of chronic inflammation. Lancet. 1990; 1: 1406–1409.
58. Burmester GR, Altstidl U, Kalden JR, Emmrich F. Stimulatory response towards the 65 kD heat shock protein and other mycobacterial antigens in patients with inflammatory joint disease. J Rheum. 1991; 18: 171.
59. Soderstrom K, Halapi E, Nilsson E, Gronberg A, Van Embden J, Klareskog L, Kiessling R. Synovial cells responding to a 65-kDa mycobacterial heat shock protein have a high proportion of a TcR $\gamma\delta$ subtype uncommon in peripheral blood. Scand J Immunol. 1990; 32: 503–515.
60. Res PCM, Orsini DLM, van Laar JM, Janson AAM, Abou-Zeid C, de Vries RRP. Diversity in antigen recognition by Mycobacterium tuberculosis reactive T cell clones from the synovial fluid of rheumatoid arthritis patients. Eur J Immunol. 1991; 27: 1297.
61. Fleming WE, Winterrowd GE, Krzesicki RF, Nickoloff BJ, Chin JE, Sanders ME. Mechanisms of CD29 T cell accumulation in rheumatoid synovium: cytokines alter phenotype and enhance adhesion of polyclonal T cells. Arthritis Rheum. 1989; 33: S58.
62. Holoshitz J, Koning F, Coligan JE, De Bruyn J, Strober S. Isolation of CD4-CD8-mycobacteria-reactive T lymphocyte clones from rheumatoid arthritis synovial fluid. Nature. 1989; 339: 226–229.
63. Chaouni I, Radal M, Simony-Lafontaine J, Combe B, Sany J, Rème T. Distribution of T cell receptor-bearing lymphocytes in the synovial membrane from patients with rheumatoid arthritis. J Autoimmun. 1990; 3: 737–745.
64. Smith MD, Broker B, Moretta L, Ciccone E, Grossi CE, Edwards JCW, Yuksel F, Colaco B, Worman C, Mackenzie L, Kinne G, Weseloh G, Gluckert K, Lydyard PM. T $\gamma\delta$ cells and their subsets in blood and synovial tissue from rheumatoid arthritis patients. Scand J Immunol. 1990; 32: 585–593.
65. Haas W, Kaufmann SHE, Martinez A-C. The development and function of γ/δ T cells. Immunol Today. 1990; 1: 340–343.
66. Kabelitz D, Bender A, Schondelmaier S, Schoel B, Kaufmann SHE. A large fraction of

human peripheral blood $\gamma/\delta+$ T cells is activated by *Mycobacterium tuberculosis* but not by its 65-kD heat shock protein. J Exp Med. 1990; 171: 667–679.

67. Sioud M, Førre O, Natvig JB. T cell receptor δ diversity of freshly isolated T lymphocytes in rheumatoid synovitis. Eur J Immunol. 1991; 21: 239–241.
68. Tsoulfa G, Rook GA, Bahr GM, Sattar MA, Behbehani K, Young DB, Mehlert A, van Embden JD, Hay FC, Isenberg DA. Elevated IgG antibody levels are characteristic of patients with rheumatoid arthritis. 1987; 30: 519–527.
69. Fischer HP, Sharrock CE, Colston MJ, Panayi GS. Limiting dilution analysis of proliferative T cell responses to mycobacterial 65-kDa heat shock protein fails to show significant frequency differences between synovial fluid and peripheral blood of patients with rheumatoid arthritis. Eur J Immunol. 1991; 21: 2937–2942.
70. Quayle AJ, Kjeldson-Kragh JK, Shu-Guang Li, Oftung F, Shinnick T, Førre O, Natvig JB. Rheumatoid synovial fluid derived T cell clones responsive to the mycobacterial antigens including the 65 kD heat shock protein. J Cell Biochem. 1989; 15A: S320.
71. Gaston JSH, Life PF, Jenner PJ, Colston MJ, Bacon PA. Fine specificity of mycobacterial 65 kD stress protein (M65kD)-specific synovial T cell clones from patients with a self limiting and persistent arthritis. Arthritis Rheum. 1990; 33: S16.
72. Palacios-Boiox AA, Estrada-G I, Colston MJ, Panayi GS. HLA-DR4 restricted lymphocyte proliferation to a Mycobacterium tuberculosis extract in rheumatoid arthritis patients and healthy individuals. J Immunol. 1988; 140: 1844–1849.
73. Silver J, Goyert SM. Epitopes are functional units of Ia molecules and form the molecular basis for disease susceptibility. In: Human Class II Histocompatibility Antigens. Springer Verlag; 1985: 32–48.
74. Gregersen PK, Silver J, Winchester RJ. The shared epitope hypothesis: an approach to understanding the molecular genetics of susceptibility to rheumatoid arthritis. Arthritis Rheum. 1987; 30: 1205–1213.
75. Lamb JR, Rees ADM, Bal V, Ikeda H, Wilkinson D, de Vries RRP, Rothbard JB. Prediction and identification of an HLA-DR-restricted T cell determinant in the 19-kDa protein of *Mycobacterium tuberculosis*. Eur J Immunol. 1988; 18: 973–976.
76. Londei M, Savill C, Verhoef A, Brennan F, Leech ZE, Duance V, Maini RN, Feldmann M. Persistence of collagen type II-specific T cell clones in the synovial fluid of a patient with rheumatoid arthritis. Proc Natl Acad Sci USA. 1989; 86: 636–640.
77. Ofosu-Appiah WA, Warrington RJ, Wilkins JA. Interleukin 2 responsive T cell clones from rheumatoid and normal subjects: proliferative responses to connective tissue elements. Clin Immunol Immunopathol. 1989; 50: 264–271.
78. Solinger AM, Schonhoft M. Collagen-reactive lines. Jap J Rheum. 1989; 1: 25–35.
79. Karlsson-Parra A, Soderstrom K, Ferm M, Ivanyi J, Kiessling R, Klareskog L. Presence of a human 65 kD heat shock protein (hsp) in inflamed joints and subcutaneous nodules of RA patients. Scand J Immunol. 1990; 31: 283–288.

Index

Immunology and Medicine Series

1. A.M. McGregor (ed.). *Immunology of Endocrine Diseases.* 1986
   ISBN: 0-85200-963-1
2. L. Ivanyi (ed.). *Immunological Aspects of Oral Diseases.* 1986   ISBN: 0-85200-961-5
3. M.A.H. French (ed.). *Immunoglobulins in Health and Disease.* 1986
   ISBN: 0-85200-962-3
4. K. Whaley (ed.). *Complement in Health and Disease.* 1987   ISBN: 0-85200-954-2
5. G.R.D. Catto (ed.). *Clinical Transplantation: Current Practice and Future Prospects.* 1987   ISBN: 0-85200-960-7
6. V.S. Byers and R.W. Baldwin (ed.). *Immunology of Malignant Diseases.* 1987
   ISBN: 0-85200-964-X
7. S.T. Holgate (ed.). *Mast Cells, Mediators and Disease.* 1988   ISBN: 0-85200-968-2
8. D.J.M Wright (ed.). *Immunology of Sexually Transmitted Diseases.* 1988
   ISBN: 0-74620-087-0
9. A.D.B. Webster (ed.). *Immunodeficiency and Disease.* 1988   ISBN: 0-85200-688-8
10. C. Stern (ed.). *Immunology of Pregnancy and its Disorders.* 1989
    ISBN: 0-7462-0065-X
11. M.S. Klempner, B. Styrt and J. Ho (ed.). *Phagocytes and Disease.* 1989
    ISBN: 0-85200-842-2
12. A.J. Zuckerman (ed.). *Recent Developments in Prophylactic Immunization.* 1989
    ISBN: 0-7923-8910-7
13. S. Lightman (ed.). *Immunology of Eye Disease.* 1989   ISBN: 0-7923-8908-5
14. T.J. Hamblin (ed.). *Immunotherapy of Disease.* 1990   ISBN: 0-7462-0045-5
15. D.B. Jones and D.H. Wright (eds.). *Lymphoproliferative Diseases.* 1990
    ISBN: 0-85200-965-8
16. C.D. Pusey (ed.). *Immunology of Renal Diseases.* 1991   ISBN: 0-7923-8964-6
17. A.G. Bird (ed.). *Immunology of HIV Infection.* 1991   ISBN: 0-7923-8962-X
18. J.T. Whicher and S.W. Evans (eds.). *Biochemistry of Inflammation.* 1992
    ISBN: 0-7923-8985-9
19. T.T. MacDonald (ed.). *Immunology of Gastrointestinal Diseases.* 1992
    ISBN: 0-7923-8961-1
20. K. Whaley, M. Loos and J.M. Weiler (eds.). *Complement in Health and Disease, 2nd Edn.* 1993   ISBN: 0-7923-8823-2